Development of Anti-asthma Drugs

Derek R. Buckle, BSc, PhD, ARCS, DIC, CChem, FRSC
Manager, Anti-allergy Project

Harry Smith, BSc, DSc
Manager, Anti-asthma Project

Beecham Pharmaceuticals—Research Division
Biosciences Research Centre
Epsom, Surrey

Butterworths
London · Boston · Durban · Singapore · Sydney · Toronto · Wellington

First published, 1984

© Butterworth & Co. (Publishers) Ltd, 1984

British Library Cataloguing in Publication Data

Development of anti-asthma drugs.
  1. Asthma—Chemotherapy
  I. Buckle, Derek R.   II. Smith, Harry, *19-- -*
  616.2'38061   RC591

  ISBN 0-408-11576-9

Library of Congress Cataloging in Publication Data
Main entry under title:

Development of anti-asthma drugs.
  Bibliography: p.
  Includes index.
  1. Antiasthmatic agents.   2. Asthma—Chemotherapy.
  I. Buckle, Derek R.   II. Smith, Harry, 1921-
[DNLM: 1. Asthma—Drug therapy.   WF 553 D489]
RC588.C45D48 1984   616.2'38061   84-7057
ISBN 0-408-11576-9

Photoset by Phoenix Photosetting, Chatham, Kent
Printed and bound by Robert Hartnoll Ltd, Bodmin, Cornwall

Development of Anti-asthma Drugs

Preface

The rapidly expanding literature relating to asthma and drugs used for its treatment has created a need for a comprehensive review of this area. This volume attempts to accomplish this objective by drawing together both the classical and current asthma therapies, grouping them in such a way that the inter-relation of the various approaches may be appreciated. Each chapter is written by acknowledged experts in that particular field, providing an authoritative account and critical evaluation of recent developments. It is expected that this will lead to a better understanding of asthma therapy and stimulate the development of improved drugs for the treatment of this debilitating disease.

Finally, the editors would like to express their thanks to Beecham Pharmaceuticals, Research Division for allowing them the facility to organize this book and to the contributors for their timely and concise chapters.

D.R. Buckle
H. Smith

Contributors

Jehan Bagli
Associate Director of Research, Department of Chemistry, Ayerst Research Laboratories, CN 8000, Princeton, New Jersey

J.R. Bantick
Team Leader, Medicinal Chemistry, Fisons p.l.c., Pharmaceutical Division, Loughborough, Leicestershire

Derek Buckle
Project Manager, Anti-allergy Project, Beecham Pharmaceuticals—Research Division, Biosciences Research Centre, Epsom, Surrey

Michael Cushley
Lecturer, Faculty of Medicine, Southampton General Hospital

Noemi Eiser
Consultant Physician, Department of Thoracic Medicine, New Cross Hospital, London

John C. Foreman
Lecturer in Pharmacology, Department of Pharmacology, University College London

Stuart M. Harding
Head, Department of Human Pharmacology, Glaxo Group Research Limited, Greenford, Middlesex

Peter M. Henson
Departments of Pathology and Medicine, National Jewish Hospital and University of Colorado Health Sciences Center, Denver, Colorado

Stephen T. Holgate
Senior Lecturer in Medicine, Faculty of Medicine, Southampton General Hospital

M.C. Holroyde
Project Leader—Pharmacology, Fisons p.l.c., Pharmaceutical Division, Bakewell Road, Loughborough, Leicestershire

A. Barry Kay
Professor and Director, Department of Allergy and Clinical Immunology, Cardiothoracic Institute, Brompton Hospital, London

T.B. Lee
Research Fellow, Fisons p.l.c., Pharmaceutical Division, Loughborough, Leicestershire

Maurice H. Lessof
Professor of Medicine, Guy's Hospital Medical School, London

J.M. Lynch
Research Associate, National Jewish Hospital and University of Colorado Health Services Center, Denver, Colorado

David M. Moran
Project Manager, Project for Specific Allergies, Beecham Pharmaceuticals—Research Division, Biosciences Research Centre, Epsom, Surrey

Gary E. Pakes
Assistant Director of International Medical Affairs, ICRMA, G. D. Searle and Co., Skokie, Illinois

Priscilla J. Piper
Reader in Pharmacology, Royal College of Surgeons of England, London

P. Sheard
Research Fellow, Fisons p.l.c., Pharmaceutical Division, Loughborough, Leicestershire

T.Y. Shen
Vice-President, Membrane and Arthritis Research, Merck Sharp and Dohme Research Laboratories, Rahway, New Jersey

Ian F. Skidmore
Head, Department of Biochemical Pharmacology, Glaxo Group Research Limited, Ware, Hertfordshire

Harry Smith
Project Manager, Anti-asthma Project, Beecham Pharmaceuticals—Research Division, Biosciences Research Centre, Epsom, Surrey

Laurie J. Smith
Assistant Chief, Allergy–Clinical Immunology Service, Department of the Army, Walter Reed Army Medical Center, Washington DC

A.N. Tischler
Research Fellow, Department of Membrane and Arthritis Research, Merck Sharp and Dohme Research Laboratories, Rahway, New Jersey

Alan W. Wheeler
Senior Biologist, Specific Allergies Project, Beecham Pharmaceuticals—Research Division, Biosciences Research Center, Epsom, Surrey

G.S. Worthen
Department of Medicine, National Jewish Hospital and University of Colorado Health Sciences Center, Denver, Colorado

Contents

Introduction

D.R. Buckle and H. Smith

The complex nature of asthma has allowed the development of a number of diverse approaches to its treatment and, as a result, the disease is controlled to some extent by existing drug regimens. A cure for asthma still remains to be discovered and it is unlikely that one will be found in the near future; however, that there will be improvements in treatment is certain. The purpose of this book is to review existing treatments and novel approaches currently under investigation, in the context of their mode of action and clinical effectiveness, in the hope that this might lead to a greater understanding of the factors involved in the expression of the disease and, therefore, in the design of better drugs.

The plan of the book is based on a concept of the causes and treatment of asthma that we have attempted to outline in *Figure 1*. Similar concepts

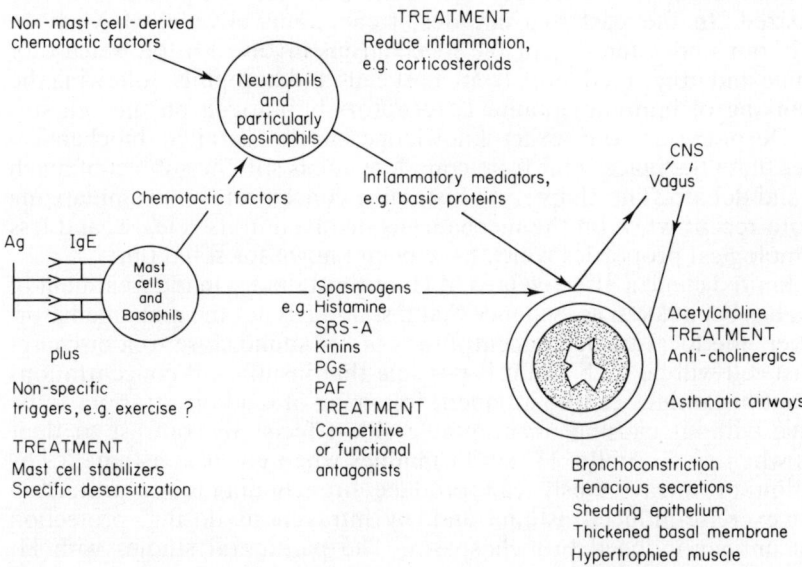

Figure 1 Causes and treatment of asthma.

1

are presented elsewhere in this book, particularly in the chapters by Professor Lessof and Professor Kay. Undoubtedly, some asthmatic attacks, especially in allergic asthmatics, are caused by the direct effect of smooth muscle constrictor materials released from the mast cell. However, there is growing evidence that an important contribution to the pathology of asthma is made by inflammatory cells, particularly eosinophilic polymorphonuclear leucocytes, infiltrating the lungs, recruited by factors from the mast cell and, probably, from other sources. The respiratory smooth muscle of an asthmatic is hypersensitive to some spasmogens which may have a direct effect on the muscle or may stimulate nerve receptors to produce an increase in cholinergic tone by a vagal reflex.

Part 1 of the book consists of a single chapter defining asthma, describing its natural history and incidence and outlining possible mechanisms that may contribute to the pathology of the disease.

Part 2 is a series of chapters each of which considers a putative mediator or group of mediators of asthma. Included in this section of the book is a chapter summarizing what is known of the involvement in the disease of the eosinophilic and the neutrophilic polymorphonuclear leucocyte. The current literature is summarized in some depth which means that, due to the lack of space, not all of the putative mediators of asthma have been considered. This has meant the omission of data on the little studied materials released from mast cells, such as proteolytic enzymes and the literature on complement and the kinins has not been reviewed.

Part 3 of the book considers the development or the attempted development of drugs for the treatment of asthma. Each chapter considers a type of drug classified according to its mode of action and this, together with the clinical effectiveness of the drug, is considered.

In Part 2 of the book, histamine is the first putative mediator of asthma to be reviewed. The involvement of histamine in allergic reactions was demonstrated early this century, at which time the compound was also synthesized. In the past two decades, tremendous advances have been made in our understanding of the mechanisms involved in the release of histamine and other mediators from mast cells and basophils, following the cross-linking of immunoglobulin E receptors by antigen on the cell surfaces. Despite this, our exact knowledge of the detailed biochemical changes that take place is far from complete and is still the subject of much effort and debate. The chapter on histamine concentrates on summarizing the more recent work on the mechanisms involved in its release, and less on its biological properties which have been known for some time.

The limited clinical effectiveness of H_1 antihistamines in the treatment of asthma has been taken as evidence that histamine is not the main mediator. However, the local tissue concentrations of histamine close to a discharging mast cell will be high and it is possible that insufficient concentrations of H_1 antihistamines can be attained, following oral administration, to be effective without causing unacceptable side-effects. In contrast to their effects when given orally, H_1 antihistamines when given to asthmatics by inhalation or intravenously can produce bronchodilatation, protection against exercise-induced asthma and, by intravenous dosing, protection against antigen-induced bronchospasm. The parenteral studies with H_1 antihistamines are, in the main, surprisingly recent, and the chapter on H_1

antihistamines considers them in some detail. When given by inhalation, the H_1 antihistamines can produce irritation and even bronchoconstriction in some asthmatics and, since about 90% of an inhaled dose is swallowed, relatively high doses have to be given which lessens the potential benefit of a reduction in side-effects. The current development of non-sedative H_1 antihistamines may allow large doses to be given to asthmatics without producing sedation and, provided that they retain sufficient potency, this may enable the importance of histamine in asthma to be established.

Since histamine is released from the mast cell, the effectiveness of mast-cell-stabilizing compounds in the treatment of asthma should contribute to our knowledge of the importance of histamine and other mast cell products in the production of asthma. The chapter on disodium cromoglycate and similar drugs considers the mechanisms by which disodium cromoglycate might stabilize mast cells and the relevance of mast cell stabilization to its clinical effects. Numerous compounds have been produced with similar mast-cell-stabilizing activity to that of disodium cromoglycate. Some have been evaluated for their effectiveness in asthma, but have failed to produce a demonstrable or worthwhile benefit when given over a period of time. This could be because of ineffective stabilization of mast cells in man, although some of the compounds have protected against provoked bronchospasm in asthmatics suggesting that, in some situations, they are capable of effective mast cell stabilization. A less orthodox explanation is that mast cell stabilization may not produce an easily measurable clinical benefit in asthma.

Since the work of Brocklehurst in the early 1950s, slow-reacting substance of anaphylaxis (SRS-A) has been a candidate for consideration as an important mediator of asthma. The recent establishment of the structure of SRS-A as a mixture of spasmogenic leukotrienes, together with the synthetic availability of these compounds, has awakened a vast amount of interest. The chapter on the leukotrienes concentrates on their biological activities. There are species differences in the responsiveness of animals to the leukotrienes, with the guinea-pig being particularly sensitive. Nevertheless, the spasmogenic leukotrienes are potent constrictors of human respiratory tissue both *in vivo* and *in vitro* and they can be released from cells other than the mast cell. Their importance in asthma should become evident when both antagonists of their action and inhibitors of their synthesis become available for evaluation in the clinic. Only one antagonist of SRS-A, the Fisons chromone FPL 55712, has been freely available for research and in Chapter 8 the development and biological activity of this compound and that of a number of congeners is discussed. The results obtained with FPL 55712 in the clinic are disappointing. When given by inhalation it has protected normal people from the reduction in respiratory function and the coughing produced by the inhalation of the leukotriene LTC_4 and yet it has provided only a modest protection against antigen-induced bronchoconstriction in asthmatics. The clinical studies with FPL 55712 are limited and a more thorough investigation of the clinical effects of this and similar compounds needs to be made before an assessment can be made of the importance of the spasmogenic leukotrienes in the aetiology of asthma.

Metabolites of arachidonic acid, other than the spasmogenic leukotrienes, may contribute to the pathology of asthma, and these include the products of the cyclo-oxygenase pathway and also the pro-inflammatory products of the lipoxygenase pathway, for example LTB_4. Work is currently being carried out in many laboratories to attempt to produce inhibitors of arachidonic acid metabolism. The published work in this area is reviewed in the chapter on non-steroidal inhibitors of arachidonic acid metabolism.

Not all the products of arachidonic acid metabolism are potentially harmful to an asthmatic. Indeed some prostaglandins, particularly those of the E series, can produce bronchodilatation and stabilize mast cells. A vast amount of effort has been expended by the pharmaceutical industry to produce analogues of the potentially beneficial prostaglandins. This work is reviewed in Chapter 12. To date, it has not been successful in terms of producing a new medicine for asthma. The compounds produce too many side-effects to be given orally and when given by inhalation they have tended to produce irritation of the upper airways.

Platelet-activating factor (PAF) is another product of lipid metabolism which can be released by antigen from sensitized tissues. It has biological activities which make it a possible mediator of some types of asthma and these properties are reviewed in Chapter 4. It can contract smooth muscle, but the bronchoconstriction produced in the rabbit by intravenous administration seems to be an indirect effect dependent upon the platelet. PAF has similarities to the pro-inflammatory LTB_4 in that it can produce similar inflammatory changes in tissues and it can produce inflammation when injected intradermally into man. It is, however, rapidly destroyed *in vivo* and there are species differences in that human platelets and neutrophilic polymorphonuclear leucocytes are less sensitive to activation with PAF than are those of the rabbit. Evaluation of the importance of PAF in asthma may be possible when a specific antagonist or inhibitor of synthesis, suitable for administration to man, has been developed; in fact a specific antagonist has been reported in the period between receiving the manuscript of Chapter 4 and the writing of this introduction[1].

The corticosteroids are an effective treatment for many forms of asthma and, when given by inhalation, they have few side-effects. As with many other effective drugs, the mode of action relevant to their therapeutic effects is far from clear, so that there is no real justification for placing them in the section under inhibitors of mediator release, other than convenience. The relevance to their clinical effects of their ability to inhibit arachidonic acid release in some experimental systems has still to be proven. At therapeutic concentrations, the corticosteroids have no demonstrable effect on the mast cell, which could be taken as further evidence that this cell might not play a central role in asthma. An important activity of the corticosteroids in asthma could be to reduce the inflammation in the lungs. The part that might be played by neutrophilic, and particularly eosinophilic, polymorphonuclear leucocytes in producing the underlying inflammation in the lungs of an asthmatic is discussed in Chapter 5.

The inflammation in the lungs of an asthmatic might increase the sensitivity of spasmogenic and nerve receptors in the airways, and the stimulation of the latter, via a vagal reflex, could increase cholinergic tone. The possibility that acetylcholine, in this sense, might be a mediator of asthma is discussed in Chapter 6. That there is an increase in cholinergic tone in the lungs of an asthmatic is shown by the bronchodilatation that can be produced by anti-cholinergic drugs in some asthmatics. The development of these drugs, in particular their evaluation in the clinic, is discussed in some detail in Chapter 9. The newer anti-cholinergic drugs when given by inhalation seem to produce few side-effects and the putative drying of mucous membranes does not seem to be a problem. The amount of bronchodilatation produced in some asthmatics is less than that produced by the inhalation of β-adrenoceptor stimulants; however, the effect can be longer lasting and of value in the prevention of an early morning attack of asthma.

The development and mode of action of β_2-adrenoceptor stimulants is discussed in Chapter 10. When given by inhalation to asthmatics, they produce bronchodilatation with very few side-effects. The one important disadvantage is that benefit does not last throughout the night. The β_2-adrenoceptor stimulants can also stabilize mast and other inflammatory cells and reduce vascular permeability. It is not certain that these activities are attained at bronchodilator doses and, if these anti-inflammatory effects are relevant, it might have been expected that the compounds would have found an application in other diseases.

Theophylline is, worldwide, the most frequently prescribed treatment for asthma, and its use has increased since the establishment of the blood levels required to produce bronchodilatation. However, at these blood levels it can produce nausea and vomiting and, more seriously, at high blood levels, convulsions and death. There is obviously room for improvement. Theophylline was introduced into therapy in 1936, and despite this it has not been superseded. Numerous compounds have been produced by the pharmaceutical industry with activities claimed to be similar, in laboratory tests, to those of theophylline; these compounds have not been listed. It was thought to be more worthwhile to review the literature on the relevant mode of action of theophylline in the hope that this might help in the design of a new drug.

The final chapter of the book reviews specific hyposensitization therapy in some detail. Although the results of this type of therapy are thought, by many, to be disappointing in the treatment of asthma, it is the one form of therapy that holds the promise of a cure. Some forms of asthma may be due to a defect in the immune system and it is hoped that, in the future, techniques of specific hyposensitization, or immunomodulation with drugs, will be developed to rectify this.

Not all existing or potential treatments of asthma are covered in this book; in particular, there is no chapter on the recent suggestion that asthma may be caused by a deficiency in calcium transport. If a successful drug can be developed based on this idea then it will form an interesting chapter in a subsequent volume.

References

1. TERASHITA, Z-i, TSUSHIMA, S., YOSHIOKA, Y., NOMURA, H., INADA, Y and NASHIKAWA, K. *Life Sciences*, **32**, 1975 (1983)

Part 1

Asthma: the nature of the disease

Chapter 1

Asthma: the nature of the disease

Maurice H. Lessof

Definition: what is asthma?

Asthma—derived from the Greek word meaning panting—was at first used to describe shortness of breath from any cause. By 1686[1] it was regarded, more specifically, as:

'difficult respiration, sometimes with and sometimes without fever, sometimes with a noise and sometimes without, arising from an obstruction of the bronchia and cells of the lungs.'

Eleven years after this description, Sir John Floyer, himself an asthmatic, made two additional observations in his *Treatise of the Asthma*[2]. The first concerned exercise-induced asthma:

'All violent exercise makes the asthmatic to breath short, because their lungs are frequently oppress'd with tubercula; and if the exercise be continued it occasions a fit, by putting the spirits to a great expansion.'

Floyer's second observation concerned the adverse effects of environmental pollution and anticipated much later work on bronchial irritability:

'Any kind of smoak offends the spirits of the asthmatic, and for that reason many of them cannot bear the air of *London*, whose smoak, like fire it self, irritates their spirits into an expansion.'

As the years passed, many further observations were made, concerning both the specific and non-specific factors which are capable of exacerbating or provoking an asthmatic attack. Until a more analytical approach developed, however, many observations of this kind remained merely as isolated records. Although Bernardina Ramazzini described a wheezing cough among grain sifters in the eighteenth century[3], the significance of asthma as an industrial disease was not recognized until the middle of the present century. By this time, the relatively small number of cases among workers who were involved in agriculture and in various types of milling or food processing were supplemented by workers in the new chemical, plastic and pharmaceutical industries. There has since been a steady increase in the number of agents which have been recognized as causing asthma.

9

Asthma has been defined[4] as:

'widespread narrowing of the bronchial airways which changes in severity over short periods of time, either spontaneously or under treatment and which is not due to cardiovascular disease.'

To this should be added the physiologist's observations that

'asthma is a disorder of airways behaviour, in which there is a persisting, overactive bronchoconstrictor response to a variety of stimuli.'

Without the physiologist's reference to bronchoconstriction any definition of asthma is incomplete. Reversible airways obstruction can be caused, not only by bronchospasm, but also by oedema of mucous membranes and by the hypersecretion of mucous glands and sputum retention. Since any or all of these factors can produce wheezing, recurring wheezing breathlessness may occur in a number of different conditions which are not only different in aetiology but require totally different types of treatment. This reservation is of practical importance in both infants and adults.

Infants

The infant's airways are narrow and, below the age of a year, it is common for episodes of bronchitis or bronchiolitis to be associated with wheezing. While bronchospasm can undoubtedly occur, objective measurements of airways resistance have not shown that sympathomimetic bronchodilators are of benefit. Both these drugs and corticosteroids usually fail to shorten the illness[5]. The possibility therefore arises that, in a substantial number of cases of bronchitis at this age, the wheezing which is so commonly observed is the result of mucosal oedema or retained secretions rather than bronchospasm. It is in keeping with this that only a small proportion of infants with wheezy bronchitis go on to develop asthma.

Since wheezing does not necessarily imply bronchospasm, its use as the sole criterion for the diagnosis of asthma will lead to overdiagnosis in some, but to a failure to identify those many asthmatic children who do not wheeze at all. The first symptom of asthma is often a recurrent cough, especially after exercise and, in children, such sputum as there may be is usually swallowed. Delay in making this diagnosis is therefore a considerable problem in this age group.

Adults

An exaggerated constriction of the airways can occur in response to a number of stimuli, including histamine, prostaglandins, cold air, sulphur dioxide and inert dusts. To justify the diagnosis of asthma, the degree of reversibility of airways obstruction therefore needs to be defined. A change of 15% (or 20%) from the baseline value is an arbitrary requirement, but can be shown to sufficiently exceed the variations found in healthy subjects to provide a useful diagnostic criterion. This is not always easy to establish. Bronchial hyper-reactivity persists but is of less importance during the more chronic phases of the disease. There is the additional paradox that a single reading may be misleading, since a transient bronchial hyper-reactivity can occur in otherwise healthy subjects during and immediately after a viral upper respiratory tract infection[6] (*Figure 1.1*). This bronchial reactivity can be partially reversed by atropine or by local anaesthesia of the pharynx, and it is therefore probable that cholinergic reflexes are involved rather than mast cell activation (*Figure 1.2*).

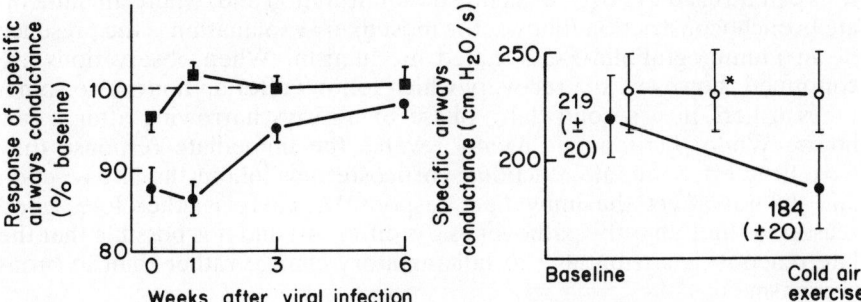

Figure 1.1 (left) Changes in airways conductance after cold air exercise in 13 patients with recent upper respiratory viral infection. ■ Cold air breathing; ● exercise with cold air. (After Aquilina *et al.*[17].)

Figure 1.2 (right) Effects of pharyngeal anaesthesia on the response to cold air exercise in 5 patients with upper respiratory tract infection. * Before this measurement was taken, the pharynx was anaesthetized with lidocaine. (After Aquilina *et al.*[17].)

In studying reversible airways obstruction, the use of the peak flow meter has achieved wide popularity because of its convenience. Nevertheless, the finding of a transient reduction in peak flow readings is open to more than one interpretation, especially in patients with chronic bronchitis and obstructive airways disease. In many such cases, a partial reversibility of airways obstruction may indicate, not the presence of bronchospasm, but of mucosal oedema and retained secretions. Since mucus secretion can be inhibited by corticosteroids[7], improvement of lung function after steroid treatment is thus insufficient evidence on which to base a diagnosis of 'missed asthma'. Due to the hazard of infection, corticosteroids should therefore be used with caution. Follow-up studies over a six-month period have indeed provided no evidence that long-term corticosteroids are beneficial in such cases[8].

The difficulty is one of definition. If it is accepted that bronchial hyperreactivity is an essential part of the asthmatic process, many of these bronchitic subjects do not have asthma at all. Instead, they often have the partially obstructed airways which result from the long-standing irritant effects of smoking, atmospheric pollution, and recurrent infection. These changes, including those of sputum retention, mucosal oedema, and other pathological changes in the bronchial wall, have been well described in patients with obstructive airways disease who come to necropsy[9].

The confusion which may arise between bronchial asthma and left-sided heart failure has also been the subject of some comment. Episodes of wheezing can occur in patients who have mitral stenosis with left atrial hypertension or 'cardiac asthma'[10]. As in other patients who wheeze, those with cardiac asthma do not necessarily have bronchospasm and may not respond to bronchodilator drugs.

Extrinsic and intrinsic asthma

In extrinsic asthma, attacks are provoked by external agents—in contrast to intrinsic asthma in which no external causative factors can be identified. The agents which are responsible are usually allergens but in some cases of occupational asthma may act as irritants. The clinical response to challenge tests can be used to provide diagnostic confirmation and, where an immediate bronchoconstriction follows, the most likely explanation is the presence of an immunoglobulin-E-associated mechanism. When observations are continued, however, the recovery which follows after an hour or so sometimes ushers in a second 'late' phase of airways narrowing after a few hours. While β-adrenergic agents reverse the immediate response they have little effect on late reactions; corticosteroids inhibit the late reaction and do not affect the immediate response[11]. There is, therefore, good reason to think that the pathogenesis is different, and it is possible that the late reaction is attributable to inflammatory change rather than to bronchospasm.

From the point of view of the patient's symptoms, the late reactions may indeed be the more important, especially because of their cumulative effect and because of the chronicity which may follow repeated antigen exposure. In a study of children with asthma who were treated with a dust mite vaccine, it was noted that clinical evidence of benefit was not accompanied by any significant change in the immediate response to a bronchial provocation test. However, the late response to a *Dermatophagoides pteronyssinus* inhalational challenge showed a significant reduction in those patients who showed the greatest improvement in symptoms[12].

It does not follow that all extrinsic asthma depends on immunological mechanisms. Irritants such as ozone or sulphur dioxide[13] can provoke asthmatic attacks, and agents used in industry such as toluene diisocyanate can also act as respiratory irritants in some cases rather than acting

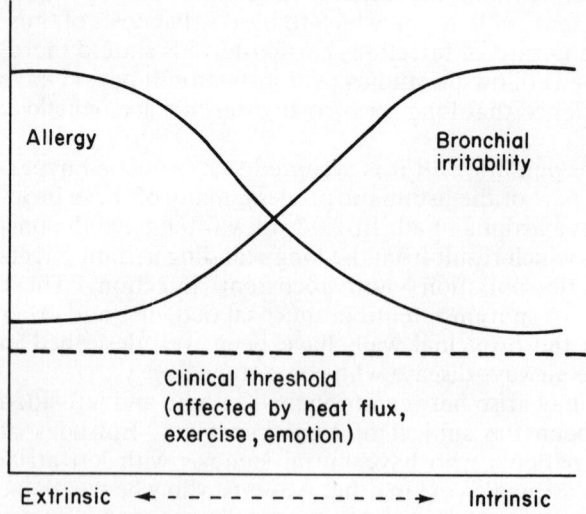

Figure 1.3 Contributory causes of asthma.

immunologically[14]. However, in the large majority of cases, immune mechanisms appear to be involved.

The distinction between extrinsic and intrinsic asthma is by no means always clear cut. Intrinsic asthma is unassociated with evidence of an IgE response and, in general, tends to develop relatively late in life[15]. In intrinsic asthma, bronchial hyper-reactivity is perhaps the most striking feature—but this cannot by itself distinguish the condition from allergic asthma, in which at least some degree of bronchial irritability is also a feature. (This could explain why 90% of grass-pollen-allergic patients merely have hay fever and only the remaining 10%, with bronchial hyper-reactivity, have asthma.) The natural history of the disease shows no respect for this classification. The man who once had allergic asthma in childhood may recover from this and lose his bronchial hyper-reactivity, only to regain it when he starts smoking cigarettes in adult life, develops chest infections and suffers the stresses of business life. He may then develop what is regarded as intrinsic asthma, based on a pattern of airways hyper-reactivity which dates back to childhood. The contributory factors (*Figure 1.3*) can thus vary in the different stages of the life of an asthmatic.

Natural history

In the United Kingdom, United States and Australia, nearly all estimates suggest that at least 40% of asthmatics have developed their illness by the age of 10 years. Atopy appears to play a considerable part in this age group, and it has been estimated that three-quarters of patients with childhood asthma are atopic, as compared with only one-third in whom asthma begins after the age of 45 years. Although the more severely affected children continue to have asthma in adult life, the prognosis for the majority is very good indeed, as has been shown in numerous follow-up studies. At least three-quarters of asthmatic children have stopped having attacks by the age of puberty and, while bronchial hyper-reactivity may still be demonstrable by exercise tests or after inhalation of methacholine, the majority (perhaps two-thirds) never have asthma again. Nevertheless, a recurrence of asthma some years later is by no means unknown.

Atopy

It is common for asthma to be associated with other manifestations of allergy. Allergic rhinitis was diagnosed in 54% of extrinsic asthmatics, but only 7% of intrinsic asthmatics, who were studied at the Brompton Hospital by Turner-Warwick. A history of infantile eczema is also common among asthmatics and was found in 26% of asthmatics of all ages at the Brompton Hospital. A familial susceptibility to atopy may thus be an important factor in many cases of asthma. This is not invariable. Eczema and other forms of allergic hypersensitivity are very uncommon among Tristan da Cunha islanders, who have a high prevalence of asthma (*see below*) with an inherited susceptibility which cannot be explained on the basis of a familial atopy. In Tristan da Cunha, it has been noted that the arrival of visiting ships is often followed by well-defined outbreaks of colds and influenza, with an increased incidence of wheeze and bronchitis. In this situation, a hyper-reactive response to respiratory tract infection appears to be by far the most common provoking cause of wheezing.

The explanation for the association between infection and bronchial hyper-reactivity remains elusive. Evidence of an association between asthma and IgE antibodies to bacterial antigens has been looked for and not found[16]. However, the relationship with viral infection still remains to be studied. When postinfective bronchial hyper-reactivity occurs in healthy subjects, it subsides within a matter of weeks[17], which could theoretically be related to the healing of a damaged mucosa or to the removal of a viral irritant. However, a similar reduction in bronchial hyper-reactivity can also occur in allergic asthma when the allergen is removed from the environment—as has been shown in dust-mite-sensitive asthmatics when the dust mite population is controlled[18].

The association between allergy and asthma involves a number of different mechanisms and the difference between early and late reactions has already been referred to. In patients with food allergy, even the smell of the offending food can be sufficient to provoke asthma by the inhalational route; but asthma may also be provoked in these subjects by blind challenge through a nasogastric tube. In some studies, but not all, oral sodium cromoglycate has been shown to prevent this type of food-induced asthma, whereas inhaled cromoglycate may fail to do so[19]. This, therefore, suggests a triggering mechanism in the bowel wall, possibly involving local mast cells.

This may apply to immediate reactions only. Food-induced late asthma can occur in isolation, without any evidence of an association with IgE mechanisms[20] and it appears that this late type of asthma cannot be prevented by oral cromoglycate[21]. It has been suggested[22] that this signifies yet another factor in food-induced asthma, such as immune complex formation. Whether this is the case remains to be established.

Environmental factors

An increased incidence of asthma is associated with residence in a damp climate and has also been noted after sudden atmospheric cooling. High altitudes are said to be beneficial and coastal resorts harmful. In virtually every case, the apparent association with meteorological factors has been explained by the presence of intermediate triggering agents, which can sometimes be clearly identified. The seasonal dispersal of mould spores in damp weather can lead to outbreaks of asthma, and Gregg[23] showed that a seasonal incidence of wheezy bronchitis in children can be correlated with a rise in the isolation rate of rhinoviruses. Other factors have also been involved. Maunsell noted the high dust mite count in damp houses and it was subsequently shown how low the mite count is in the beneficial climate of the Swiss Alps. Mites can also cause seasonal asthma, as Pickering and Gabriel found in Hong Kong, where asthma during the winter months may result from contact with mite-infested bed quilts.

The effects of urbanization and of affluence are less clearly documented. A higher incidence in African townships than in the country has led to speculation about the possible role of parasites, either in provoking asthma or in providing protection. No clear-cut evidence has been produced, and among Western communities it has been noted that the disease is more common in overcrowded, damp and badly heated houses, where there may be both a high exposure to house dust mites and an increased risk of respiratory tract infection.

Other types of environmental exposure are seen in industry, and it has been estimated that 10–20% of bakers eventually develop respiratory tract symptoms following exposure to flour. Although environmental control measures can be of considerable benefit, those involved in the colour printing trade or in the platinum industry tend to have an even higher incidence of industrial asthma, and those who work with animals or who manufacture plastic or pharmaceutical materials also encounter a similar problem. Nevertheless, occupational asthma represents only a small percentage of all cases in Britain. In other countries, for example in Japan, up to 15% of all male cases of asthma have been suspected as being of an industrial origin.

It is now clear that there are a number of powerful sensitizers which can provoke asthma both in atopic and in non-atopic individuals (*see Table 1.1*). These include the enzymes of *Bacillus subtilis* which are present in biological washing powders and the dust of the Western Red Cedar and other veneers used by woodworkers. Asthma can also be provoked by the dust from castor bean mills or grain mills and, in the case of toluene diisocyanate, a case of sensitization has been reported in a man who was exposed to the ventilation fumes from a nearby factory.

TABLE 1.1. Occupational causes of asthma*

Biological causes	Industrial process
Bacillus subtilis enzymes	Enzyme manufacture
Small mammals' urine	Laboratory work, pig breeding
Soft solder flux (colophony)	Electronic industry soldering
Grain, flour, moulds and mites	Farming, grain handling, baking
Antibiotics and other drugs	Manufacture of pharmaceuticals
Wood dust	Forestry and wood handling
Chemical causes	*Industrial process*
Diisocyanates	Polyurethane manufacture, spray painting, some printing
Acid anhydrides and hardening agents	Manufacture and use of adhesives and surface coatings
Complex platinum salts	Platinum refining

* After Newman Taylor, 1982[24].

In each case of industrial exposure, the atopic individual is likely to be affected at an early stage. In one study in a platinum refinery[24], 40% of new employees left within 18 months because they developed occupational asthma. Although the prevalence of occupational asthma is much lower in other industries, between 5 and 10% of those who work with laboratory animals are affected and perhaps 3% of those who manufacture enzyme detergents.

Symptoms of occupational asthma tend to begin late, some hours after contact with the offending material. Cough may predominate rather than wheeze, and the effect may be worse at home in the evenings or be cumulative throughout a working week, until the prolonged episodes of bronchial narrowing no longer seem to have any relationship to their occupational origin. At a time of rapid increase in the use of highly reactive industrial chemicals, the potential role of these agents in provoking asthmatic attacks may be insufficiently appreciated.

Exercise-induced asthma

In asthmatics, the response to exercise depends on its duration, on the frequency with which it is repeated and on the heat flux across the mucous membranes of the respiratory tract. The degree of heat flux appears to be of crucial importance in provoking bronchospasm, and hyperventilating in cold dry air can achieve a similar result. In asthmatics who take exercise, estimates of heat flux, based on differences of temperature and water content of inspired and expired air, show a close correlation with the one-second forced expiratory volume (FEV_1)[25].

The response to exercise is not a simple one. Exercise of one or two minutes duration is likely to cause bronchodilatation, but after five to eight minutes bronchoconstriction occurs[26]. The maximum bronchoconstriction is achieved five minutes or more after the end of the exercise, and residual changes may still be detectable after one hour or more.

When exercise is repeated every 30–40 minutes, the bronchoconstrictor effect diminishes and a reduced effect is still noted when the exercise is repeated after one hour but not after two[27]. It has been suggested that this time delay is highly significant, and that a full response to exercise is able to occur again only after the time it takes for the chemical mediators of the response to be replenished. Allergen challenge can, however, sometimes provoke bronchospasm in subjects who have ceased to respond to exercise[28].

Sodium cromoglycate is capable of preventing exercise-induced asthma, and the simplest explanation of this effect is that this drug prevents the release of mast cell products, so interfering with the mediating mechanism. As in all discussions concerning cromoglycate, this may be an over-simplification, since it is possible that cromoglycate also has an inhibitory affect on neural reflexes, as suggested by its ability to prevent sulphur-dioxide-induced asthma[13] and by its effect on the afferent C fibres of dog lung[29].

It does not necessarily follow that the mechanism is the same in all subjects. When maximal expiratory flow–volume curves are recorded, breathing either air or a 20% : 80% mixture of oxygen in helium, the flow rate in the larger airways is disproportionately dependent on the density of the mixture breathed. After exercise, McFadden and his colleagues[30] found that this dependence on density was reduced in seven out of twelve asthmatics, suggesting that the changes were mainly those of small airways obstruction. Prophylactic cromoglycate reduced the constrictor effect of exercise in these seven, conceivably by preventing the non-specific release of mediators from mast cells. While this interpretation remains speculative, the effect of exercise in the remaining five was different and resulted in an increased dependence of flow upon changes in density, suggesting that the obstruction was mainly in the larger airways. In these five, cholinergic blockade was able to prevent postexertional air-flow obstruction, suggesting that the obstruction in these cases may have been neurogenic.

The role of mediators has been further investigated by Barnes and Brown[31], who found a rise in plasma histamine levels in those subjects who develop exercise-induced asthma, and in the work of Lee and his colleagues[32], who found a rise in plasma levels of neutrophil chemotactic activity. While exercise-induced asthma may thus show features which are compatible with a vagal reflex origin in some cases and a dependence of mediators in others, both factors may well play some part in the majority.

Psychological factors

The French physician Trousseau was an asthmatic who knew that he was sensitive to horses but could go into the stables without incident. He often lost his temper with his coachman but found that he could do this with impunity provided that it was in the open air. What he learned was that he had to avoid losing his temper with his coachman in the stable. This combination of circumstances always provoked an attack of asthma. Trousseau thus proved, to his own satisfaction, what many asthmatics know instinctively—that emotion can act as an exacerbating factor in asthma.

There are probably several pathways by which emotion can provoke an asthmatic attack. Emotionally induced asthma has been mimicked by asking patients to imagine a frightening experience. In these circumstances, hyperventilation can be shown to form a part of the early response, followed shortly afterwards by bronchospasm. In one study, the response was abolished by atropine.

The question of whether emotion can play a more fundamental part in the aetiology of asthma remains uncertain. None of the studies which have attempted to establish this have given clear-cut results. These negative findings do not, however, diminish the importance of emotion as a conditioning factor in this disease.

Asthma deaths

Despite the development of effective and safe anti-asthma drugs, more than 1000 asthma deaths occur each year in England and Wales. A sudden rise in deaths from asthma in Britain, Australia and New Zealand in the mid-1960s, after years of relatively stable mortality rates, suggested a new factor in the treatment of asthma. At the time, suspicion fell on the insufficient use of corticosteroids in an acute attack and, more importantly, on an increased use of nebulized isoprenaline in doses which were relatively uncontrolled and were suspected of causing cardiac arrhythmia. In West Germany, Canada and the United States, where the mortality rate for asthma was in any case low and where this form of treatment had not been adopted, the death rate did not show any significant variation during the same period.

From 1975 to 1979, mortality figures from New Zealand showed a further sharp increase in deaths from asthma in young people which has not appeared in any other country studied and cannot be explained by changes in certification or in the populations studied[33]. This change has almost certainly been due to an increase in case fatality rate. Among other possible explanations, the additive toxicity of β agonists and oral theophylline has been suggested as a cause[34], although firm conclusions cannot yet be drawn.

Pathology

The histology of the relatively early changes seen in lung biopsy specimens and the relatively acute necropsy changes of status asthmaticus, throw some added light on the subject. In status asthmaticus, the lungs are over-inflated and the air is 'trapped' within them by the blockage of large and small airways with tenacious secretions. The alveoli may be affected by impacted mucus, by oedema or by inflammatory consolidation. The ciliary action which clears mucus from the bronchi has failed, and beneath the impacted mucus are layers of cells, particularly eosinophils[35]. Below the shedding layers of surface epithelium the membrane is thickened and there is an inflammatory cell infiltrate (sometimes modified by corticosteroid treatment) in which, again, the eosinophils have a prominent place. The muscle of the bronchial wall is hypertrophied, and as in chronic bronchitis, there may be hypertrophy of the mucus-secreting glands[9], but this is by no means an invariable feature. This is consistent with the observation of Lynne Reid that, whereas the hallmark of chronic bronchitis is the regular and persistent production of sputum, the hallmark of asthma is rapidly reversible airways obstruction.

In those patients who, instead of dying of status asthmaticus, make a satisfactory recovery, it is likely that the clearance of retained secretions is impaired until, within a week or two, normal ciliated epithelium regenerates. While, to some extent, cough may replace ciliary action in clearing retained secretions, there appears to be a structural basis for the increased susceptibility to infection which is commonly noted. Oedema and inflammation of the bronchial or bronchiolar wall adds to the airways obstruction and may take some time to subside.

After severe and long-lasting disease, recurrent bronchospasm, with bronchial obstruction, secondary infection and inflammatory reaction can lead on to the secondary changes of recurrent bronchial damage and of chronic bronchitis. These are then added to the earlier features of asthma. In addition, there may occasionally be such additional developments as plastic bronchitis, in which the patient coughs up casts, or blockage of the large airways which can lead to massive collapse; there may be secondary aspergillosis, with eosinophilia, vasculitis, and the development of 'cystic' regions.

Epidemiology

Most of the epidemiological studies of asthma have been conducted among children. Most have reported cumulative prevalence rates, but the diagnostic criteria have differed so much that some of the differences, especially between one country and another, have related as much to the different criteria used as to the differing incidence of the disease.

In the United Kingdom among school children, prevalence rates have ranged from 1.6% to 4.8% in different studies[23]. If, on the other hand, the prevalence of wheeze or 'wheezy bronchitis' is studied, a much higher range is reported, varying between 9.9% and 24.9%. Similar figures have been noted for the United States and a rather higher incidence of asthma among school children in Australasia. The higher figures from Australasia may represent a difference in diagnostic custom, since the breakdown into unequivocal asthma, asthmatic bronchitis and occasional mild wheezy bronchitis has, in one series[36], given figures which seem comparable to those reported in Britain.

It has been noted that, in Singapore, 86% of all asthma begins before the age of 20 years, as compared with 31.1% in Zaria, Nigeria and only 11.5% in Misurata, Libya[37]. To some extent, different diagnostic criteria may have influenced these figures, but they could hardly explain such gross discrepancies. There are also other national differences which would be even more difficult to explain on the assumption that different diagnostic criteria have been used. At least five separate Scandinavian studies have indicated an incidence below 1%. It is also possible that there is a low prevalence rate in Japan, in Papua New Guinea, and in rural India.

An interesting study has been carried out by Morrison-Smith and his colleagues[38], who estimated the prevalence of asthma among a multiracial population of school children in Birmingham. Negro children who had been born in the West Indies but had come to this country when young had significantly less asthma than English children or Negro children who were born in England. Asian children born in England or in Asia also had a low prevalence, but Asian children born in Kenya had as high a prevalence as English children. There thus appeared to be differences between different groups of children of the same racial origin, apparently related in some way to environmental factors.

It is notable that Asians in Kenya enjoyed a high standard of living conditions before leaving their country to come to Britain. Since they were alone among Asians in having a high prevalence of asthma, this suggested that there might be environmental factors in those with improved living conditions which favoured the development of childhood asthma. This remains unproven but, as in the case of eczema[39], it has been argued that the abandonment of breast feeding and a high exposure to dust mite and other environmental allergens might conceivably result in an increased susceptibility to allergic reactions.

The problem of identifying asthma among adults is even greater than in children, because of the different diagnostic labels that are attached to patients with chronic obstructive bronchitis who wheeze. Some impressive geographical variations have, however, been reported. North American Indians and Eskimos rarely develop asthma. Fifty years ago, some hospitals in the Indian reservations had never seen a case. More recently, a review of all hospital admissions among Eskimos in the Mackenzie Delta showed only three certain cases of asthma during a 12-year period.

In striking contrast to these populations in which the prevalence of asthma is low, reference has already been made to the remarkably high prevalence among the closely inbred population of Tristan da Cunha. Three of the 15 original settlers suffered from asthma, and when Citron and Pepys studied this small community of about 70 families in 1963, three-quarters of the population had a family history of the disease. It seems, however, that the prevalence of asthma has decreased in this island from 1946, when it was estimated that 49% of the population had active asthma. In 1971, a further survey established that active asthma was present in only 32% of the population.

Sex distribution

In Tristan da Cunha, active asthma was found to be four times more common in women than in men aged 13–39 years. This may, however, represent a special case, since the three original settlers who had asthma were all women. In other countries, surveys carried out among school children have suggested that asthma is more common among boys than among girls, by factors of as much as 2.5:1 and 3.3:1 in Aberdeen school children of various ages; the reason for this higher incidence among male children is unknown. There is no evidence of a sex difference in sensitization to common allergens. On the other hand, boys are more susceptible to development of lower respiratory tract infection, and behavioural differences may also make them more prone to the development of exercise-induced symptoms.

When the sex distribution among adult asthmatics has been analysed, the difference has been much less prominent. In some Scandinavian series, women have been more frequently affected. A genetic component has been suggested by the finding that the concordance of asthma is much higher in monozygotic than in dizygotic twins, but the fact that monozygotic twins do not always behave in the same way suggests that, regardless of an inherited predisposition, environmental factors also play a part.

Pathological mechanisms

In extrinsic asthma, it is assumed that antigens are deposited in the airways and react with antibody on the surface of mast cells. In keeping with this, in both man and primates, it has been shown that mast cells are present above the epithelial membrane, close to the bronchial lumen. When stimulated, they release chemical mediators and this is followed by the development of bronchospasm, together with insidious changes in the mucosal lining of the bronchi and in the mucous secretions which are responsible for the late reaction. While the normal bronchial epithelium is virtually impermeable to high-molecular-weight proteins[40], histamine release increases the permeability of the surface epithelium and allows antigen to penetrate. In this way further reactions may be stimulated.

In addition to this mechanism, it has been shown that vagal reflexes are involved in some types of acute allergic bronchoconstriction[41]. Direct stimulation of irritant receptors by histamine can also lead to bronchoconstriction, which can be effectively blocked with atropine or with inhaled hexamethonium[42]. The importance of a vagal reflex mechanism is also suggested by the fact that non-immunological factors such as cold air, exercise and sulphur dioxide are all capable of causing bronchoconstriction, not only in allergic individuals, but also in patients with intrinsic asthma. Without the vagal reflex it is, indeed, difficult to explain why asthma should be provoked by large particles of grass pollen or dust mite faeces, which do not appear to penetrate beyond the larger airways.

The role of the vagal pathway is, however, limited. This is much more evident in clinical asthma than it is in the experimental situation. Drugs with atropine-like activity have little clinical value in patients with asthma. Even in acute provocation tests, blocking the vagal pathway does not prevent a bronchoconstrictor response to methacholine[42], and only about 60% of cases of exercise-induced asthma are blocked by ipratropium in doses up to 2 mg[43].

Many attempts have been made to identify the site of narrowing in bronchial asthma. Like everything else in this multifactorial disease, this problem evades a simple answer. Both larger and smaller airways are involved, and the relative importance of each may vary from time to time in the same individual. The newer techniques for recording flow–volume loops have suggested that it is the larger airways which mainly determine air-flow resistance, and it is the constriction of these larger airways which appears to be mainly responsible for acute episodes in which the forced expiratory volume falls suddenly and then recovers equally rapidly. Even when asthmatics are thought to be in remission, however, reduced air-flow at low lung volumes suggests that there may be small airways narrowing in the absence of clinical asthma.

The role of mediators

It is clear that no simplistic view of the mechanism of asthma can stand up to examination. The prominence which has been given to the role of histamine in the past can be seen to explain only a part of a very complex picture. Plasma histamine levels are raised in patients admitted to hospital with severe asthma, and these levels fall to normal during therapy[44]. Diurnal changes in peak expiratory flow rates in many patients with asthma can also be correlated with venous plasma levels of histamine[45]. However, antihistamines are not, in general, effective in the treatment of this disease. This suggests that histamine levels may represent merely a marker of mast cell activity. As compared to the leukotrienes which have much more potent bronchoconstrictor activity, the role of histamine in asthma is probably a relatively minor one. As illustrated in *Figure 1.4*, the triggering of mast cells involves the cascading effects, not of a single mediator, but of a complex system which leads to smooth muscle spasm, mucus production, mucosal oedema, and eventually to complex inflammatory changes.

The effects of mediators have now come to be analysed in some detail. Prostaglandins and thromboxanes are derived from arachidonic acid through the cyclo-oxygenase pathway. Of the prostaglandins, only PGD_2 has been identified as originating from the mast cell. However, prostaglandin $F_{2\alpha}$ and thromboxane A_2 have similar constrictor effects on bronchial smooth muscle, and it is possible that all three contribute to the complex reactions which are involved in an anaphylactic response. Arachidonic acid also acts as a raw material for the production of the lipidopeptide substances known as leukotrienes. The lipoxygenase pathway of arachidonic acid metabolism leads to the production of leukotrienes C_4 and D_4, which also have powerful effects in increasing muscle reactivity and in stimulating

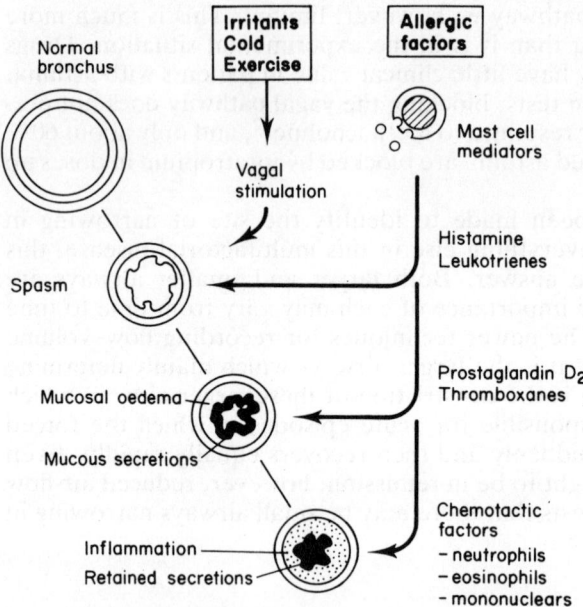

Figure 1.4 Pathogenesis of asthma.

contraction. The complex interaction of these different substances is still not fully understood. When the cyclo-oxygenase pathway is blocked by aspirin or other non-steroidal anti-inflammatory drugs, a diversion to the lipoxygenase pathway may occur and it is possible that inhibition of the synthesis of one type of mediator may lead to the increased production of another. In addition, the homeostatic balance between bronchodilator prostaglandins of the E series and bronchoconstrictor prostaglandins appears to vary in different subjects. This may help to explain the observation that, in some non-atopic asthmatic subjects, aspirin relieves an asthmatic attack, in contrast to a rather larger number of asthmatics who note that their attacks can be provoked by a variety of aspirin-like drugs.

In most healthy people, aspirin is well tolerated and causes neither bronchodilatation nor bronchoconstriction, neither vasodilatation nor vasoconstriction, and neither platelet aggregation nor any gross bleeding tendency. Depressed synthesis of arachidonic acid metabolites, whether due to malnutrition and arachidonic acid deficiency or to drug effects on cyclo-oxygenase activity, may therefore have the effect of depressing what is already a self-balanced system. The consequence may be the loss of powerful regulating mechanisms, but there are no catastrophic changes in the short term. The homeostatic balance may, nevertheless, be disturbed by drugs which inhibit some or all of the arachidonic acid metabolic pathways. What is surprising is that this does not occur more often.

The role of leukotrienes in asthma has still to be evaluated. In experimental situations, the potent effect on smooth muscle of even pico-gram amounts of leukotrienes C_4 and D_4 has suggested that these subst-ances can have a powerful role in asthma. Paradoxically, drugs such as benoxaprofen which have been claimed to inhibit the lipoxygenase path-way have, as yet, had little effect on asthma. Several explanations have been offered but it seems possible that, as with histamine and the prosta-glandins, we may be examining a series of mediators of which no single one is of over-riding importance. In the lipoxygenase pathway, as in the cyclo-oxygenase pathway, there may be a balanced system of products with opposite effects, some of which have yet to be identified. If so, this would explain why the results of interference with any of the arachidonic acid metabolic pathways is essentially neutral and containable. Not surpri-singly, the loss of a powerful fine-adjusting system could nevertheless cause occasional clinical problems.

The effects of mast cell mediators do not terminate with the end of the immediate response. The increased vascular permeability caused by such mediators as histamine sets the scene for subsequent inflammatory changes, and the release of eosinophil and neutrophil chemotactic factors attracts an inflammatory infiltrate which, in turn, releases proteolytic enzymes and causes further tissue damage. Platelet-activating factor also has an inflammatory role and it is possible that, in some circumstances, the complement enzymes may be activated.

The processes which have so far been considered are mainly concerned with the triggering of bronchoconstriction. Cut-off mechanisms are equally important. Indeed, it is the speed of mediator breakdown by the body's complex enzyme systems that has made it so difficult to isolate and char-acterize these very powerful substances. The attraction to the area of eosi-nophil and mononuclear cells reinforces the breakdown mechanisms by providing a fresh supply of enzymes, including histaminases. In addtion to its reaction-limiting role, however, the eosinophil is itself able to cause tis-sue damage by releasing granules of major basic protein[46]. This could explain why, in diseases such as polyarteritis nodosa, the presence of pul-monary eosinophilia is not infrequently associated with asthma.

Adrenergic and cholinergic influences

Adrenergic mechanisms are also an intimate part of the switch-off appar-atus which limits the duration of bronchospasm. Mast cells have both adrenergic and cholinergic receptors, and by increasing intracellular levels of adenosine cyclic $3':5'$-monophosphate (cyclic AMP or cAMP) β-adrenergic agents such as isoprenaline can be shown to suppress mediator release, and circulating catecholamines can cut short the broncho-constrictor response. α-Adrenergic agents reduce cyclic AMP concentra-tions and have the reverse effect. It has been suggested that a 'Yin-Yang' relationship may exist between cyclic AMP and cyclic GMP (guanosine cyclic 3':5'-monophosphate) and that cholinergic stimulation, by causing a rise in cyclic GMP and a fall in cyclic AMP, may have the opposite effect to β-adrenergic stimulation. This view has been challenged but the situation is far from clear.

Apart from adrenergic and cholinergic effects upon mediator release from mast cells, and hence upon smooth muscle contraction, the tone of airways smooth muscle is also regulated more directly by the vagus and by cholinergic stimulation which can cause contraction. In addition, although sympathetic nerve endings have never been demonstrated in smooth muscle, β-adrenergic stimulation leads to relaxation. By its controlling influence on submucosal glands and blood vessels, the autonomic nervous system can also stimulate excessive mucus secretion and help to provoke bronchial mucosal oedema, both of which are additional features of asthma.

Szentivanyi[47] suggested that β-adrenoceptor blockade might be responsible for the hyper-reactivity of the airways in asthmatics, and there is evidence that asthmatics have a decreased β-adrenergic response but an increased responsiveness to cholinergic stimuli. It is still uncertain whether this represents a basic defect in asthmatic individuals, or whether it results from adrenergic treatment or the excessive release of endogenous catecholamines. Although some asthmatics possess autoantibodies to β_2-adrenergic receptors[48], suggesting a mechanism by which this blockade could operate, this could account for only a minority of cases in which this antibody is detectable. Furthermore, when adrenergic treatment is withdrawn, the observed reduction in both β-adrenergic responsiveness and β-receptor density disappears within a few days, suggesting merely a secondary effect of treatment, possibly the result of tachyphylaxis[49].

The airways of asthmatics are also hyper-reactive to cholinergic agonists and, in the presence of β blockade, inhaled α-adrenergic agents can also cause bronchoconstriction. While the significance of α-adrenergic responses is still debatable, there is some evidence that atopic subjects, in general, show a reduced response to β-adrenergic stimulation and an increased cholinergic response, even apart from asthma[50].

There is little evidence to suggest that an imbalance of autonomic control is a primary defect in asthma. It seems likely, however, that mast cell excitability and bronchial smooth muscle responsiveness are influenced by a number of different homeostatic mechanisms, including some which are concerned with autonomic receptors or with autonomic neurotransmitters. Any modulation or failure of the homeostatic apparatus may, therefore, add to the complexity of the asthmatic response.

References

1. SALMON. *Compleat System of Physic*, London (1686)
2. FLENLEY, D. C. Quoted in *The Current Role of Intal in the Management of Asthma*, Medical Education Services. Oxford: Medicine Publishing Foundation (1982)
3. RAMAZZINI, M. *De Morbus Artificum Diatriba* 1713. Trans. W. C. Wright. Chicago: University Chicago Press (1940)
4. CIBA GUEST SYMPOSIUM. *Thorax*, **14**, 286 (1959)

5. GODFREY, S. In *Asthma*. Eds. T. J. H. Clark and S. Godfrey. p. 324. London: Chapman and Hall (1977)

6. EMPEY, D.W., LAITINEN, L.A., JACOBS, L., GOLD, W.M. and NADEL, J.A. *American Review of Respiratory Diseases,* **113,** 131 (1976)

7. SHELHAMER, J.H., MAROM, Z. and KALINER, M. *American Academy of Allergy*, Abstracts **6,** 24 (1981)

8. STOKES, T.C., SHAYLOR, J.M., O'REILLY, J.F. and HARRISON, B.D.W. *Lancet*, **ii**, 345–348 (1982)

9. DUNNILL, M.S., MASSARELLA, G.R. and ANDERSON J. *Thorax*, **24,** 176 (1969)

10. ROSS, J. In *Textbook of Medicine*, 16th ed. Eds J.B. Wyngaarden and L.H. Smith. p. 196. Philadelphia: W.B. Saunders (1982)

11. DAVIES, R.J. In *Immunological and Clinical Aspects of Allergy*. Ed. M.H. Lessof. p. 217. Lancaster: MTP Press (1981)

12. WARNER, J.O., PRICE, J.F., SOOTHILL, J.F. and HEY, E.N. *Lancet*, **ii,** 912 (1978)

13. HARRIES, M.G., PARKES, P.E.G., LESSOF, M.H. and ORR, S.T.C. *Lancet*, **i,** 5 (1981)

14. DAVIES, R.J. and PEPYS, J. In *Asthma*. Eds T.J.H. Clark and S. Godfrey. p. 190. London: Chapman and Hall (1977)

15. RACKERMANN, F.M. *Archives of Internal Medicine*, **22,** 517 (1981)

16. TEE, R.D. and PEPYS, J. *Clinical Allergy*, **12,** 439–450 (1982)

17. AQUILINA, A.T., HALL, W.J., DOUGLAS, R.J. Jr and UTELL, M.J. *American Review of Respiratory Diseases*, **122,** 3 (1980)

18. MURRAY, A.N. and FERGUSON, A.C. *Lancet*, **ii,** 1212 (1982)

19. DAHL, R. *Allergy*, **36,** 161 (1981)

20. LESSOF, M.H., WRAITH, D.G., MERRETT, T.G. and BUISSERET, P.D. *Quarterly Journal of Medicine,* **49,** 259 (1980)

21. PAPAGEORGIOU, N., LEE, T.H., NAGAKURA, T., WRAITH, D.G. and KAY, A.B. *Journal of Allergy and Clinical Immunology*, **72,** 75–82 (1983)

22. BROSTOFF, J., CARINI, C. and WRAITH, D.G. In *The Mast Cell: Its Role in Health and Disease*. Eds J. Pepys and A.M. Edwards. p. 380. London: Pitman Medical (1979)

23. GREGG, I. In *Asthma*. Eds T.J.H. Clark and S. Godfrey. p. 214. London: Chapman and Hall (1977)

24. NEWMAN TAYLOR, A. *Medicine International*, **1,** 1007 (1982)

25. DEAL, E.C. McFADDEN, E.R. Jr, INGRAM, R.H. Jr, HAYNES, R.L. and WELLMAN, J.J. *Journal of Applied Physiology*, **2,** 746 (1977)

26. SLY, R.M. *Annals of Allergy*, **49,** 16–19 (1982)

27. JAMES, L., FACIANE, J. and SLY, R.M. *Journal of Allergy and Clinical Immunology*, **57,** 408–416 (1976)

28. WEILER-RAVELL, D. and GODFREY, S. *Journal of Allergy and Clinical Immunology*, **67,** 391 (1980)

29. DIXON, M., JACKSON, D.M. and RICHARDS, I.M. *British Journal of Pharmacology*, **70,** 11 (1980)

30. McFADDEN, E.R. Jr, INGRAM, R.H. Jr, HAYNES, R.L. and WELLMAN, J.J. *Journal of Applied Physiology*, **46,** 467 (1977)

31. BARNES, P.J. and BROWN, M.H. *Clinical Science*, **61,** 159 (1981)

32. LEE, T.H., NAGY, L., NAGAKURA, T., WALPOST, M.H. and KAY, A.B. *Journal of Clinical Investigation*, **69,** 889 (1982)

33. JACKSON, R.T., BEAGLEHOLE, R., REA, H.H. and SUTHERLAND, D.C. *British Medical Journal*, **285,** 771 (1982)

34. WILSON, J.D., SUTHERLAND, D.C. and THOMAS, A.C. *Lancet*, **i,** 1235 (1981)

35. REID, L. In *Asthma*. Eds T.J.H. Clark and S. Godfrey. p. 79. London: Chapman and Hall (1977)

36. WILLIAMS, H.E. and McNICHOL, K.N. *British Medical Journal*, **4,** 321 (1969)

37. WARRELL, D.A., FAWCETT, I.W., HARRISON, R.D.W., AGAMCH, A.J., IBU, J.O., PEPE, H.M. *et al.* *Quarterly Journal of Medicine*, **44,** 325 (1975)

38. MORRISON-SMITH, J., HARDING, L.K. and CUMMING, G. *Clinical Allergy*, **1,** 57 (1971)

39. SOOTHILL, J.F., STOKES, C.R., TURNER, M.W. and NORMAN, A.P. *Clinical Allergy*, **6,** 305 (1976)

40. PANE, P.D. and HOGG, J.C. In *Asthma and Bronchitis*. Eds N. Mygind and T.J.H. Clark. Eastbourne: Baillière Tyndall (1980)

41. NADEL, J.A. In *Physiology and Pharmacology of the Airways*. Ed. J.A. Nadel. New York: Marcel Dekker (1980)

42. HOLTZMANN, M.J., SHELLER, J.R., DIMED, M., NADEL, J.A. and BOUSHEY, H. *American Review in Respiratory Diseases*, **122**, 17 (1980)
43. THOMSON, N.C., PATEL, K.R. and KERR, J.W. *Thorax*, **33**, 694 (1978)
44. BRUCE, C., WEATHERSTONE, R., SEATON, A. and TAYLOR, W.H. *Thorax*, **31**, 724 (1976)
45. BARNES, P., FITZGERALD, G., BROWN, M. and DOLLERY, C. *New England Journal of Medicine*, **303**, 263 (1980)
46. FILLEY, W.V., HOLLEY, K.E., KEPHART, G.M. and GLEICH, G.J. *Lancet*, **ii**, 11 (1982)
47. SZENTIVANYI, A. *Journal of Allergy*, **42**, 203 (1968)
48. VENTER, J.C. and FRASER, C.M. *Science*, **207**, 1361 (1980)
49. Editorial. *Lancet*, **i**, 1224 (1982)
50. KALINER, M., SHELHAMER, J., DAVIS, P.B., SMITH, L.J. and VENTER, J.C. *Annals of Internal Medicine*, **96**, 349 (1982)

Part 2

Mediators

Chapter 2
Histamine
John C. Foreman

Introduction

Histamine is a classical mediator of acute hypersensitivity and inflammatory reactions and, while it is now clear that it is not the sole mediator of these reactions, it serves as a useful model upon which to base studies of other putative mediators. There is no shortage of information about histamine, although some important questions about its role in inflammatory and hypersensitivity reactions remain to be answered. In this chapter, a brief review of the historical aspects of histamine research will be followed by a statement of the criteria to be satisfied if histamine is to be considered as a mediator of asthma. A discussion of histamine release and actions will be based upon these criteria in order to evaluate its role in asthma.

Historical aspects

In the first decade of this century histamine was discovered independently from two sources. Windaus and Vogt[1] prepared it synthetically and Kutscher[2] identified it as a base isolated from ergot. Barger and Dale[3] described the biological actions of the material derived from ergot and this was followed by an extensive study of the biological actions of histamine carried out by Dale and Laidlaw[4,5]. In fact, Dale and Laidlaw[4] drew attention to the parallel between the actions of histamine in animals and the response of an animal to a protein, normally inert, but to which the animal had been sensitized by prior injection. Here, then, was probably the earliest realization that release of histamine in tissues was responsible, at least in part, for an acute hypersensitivity reaction or anaphylactic shock. Dale went on, in fact, to show that it was possible to produce shock in animals by injection of histamine alone[6].

The term 'anaphylaxis' (decreased protection) was used by Portier and Richet[7] to describe the phenomenon in which a second dose of toxin or protein into an animal produced a greater reaction than the first. It was realized that toxins generally induced immunity or protection (phylaxis), but the anaphylactic reaction to a toxin or protein upon second injection into

29

a previously sensitized animal appeared to be the opposite of normal immunity or protection. Dale and Schultz were responsible independently[8,9] for the demonstration of an anaphylactic reaction in isolated smooth muscle. Dale showed that the anaphylactic contraction of smooth muscle was due to an interaction between antigen and specific antibody fixed to the tissue. Passive sensitization of the smooth muscle tissue with antibody was demonstrated and it was noted that the antigen–antibody reaction produced, in the muscle, a response similar to and as rapid as that produced directly by histamine.

Not long after this pioneering work of Dale and others. Feldberg and colleagues[10] demonstrated that challenge of the lung from a sensitized animal with the appropriate antigen caused the release of histamine from the lung tissue. Lewis[11] also showed that the injection of histamine into skin produced a 'triple response', characteristically seen after injury to a point in the skin. Furthermore, it was shown that injury to the skin causes the release of histamine.

It was becoming clear that an immune reaction or injury could liberate histamine from tissues and also that injection of histamine could mimic injury in the skin or an anaphylactic reaction in the whole animal. In a unique experiment with bronchial tissue from an allergic human, it was shown[12] that histamine caused the muscle to contract and that application of antigen (pollen in this case) caused a similar contraction in the tissue.

It was some years after the work implicating histamine as the mediator of anaphylaxis that its source in tissues was identified. Ehrlich had first described the mast cell calling it 'mastzellen' (well-fed cell) because it was stuffed with granules. The metachromatic staining of these mast cell granules was demonstrated and the mast cell identified as a source of heparin. Rocha e Silva[13] showed that histamine was released simultaneously with heparin from dog liver during anaphylaxis and, since this organ is rich in mast cells, this was the first indication that histamine might be located in mast cells. MacIntosh and Paton[14] described some basic compounds, such as Compound 48/80, which liberated histamine from tissues, and Riley and West[15] went on to show that the release of histamine from tissues by these histamine liberators was paralleled by a degranulation of mast cells. It was appreciated in this early work that not all histamine could be accounted for by mast cell stores: important non-mast-cell sources being blood basophil leucocytes, platelets, enterochromaffin cells of the gut and some neurones. Furthermore, it appeared that some histamine was not stored preformed in granules, but was synthesized *de novo* by histamine decarboxylation especially in areas of rapid proliferation[16].

This brief historical excursion has set the scene for the description of the role of the mast cell and histamine in an acute allergic reaction. The mast cell is the store of tissue histamine and the target for the antigen–antibody reaction. Before going to look in detail at mast cell function and the actions of histamine, it may be helpful briefly to state the criteria by which one can judge a putative mediator of an immediate hypersensitivity reaction. The criteria are, in fact, based on those drawn up by Dale and it is ironic that they have been applied more often to putative neurotransmitters than to putative mediators of inflammation and hypersensitivity, where Dale did so much fundamental and important work.

Criteria of mediator action

A putative mediator of inflammation or hypersensitivity should fulfill the following criteria:
(a) The substance when given at appropriate doses *in vivo* and *in vitro* should produce the effects seen in the inflammatory or hypersensitivity reaction
(b) The inflammatory or hypersensitiviy reaction should lead to the formation or release of the mediator
(c) The enzymes necessary for the production of the mediator should be present at the site of its formation and such enzyme activity should increase when the inflammatory stimulus causes increased turnover of the mediator
(d) A mechanism, such as metabolism, uptake or desensitization, must be available to terminate the actions of the mediator so that its effects do not persist indefinitely
(e) Pharmacological interference with release, metabolism, storage, synthesis or action of the mediator should give rise to the predictable changes in the inflammatory or hypersensitivity reaction
(f) Clinical or experimental conditions involving deficiencies of the mediator or its metabolizing enzymes should give rise to appropriate alterations in the hypersensitivity or inflammatory reaction
(g) Receptors or other recognition–transduction systems should be demonstrable on relevant cells, by pharmacological techniques and binding experiments
These criteria will not be considered formally, but they should be borne in mind when assessing histamine, or any other putative mediator, for the part that it, or they, may play in the pathogenesis of asthma.

Histamine release

Mast cells and basophil leucocytes

Mast cells are the principal stores of histamine in most tissues, whilst the histamine in blood is found in basophil leucocytes[17] except in some species, such as rabbit, where histamine is also contained in the platelets. The histamine is stored in granules contained within the cytoplasm (*Figure 2.1*), each granule being limited by a membrane. Apart from the granules and the nucleus, the cytological features of the mast cell or basophil are not noteworthy. There are few mitochondria and the Golgi bodies are not prominent. Microfilaments and microtubules are identifiable and some cells contain cytoplasmic inclusions that resemble many layers of membrane packed together. The cell membrane shows numerous microvillar projections and these are evident in *Figure 2.1*.

The granules of mast cells and basophils differ both morphologically and chemically depending on the species and site of origin of the cell. For example, human mast cells have a regular crystalline structure when examined with the electron microscope[18] and the mucopolysaccharide (proteoglycan) content of the granules is different in the rat from that in man[19,20]. The matrix of the granule is essentially protein to which

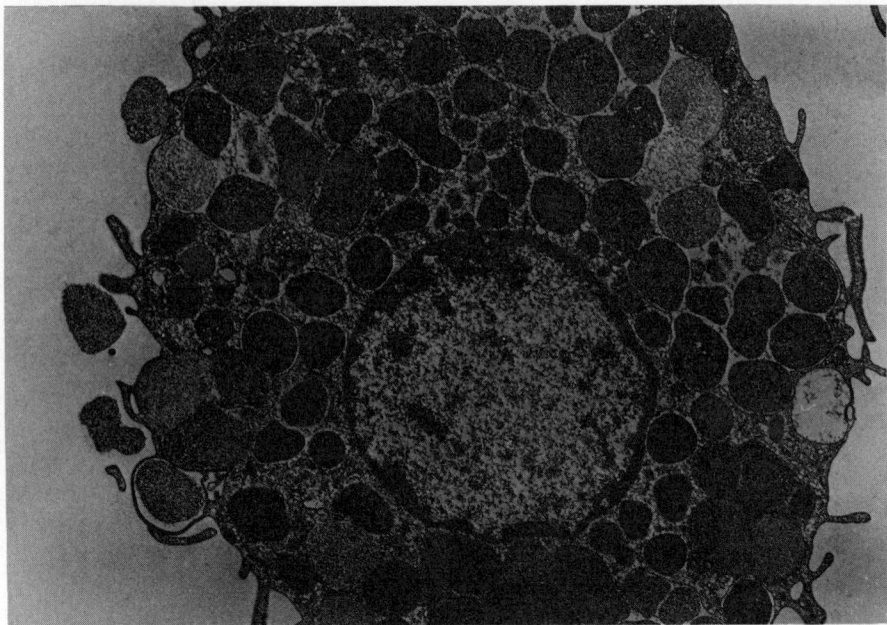

Figure 2.1 Transmission electron micrograph of a degranulating mast cell. The nucleus is apparent surrounded by electron dense histamine-containing granules. At the periphery are less dense or 'altered' granules which are extracytoplasmic and have released histamine. Microvilli are visible on the cell membrane. One or two mitochondria are visible. Magnification × 4875.
(The electron micrograph was prepared and kindly supplied by Dr D. Lawson, University College London.)

histamine and heparin are bound ionically[21]. In contrast to, for example, chromaffin granules from the adrenal medulla, mast cell granules seem to have little adenosine triphosphate (ATP) or divalent cation though they do have a high affinity for divalent cations such as calcium[22]. The protein matrix displays a number of enzyme activities including β-hexosaminidase, β-glucuronidase, arylsulphatase, chymase and carboxypeptidase A[23].

The origin of mast cells and basophils is a matter of considerable interest and speculation. Mast cells and basophils clearly differ both morphologically and biochemically, but so do mast cells from different sites[24–26] and the reasons for this heterogenicity appear, at present, to be the result of the environment the cell finds itself in rather than being due to different origins. The basophil is presumed to originate, along with other leucocytes, from a stem cell in the bone marrow, but the evidence for this seems largely to depend on histology. Burnet[27] was the first to suggest that the mast cell originated from the thymus and several studies have shown that mast cells can be derived from cultures of thymocytes[28,29]. However, mast cells are present in athymic mice and humans[30]. Recent work has shown that a bone marrow cell, called by one group a 'persisting' or 'P' cell, can give rise to both mast-cell-like and leucocyte-cell-like cells[31,32]. These P cells can be cloned and are deficient in Thy 1, Lyt 2, and Ia antigens[33]. P cells are not derived from T lymphocytes, nor are T cells required for P-cell production but there does appear to be a T-cell-derived factor which supports P-cell growth. At present, it is possible to say little more than that mast cells and basophils may originate from a common precursor in bone marrow which interacts with T lymphocyte products. A further recent development on the origin of mast cells[34] has suggested that they may have a common origin with a line of mononuclear phagocytes. Bone marrow precursor cells with phagocytic activity develop in culture into histamine-containing, IgE-bearing cells which display phagocytic activity. It has long been known that mast cells can phagocytose particles[35] and recent evidence has indicated that macrophages can bind IgE[36].

Immunoglobulin E and its receptors

The link between the environmental agent, for example pollen or house dust mite in asthma, and the release of histamine from mast cells is immunoglobulin E (IgE). IgE differs from IgG in having one additional heavy chain domain in the Fc region and about three times more associated carbohydrate. Other differences are that IgE is destroyed by heating to 56°C and that it does not fix complement like IgG. However, the most important feature of IgE is its unique ability to bind with high affinity to receptors on mast cells and basophils.

Whilst individuals with allergies, such as asthma, may have raised circulating levels of IgE, normal individuals also have circulating IgE. The factor which is important, although not the sole determining feature in the generation of allergy, is the formation of antigen-specific IgE and the fixing of this to mast cell receptors for IgE. The initial access of antigen permits it to interact with a specific receptor (surface immunoglobulin) on a B lymphocyte and this, in turn, leads to B-cell proliferation and differentiation. B memory cells are generated, but other B cells differentiate into IgE-secreting plasma cells. Antigen also interacts with T lymphocytes to produce suppressor cells which limit IgE production from stimulated B cells[37]. Other T cells interact with macrophages stimulated by antigen and this gives rise to T helper cells which augment the B cell response to antigen[38]. T suppressor cells may be either antigen specific or not specific for a particular antigen and, in addition to these various cellular interactions, T cells can produce soluble factors which suppress IgE production[39–41].

It is important to point out that a particular antigen will generate IgG as well as IgE responses and the proportion of the two classes formed can be influenced in several ways[42,43]. Also it should be mentioned that, whilst in rat and man IgE appears to be the principal antibody class involved in the pathogenesis of allergic reactions, in other species, such as guinea-pig, subclasses of IgG are the main antibodies involved in such reactions[44]. Furthermore, there is evidence that, in rat, the IgG subclass IgG_{2a} can bind with low affinity to IgE receptors and can activate histamine secretion when the appropriate antigen is used[45].

Having stated that IgE binds to a receptor on mast cells and basophils, it is pertinent to ask which part of the IgE binds to the receptor and also to examine the nature of the receptor to which the IgE binds. Using fragments of IgE antibody to compete with intact IgE for binding to the receptor, it has been shown that it is the Fc region of IgE which binds to the receptor[46] and more specifically the C3 domain of the Fc region[47]. IgE labelled with ^{125}I has been shown by autoradiography to bind almost exclusively to mast cells and basophil leucocytes[48]. Macrophages, monocytes, neutrophil leucocytes, eosinophil leucocytes and lymphocytes bind little or no IgE. Such autoradiographic and direct radioassays of ^{125}I-labelled IgE binding to cells have demonstrated the presence of about 10^5 Fc receptors on each mast cell or basophil. The rat basophil leukaemic cells possess about 10^6 Fc receptors per cell[49,50].

The Fcε receptor isolated from rat basophilic leukaemia cells has been solubilized and purified[51,52] and it appears to be a glycoprotein with a molecular weight of about 80 000. Each receptor consists of two subunits: one of molecular weight 50 000 (α) and one of 30 000 (β)[53]. Polyacrylamide gel electrophoresis, amino acid analysis and radiation inactivation analysis yield slightly different molecular weight estimates for the receptor, but the binding of IgE is to the larger subunit. The smaller subunit is of unknown function and its presence or absence does not influence the binding of IgE to the larger subunit. No enzyme activities or ion conductances are known to be associated with the receptor, but recent studies reveal that phosphorylation is associated with activation. Cross-linking IgE receptors results in phosphorylation of the β subunit at a serine residue on the cytoplasmic face of the receptor[54]. Other studies[55] have shown α subunit phosphorylation in response to the action of a calcium ionophore. The significance of both these observations is at present unknown.

The binding of IgE molecules to the receptors has a rate constant of about 10^5 M^{-1}·s^{-1} while the reverse reaction has a rate constant of about 10^{-7} M^{-1}·s^{-1}. The equilibrium dissociation constant for the binding of IgE to the Fcε receptor is approximately 10^{-11} M[56]. It seems that the valency of the Fcε receptor is unity and this is based on experiments in which free receptors were exposed to equimolar mixtures of IgE labelled with rhodamine and IgE labelled with fluorescein. Anti-IgE treatment of cells exposed to these labelled IgE molecules caused the two colours of fluorescence to co-cap on the membrane, but anti-fluorescein-labelled antibody produced only green cap formation indicating that IgE–fluorescein-bearing receptors had no IgE–rhodamine attached[57]. Additional evidence favouring univalency of the receptor also demonstrated mobility of the receptor within the lateral plane of the membrane. Membrane bearing IgE–fluorescein and IgE–rhodamine attached to Fc receptors was photobleached at a point with a laser beam and the fluorescence recovery time of the bleached area was measured. Immobilization of IgE–fluorescein prevented recovery of green fluorescence without altering the mobility of IgE–rhodamine[58]. The rate of diffusion of the IgE-bearing Fc receptor in the membrane was calculated to be 2×10^{-10} cm^2·s^{-1} which is similar to that for a lipid probe in the same membrane (8×10^{-9} cm^2·s^{-1}) and indicates the fluid nature of the membrane at physiological temperatures.

Mast cell activation

Simple binding of the IgE molecule to its Fcε receptor on a mast cell or basophil leucocyte does not activate the cell to secrete histamine. It is the binding of specific antigen to the cell-fixed IgE which activates the cell.

One suggestion for the mechanism by which antigen binding to IgE activates the cell is that such binding produces conformational change in the antibody molecule and the cross-linking of the IgE antibody, and therefore its receptor, by antigen is only of importance in that it produces this change. The conformational change is supposed to be the exposure of a basic peptide in the Fc region of the IgE molecule and it is suggested that this basic peptide then produces changes in the mast cell or basophil membrane to induce mediator release[59]. An active peptide has been isolated from the IgE molecule[60] and there is experimental work demonstrating that analogues of this peptide can inhibit allergic reactions by preventing mast cell activation[61]. However, the majority of experimental work favours an alternative explanation of the role of IgE receptors in mast cell activation, in that cross-linking of the IgE receptor is itself the trigger for activation and mediator release (*Figure 2.2*).

Monovalent antigens do not activate mast cells or basophils[62,63]. Early work suggesting that they did may well have been misleading because of the spontaneous association of monomers into larger units. Bivalent or polyvalent signals are needed to activate the cells. Polyvalent antigens cross-link adjacent IgE molecules by bridging Fab regions of neighbouring

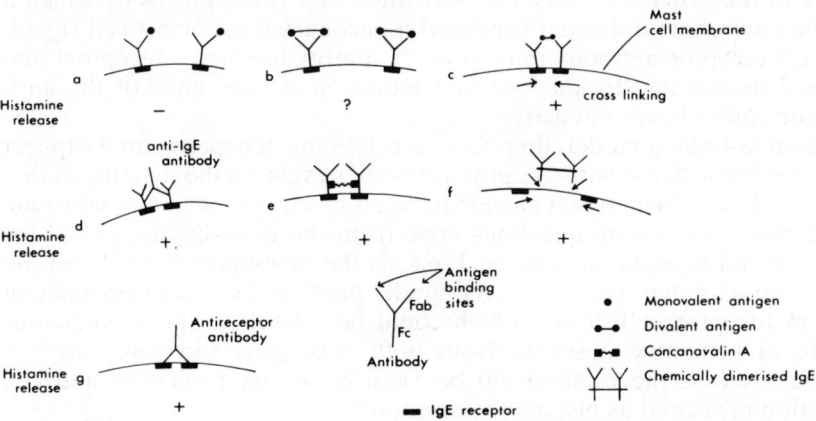

Figure 2.2 Diagrammatic representation of the various ways of inducing mast cell or basophil activation (histamine release) by aggregating Fcε receptors in the membrane.

IgE molecules (*Figure 2.2c*); the Fab region containing the specific antigen-combining site. Anti-IgE, which is an IgG antibody directed against determinants in the Fcε heavy chains of IgE, aggregates membrane-bound IgE as shown in *Figure 2.2d*[64]. The Fab' fragments of such an anti-IgE are, being monovalent, inactive. Several lectins induce histamine release from mast cells or basophils. The action of concanavalin A is probably the best characterized[65–67] and appears to cross-link IgE molecules by binding to the associated carbohydrate of the immunoglobulin (*Figure 2.2c*). Concanavalin A is tetrameric and dissociation of the tetramer using trypsin results in a loss of the histamine-releasing activity of the lectin[65]. Also, α-methyl-D-mannoside competes with concanavalin A for carbohydrate binding and prevents the release of histamine induced by this lectin[67]. IgE molecules can be chemically polymerized using suberimidate and the dimers induce histamine release by cross-linking IgE receptors[68].

The experiments are important in two ways. First they imply that cross-linking receptors is the signal to the cell and that IgE does not have to be bound before cross-linking. Second, the signal to the cell is a simple bridging of two receptors and need not be a complex aggregation or lattice formation (*Figure 2.2f*). In fact, in the passive cutaneous anaphylactic reaction and in rat mast cells, trimers and larger oligomers were equipotent with dimers[69]. Interestingly, in the rat basophilic leukaemia (RBL), the larger oligomers were more active than the dimers but the reason for this is not known though it was probably not a matter of different extents of binding. A most elegant demonstration that mast cell activation is the result of cross-linking *two* receptors is provided by experiments with antibody (IgG) directed against IgE receptors themselves[70]. The antibody was raised against purified IgE receptor from RBL cells and its action is shown in *Figure 2.2g*. It is clear from these experiments that IgE antibody is unnecessary for mast cell activation. In fact, if IgE is present on the Fcε receptors, the antigenic determinants of the receptors are masked and the anti-receptor antibody is inactive[70]. Thus, IgE merely serves to convey specificity in the process of mast cell activation and is the means by which a specific environmental agent (antigen) is recognized as a mast cell signal. The anti-receptor antibody must provide a cross-linking of receptors and this is demonstrated by the fact that monovalent Fab′ units of the anti-receptor antibody are not active.

The cross-linking model, therefore, receives much experimental support and the work with the anti-receptor antibodies excludes the hypothesis that an antibody conformational change induced by antigen is the signal to the cell. Several interesting questions arise from the cross-linking model for mast cell and basophil activation. First, as the membrane is fluid and the Fcε receptors move freely in it, the model predicts a certain frequency of random receptor collisions[71] which could be related to the spontaneous release of histamine observed from both mast cells and basophils[72,73]. Second, what is the relationship between cross-link formation and cell activation measured as histamine secretion?

A thermodynamic model[74] for cross-linking of membrane-bound IgE by a simple bivalent hapten has been developed in which it is assumed that IgE molecules are two-dimensional discs free to diffuse in the plane of the membrane and unable to intersect with each other. Each disc bears two hapten-binding sites. The hapten is considered to be a flexible chain and, when one end is bound, the other end is freely distributed over the surface of a sphere with a radius equivalent to the hapten chain length. From these assumptions, it may be shown that the number of cross-links comprising two or more antibody molecules approaches zero at *high* and at low hapten concentrations (*Figure 2.3*) and a plot of the number of cross-links against the logarithm of the hapten concentration is symmetrical about a maximum value for the number of cross-links. The model fits the data remarkably well in a basophil system, from rabbits with antibodies to the benzylpenicilloyl group, challenged with benzylpenicilloyl-NH-$(CH_2)_n$-NH-benzyl-penicilloyl (*Figure 2.3*)[75]. The degree of histamine release appears to be controlled by the number of cross-links formed.

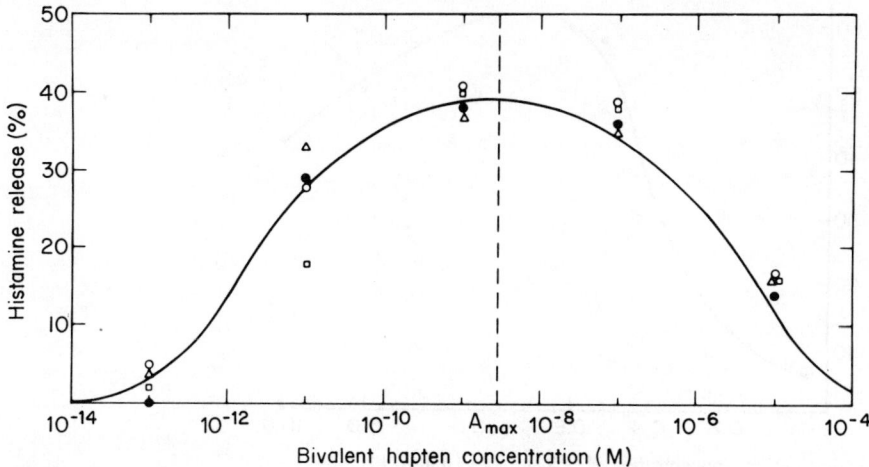

Figure 2.3 Histamine release induced by (benzylpenicilloyl-NH)$_2$-(CH$_2$)$_n$ hapten from human basophils. Each type of symbol represents a different experiment. The curve is the theoretical fit obtained from a thermodynamic model of hapten–IgE binding—*see text*. Reproduced from Dembo M., Goldstein, B., Sobotka, A.K. *et al.*, 1978, *Journal of Immunology*, Vol. 121, p. 354, by courtesy of the authors and publisher.

Although the thermodynamic model provides a structure for thinking about mast cell and basophil activation, some problems remain unsolved. It has already been pointed out above that in RBL cells, trimeric and larger oligomeric signals are more effective than dimeric ones. Also, in certain human subjects, basophils known to possess IgE bound to Fcε receptors fail to release histamine when cross-linking is induced[76]. About one-fifth of all human subjects yield such non-releaser cells and the failure of cells to secrete histamine appears to be the result of some uncoupling between IgE-receptor cross-linking and later stages in cellular biochemsitry which lead to histamine secretion.

It is now pertinent to consider the events leading to histamine secretion that follow the cross-linking of Fcε receptors.

Calcium requirement

Antigen-induced histamine secretion from mast cells and basophils is affected by calcium in the extracellular medium (*Figure 2.4*)[77, 78]. Calcium 0.1–1 mM activates antigen-induced histamine secretion, but in the presence of zero extracellular calcium, a small amount of histamine secretion still occurs following antigen stimulation[79].

Attention has been drawn to the similarities between excitation–contraction coupling in muscle and stimulus–secretion coupling in various cells which release materials stored in granules within the cytoplasm[80]. It has been proposed that a rise in the level of free calcium within the cytosol is the second messenger coupling the IgE-receptor cross-linking to the subsequent secretion of histamine-containing granules. There are several pieces of experimental evidence consistent with this hypothesis. First, of course, the dependence of antigen-induced histamine release on extracellular

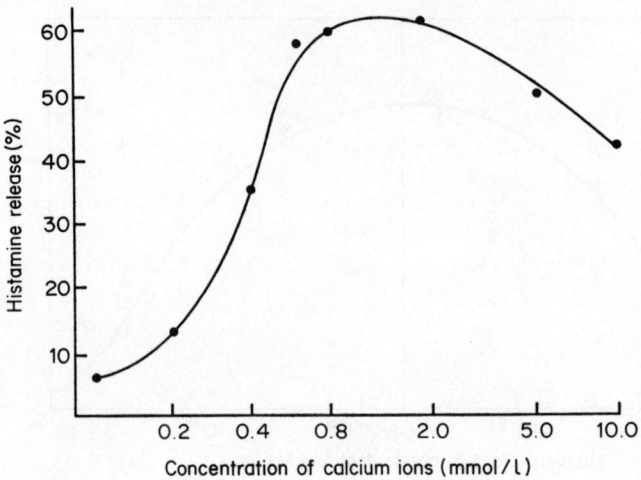

Figure 2.4 Effect of calcium concentration in the extracellular medium on histamine release from rat mast cells stimulated by an antigen–antibody reaction.

calcium. Second, the calcium ionophores A23187 and ionomycin transport calcium from the extracellular medium into the cell and induce the exocytotic secretion of histamine[81,82]. It is worth nothing that the calcium ionophore A23187 induces histamine release in the absence of extracellular calcium under certain conditions and this is presumed to be due to the release of intracellular stores of calcium[83]. Third, microinjection of calcium into mast cells causes degranulation of the cells[84]. Fourthly, fusion of calcium-loaded liposomes with rat mast cells leads to histamine secretion, presumably because the calcium in the liposomes is released into the mast cell[85]. Another technique of raising the cytosolic calcium level is to make the cell membrane freely permeable using ATP or Sendai virus[86] and to control the cytosolic calcium by using calcium buffers in the extracellular medium. Increasing extracellular free calcium in such permeable cells leads to increasing histamine release. The experiments also indicate that mast cell cytosolic calcium is normally maintained around the micromolar level and increases above this resting level lead to histamine secretion. The final piece of evidence to be mentioned is the inhibitory action of lanthanum, a rare earth ion which competes for calcium binding sites in many biological systems and prevents membrane transport of calcium. Lanthanum inhibits antigen-induced histamine secretion by competition with calcium for what is believed to be a calcium channel in the mast cell or basophil membrane[87, 88].

Considering the experimental evidence discussed above, it might be expected that the cross-linking of Fcε receptors would lead to an increase in the membrane permeability of mast cells and basophils towards calcium. It is also possible that such membrane activation could release some calcium from internal stores. Indeed, it has been shown that antigen–IgE and anti-receptor activation of mast cell membrane leads to an increased uptake of radiolabelled calcium (^{45}Ca) by the cell[89,90]. Such stimulated increases in ^{45}Ca uptake by mast cells consist of several components, including one which represents increased calcium binding to the cell surface[90]. However, it is possible to show that part of the stimulated uptake of ^{45}Ca is due to the movement of the label across the cell membrane and hence it is inferred that the cross-linking stimulus induces an increase in the cell membrane permeability to calcium.

It has already been stated that some secretion appears to depend on internal stores of calcium. For ligands such as Compound 48/80, peptide 401 and polylysine, a large proportion of the histamine secretion is independent of extracellular calcium, but it can be reduced by a prolonged preincubation of the cells with the calcium-chelating agent, ethyleneglycol bis(2-aminoethyl-N,N'-tetraacetic acid) (EGTA), which is supposed to deplete internal calcium stores[91]. Changes of extracellular pH also affect the response of mast cells to calcium. Shifting the pH to a lower level increases the proportion of stimulated histamine secretion which is independent of extracellular calcium, possibly by increasing mobilization from internal stores of calcium[92].

It has already been pointed out that there are theoretical reasons for anticipating a certain level of spontaneous secretion from mast cells and basophils in the absence of any membrane activation by a ligand–receptor interaction. Spontaneous histamine release from mast cells increases very little over a period of up to 2 hours incubation at 37°C and extracellular calcium has no apparent effect on this spontaneous release. However, it could be that any calcium permeability induced by spontaneous receptor aggregations is too low to give rise to histamine secretion and there is some support for this. It has been shown that the calcium channel operated by Fcε receptor cross-linking is more permeable to strontium than calcium[88,93,94] and so this ion can be used in place of calcium as a more sensitive probe for available calcium channels. Replacement of extracellular calcium with strontium produces spontaneous secretion which increases with incubation time, is dependent on the ion concentration and is associated with accumulation of the ion within the cell. The resting mast cell permeability to calcium is low at 8 fmol·cm^{-2}·s^{-1} whereas the resting strontium permeability is 38 fmol·cm^{-2}·s^{-1}. Thus, there is some evidence for the presence of calcium channels in the unstimulated membrane of mast cells.

Strontium has also been used to show that Fcε receptors may be uncoupled from membrane ion permeability changes. It was pointed out above that in some populations of human basophils, Fcε receptor cross-linking fails to elicit histamine secretion[76]. Interestingly, this failure is overcome by substituting strontium for calcium and this has been used to argue that, in these non-releaser cells, there is an uncoupling of Fcε receptor aggregation from calcium channel opening, and hence a failure of the membrane signal to elicit secretion[88]. In the same context there is some evidence that the non-secreting line of RBL cells[95] which do bear IgE receptors, fail to secrete because they lack calcium channels[96].

Whereas increased levels of cytosolic calcium initiate secretion, it is also necessary to reverse such changes in order to maintain cellular homeostasis. Thus, increases in membrane permeability to calcium initiated by receptor cross-linking must be reversed and calcium in the cytosol sequestered in an inactive form. Like many other secretory cells, mast cells and basophils show inactivation of receptor-triggered membrane permeability to calcium. If the cells are stimulated by a cross-linking stimulus in the absence of extracellular calcium, little or no histamine secretion occurs (*see above*) until calcium is added back to the extracellular medium[97,98]. The cells show a decreasing response to calcium as the interval between stimulus and calcium addition is increased (*Figure 2.5a*). At the same time as the secretory response is decaying or desensitizing with respect to calcium, the increased calcium permeability of the membrane following stimulation also decays (*Figure 2.5b*). Furthermore, cells whose response to calcium has decayed remain fully responsive to the calcium ionophore A23187[97] and the response to A23187 does not decay in this way.

When mast cells bearing IgE against two different antigens are examined, it has been shown that the inactivation which follows stimulation with one of the antigens does not result in inactivation to the other antigen[99]. However, this is only true when a relatively small fraction of Fcε receptors are cross-linked. An anti-IgE stimulus involving the cross-linking of a large fraction of the occupied Fcε receptors induces inactivation which makes the cell refractory to cross-linking of the remaining receptors[100].

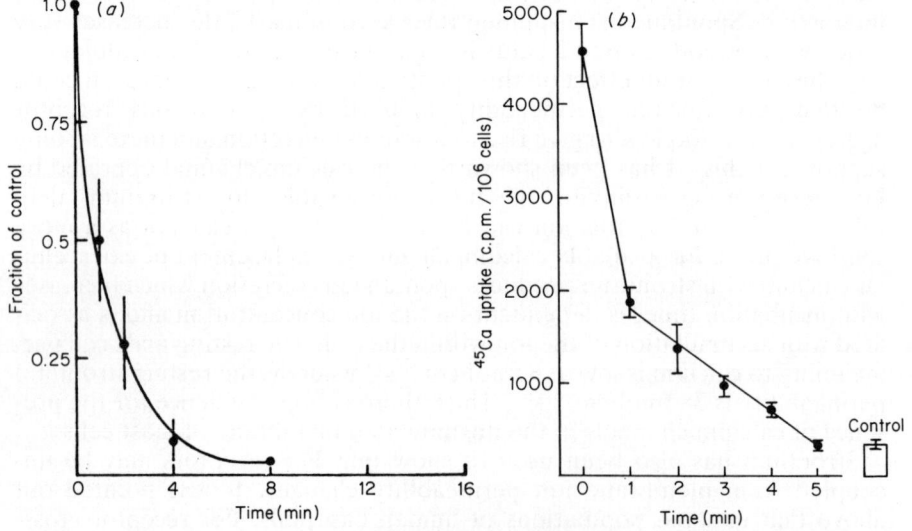

Figure 2.5 (a) Rate of decay of the response of rat mast cells to calcium added following the antigen–IgE stimulus. Histamine release is measured as a function of increasing interval between stimulating the cells and adding calcium. (*b*) Rate of change of ^{45}Ca uptake after antigen stimulation. Cells were either challenged with antigen in the presence of ^{45}Ca ($t = 0$) or were challenged with antigen in the presence of non-labelled calcium and then the ^{45}Ca was added t minutes after the stimulus. The control is the ^{45}Ca uptake with no antigen stimulus.

The reasons for this non-specific desensitization are not known, but it has been suggested that the number of available calcium channels is exceeded by the number of receptors to which they may be coupled. Then, if a large fraction of receptors is cross-linked all available channels may be opened and inactivated so that remaining Fcε receptors cannot be linked to channels. It is assumed that calcium channel inactivation is either irreversible or very slowly reversible. Hence, the inactivation process appears to represent a mechanism by which stimulus-operated calcium conductance is shut down after initiation of histamine secretion, thereby limiting calcium entry and maintaining cellular homeostasis with respect to calcium.

Phospholipid and fatty acid metabolism

Recently, considerable interest has been focused on the roles of membrane phospholipids in mast cell and basophil responses. Such interest is mainly at two levels: (*a*) the function of phospholipid metabolism in operating calcium channels and (*b*) the generation of fatty acid such as arachidonic acid as a substrate for cyclo-oxygenase and lipoxygenase. It is likely that the two processes are very closely coupled since it has long been appreciated that IgE-mediated histamine release and slow-reacting substance generation (SRS-A, now known to be leukotrienes) are difficult to separate.

In several systems, evidence has been gathered which supports the hypothesis that receptor–ligand interaction in the membrane stimulates the turnover of phosphatidylinositol and it is that turnover which leads to the formation of calcium channels in the membrane[101]. It appears that stimulation of rat mast cells with antigen, anti-IgE, concanavalin A, Compound 48/80 and the ionophore A23187 produces increased turnover of phosphatidylinositol[102,103]. However, if such phospholipid turnover is required for calcium channel formation, it is not clear why A23187 should induce such turnover since it itself is a calcium transporter. In fact, the experiments with A23187[103] may be criticized for not measuring phosphatidylinositol breakdown, since studies were done with [^{32}P]phosphatidylinositol and not with cells prelabelled with [^{3}H]inositol. It is clear that the cross-linking stimulus to mast cells produces phosphatidylinositol turnover which is independent of calcium and has a time-course similar to that for secretion[102]. As might be expected, concentrations of ligand/inducing phospholipid turnover are somewhat lower than those inducing histamine secretion, indicating that a certain level of turnover has to be achieved before a secretory response is manifest. It was pointed out above that a certain level of calcium entry needs to be achieved before secretion occurs. Apart from phosphatidylinositol, phosphatidic acid and phosphatidylcholine also have been reported to be turned over at increased rates in the stimulated mast cells, but phosphatidylserine, phosphatidylethanolamine and sphingomyelin do not show such increased turnover[103,104].

Another hypothesis which has been put forward to explain the relationship between phospholipid metabolism and calcium in the activation of histamine secretion concerns the methylation of phosphatidylethanolamine in the membrane[105]. It has been suggested that phosphatidylserine in the membrane, or perhaps from an exogenous source (*see below*), is decarboxylated by mast cells, when a cross-linking stimulus is applied, to yield phosphatidylethanolamine. The phosphatidylethanolamine then acts as a substrate for two methyltransferase enzymes which appear to be present in the mast cell and other cell membranes. Methyltransferase I, located on the inner surface of the membrane, transfers a methyl group from *S*-adenosylmethionine to phosphatidylethanolamine. A second enzyme methyltransferase II, located on the external surface of the membrane

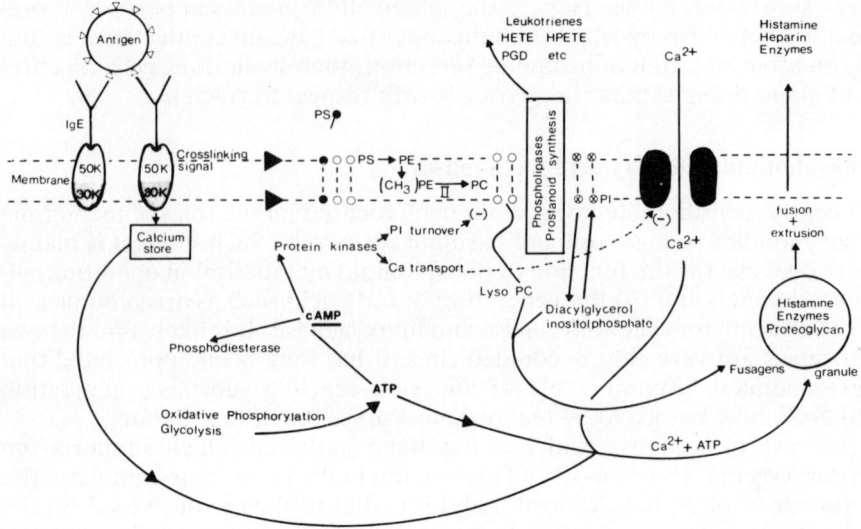

Figure 2.6 The membrane events of mast cell activation. Receptor cross-linking initiates changes in membrane phospholipid composition, arachidonate is released by a phospholipase A_2 and calcium channels open. Cyclic AMP levels, which may be controlled by the receptor aggregation (adenylate cyclase not shown), activate a protein kinase which may interact with calcium channels or stores to control the secretory process. Oxidative phosphorylation and glycolysis supply an essential source of ATP.

further methylates the *N*-monomethylphosphatidylethanolamine to generate phosphatidylcholine. In this process the phospholipid is transferred from the inner leaflet of the membrane to the outer leaflet as it is metabolized. It is then supposed that a calcium-independent phospholipase A_2, also activated by the cross-linking stimulus, acts on the phosphatidylcholine formed from the methylations to yield arachidonic acid and lyso-phosphatidylcholine. The arachidonic acid can, of course, be a substrate for cyclo-oxygenase and lipoxygenase yielding prostaglandins, thromboxanes, prostacyclin, hydroxy-, hydroperoxy-arachidonate and leukotrienes (*see Figure 2.6*). The whole process is said to lead to increased membrane fluidity which favours the formation of calcium channels[105]. The experimental evidence has shown that anti-Fcε receptor antibody and other cross-linking agents produce an early rapid methylation of membrane phospholipids which is followed by increased [45]Ca uptake and histamine secretion[106]. The secreting RBL cells show these changes, but the non-secreting RBL cells do not[96]. Furthermore, phosphatidylserine, the proposed initial substrate which may be limiting, can, when added exogenously, increase antigen-stimulated [45]Ca uptake and histamine secretion in rat mast cells[89,107]. Interestingly, phosphatidylserine derivatives which are N substituted are not metabolized and do not have these effects on histamine secretion[108].

There has been considerable debate about the phospholipid metabolism hypothesis and critics point out that the degree of methylation is very small and the changes of membrane fluidity insignificant. Also, *S*-isobutyryl-3-

deaza-adenosine, an inhibitor of S-adenosylmethionine-dependent methylations, inhibits the methylation reactions in mast cells at concentrations which are about ten times less than those required to inhibit histamine secretion and three times less than those needed to prevent ^{45}Ca uptake[106]. Theophylline, another inhibitor, behaves similarly[109]. It appears, therefore, that phospholipid methylation is not essential for calcium movement or histamine secretion in response to a cross-linking stimulus. Perhaps the use of other drugs as inhibitors of the process would help to resolve the problem of whether or not methylation of membrane phospholipids plays a key role in histamine secretion following aggregation of $Fc\varepsilon$ receptors.

Another product of phospholipid methylation which may play a part in histamine release is diacylglycerol. It has been suggested that its presence may be necessary for the fusion of cell and membrane granules in the process of exocytosis[110]. As with all the hypotheses relating membrane phospholipid turnover to histamine secretion, there is no evidence that diacylglycerol formation by mast cells is anything more than an epiphenomenon and what is needed is convincing data that prevention of its formation by specific inhibitors actually prevents the secretion of histamine from occurring.

Mast cells and basophils incorporate labelled arachidonate which can be metabolized by either lipoxygenase or cyclo-oxygenase pathways[111]. The principal prostaglandin produced by mast cells and basophilic leukaemia cells is PGD_2, with little or no PGE_2 and $PGF_{2\alpha}$ being formed[112,113]. Inhibition of cyclo-oxygenase by indomethacin does not alter histamine secretion and so it seems unlikely that these prostaglandins participate in the release process[113]. It should be pointed out that PGD_2 and PGE_1 both increase adenylate cyclase activity in mast cells and PGE_1 can inhibit histamine secretion when applied exogenously[113–116].

Mast cells and RBL cells can produce leukotrienes when stimulated with the ionophore A23187, although it is not clear that leukotrienes are produced in response to an immunological stimulus[117,118]. Thus, an interesting question arises as to how the immunological reaction of antigen with IgE— a process apparently specific for mast cells—brings about the release of SRS-A (leukotrienes C and D)[119].

It has been suggested that lipoxygenase products play a part in the histamine release reaction, based upon the observation that ETYA (5,8,11,14-eicosatetraynoic acid) inhibits lipoxygenase and histamine secretion[120]. However, this has been called into question since the concentrations of the inhibitor required to inhibit histamine release are larger than those affecting arachidonate lipoxygenation[121].

No firm conclusion about the role of phospholipids and arachidonate metabolism in histamine release can be drawn, but it seems that these molecules are involved and some interesting hypotheses are available for examination.

Cyclic nucleotides and kinases

The starting point for the study of the role of cyclic nucleotides in the release of histamine was the observation that antigen-induced histamine release from lung was inhibited by adrenaline[122.] A similar observation was later made in human basophils[123]. In human and guinea-pig lung there is good evidence that a β-adrenergic receptor, when activated, inhibits immunologically triggered histamine release[124]. Quantitatively, the evidence in human basophils is not so good[125] and in the rat mast cell it is clear that the activation of a β-adrenergic receptor has no effect on histamine secretion[126]. Of course, the failure of cells to respond to β agonists may reflect the absence of a receptor or an uncoupled receptor.

In all histamine-containing cells examined, there is some evidence that increased levels of intracellular cyclic AMP (cAMP) are associated with inhibition of histamine release induced by cross-linking stimuli. Dibutyryl-cAMP can invariably be used to inhibit immunologically mediated histamine secretion from both mast cells and basophils[125.127]. Activation of adenylate cyclase by β agonists has already been discussed, but other receptors activating this enzyme, including receptors for PGE_1, PGD_2 and adenosine, have been reported to lead to inhibition of histamine release[113–116,128].

Cholera toxin, a direct activator of adenylate cyclase, inhibits histamine release induced by a cross-linking stimulus[129] and the cyclic AMP analogue, adenosine phosphorothioate, inhibits antigen-induced histamine release[130].

Inhibitors of phosphodiesterase, the enzyme destroying cyclic AMP, also inhibit histamine release. Such drugs include isobutylmethylxanthine and theophylline, but in the case of theophylline there is debate about how it inhibits histamine release[114,115,123]. Whereas, in basophils, adenosine inhibits histamine release, in rat mast cells, adenosine enhances histamine release[131]. These opposite effects may still be mediated through adenylate cyclase as is explained below. However, theophylline may inhibit histamine release, especially in whole tissues, by preventing the enhancing action of adenosine on mast cells[132,133].

Accepting, in general terms, the evidence so far presented that increased levels of cyclic AMP inhibit immunologically stimulated histamine release, it is important to examine what happens to cyclic AMP levels in mast cells and basophils when they are so triggered. Following a cross-linking stimulus, cyclic AMP levels show a rapid rise (first 10 seconds) above basal levels followed by a fall either below or back to basal levels in the following 60 seconds[113,134,135]. To consider the implications of this it is necessary to introduce some more experimental evidence.

It has been shown that rat mast cells contain a cAMP-dependent protein kinase which is activated by cross-linking stimuli and which accounts for the majority of protein kinase activity in these cells[136]. It has already been pointed out that the β subunit of the Fcε receptor is phosphorylated during activation of RBL cells and there are other studies demonstrating association between histamine release and phosphorylation of membrane proteins[137]. Thus, there appears to be a link between phosphorylation and secretion, and this could include the cAMP-dependent protein kinase activated by the early rise of cyclic AMP. Of course, these phosphorylations could be involved in activating the cell or in bringing about a homeostatic inactivation to control the secretory process.

In basophils, it has been shown that cyclic AMP can have two opposite actions, depending on how the cell is stimulated[138]. Cross-linking stimuli result in histamine secretion whose rate is increased by cyclic AMP, whereas the maximum degree of secretion is reduced. In contrast, non-cross-linking stimulation produces secretion, the maximum of which is not changed by cyclic AMP, although the rate is increased.

The exact nature of the role of cyclic AMP in mast cells and basophils may only come to light when it is possible to study compartmentalization of the nucleotide within the cell and its effects on different aspects of the histamine release mechanism. So far it seems that cyclic AMP can influence the biochemistry of mast cells in two ways: (i) activation of protein kinase leading to phosphorylation, (ii) reduction of calcium permeability of the membrane[139].

Little is known about the role of cyclic GMP in mast cells and basophils. Indeed, the nucleotide may have no function in terms of histamine secretion. In lung mast cells it has been reported that α-adrenergic agonists and cholinergic (muscarinic) agonists potentiate immunologically mediated histamine secretion[140]. The evidence for α-adrenergic or muscarinic receptors on mast cells is poor. Similarly, the report that 8-bromo-cGMP potentiates histamine release in lung has not been confirmed[140]. The report that acetylcholine itself releases histamine[141] has not been reproduced in any laboratory in which, to my knowledge, it has been tried and the workers themselves find the effect inconsistent[142].

Cellular metabolism and ATP supply

So far, the early membrane-associated events of histamine release have been discussed. Very little is known about how these membrane events are transformed into the secretion of histamine-containing granules. It is clear, however, that an intracellular supply of ATP is needed for histamine secretion[143]. There is no apparent increase in oxygen consumption when mast cells are stimulated to secrete[144] and anoxia has little inhibitory effect on the cell's ability to secrete[145]. Also, inhibitors of oxidative phosphorylation, such as cyanide or antimycin A, only partially inhibit histamine release induced by aggregation of Fcε receptors[146,147]. It has already been stated that mast cells and basophils possess relatively few mitochondria but they seem to be active glycolytic metabolizers[148]. Removal of glucose from the extracellular medium will partly inhibit histamine release mediated via Fcε receptors and, if both glycolytic and oxidative metabolism is prevented, secretion is totally suspended. Provision of glucose will overcome the inhibition of secretion which occurs when glucose-deprived cells are treated with inhibitors of oxidative metabolism, such as antimycin A. The interpretation placed on these results is that ATP is required for secretion and it has been shown that depletion of ATP is associated with reduced histamine secretion. Furthermore, when histamine secretion is stimulated by Fcε receptor cross-linking ATP is consumed[149,150].

The role of the cytoskeleton

Given the central role played by calcium in histamine secretion and the observed need for ATP, it is clear why speculation has arisen about the role of contractile proteins in histamine secretion. Of course ATP consumption may not be related to the role of calcium, since ATP is required by many processes other than the calcium ATPase system of contractile proteins, the generation of cyclic AMP being just one example.

Two models for the role of contractile microfilaments in histamine secretion have been proposed: one in which the filaments contract and move the granules towards the cell membrane to allow fusion of cell and granule membranes to occur and a second in which it has been suggested that a network of filaments just below the cell membrane normally prevents granule membranes from coming into contact with the cell membrane[151]. Contraction of these filaments would allow such contact to occur as a prerequiste for the fusion of membranes in the secretion of granule contents.

Actin has been demonstrated in mast cells both chemically[152] and by inference from the observation of microfilaments in the cytoplasm of mast cells and basophils[18,153]. Attempts to inhibit microfilament function with cytochalasins have yielded results which do not lead to any firm conclusion. In rat mast cells, cytochalasin B inhibits histamine release induced by Fcε receptor aggregation[154] but much, if not all, of this inhibition may be due to prevention of glucose utilization by mast cells[155]. In basophils from human blood, cytochalasin B enhances histamine secretion induced by an immunological stimulus[156].

Microtubules are also visible in mast cells and basophils[153,157] and it has been suggested, on the basis that colchicine and vinblastine inhibit histamine release[158,159], that microtubules are necessary for histamine secretion. However, it is quite clear that concentrations of colchicine which causes complete disruption of microtubules do not inhibit histamine release[157]. It has also been argued that potentiation of histamine release by heavy water is due to the stabilizing action of D_2O on microtubules[158,159]. D_2O is, in fact, unlikely to be a specific agent and hence this argument should be viewed cautiously.

Exocytosis

Having dealt with aspects of the activation of mast cells and basophils it is necessary to say a few words about the final event: release of preformed granules containing histamine. Studies have shown that, during the release process, the granule and cell membranes fuse specifically to release the contents of the granule and conserve the cytoplasm[160]. At the point of fusion between the two membranes there is exclusion of membrane protein[161]. During exocytosis, vacuoles form, apparently within the cell, but these have been shown to communicate with the extracellular medium and so, during the secretory event, the cell becomes rather like a sponge, the granule contents being poured into the canicular spaces[162,163]. Clearly there is expansion of the cell membrane during this process[164] and redundant membrane may be either budded off from the cell in 'blebs'[161,165] or internalized in condensed lamellar packages[161].

It is not clear what the fate of the mast cell is *in vivo* after it has secreted, though *in vitro* there is some evidence that regeneration of granules can occur[166–170].

Actions of histamine

Bronchial smooth muscle

Having looked at the cell involved in storing and releasing histamine and how it is activated, it is now relevant to ask what actions it has which are relevant to the pathogenesis of asthma.

Schild and others were responsible for the first demonstration that human bronchial smooth muscle *in vitro* contracted in response to histamine[12]. They were also fortunate to have human lung tissue from a pollen-sensitized individual and showed that the bronchial smooth muscle contracted, not only to histamine but also to pollen antigens. Furthermore, they showed that the contraction of the muscle induced by pollen was inhibited by the antihistamine mepyramine. It was clear, therefore, that histamine released from tissue mast cells by appropriate antigen contributed to the contraction of bronchial smooth muscle. The observation has been confirmed more recently using passively sensitized human bronchial tissue[171]. In this latter study, it was shown that antagonists of histamine at H_1-receptors delayed and reduced the magnitude of an anaphylactic contraction of human bronchial smooth muscle. The effect was only seen if the antihistamine was present before antigen challenge of the tissue and the drug was inactive if added after the challenge. It was clear that the component of anaphylactic bronchoconstriction in this system which was insensitive to H_1 histamine antagonists was almost completely suppressed by the slow-reacting substance antagonist, FPL 55712.

In addition to producing contraction of bronchial smooth muscle, histamine also contracts lung strip preparations[172,173] which contain much smaller airways and where it is not clear precisely which elements of the tissue display a contractile response to histamine[174].

Apart from the *in vitro* studies, there have been a number of *in vivo* studies of histamine as a bronchoconstrictor agent. Inhalation of a histamine aerosol by asthmatics induces a fall in FEV_1 and this effect may be blocked by an H_1 antagonist of histamine[175]. However, falls in FEV_1 produced by bronchial challenge of allergic individuals with antigen cannot be modified by H_1 antagonists of histamine given orally[176], although protection was obtained when the compounds were given intravenously or by inhalation (Chapter 7). Thus, one is left with clear evidence that contractile elements in small and large airways of man contract in response to histamine and this effect is mediated through H_1-receptors. However, *in vitro* H_1 antihistamines only modify the anaphylactic contraction of bronchial smooth muscle and *in vivo* H_1 antihistamines have limited effectiveness in asthma. One reason why H_1 antihistamines have little effect in asthma could be the involvement of other mediators such as leukotrienes (SRS-A). However, histamine probably does play a significant part in the pathogenesis of asthma and the ineffectiveness of H_1 antihistamines when given orally may reflect the fact that the concentrations of these drugs which can be achieved without untoward side-effects is low compared with histamine levels likely to be achieved in tissues. It should be remembered that most H_1 antihistamines are competitive antagonists and it can be calculated that the histamine concentration in a single mast cell granule is about 1 molar.

It should be emphasized that the discussion has been centred on human tissue and there are marked species variations in response to histamine[177].

Whilst H_1-receptors in human lung are involved in smooth muscle contraction, there is now evidence that H_2-receptors are also present and mediate relaxation of bronchial smooth muscle[178]. Although, *in vitro*, H_2 antagonists potentiate the action of histamine and also anaphylactic contraction of bronchial smooth muscle, *in vivo* there is no evidence that cimetidine alters either histamine-induced bronchospasm or bronchospasm induced by antigen challenge[175,176,178,179]. Again there are marked species variations in the extent of the H_2-receptor effect in lung[177].

Mucus production

One feature of asthma is the bronchial plugging with mucus. Some recent work with human bronchial tissue has reported that histamine induces mucus production and that the effect was blocked by H_2-receptor antagonists. The work can be critized for using very high doses of histamine and also failing to investigate whether the applied histamine was acting directly to increase mucus production or indirectly through neuronal release mechanisms[180]. Mucus production is mainly under the control of the parasympathetic nervous system through muscarinic receptors on mucus-secreting cells. It should be added that other work[181] failed to demonstrate any effect of histamine on mucus production in human bronchial tissue. Also, there is no evidence as to whether an antigen–antibody reaction can induce increased mucus production either directly or indirectly[182].

Pulmonary vasculature

In general terms histamine has two actions on vessels: (*a*) to alter vessel diameter and therefore flow, and (*b*) to alter vessel permeability. There is almost no information about the actions of histamine on pulmonary vessels of man although a considerable amount of experimental work has been done in animals[177]. It is, therefore, difficult to draw any conclusion about whether histamine release in asthma has any action on lung vessels which contributes to the pathogenesis of asthma. Pulmonary hypertension and hypoxia are both features of asthma, although pulmonary oedema is not. If one uses results from the higher species of animal, it is clear that histamine, acting through H_1-receptors, constricts pulmonary vessels and induces pulmonary hypertension[183,184]. There is some evidence for the existence of H_2-receptors which cause relaxation of pulmonary vessels and lower pulmonary artery pressure[185,186]. All of this, however, cannot be fitted into the context of asthma since it has not been established what the effects are of histamine released by antigen challenge on pulmonary vasculature.

Concluding remarks

It should be apparent that, despite being the first proposed mediator of anaphylactic bronchoconstriction, there is still much to be learnt about histamine's role in the pathogenesis of asthma. It is clear that the immunological mechanisms that are activated in asthma bring about the release of histamine in lung and this histamine exerts various actions. The important questions that remain are to what extent histamine mediates the various pathological processes in asthma and how it interacts with other mediators which are released.

References

1. WINDAUS, A. and VOGT, W. *Berichte der Deutschen chemischen Gesellschaft,* **40,** 3691 (1907)
2. KUTSCHER, F. *Zentralblatt für Physiologie,* **24,** 163 (1910)
3. BARGER, G. and DALE, H.H. *Journal of Physiology,* **60,** 38p (1910)
4. DALE, H.H. and LAIDLAW, P.P. *Journal of Physiology,* **41,** 318 (1910)
5. DALE, H.H. and LAIDLAW, P.P. *Journal of Physiology,* **43,** 182 (1911)
6. DALE, H.H. and LAIDLAW, P.P. *Journal of Physiology,* **52,** 355 (1919)
7. PORTIER, P. and RICHET, C. Comptes Rendus des Seances de la Société de Biologie et de ses Filiales, **54,** 170 (1902)
8. DALE, H.H. *Journal of Pharmacology and Experimental Therapeutics,* **4,** 167 (1913)
9. SCHULTZ, *Journal of Pharmacology and Experimental Therapeutics,* **1,** 549 (1910)
10. BARTOSCH, R., FELDBERG, W. and NAGEL, E. *Pflügers Archiv für die Gesamte Physiologie,* **230,** 129 (1932)
11. LEWIS, T. *The Blood Vessels of the Human Skin and their Responses.* London: Shaw & Son Ltd (1927)
12. SCHILD, H.O., HAWKINS, D.F., MONGAR, J.L. and HERXHEIMER, H. *Lancet,* **ii,** 376 (1951)
13. ROCHA E SILVA, M., SCROGGIE, A.E., FIDLAR, E. *et al. Proceedings of the Society for Experimental Biology and Medicine,* **64,** 141 (1947)
14. MacINTOSH, F.C. and PATON, W.D.M. *Journal of Physiology,* **109,** 190 (1949)
15. RILEY, J.F. and WEST, G.B. *Journal of Physiology,* **120,** 528 (1953)
16. SCHAYER, R.W. In *Handbook of Experimental Pharmacology.* Ed. M. Rocha e Silva. Vol. 18(1), p. 672. Berlin: Springer Verlag (1966)
17. GRAHAM, H.T., LOWRY, O.H., WHEELWRIGHT, F. *et al. Blood,* **10,** 407 (1955)
18. TROTTER, C.H. and ORR, T.S.C. *Clinical Allergy,* **4,** 421 (1974)
19. METCALFE, D.D., LEWIS, R.A., SILBERT, J.E. *et al. Journal of Clinical Investigation,* **64,** 1537 (1979)
20. METCALFE, D.D., SMITH, J.A. and AUSTEN, K.F. *Journal of Biological Chemistry,* **255,** 11 753 (1980)
21. ABORG, C.H. and UVNAS B. *Acta Physiologica Scandinavica,* **74,** 552 (1968)
22. BERGENDORFF, A. and UVNAS, B. *Acta Physiologica Scandinavica,* **87,** 213 (1973)
23. SCHWARTZ, L.B. and AUSTEN, K.F. In *Biochemistry of the Acute Allergic Reaction.* Eds E.L. Becker, A. Stolper Simon and K.F. Austen. p. 103. New York: Alan Liss Inc. (1981)
24. BLOOM, G.D. In *The Inflammatory Process,* 2nd edn. Vol. 1, Chap. 10, p. 545. New York: Academic Press (1974)
25. HASTIE, R. *Laboratory Investigation,* **31,** 223 (1974)
26. PEARCE, F.L. *Trends in Pharmacological Sciences,* **4,** 165 (1983)
27. BURNET, F.M. *Journal of Pathology and Bacteriology,* **89,** 271 (1965)
28. GINSBURG, H., NIR, I., HAMMEL, I. *et al. Immunology,* **35,** 485 (1978)
29. ISHIZAKA, T., OKUDAIRA, H., MAUSER, L.E. and ISHIZAKA, K. *Journal of Immunology,* **116,** 747 (1976)
30. KELLER, R. *et al. Experientia,* **32,** 171 (1970)
31. KITAMURA, Y., YOKOYAMA, M., MATSUDA, H. and OHNO, T. *Nature,* **291,** 159 (1981)
32. SCHRADER, J.W. *Journal of Immunology,* **126,** 452 (1981)
33. SCHRADER, J.W., LEWIS, S.J., CLARK-LEWIS, I. *et al. Proceedings of the National Academy of Sciences of the United States of America,* **78,** 323 (1981)
34. CZARNETSKI, B., STERRY, W., BAZIN, H. and KALVERAM, K.J. *International Archives of Allergy and Applied Immunology,* **67,** 44 (1982)
35. PADAWER, J. *Laboratory Investigation,* **25,** 320 (1971)
36. DESSAINT, J-P., TORPIER, G., CAPRON, M. *et al. Cellular Immunology,* **46,** 12 (1979)
37. DIXON, F.J. and McCONAHEY, R.W. *Journal of Experimental Medicine,* **117,** 833 (1963)

38. ISHIZAKA, K. and ADACHI, T. *Journal of Immunology*, **117**, 40 (1976)
39. CHIORAZZI, N., FOX, D.A. and KATZ, D.M. *Journal of Immunology*, **118**, 48 (1977)
40. WATANABE, N., KOJIMA, S., SHEN, F.W. *et al. Journal of Immunology*, **118**, 485 (1977)
41. TUNG, A.S., CHIORAZZI, N. and KATZ, D.M. *Journal of Immunology*, **120**, 2050 (1979)
42. MOTA, I. *Immunology*, **7**, 681 (1965)
43. KATZ, D.M. *Journal of Allergy and Clinical Immunology*, **62**, 44 (1978)
44. MONGAR, J.L. and WINNE, D. *Journal of Physiology*, **182**, 79 (1966)
45. HALPER, J. and METZGER, H. *Immunochemistry*, **13**, 907 (1976)
46. STANWORTH, D.R., HUMPHREY, J.H., BENNICH, H. *et al. Lancet*, **ii**, 17 (1968)
47. DORRINGTON, K.J. and BENNICH, H. *Journal of Biological Chemistry*, **248**, 8378 (1973)
48. ISHIZAKA, T., TOMIOKA, H. and ISHIZAKA, K. *Journal of Immunology*, **105**, 1459 (1970)
49. CONRAD, D.H., BAZIN, H., SEHON, A.H. *et al. Journal of Immunology*, **114**, 1688 (1975)
50. KULCZYCKI, A. and METZGER, H. *Journal of Experimental Medicine*, **140**, 1676 (1974)
51. CONRAD, D.H., BERCZI, I. and FROESE, A. *Immunochemistry*, **13**, 329 (1976)
52. CONRAD, D.H. and FROESE, A. *Journal of Immunology*, **120**, 429 (1978)
53. HOLOWKA, D., HARTMANN, H., KANELLOPOULOS, J. *et al. Journal of Receptor Research*, **1**, 41 (1980)
54. FEWTRELL, C., GOETZ, A. and METZGER, H. (1982) *Biochemistry*, **21**, 2004 (1982)
55. HEMPSTEAD, B.L., KULCZYCKI, A. and PARKER, C.W. *Biochemical and Biophysical Research Communications*, **98**, 815 (1981)
56. METZGER, H. In *Receptors and Recognition*. Eds P. Cuatrecasas and M.F. Greaves. Vol. 4, p. 73. London: Chapman Hall (1977)
57. MENDOZA, G. and METZGER, H. *Nature*, **264**, 548 (1976)
58. SCHLESSINGER, J., WEBB, W.W., ELSON, E.L. *et al. Nature*, **264**, 550 (1976)
59. STANWORTH, D.R. *Nature*, **233**, 310 (1971)
60. STANWORTH, D.R., KINGS, M., ROY, P.D. *et al. Biochemical Journal*, **180**, 665 (1979)
61. HAMBURGER, R.N. *Science*, **189**, 389 (1975)
62. LANDSTEINER, K. *Journal of Experimental Medicine*, **39**, 631 (1924)
63. SIRAGANIAN, R.P., HOOK, W.A. and LEVINE, B. *Immunochemistry*, **12**, 149 (1975)
64. ISHIZAKA, K. and ISHIZAKA, T. *Journal of Immunology*, **103**, 588 (1969)
65. KELLER, R. *Clinical and Experimental Immunology*, **13**, 139 (1973)
66. MAGRO, A.M. *Nature*, **249**, 572 (1974)
67. SIRAGANIAN, R.P. and SIRAGANIAN, P.A. *Journal of Immunology*, **114**, 886 (1975)
68. SEGAL, D.M., TAUROG, J.D. and METZGER, H. *Proceedings of the National Academy of Sciences of the United States of America*, **74**, 2993 (1977)
69. FEWTRELL, C. and METZGER, H. *Journal of Immunology*, **125**, 701 (1980)
70. ISHIZAKA, T. and ISHIZAKA, K. *Journal of Immunology*, **120**, 800 (1978)
71. DELISI, C. *Nature*, **289**, 322 (1981)
72. FOREMAN, J.C. *Journal of Physiology*, **271**, 215 (1977)
73. FOREMAN, J.C. and LICHTENSTEIN, L.M. *Journal of Pharmacology and Experimental Therapeutics*, **210**, 75 (1979)
74. DEMBO, M. and GOLDSTEIN, B. *Journal of Immunology*, **121**, 345 (1978)
75. DEMBO, M., GOLDSTEIN, B., SOBOTKA, A.K. *et al. Journal of Immunology*, **121**, 354 (1978)
76. CONROY, M.C., ADKINSON, N.F. and LICHTENSTEIN, L.M. *Journal of Immunology*, **118**, 1317 (1977)
77. MONGAR, J.L. and SCHILD, H.O. *Journal of Physiology*, **140**, 272 (1958)
78. GREAVES, M.W. and MONGAR, J.L. *Immunology*, **15**, 743 (1968)
79. FOREMAN, J.C. and MONGAR, J.L. *Journal of Physiology*, **224**, 753 (1972)
80. DOUGLAS, W.W. *British Journal of Pharmacology*, **34**, 451 (1968)
81. FOREMAN, J.C., MONGAR, J.L. and GOMPERTS, B.D. *Nature*, **245**, 249 (1973)
82. BENNETT, J.P., COCKROFT, S. and GOMPERTS, B.D. *Nature*, **282**, 851 (1979)
83. JOHANSEN, T. *European Journal of Pharmacology*, **62**, 329 (1980)
84. KANNO, T., COCHRANE, D.E. and DOUGLAS, W.W. *Canadian Journal of Physiology and Pharmacology*, **51**, 1001 (1973)
85. THEOHARIDES, T.C. and DOUGLAS, W.W. *Science*, **201**, 1143 (1978)
86. BENNETT, J.P., COCKROFT, S. and GOMPERTS, B.D. *Journal of Physiology*, **317**, 335 (1981)
87. FOREMAN, J.C. and MONGAR, J.L. *British Journal of Pharmacology*, **48**, 527 (1973)
88. FOREMAN, J.C., SOBOTKA, A.K. and LICHTENSTEIN, L.M. *Journal of Immunology*, **231**, 153 (1979)
89. FOREMAN, J.C., HALLETT, M.B. and MONGAR, J.L. *Journal of Physiology*, **271**, 193 (1977)

90. ISHIZAKA, T., FOREMAN, J.C., STERK, A.R. *et al. Proceedings of the National Academy of Sciences of the United States of America*, **76**, 5858 (1979)
91. PEARCE, F.L., ENNIS, M. TRUNEH, A. *et al. Agents and Actions*, **11**, 51 (1981)
92. FOREMAN, J.C. In *Biochemistry of the Acute Allergic Reaction*. Eds E.L. Becker, A. Stolper Simon and K.F. Austen. New York: Alan Liss Inc., p. 315. (1981)
93. FOREMAN, J.C. and MONGAR, J.L. *Journal of Physiology*, **230**, 493 (1973)
94. FOREMAN, J.C., HALLETT, M.B. and MONGAR, J.L. *Journal of Physiology*, **271**, 233 (1977)
95. SIRAGANIAN, R.P., KULCZYCKI, A., MENDOZA, G. *et al. Journal of Immunology*, **115**, 159 (1975)
96. McGIVNEY, A., CREWS, F., HIRATA, F. *et al. Proceedings of the National Academy of Sciences of the United States of America*, **78**, 617 (1981)
97. FOREMAN, J.C. and GARLAND, L.G. *Journal of Physiology*, **239**, 381 (1974)
98. LICHTENSTEIN, L.M. *Journal of Immunology*, **107**, 1122 (1971)
99. SIRAGANIAN, R.P. and HAZARD, K.A. *Journal of Immunology*, **122**, 1719 (1979)
100. SOBOTKA, A.K., DEMBO, M., GOLDSTEIN, B. *et al. Journal of Immunology*, **122**, 511 (1979)
101. MICHELL, R.H. and KIRK, C.J. *Trends in Pharmacological Science*, **2**, 86 (1981)
102. COCKROFT, S. and GOMPERTS, B.D. *Biochemical Journal*, **178**, 681 (1979)
103. KENNERLY, D.A., SULLIVAN, T.J. and PARKER, C.W. *Journal of Immunology*, **122**, 152 (1979)
104. STRANDBERG, K., SYDBOM, A. and UVNAS, B. *Acta Physiologica Scandinavica*, **94**, 54 (1975)
105. HIRATA, F., AXELROD, J. and CREWS, F. *Proceedings of the National Academy of Sciences of the United States of America*, **76**, 4813 (1979)
106. ISHIZAKA, T., HIRATA, F., ISHIZAKA, K. *et al. Proceedings of the National Academy of Sciences of the United States of America*, **77**, 1903 (1980)
107. MONGAR, J.L. and SVEC, P. *British Journal of Pharmacology*, **46**, 741 (1972)
108. MARTIN, T.W. and LAGUNOFF, D. *Science*, **204**, 631 (1979)
109. ISHIZAKA, T., HIRATA, F., STERK, A.R. *et al. Proceedings of the National Academy of Sciences of the United States of America*, **78**, 6812 (1981)
110. KENNERLY, D.A., SULLIVAN, T.J., SYLWESTER, P. *et al. Journal of Experimental Medicine*, **150**, 1039 (1979)
111. JAKSCHIK, B.A., FALKENHEIM, S. and PARKER, C.W. *Proceedings of the National Academy of Sciences of the United States of America*, **74**, 4577 (1977)
112. STRANDBERG, K., MATHE, A.A. and YEN, S-S. *International Archives of Allergy and Applied Immunology*, **53**, 520 (1977)
113. LEWIS, R.A., HOLGATE, S.T., ROBERTS, L.J. *et al. Journal of Immunology*, **123**, 1663 (1979)
114. LOEFFLER, L.J., LOVENBERG, W. and SJOERDSMA, A. *Biochemical Pharmacology*, **20**, 2287 (1971)
115. TAYLOR, W.A., FRANCIS, D.H., SHELDON, D. *et al. International Archives of Allergy and Applied Immunology*, **46**, 104 (1974)
116. BOURNE, H.R. and MELMON, K.L. *Journal of Pharmacology and Experimental Therapeutics*, **178**, 1 (1971)
117. BACH, M.K. and BRASHLER, J.R. *Journal of Immunology*, **120**, 998 (1978)
118. JAKSCHLIK, B.A., KULCZYCKI, A., MacDONALD, H.H. *et al. Journal of Immunology*, **119**, 618 (1977)
119. BACH, M.K., BRASHLER, J.R., JOHNSON, M.A. *et al.* In *Biochemistry of the Acute Allergic Reaction*. Eds. E.L. Becker, A. Stolper Simon and K.F. Austen, p. 37. New York: Alan Liss Inc. (1981)
120. MARONE, G., HAMMERSTROM, S. and LICHTENSTEIN, L.M. *Journal of Immunology and Immunopathology*, **17**, 117 (1980)
121. McGIVNEY, A., MORITA, Y., CREWS, F.T. *et al. Archives of Biochemistry and Biophysics*, **212**, 527 (1981)
122. SCHILD, H.O. *Quarterly Journal of Physiology*, **26**, 165 (1936)
123. LICHTENSTEIN, L.M. and MARGOLIS, S. *Science*, **161**, 902 (1968)
124. ASSEM, E.S.K. and SCHILD, H.O. *British Journal of Pharmacology*, **46**, 62 (1971)
125. LICHTENSTEIN, L.M. and DE BERNARDO, R. *Journal of Immunology*, **107**, 1131 (1971)
126. JOHNSON, A.R. and MORAN, N.C. *Journal of Pharmacology and Experimental Therapeutics*, **175**, 632 (1970)
127. FOREMAN, J.C., MONGAR, J.L., GOMPERTS, B.D. *et al. Biochemical Pharmacology*, **24**, 538 (1975)
128. MARONE, G., FINDLAY, S.R. and LICHTENSTEIN, L.M. *Journal of Immunology*, **123**, 1473 (1979)

129. LICHTENSTEIN, L.M., HENNEY, C.S., BOURNE, H.R. *et al. Journal of Clinical Investigation*, **52,** 691 (1973)
130. ECKSTEIN, F. and FOREMAN, J.C. FEBS *Letters*, **91,** 182 (1978)
131. MARQUARDT, D.L., PARKER, C.W. and SULLIVAN, T.J. *Journal of Immunology*, **120,** 871 (1978)
132. WELTON, A.F. and SIMKO, B.A. *Biochemical Pharmacology*, **29,** 1085 (1980)
133. FREDHOLM, B.B. and SYDBOM, A. *Agents and Actions*, **10,** 145 (1980)
134. SULLIVAN, T.J., PARKER, C.W., EISEN, S.A. *et al. Journal of Immunology*, **114,** 1480 (1975)
135. KALINER, M. and AUSTEN, K.F. *Journal of Immunology*, **112,** 664 (1974)
136. HOLGATE, S.T., LEWIS, R.A. and AUSTEN, K.F. *Journal of Immunology*, **124,** 2093 (1980)
137. SIEGHART, W., THEOHARIDES, T.C., DOUGLAS, W.W. *et al. Nature*, **275,** 329 (1978)
138. FOREMAN, J.C., SOBOTKA, A.K. and LICHTENSTEIN, L.M. *European Journal of Pharmacology*, **63,** 314 (1980)
139. FOREMAN, J.C., HALLETT, M.B. and MONGAR, J.L. *British Journal of Pharmacology*, **59,** 473P (1977)
140. KALINER, M., ORANGE, R.P. and AUSTEN, K.F. *Journal of Experimental Medicine*, **136,** 556 (1972)
141. BLANDINA, P., FANTOZZI, R., MANNAIONI, P.F. *et al. Journal of Physiology*, **301,** 281 (1980)
142. MONGAR, J.L. Personal communication
143. DIAMANT, B. *International Archives of Allergy and Applied Immunology*, **49,** 155 (1975)
144. MONGAR, J.L. and PERERA, B.A.V. *Nature*, **202,** 93 (1964)
145. PERERA, B.A.V. and MONGAR, J.L. *Immunology*, **8,** 519 (1965)
146. CHAKRAVARTY, N. *Acta Physiologica Scandinavica*, **72,** 425 (1968)
147. YAMASAKI, H. and ENDO, K. *Japanese Journal of Pharmacology*, **15,** 48 (1965)
148. CHAKRAVARTY, N. and SORENSEN, H.J. *Acta Physiologica Scandinavica*, **91,** 339 (1974)
149. JOHANSEN, T. and CHAKRAVARTY, N. *Naunyn-Schmiedeberg's Archives of Pharmacology*, **275,** 457 (1972)
150. DIAMANT, B., NORN, S., FELDING, P. *et al. International Archives of Allergy and Applied Immunology*, **47,** 894 (1974)
151. ALLISON, A.C. In *Locomotion of Tissue Cells*. Ciba Foundation Symposium 14. p. 109. Amsterdam: Associated Scientific Publishers (1973)
152. ROHLICH, P. *Experimental Cell Research*, **93,** 293 (1975)
153. ZUCKER-FRANKLIN, D. *Blood*, **29,** 878 (1967)
154. ORR, T.S.C., HALL, D.E. and ALLISON, A.C. *Nature*, **236,** 350 (1972)
155. NEMETH, E.F. and DOUGLAS, W.W. *Naunyn-Schmiedeberg's Archives of Pharmacology*, **302,** 153 (1978)
156. COLTEN, H. and GABBAY, K.H. *Journal of Clinical Investigation*, **51,** 1927 (1972)
157. LAGUNOFF, D. and CHI, E.Y. *Journal of Cellular Biology*, **67,** 231 (1975)
158. GILLESPIE, E. and LICHTENSTEIN, L.M. *Journal of Clinical Investigation*, **51,** 2941 (1972)
159. GILLESPIE, E., LEVINE, R.J. and MALAWISTA, S.E. *Journal of Pharmacology and Experimental Therapeutics*, **164,** 158 (1968)
160. ROHLICH, P., ANDERSON, P. and UVNAS, B. *Journal of Cellular Biology*, **51,** 465 (1971)
161. LAWSON, D., RAFF, M.C., GOMPERTS, B.D. *et al. Journal of Cellular Biology*, **72,** 242 (1977)
162. ANDERSON, P., SLORACH, S.A. and UVNAS, B. *Acta Physiologica Scandinavica*, **88,** 359 (1973)
163. LAGUNOFF, D. *Journal of Investigative Dermatology*, **58,** 296 (1972)
164. KINSOLVING, C.R., JOHNSON, A.R. and MORAN, N.C. *Journal of Pharmacology and Experimental Therapeutics*, **192,** 654 (1975)
165. BURWEN, S.J. and SATIR, B. *Journal of Cellular Biology*, **74,** 690 (1977)
166. PADAWER, J. *Experimental and Molecular Pathology*, **20,** 269 (1974)
167. DROBIS, J.D. and SIRAGANIAN, R.P. *Journal of Immunology*, **117,** 1049 (1976)
168. BYTZER, P., HOLMNIELSEN, E. and CLAUSEN, J. *Cell Tissue Research*, **216,** 647 (1981)
169. HOLMNIELSEN, E., BYTZER, P., CLAUSEN, J. *et al. Cell Tissue Research*, 216, 635 (1981)
170. WEILL, B.J. and RENOUX, M.L. *Cellular Immunology*, **68,** 220 (1982)
171. ADAMS, G.K. and LICHTENSTEIN, L.M. *Journal of Immunology*, **122,** 555 (1979)
172. DRAZEN, J.M. and SCHNEIDER, M.W. *Journal of Clinical Investigations*, **61,** 1441 (1978)
173. BRINK, C., DUNCAN, P.G. and DOUGLAS, J.S. *Journal of Pharmacology and Experimental Therapeutics*, **219,** 1 (1981)
174. EVANS, J.N., PREVITI, R., ADLER, K.B. *et al. Physiologist*, **21,** 35 (1978)
175. MACONOCHIE, J.G., WOODINGS, E.P. and RICHARDS, D.A. *British Journal of Clinical Pharmacology*, 7, 231 (1979)

176. LEOPLOLD, J.D., HARTLEY, J.P.R. and SMITH, A.P. *British Journal of Clinical Pharmacology*, **8,** 249 (1979)
177. CHAND, N. *Advances in Pharmacology and Chemotherapy*, 17, 103 (1980)
178. DUNLOP, L.S. and SMITH, A.P. *British Journal of Pharmacology*, **59,** 475P (1977)
179. NATHAN, R.A., SEGALL, N. and SCHOCKET, A.L. *Journal of Allergy and Clinical Immunology*, **67,** 171 (1981)
180. SCHELHAMER, J.H., MAROM, Z. and KALINER, M. *Journal of Clinical Investigations*, **66,** 1400 (1980)
181. STURGESS, J. and REID, L. *Clinical Sciences*, **43,** 533 (1972)
182. RICHARDSON, P.S., PHIPPS, R.J., BALFRE, K. *et al.* In *Respiratory Tract Mucus*. Ciba Foundation Symposium 54. p. 111. Amsterdam: Elsevier (1978)
183. EYRE, P. *British Journal of Pharmacology*, **43,** 302 (1971)
184. TUCKER, A., WEIR, E.K., REEVE, J.T. *et al. American Journal of Physiology*, **229,** 1008 (1975)
185. EYRE, P. and WELLS, P.W. *British Journal of Pharmacology*, **49,** 364 (1973)
186. CHAND, N. and EYRE, P. *European Journal of Pharmacology*, **45,** 213 (1977)

Chapter 3

Leukotrienes

Priscilla J. Piper

Introduction

When Feldberg and Kellaway[1] injected cobra venom into guinea-pig perfused lungs they observed the release of a substance into the perfusate
which contracted guinea-pig jejunum. This material differed from histamine in that the contraction was slow in onset and of long duration. On
account of its action this material was referred to as 'slow-reacting substance'. Two years later the release of a similar slow-reacting substance was
demonstrated during anaphylactic shock in guinea-pig perfused lungs by
Kellaway and Trethewie[2]. The study of the slow-reacting substances
(SRSs) was revived in the 1950s by Brocklehurst who coined the term
'slow-reacting substance of anaphylaxis' or 'SRS-A' to describe the material released during anaphylactic shock. SRS-A was characterized by its
potent contraction of various types of smooth muscle: guinea-pig ileum,
several other types of gastrointestinal smooth muscle, guinea-pig trachea
and human bronchus. The availability of antihistamines enabled
Brocklehurst[3] to distinguish SRS-A from histamine. The difference
between the fast response to histamine and the slower response to SRS-A
is shown in *Figure 3.1*.

In addition to guinea-pig lung, further sources of SRS-A were detected.
It was released during antigen challenge of passively sensitized human
lung[3], from rat peritoneum during immunological challenge[4] and Chakravarty and colleagues[5] showed the release of a similar slow-reacting substance from cat paws perfused with the histamine releaser Compound
48/80. Considerably later, Jakshik and colleagues[6] and Bach and Brashler[7]
showed that rat basophilic leukaemia cells and rat mononuclear cells stimulated with the calcium ionophore A23187 were also rich sources of SRS.
All these SRSs appeared to be very similar and possessed the same type of
biological activity.

Although SRS-A possessed extremely potent biological activity, the
determination of its chemical structure proved to be an onerous task
because it became clear that it was released in only very small quantities. A
number of groups made important contributions to the study of the structure of SRS-A which formed a valuable background to the ultimate elucidation of its structure as a leukotriene(s). For instance, Orange, Murphy

55

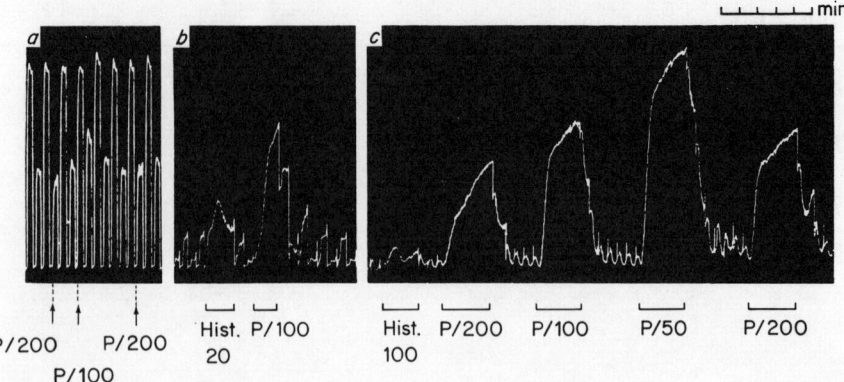

Figure 3.1 The use of mepyramine to demonstrate the presence of both histamine and SRS-A in the perfusate (P) from shocked guinea-pig lung. The record shows the contractions of guinea-pig ileum suspended in Tyrode solution containing atropine 5×10^{-7}M. The kymograph began to move just before the dose of active substances was placed in the bath, and stopped when the bath was drained. (*a*) Unlabelled contractions were produced by histamine 5 and 10 ng/ml with a normal contact time (25 s). (*b*) In the presence of mepyramine 2×10^{-10}M, histamine 10 and 20 ng/ml; at 'Hist.20' the dose was left in the bath for a longer time. (*c*) In the presence of mepyramine 10^{-6}M. Movements recorded on base line are due to washing and refilling bath. The concentrations of mepyramine used in (*b*) and (*c*) were present in the bath for 15 min beforehand, and at all times during the record. Reproduced with permission from Brocklehurst, W.E., 1960, *Journal of Physiology*, **151**, 416–435, by courtesy of the author and publisher.

and Austen[8] showed the inactivation of SRS-A by arylsulphatase; together with mass spectrometric observations, this suggested the possible presence of sulphur in the molecule. Orange and Chang[9] showed that various thiols enhanced the generation of SRS. Walker[10] showed that inhibition of cyclo-oxygenease in human lung tissue enhanced the release of SRS-A during antigen challenge, thus suggesting a link between arachidonic acid and SRS-A, and Parker, Huber and Falkenheim[11] suggested that SRS might be a fatty acid thioether. The development of an antagonist to SRS-A, FPL 55712, by workers at Fisons laboratories[12] further facilitated study of SRS-A for, although it was not truly competitive, its selectivity allowed distinction of the biological activity of SRS-A from that of other naturally occurring substances. The observation that SRS-A possessed u.v. absorbance with λ_{max} of 280 nm, showing the presence of a conjugated triene chromophore[13], was of paramount importance in the elucidation of the structure of SRS-A which is described below.

Structure, formation and metabolism of leukotrienes

Investigation by Samuelsson and his colleagues at the Karolinska Institute in Sweden, of the metabolism of arachidonic acid by rabbit poly-morphonuclear leucocytes (PMNs) led to the discovery of a family of arachidonic acid metabolites (hydroxy acids) whose formation was initiated by the action of a 5-lipoxygenase[14–16]. Like SRS-A, the hydroxy acid molecules possessed triene chromophores and an unstable epoxide, 5,6-oxido-7,9,11,14-eicosatetraenoic acid, was intermediate in their formation[16]. Samuelsson and colleagues[17] introduced the term leukotriene (LT) to describe compounds produced by this metabolic pathway and which possessed conjugated triene chromophores. Since analogous compounds can be derived from 5,8,11-eicosatrienoic acid, and 5,8,11,14,17-eicosapentaenoic acid, as well as 5,8,11,14-eicosatetraenoic acid (arachidonic acid), a subscript has been used to describe the total number of double bonds in the molecule[18].

Leukotrienes account for the activity of the slow-reacting substances. The SRS generated from murine mastocytoma cells by the calcium ionophore A23187 was characterized by degradative studies and comparison with pure synthetic materials and shown to be LTC_4[17,19,20]. SRS from rat basophilic leukaemia (RBL-1) cells was purified to homogeneity and characterized by electron impact mass spectrometry in conjunction with techniques used in protein chemistry and shown to be LTD_4[21]. By the use of similar techniques, the major biological activity (assayed on guinea-pig ileum) of SRS-A from guinea-pig lung was also shown to be LTD_4[22]. In addition, SRS-A from guinea-pig lung also contained appreciable amounts of LTB_4[23] (which does not contract guinea-pig ileum).

The unstable intermediate LTA_4 may be converted enzymatically into LTB_4 (*Figure 3.2*) or non-enzymatically into the isomers of LTB_4[24]. Alternatively, LTA_4 may be acted upon by enzymes involved in the glutathione detoxification pathway[25] and undergo nucleophilic attack resulting in the incorporation of a sulphur linkage and amino acid residues at C-6. Leukotriene C_4 is the first peptidolipid leukotriene to be formed and may then be converted to the cysteinylglycinyl derivative, LTD_4, by the action of γ-glutamyltranspeptidase (γ-GT). This conversion can occur sufficiently rapidly in guinea-pig isolated ileum to modify the activity of LTC_4[25,26]. A similar conversion of LTC_3 to LTD_3 occurs rapidly in guinea-pig lung homogenates[27]. Cleavage of glutamic acid from LTC_4 to form LTD_4 does not occur in all cells capable of generating LTC_4. For instance, A23187-stimulated mouse mastocytoma, bone marrow-derived mast cells, zymosan-activated mouse peritoneal or pulmonary macrophages do not substantially convert LTC_4 to LTD_4[20,28–30]. Leukotriene D_4 is further metabolized to the cysteinyl derivative LTE_4, by the action of a dipeptidase[31,32]. Recently, it was shown that incubation of LTE_4 with γ-GT in the presence of glutathione results in the reincorporation glutamic acid into the molecule and the formation of LTF_4[33]. Leukotriene F_4 has comparable activity with LTD_4 on guinea-pig trachea, but is less active on guinea-pig ileum[34]. Generation of LTF_4 from tissues has not yet been demonstrated. It is not known, therefore, whether the transformation to LTF_4 represents the normal metabolism of the peptidoleukotrienes, especially as the final product retains considerable biological activity.

Leukotriene C_4 can undergo metabolic inactivation in human PMNs, stimulated with phorbol myristate acetate, by an oxidative process dependent on the respiratory burst. In human PMNs, LTC_4 is converted to LTC_4 sulphoxides, $(5S,12S)$- and $(5S,12R)$-6-*trans*-LTD_4, which have much less

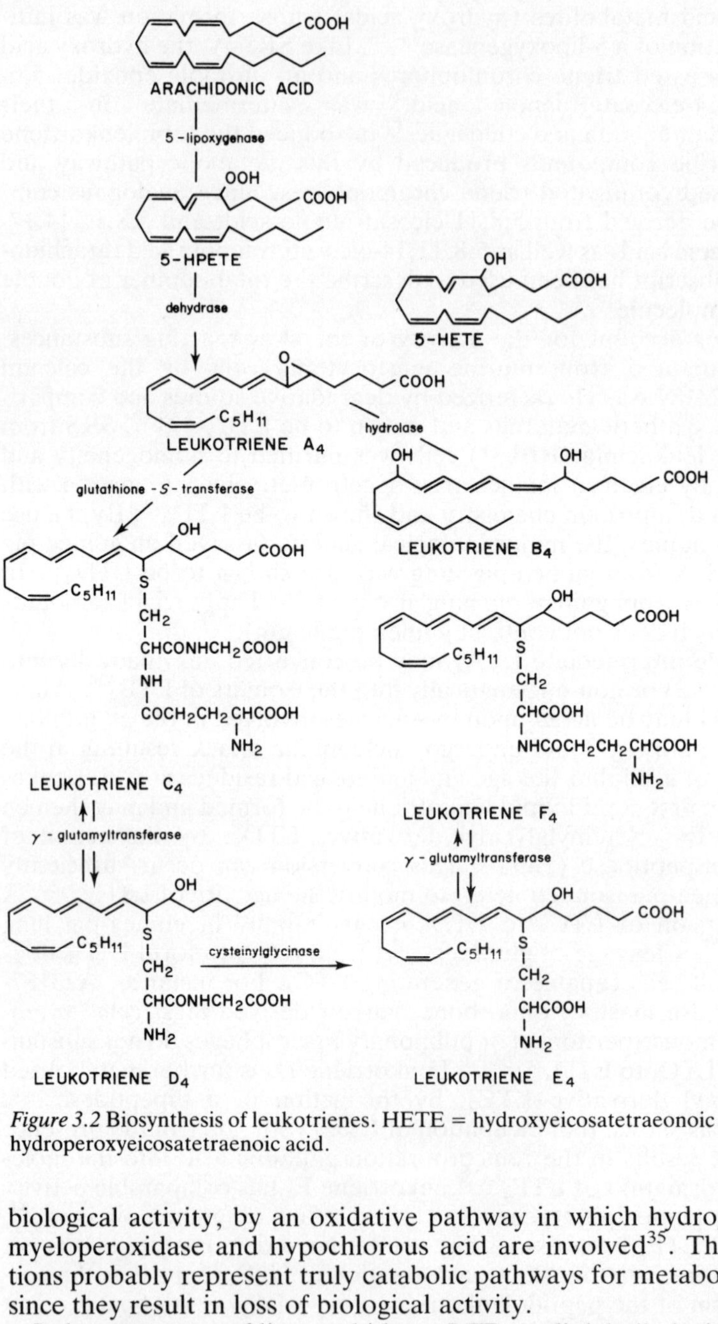

Figure 3.2 Biosynthesis of leukotrienes. HETE = hydroxyeicosatetraeonoic acid; HPETE = hydroperoxyeicosatetraenoic acid.

biological activity, by an oxidative pathway in which hydrogen peroxide, myeloperoxidase and hypochlorous acid are involved[35]. The above reactions probably represent truly catabolic pathways for metabolism of LTC$_4$, since they result in loss of biological activity.

In homogenates of liver or kidney, LTD$_3$ radiolabelled with ^{3}H is extensively metabolized to LTC$_3$ and LTE$_3$ showing that glutamic acid can be reincorporated into LTD$_3$[36]. In these systems, leukotriene B$_4$ is converted firstly to 20-hydroxy- and then to 20-carboxy-LTB$_4$ and both of these metabolites possess potent biological activity[37].

The generation of leukotrienes has been described in a number of tissues or cell suspensions as shown in *Table 3.1*. The leukotrienes formed by individual cells or tissues depend on the enzymes present in the tissue and the incubation conditions used. For example, RBL-1 cells incubated with the calcium ionophore A23187 are a rich source of LTD_4, but alteration of incubation conditions yields LTB_4, the $(5S,12R)$-*cis,trans,trans* isomer and its isomers $(5S,12S)$-all-*trans*-LTB_4 and $(5S,12R)$-all-*trans*-LTB_4, but little LTD_4[21,38]. In incubations of RBL-1 cells, inclusion of serine borate to inhibit γ-GT results in the generation of LTC_4[39] and LTD_4[40]. Murine mastocytoma cells on the other hand lack γ-GT and form only LTC_4[20]. Rat SRS-A contains LTC_4, LTD_4 and LTE_4[41,42]. It is of interest that, in addition to LTD_4, effluent from guinea-pig lungs during antigen challenge also contained appreciable amounts of LTB_4[23]. Guinea-pig lung contains sufficient γ-GT to convert tens of nanomoles of LTC_4 to LTD_4 per minute, which probably accounts for the fact that the major biological activity of guinea-pig SRS-A (assayed on guinea-pig ileum) is LTD_4[22,26].

TABLE 3.1. Release of leukotrienes (LTs)

Cellular source	LT released
Guinea-pig lung*[22,23]	LTB_4, LTD_4
Human lung*[42]	LTC_4, LTD_4
Rat alveolar macrophages*[106]	LTC_4
Rat peritoneal cells*[41,42]	LTC_4, LTD_4, LTE_4
Human polymorphonuclear leucocytes (PMNs)[15]	LTB_4, LTC_4
Rabbit PMNs[16]	LTB_4
Rat basophilic leukaemia (RBL-1) cells, [21,38,39]	LTB_4, LTD_4
Rat macrophages[107]	LTB_4
Rat mononuclear cells[108]	LTC_4, LTD_4
Rat PMNs[82]	LTB_4
Mouse macrophages[29]	LTC_4
Mouse mastocytoma cells[20]	LTC_4
Cat paw[109]	LTD_4, LTE_4

* Immunological challenge.

In addition to 5-lipoxygenase, preparations of human leucocytes contain enzymes which catalyse the introduction of oxygen into arachidonic acid at C-12 and C-15. Under appropriate conditions this can lead to the formation of novel leukotrienes, such as 14,15-LTB_4 and 14,15-LTC_4[43], but the biological actions of these leukotrienes have not yet been determined.

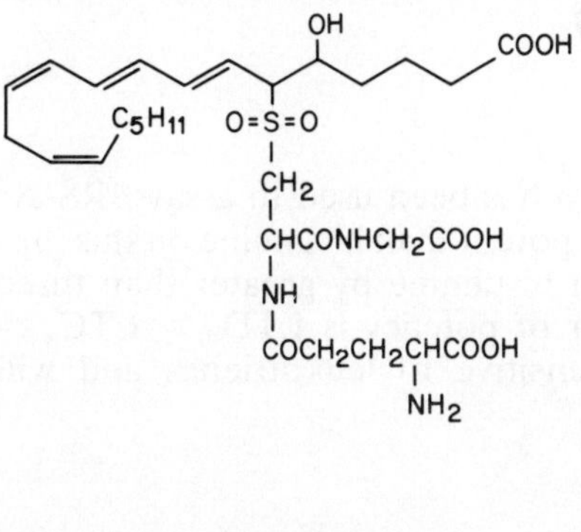

Figure 3.3 Structure of leukotriene D_4 sulphone.

As discussed above, there is some variation in the peptidolipid leukotrienes present in different SRSs, and Ohnishi and colleagues[44] identified the SRS produced from rat peritoneal cells as a leukotriene with a sulphone rather than a sulphide linkage at C-6 (*Figure 3.3*).

Leukotriene sulphones have recently been chemically synthesized[45] and shown to possess biological activity which closely resembles that of the leukotriene sulphides and is antagonized by FPL 55712[46], but to date the natural occurrence of leukotriene sulphones has not been confirmed.

Biological activities of the leukotrienes

Leukotrienes have potent biological actions which appear to broadly divide into two groups: those involving contraction of smooth muscle which are exhibited by the peptidolipid leukotrienes and the actions on cell motility which are shown by the dihydroxy acids, LTB_4 and its isomers (*see Table 3.2*).

TABLE 3.2. Leukotrienes

Dihydroxy acid	*S-linkage and amino acid residues at C-6*
LTB_4	LTC_4, LTD_4, LTE_4, LTF_4 (SRSs)
Chemotaxis	Contraction of smooth muscle
Chemokinesis	Bronchoconstriction
Aggregation of PMNs	Vasoconstriction
Exudation of plasma	Exudation of plasma
Contraction of guinea-pig parenchymal strip*	Secretion of mucus
	Activation of phospholipase A_2
Contraction of human bronchial strip*	
Translocation of Ca^{2+}	
Activation of phospholipase A_2	Antagonized by FPL 55712

* Show tachyphylaxis.

The action of leukotrienes occurs at various receptor sites in tissues and, as shown by different pharmacological actions and experiments in which tissues have been made tachyphylactic to leukotrienes, the receptors occupied by LTB_4 clearly differ from those for LTC_4, LTD_4 and LTE_4[47,48]. Using the antagonist presently available (FPL 55712), the receptors for the peptidolipid leukotrienes have been partially characterized[49,50]. So far, there is evidence for three types of receptors for LTD_4 in the guinea-pig, one in the ileum and two in the trachea.

Gastrointestinal smooth muscle

For many years, guinea-pig ileum *in vitro* has been used to assay SRS-A[3] and leukotrienes C_4, D_4 and E_4 are more potent than histamine on this preparation, LTD_4 being more potent than histamine by greater than three orders of magnitude. The relative order of potency is $LTD_4 > LTC_4 > LTE_4$[40,51]. Guinea-pig ileum is very sensitive to leukotrienes and will respond to picomole doses.

Rat stomach strip[52] and guinea-pig gall bladder strips are also contracted by leukotrienes but tend to be less sensitive than guinea-pig ileum[53]. These contractile responses are all antagonized by the SRS-A leukotriene antagonist, FPL 55712.

Respiratory smooth muscle

Leukotrienes are formed in the lung and have potent actions in the airways.

Leukotrienes are generated in lung tissue during anaphylaxis and collectively account for the biological activity of SRS-A from human and guinea-pig lung. They contract isolated respiratory smooth muscle *in vitro*, being active both in large and medium-sized airways such as guinea-pig trachea and human bronchus and in parenchymal strips which consist of small airways also containing small blood vessels. There is considerable species variation in the responses of airways to leukotrienes—they are thousands of times more active than histamine in respiratory smooth muscle from human and guinea-pig lung[40,54,55], but are less active on monkey trachea[56] and have little or no action in rat, cat or dog[57]. Leukotrienes C_4 and D_4 are about equiactive in contracting human isolated bronchial smooth muscle, guinea-pig trachea and parenchymal strips, but less active on parenchymal strips from human lung[48,54]. LTE_4 is less potent than LTC_4 or LTD_4 in all preparations. Human isolated bronchus is also contracted by LTB_4 but tachyphylaxis rapidly develops[48]. In guinea-pig isolated perfused lung, or superfused parenchymal strips, leukotrienes B_4, C_4, D_4, E_4 and F_4 stimulate the release of cyclo-oxygenase products, probably as a result of activating a phospholipase[48,52]. Thromboxane A_2 (TxA_2) is the main cyclo-oxygenase product released by leukotrienes, but other prostaglandin-like substances are also formed. The released TxA_2 plays an important role in the bronchoconstrictor actions of leukotrienes in some *in vivo* or *in vitro* preparations of guinea-pig tissues: TxA_2 is a potent bronchoconstrictor and augments the constrictor actions of the leukotrienes in superfused parenchymal strips *in vitro* (*Figure 3.4*) and when given by the intravenous route *in vivo*. In these preparations, leukotriene-induced bronchoconstriction is inhibited by the cyclo-oxygenase inhibitor indomethacin; however, when guinea-pig parenchymal strips are suspended in a conventional organ bath and cumulative doses of leukotrienes given, inhibition of leukotriene-induced contractions by indomethacin does not occur[58]. The actions of leukotrienes on guinea-pig parenchymal strips are also inhibited by thromboxane sythetase inhibitors or the phospholipase inhibitor mepacrine[52]. However, when leukotrienes are administered by aerosol to guinea-pigs, they appear to have a direct action which is not reduced by indomethacin[59,60] and may even be potentiated[58]. Leukotriene B_4 is a potent constrictor of guinea-pig parenchymal strip *in vitro*[47], an action which is dependent on the generation of TxA_2[52,61]. It also causes bronchoconstriction in guinea-pig *in vivo* which is blocked by indomethacin[62]. Leukotriene B_4-induced constriction differs from that of LTC_4 and LTD_4 in that it easily develops tachyphylaxis and is not antagonized by FPL 55712. Although the contraction of guinea-pig parenchyma induced by

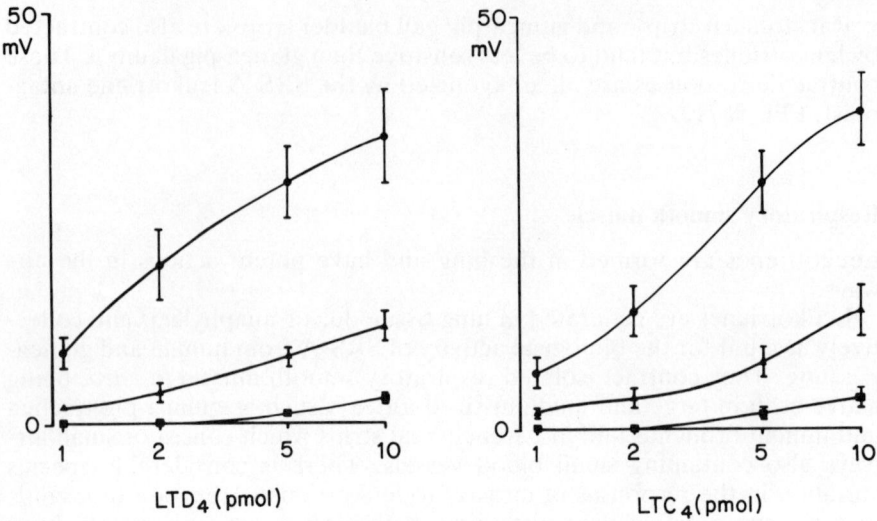

Figure 3.4 Inhibition of contractions of guinea-pig parenchymal strips due to 1–10 pmol of LTD$_4$ and LTC$_4$ (left and right-hand panels, respectively) by the thromboxane synthetase inhibitor carboxyheptylimidazole 24 μM, alone (▲) and with FPL 55712 1.9 μM (■). Bars represent s.e. from 8 experiments. Reproduced from Piper, P.J. and Samhoun, M.N. 1982, *British Journal of Pharmacology*, Vol. 77, pp. 267–275, by courtesy of the authors and publisher.

LTE$_4$ is dependent on the generation of TxA$_2$, it is of much longer duration than contraction due to LTC$_4$ and LTD$_4$[48]. Recent investigations show that LTF$_4$-induced contractions of guinea-pig parenchymal strips are also long lasting (Piper and Samhoun, unpublished observations) and raises the possibility that these leukotrienes either bind firmly to receptors or are metabolized more slowly than the other leukotrienes.

The findings discussed above show that, in certain guinea-pig preparations, leukotrienes stimulate the metabolism of arachidonic acid, probably by activating phospholipase A$_2$. Leukotriene B$_4$ has been shown to increase neutrophil membrane permeability to calcium, to enhance calcium influx and evoke a release of intraneutrophil calcium[63]. The action of phospholipase A$_2$ is calcium dependent and the activation of this enzyme by all leukotrienes in guinea-pig lung could be due to similar effects on translocation of calcium in this tissue.

The involvement of TxA$_2$ in the actions of leukotrienes does not occur when they are given to guinea-pigs by aerosol[59,60], probably because TxA$_2$ is released by guinea-pig lung parenchyma but not by the trachea[64]. There is no evidence for potentiation of leukotriene actions by TxA$_2$ in parenchyma from human, rabbit or rat lung[48], which probably accounts for these tissues being less sensitive to leukotrienes than guinea-pig lung parenchyma. In guinea-pig trachea, leukotriene-induced contractions are potentiated in the presence of indomethacin, perhaps on account of the release of a constrictor lipoxygenase product or inhibition of release of dilator prostaglandins[65,66].

Investigations *in vivo* have shown that leukotrienes C_4 and D_4 have selective actions on the small airways of the lung and cause a preferential reduction in compliance, although they also produce a modest fall in specific airways conductance[49]. In one study, when given by aerosol to two normal human volunteers, LTC_4 and LTD_4 caused bronchoconstriction and coughing[67]. In another study, inhaled LTC_4 was more potent than histamine in causing long-lasting respiratory effects, as measured by a reduction in expiratory maximum air-flow rate at 30 per cent of the vital capacity above residual volume (V_{max30}), and caused wheezing and tightness of the chest. There was evidence that LTC_4 had less effects on the central airways than shown by histamine[68]. Inhalation of LTD_4 by asymptomatic asthmatics again caused prolonged reduction of V_{max30}, wheezing and tightness in the chest. Leukotriene D_4 was more than one hundred times more potent than histamine and, although the asthmatics showed hyper-reactivity to histamine, they did not show marked increase in sensitivity to LTD_4[69].

The long duration of the leukotriene-induced effects resembles those seen in asthma and suggests a role for these substances as mediators of allergic airways constriction. Leukotrienes sensitize guinea-pig ileum to other agonists, such as histamine, and in a similar way leukotrienes may sensitize the airways to the actions of other bronchoconstrictor agonists.

Secretion of mucins

Indirect evidence based on the ability of the leukotriene antagonist FPL 55712 to reverse the slowing of mucociliary transport in patients undergoing antigen provocation, suggested that leukotrienes might impair airways clearance by stimulating mucus secretion[70]. Leukotrienes C_4 and D_4 caused secretion of mucins into the lumen of the cat trachea *in vivo*, but these effects could only be demonstrated with concentrations greater than those required to cause exudation of plasma in the skin[71,72]. The effects of LTC_4 and LTD_4 were weaker than those of other agonists such as adrenoceptor or cholinergic agonists or prostaglandins. Even in high doses, leukotrienes did not stimulate mucus secretion from cat trachea *in vitro*[71]. This suggested that a reflex or indirect mechanism might be involved in the leukotriene-induced secretion of mucus *in vivo*, but no changes in blood pressure or respiration indicative of reflex action were seen during administration of leukotrienes. From these observations, it seems that leukotrienes are not potent agonists of mucus secretion in the cat, but species differences obviously exist and LTC_4 and LTD_4 stimulate output of mucins from human bronchial strips cultured *in vitro*[73]. These leukotrienes are also two orders of magnitude more potent than methacholine in stimulating secretion of macromolecular glycoproteins, which are likely to be mucous glycoproteins, from human bronchial mucosa[74]. A possible explanation for this is that the human bronchus was taken from patients with bronchial carcinoma who may also have had bronchitis, and thus the bronchial mucous glands could have an increased number of receptors for agonists and an altered spectrum of sensitivity to agonists or they would have produced other mediators which might have acted synergistically with leukotrienes[72], whereas the cat studies were carried out in specific pathogen-free animals.

Microvasculature

Leukotrienes C_4 and D_4 cause exudation of plasma as measured by extra-vasation of ^{131}I-labelled albumin and of Evans' or Coomassie blue dye when injected intradermally into guinea-pig skin[75,76]. Leukotriene C_4 was much weaker than LTD_4 in stimulating plasma exudation on account of its vasoconstrictor action (*see below*). Leukotriene E_4 also induces exudation of plasma but is less potent than LTC_4 and LTD_4. The leukotriene-induced exudation of plasma in guinea-pig skin is potentiated by vasodilator pros-taglandins such as prostaglandins E_2 or I_2[76]. Leukotrienes C_4 and D_4 are unusual compounds in having a vasoconstrictor action in guinea-pig skin, in addition to causing plasma leakage. Leukotriene C_4 is the most active constrictor and causes blanching at injection sites[49,76], and the LTC_4-induced vasoconstriction is sufficient to mask the exudation of plasma. The potentiation of plasma exudation by vasodilator prostaglandins is probably due to reversal of leukotriene-induced vasoconstriction.

Considerable species variation occurs in the action of leukotrienes in the microvasculature of the skin; in human skin, LTC_4 and LTD_4 are potent vasodilators and produce wheal and flare responses at low concentrations[77,78]. Leukotriene B_4 also produces vascular permeability changes when injected into rabbit, rat and guinea-pig skin in the presence of a vasodilator prostaglandin[79]. This action of LTB_4 is dependent upon the presence of neutrophils and may result from the interaction of PMNs with the vascular endothelium[80].

The C-6-amino acid substituted leukotrienes LTC_4, LTD_4, and LTE_4 are also active in the terminal vascular bed of the hamster cheek pouch *in vivo*, where they cause plasma leakage from postcapillary venules and vasocon-striction in the terminal arterioles[81]. In this preparation, the leukotriene-induced vasoconstriction is equivalent to that of angiotensin II. However, leukotrienes are most active in causing plasma leakage since leukotrienes have virtually no vasoconstrictor action at doses which cause near maxi-mum plasma exudation. Leukotrienes are at least three orders of magni-tude more active than histamine in causing plasma leakage which is thought to be due to a direct action on the endothelial lining in the post-capillary venules.

Leukotriene B_4 is a potent chemotactic and chemokinetic agent for PMNs, its isomers, (5S,12R)-all-*trans*-LTB_4, and (5S,12S)-all-*trans*-LTB_4 being less active[82-84]. The peptidolipid leukotrienes do not show chemotac-tic or chemokinetic action. Leukotrienes B_4 have comparable biological activity to other potent chemotactic agents, such as the synthetic formyl-methionyl-leucyl-phenylalanine, the completment-derived peptide C5a and platelet-activating factor. Leukotriene B_4 also caused exudation of plasma, but was less active than LTC_4, LTD_4 and LTE_4. The response to LTB_4 was slow in onset and, as in the skin, dependent on adhering PMNs in the vascular bed[85]. In addition to PMNs, leukotriene B_4 is also chemo-tactic for eosinophils and monocytes[84], and might contribute to the eosi-nophilia which occurs in asthma. The accumulation of leucocytes also occurs when LTB_4 is administered *in vivo* into rabbit skin[86], guinea-pig peritoneal cavity[84], rabbit eye[87], hamster cheek pouch[86] and into abraded skin of human forearm[86]. Chemoattraction of leucocytes appears to be the main action of LTB_4 in the microvasculature, since exudation of plasma usually requires higher concentrations of LTB_4 and is dependent on the presence of PMNs. It is of interest that LTD_4 has no action on cell migration *in vitro*, but that falls in leucocyte counts occur in rats and monkeys following administration of LTD_4[56,88,89].

Cardiovascular system

Leukotrienes C_4 and D_4 have potent effects in the cardiovascular system and, as described previously for other activities, there are species differences in these actions: sometimes leukotrienes invoke release of cyclo-oxygenase products and their actions differ according to the route of administration. When given intravenously (i.v.) in the guinea-pig, LTC_4 and LTD_4 cause an initial hypertensive response, which is probably reflex in origin, resulting from bronchoconstriction, followed by long-lasting hypotension[49,55]. When leukotrienes are given into the aortic arch (a.a.), the hypotension is more prolonged while the hypertensive phase is less marked. Cyclo-oxygenase products are probably involved in this response, since indomethacin inhibits the hypertension and shortens the duration of the hypotension. In conscious guinea-pigs, after a brief pressor phase, LTD_4 (given intravenously) causes a long-lasting hypotensive effect which is accompanied by reflex bradycardia[90]. However, in this preparation indomethacin prolonged the hypotensive phase. In spontaneously hypertensive rats, LTD_4 caused an initial hypotension, brief hypertension, followed by prolonged hypotension in doses which did not reduce the blood pressure of normotensive rats[88]. Changes in blood pressure were accompanied by changes in heart rate. The long-lasting hypotension was attenuated by indomethacin. Leukotrienes had different effects in the cardiovascular system of the cat; when given intravenously, LTC_4 and LTE_4 all caused dose-related increases in blood pressure, LTE_4 being less potent than LTC_4 or LTD_4[91]. In primates (*Macaca irus*), LTC_4 administered into the right atrium caused a transient rise in mean arterial pressure followed by long-lasting hypotension which was accompanied by reduced cardiac output. Right and left atrial pressures were also increased reflecting increased resistance in both pulmonary and systemic vascular beds[56]. Although histamine had similar actions, these were of much shorter duration than LTC_4 effects. When given by aerosol, LTC_4 evoked long-lasting changes in pulmonary function, including increase in pulmonary arterial pressure, but had only small pressor effects on systemic arterial pressure[56]. In another species of monkey (*Macaca mulatta*), LTD_4 given by inhalation had less effect but showed a decrease in mean arterial pressure after intravenous injection[89]. LTD_4 is a potent pulmonary and systemic vasoconstrictor in the new-born lamb, but causes an initial hypotensive response which is probably mediated by a cyclo-oxygenase product(s)[92].

Leukotrienes have actions on cardiac function and are potent vasoconstrictors in the coronary circulation *in vivo* and *in vitro* and, as with other actions of leukotrienes, species differences occur. In guinea-pig isolated hearts perfused under constant pressure, LTC_4 and LTD_4 caused marked reduction in coronary flow (*Figure 3.5*)[93,94].

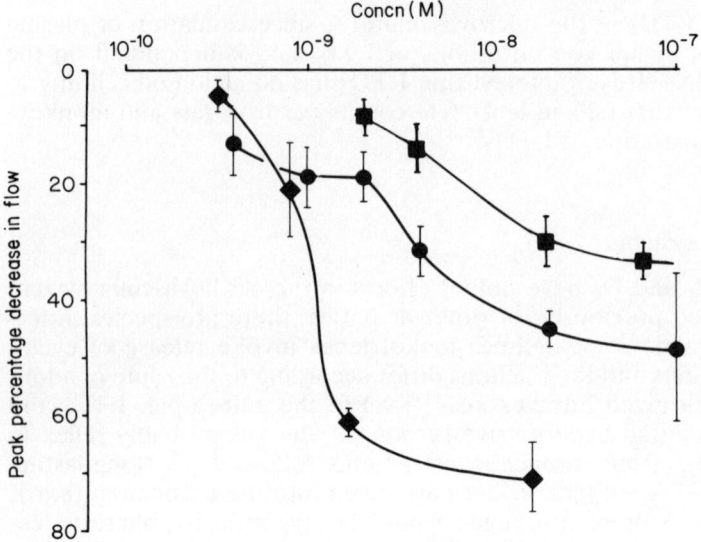

Figure 3.5 Actions of LTC$_4$ (◆), LTD$_4$ (●) and LTE$_4$ (■) on guinea-pig isolated heart. All three caused dose-related reduction in coronary flow. LTC$_4$ 2.0×10^{-8} M caused a maximum reduction of $71\pm6\%$, the maximum reduction produced by LTD$_4$ 1.6×10^{-8} M was $45\pm2\%$ while LTE$_4$ 9.1×10^{-8} M caused a maximum reduction of $33\pm3\%$. Vertical bars show s.e.m. ($n=3$–5 per dose). (Reproduced from Letts and Piper[94] with permission of the authors and publishers.)

A decrease in contractility occurred with the reduction in flow, but there were no arrhythmias or changes in heart rate. The reduction in flow was due to a direct vasoconstrictor action in the coronary circulation, since neither LTC$_4$ nor LTD$_4$ had any direct action on spontaneously beating atria or driven ventricular strips[94]. As in the skin of this species, LTC$_4$ was the most active vasoconstrictor. LTD$_4$ caused a similar reduction in flow in rat isolated hearts perfused under constant pressure, but reduced the spontaneous heart rate to a greater extent than contractility, indicating an action on conductivity in this species[95]. Leukotriene E$_4$ had similar actions in guinea-pig and rat hearts, but was 10–15 times less active[95]. Leukotriene F$_4$ caused an increase in perfusion pressure in guinea-pig hearts (perfused under constant flow), reduced contractility and was more potent than LTE$_4$ but less active than LTD$_4$[96]. In rabbit and cat isolated hearts, LTC$_4$ and LTD$_4$ were also potent constrictors of the coronary circulation[95]. Even in high doses, LTB$_4$ had no detectable action in perfused hearts of any species. In high doses (3.8×10^{-6} M), FPL 55712 antagonized the actions of leukotrienes in guinea-pig and rat hearts. Indomethacin partially inhibited the actions of LTC$_4$, and LTD$_4$ in guinea-pig hearts, but had no action in rat, rabbit or cat[94,97]. This action of indomethacin in guinea-pig hearts suggests the involvement of a cyclo-oxygenase product(s), but the vasoconstrictor cyclo-oxygenase product generated by leukotrienes in guinea-pig heart is unidentified since there was no evidence of release of thromboxane A$_2$ into the heart effluent, and a thromboxane synthetase inhibitor did not affect leukotriene actions in the heart[95]. The effects of LTC$_4$ and LTD$_4$ on coronary circulation of guinea-pig hearts may contribute to their hypotensive effects *in vivo*.

In anaesthetized greyhounds where the left anterior descending coronary artery was perfused with carotid blood, intracoronary injections of LTD_4 caused long-lasting dose-related reduction in mean coronary flow[97]. Leukotriene D_4 administered by this route had little effect on systemic arterial blood pressure, heart rate and cardiac output, although LTD_4-induced falls in coronary flow were associated with slight increases in the rate of pressure change (dP/dt). After administration of LTD_4 small discrete haemorrhages developed on the surface of the heart, mainly along the large coronary arteries, although there was no evidence of generalized vascular leakage (Evan's blue dye) or structural damage. Intracoronary injections of LTC_4 and LTD_4 in similar preparations of pig were more potent in causing prolonged reduction in coronary flow (*Figure 3.6*) than in the dog, but did not produce the surface haemorrhages described above[97].

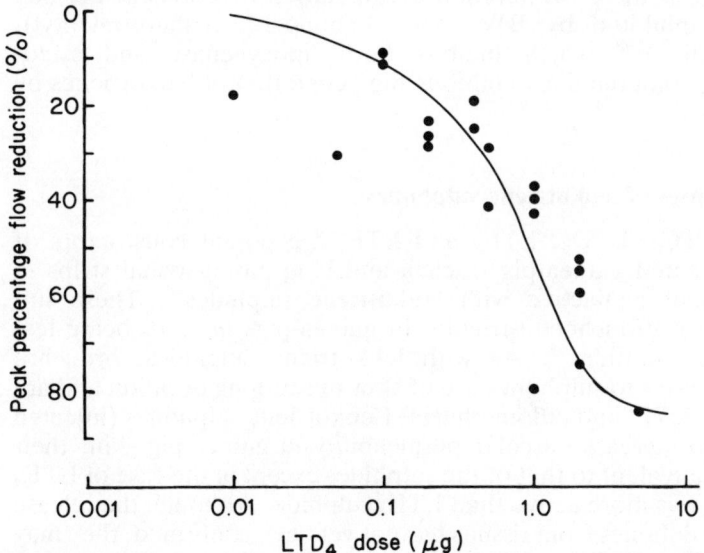

Figure 3.6 Percentage reduction in flow in the anterior descending coronary artery of the pig following bolus injections of LTD_4 into the blood perfusing the artery. From Letts, L.G., Piper, P.J. and Newman, D.L. 1983, *Leukotrienes and other Lipoxygenase Products*, Ed. P.J. Piper, Research Studies Press, John Wiley and Sons, Chichester and by courtesy of the authors and publishers.

Leukotrienes caused a slight transient decrease in dP/dt, but had little other action on cardiovascular parameters. Indomethacin did not affect leukotriene-induced reduction in coronary flow in either dogs or pigs, indicating that cyclo-oxygenase products were not involved in the actions of leukotrienes in these species[97]. In both dog and pig, LTD_4 was more active than angiotensin in constricting the coronary artery. Leukotriene D_4 also showed very potent vasoconstrictor actions in the coronary circulation of the sheep and produced local coronary constriction and impaired ventricular contraction resulting from the myocardial ischaemia[98].

The blood-bathed organ technique has been used in guinea-pigs to show that the biological activity of LTD_4 rapidly disappears in contact with circulating blood (Piper, unpublished observations). Leukotriene C_3 has also been shown to be rapidly degraded in monkeys and guinea-pigs *in vivo*[36]. These facts indicate that leukotrienes are not circulating hormones, which makes their local actions in individual vascular beds of special interest. For instance, the C-6-amino acid substituted leukotrienes exhibit potent vaso-constrictor actions in the coronary circulation of all species so far investigated and they have been shown to act directly on isolated coronary arteries from rabbit[99]. A 5-lipoxygenase system is present in porcine coronary arteries and the vessels and adjacent adventitia generate a leukotriene-like substance when challenged by A23187[100,101]. Since leukotrienes (SRS-A) are also generated from guinea-pig blood vessels during antigen challenge[3], the possibility exists of leukotrienes being generated from vascular tissue in pathological conditions and acting locally to cause vaso-constriction. Another indication of generation of 5-lipoxygenase products in tissue damage is the postinfarction accumulation of PMNs in the dog which can be inhibited by BW 755c (3-amino-1-[3-(trifluoromethyl)-phenyl]pyrazolidine)[102] which inhibits both lipoxygenase and cyclo-oxygenase. This compound also inhibits the generation of leukotrienes by porcine vascular tissue[101].

Biological responses of leukotriene sulphones

Sulphones of LTC_4, LTD_4, LTE_4 and LTF_4 are potent constrictors of indomethacin-treated guinea-pig trachea and lung parenchymal strips *in vitro*, being about equiactive with leukotriene sulphides[46]. These sulphones also cause bronchoconstriction in guinea-pigs *in vivo*, being less active than the sulphides[34]. As with leukotriene sulphides, broncho-constrictor responses to sulphones are of slow onset, long duration and are blocked by FPL 55712 and indomethacin. Leukotriene sulphones (injected with PGE_2) also increase vascular permeability in guinea-pig skin, their activity being equivalent to that of the sulphides except in the case of LTE_4 sulphone which was more active than LTE_4 sulphide. Although the release of leukotriene sulphones from tissues has not yet been confirmed, they may be released in and contribute to the signs of various allergic conditions.

Conclusions

Leukotrienes are a novel group of arachidonic acid metabolites which have a variety of biological actions. These actions (*see Table 3.2*) suggest that leukotrienes may have a role in various pathological conditions. The potent chemotactic and chemokinetic actions of LTB_4, which are dependent on the presence of PMNs, suggest that this leukotriene has an important role in inflammatory conditions and in tissue damage. Evidence has been provided for this by the detection of LTB_4 in synovial fluid from patients with rheumatoid arthritis[83] and gout[103] and the release of LTB_4, together with monohydroxyeicosatetraenoic acids (mono-HETEs) from abraded lesional areas of skin of psoriatics[104]. The generation of LTB_4 from human alveolar macrophages has also been detected[105] suggesting that LTB_4 is involved in inflammatory conditions of the lung as well as of peripheral tissues. Leukotrienes C_4 and D_4 cause changes in pulmonary mechanics of normal and asymptomatic asthmatic volunteers, including reduction in expiratory flow, tightness of the chest and wheezing which are of slow onset and long duration and suggest these leukotrienes may have a role in respiratory diseases such as asthma. Leukotrienes stimulate mucus secretion from human bronchus and may also act with other mediators to provoke generation of mucins in inflamed airways. The vasoconstrictor actions of LTC_4 and LTD_4 in the coronary circulation of various species suggest that they may be involved in conditions such as myocardial ischaemia and angina, and may perhaps be generated locally by vascular tissue. Another possibility is that interaction of the potent vasodilator prostacyclin, formed by vascular endothelial cells, and leukotrienes, formed by the outer layers of blood vessel walls and adventitia, may represent a homeostatic mechanism. As discussed above, compounds which prevent release of leukotrienes by inhibiting various stages of their synthesis are being developed and it will be of interest to investigate their action in pathological conditions where leukotrienes may have a role.

References

1. FELDBERG, W. and KELLAWAY, C.H. *Journal of Physiology*, **94,** 187 (1938)
2. KELLAWAY, C.H. and TRETHEWIE, E.R. *Quarterly Journal of Experimental Physiology*, **30,** 121 (1940)
3. BROCKLEHURST, W.E. *Journal of Physiology*, **151,** 416 (1960)
4. ORANGE, R.P., VALENTINE, M.D. and AUSTEN, K.F. *Journal of Experimental Medicine*, **127,** 767 (1968)
5. CHAKRAVARTY, N., HÖGBERG, B. and ÜVNAS, B. *Acta Physiologica Scandinavica*, **45,** 255 (1959)
6. JAKSHIK, B.A., KULCZYCKI, A., MacDONALD, H.H. and PARKER, C.W. *Journal of Immunology*, **119,** 618 (1977)
7. BACH, M.K. and BRASHLER, J.R. *Journal of Immunology*, **113,** 2040 (1974)
8. ORANGE, R.P., MURPHY, R.C. and AUSTEN, K.F. *Journal of Immunology*, **113,** 316
9. ORANGE, R.P. and CHANG, P.L. *Journal of Immunology*, **115,** 1072 (1975)
10. WALKER, J.L. *Advances in the Biosciences*, **9,** 235 (1973)
11. PARKER, C.W., HUBER, M.G. and FALKENHEIM, S.F. *Clinical Research*, **473,** 27 (1979)
12. AUGSTEIN, J., FARMER, J.B., LEE, T.B., SHEARD, P. and TATTERSALL, M.L. *Nature New Biology*, **245,** 215 (1973)
13. MORRIS, H.R., TAYLOR, G.W., PIPER, P.J., SIROIS, P. and TIPPINS, J.R. *FEBS Letters*, **87,** 203 (1978)
14. BORGEAT, P., HAMBERG, M. and SAMUELSSON, B. *Journal of Biological Chemistry*, **251,** 7816 (1976)
15. BORGEAT, P., and SAMUELSSON, B. *Journal of Biological Chemistry*, **254,** 7865 (1979)
16. BORGEAT, P. and SAMUELSSON, B. *Proceedings of the National Academy of Sciences of the United States of America*, **76,** 3213 (1979)
17. SAMUELSSON, B., BORGEAT, P., HAMMARSTRÖM, S. and MURPHY, R.C. *Prostaglandins*, **17,** 785 (1979)
18. SAMUELSSON, B. and HAMMARSTRÖM, S. *Prostaglandins*, **19,** 645 (1980)
19. HAMMARSTRÖM, S., MURPHY, R.C., SAMUELSSON, B., CLARK, D.A., MIOSKOWSKI, C. and COREY, E.J. *Biochemical and Biophysical Research Communications*, **91,** 1266 (1979)
20. MURPHY, R.C., HAMMARSTRÖM, S. and SAMUELSSON, B. *Proceedings of the National Academy of Sciences of the United States of America*, **76,** 4275 (1979)
21. MORRIS, H.R., TAYLOR, G.W., PIPER, P.J., SAMHOUN, M.N. and TIPPINS, J.R. *Prostaglandins*, **19,** 185 (1980)
22. MORRIS, H.R., TAYLOR, G.W., PIPER, P.J. and TIPPINS, J.R. *Nature*, **285,** 104 (1980)
23. MORRIS, H.R., TAYLOR, G.W., PIPER, P.J. and TIPPINS, J.R. In *Prostaglandins and Inflammation*. Eds K.D. Rainsford and A.W. Ford-Hutchinson, *Agents and Actions*, Suppl. 6, p. 27. Basel: Birkhäuser (1979)

24. SAMUELSSON, B. *Advances in Prostaglandin, Thromboxane and Leukotriene Research*, **9**, 1 (1982)
25. GRIFFITH, O.W. and MEISTER, A. *Proceedings of the National Academy of Sciences of the United States of America*, **76**, 268 (1979)
26. MORRIS, H.R., TAYLOR, G.W., JONES, C.M., PIPER, P.J., SAMHOUN, M.N. and TIPPINS, J.R. *Proceedings of the National Academy of Sciences of the United States of America*, **79**, 4838 (1982)
27. HAMMARSTRÖM, S. *Journal of Biological Chemistry*, **256**, 7712 (1981)
28. RAZIN, E., MENCIA-HUERTA, J.M., LEWIS, R.A., COREY, E.J. and AUSTEN, K.F. *Proceedings of the National Academy of Sciences of the United States of America*, **79**, 4665 (1983)
29. ROUZER, C.A., SCOTT, W.A., COHN, Z.A., BLACKBURN, P. and MANNING, J.M. *Proceedings of the National Academy of Sciences of the United States of America*, **77**, 4928 (1980)
30. ROUZER, C.A., SCOTT, W.A., HAMILL, A.C. and COHN, Z.A. *Journal of Experimental Medicine*, **155**, 720 (1982)
31. PARKER, C.W., FALKENHEIN, S.F. and HUBER, M.M. *Prostaglandins*, **20**, 863 (1980)
32. SOK, D.E., PAI, J.K., ARRACHE, V., KUNG, V.C. and SIH, C.J. *Biochemical and Biophysical Research Communications*, **101**, 222 (1981)
33. ANDERSON, M.E., ALLISON, D.R.D. and MEISTER, A. *Proceedings of the National Academy of Sciences of the United States of America*, **79**, 1088 (1982)
34. DENIS, D., CHARLESON, S., ROKACH, A., JONES, T.R., FORD-HUTCHINSON, A.W., LORD, A. *et al. Prostaglandins*, **24**, 801 (1982)
35. LEE, C.W., LEWIS, R.A., COREY, E.J., BARTON, A., Oh, H., TAUBER, A.I. *et al. Proceedings of the National Academy of Sciences of the United States of America*, **79**, 4166 (1982)
36. HAMMARSTRÖM, S. *Advances in Prostaglandin, Thromboxane and Leukotriene Research: Leukotrienes and other Lipoxygenase Products*, **9**, 83 (1982)
37. LINDGREN, J.A., HANSSON, G., CLAESSON, H.E. and SAMUELSSON, B., *Advances in Prostaglandin, Thromboxane and Leukotriene Research*, **9**, 53 (1982)
38. FORD-HUTCHINSON, A.W., PIPER, P.J. and SAMHOUN, M.W. *British Journal of Pharmacology*, **76**, 215 (1982)
39. ÖRNING, L. and HAMMARSTRÖM, S. *Journal of Biological Chemistry*, **255**, 8023 (1980)
40. LEWIS, R.A., DRAZEN, J.M., AUSTEN, K.F., CLARK, D.A. and COREY, E.J. *Biochemical and Biophysical Research Communications*, **96**, 271 (1980)
41. LEWIS, R.A., DRAZEN, J.M., COREY, E.J. and AUSTEN, K.F. In *SRS-A and Leukotrienes*. Ed. P.J. Piper. p. 101 Chichester: Research Studies Press, John Wiley and Sons (1981)
42. LEWIS, R.A., AUSTEN, K.F., DRAZEN, J.M., CLARK, D.A., MARFAT, A. and COREY, E.J. *Proceedings of the National Academy of Sciences of the United States of America*, **77**, 3710 (1980)
43. SAMUELSSON, B. *Advances in Prostaglandin, Thromboxane and Leukotriene Research*, **11**, 1 (1983)
44. OHNISHI, H., KOSUZUMA, H., KITAMURA, Y., YAMAGUCHI, K., NOBUHARA, M. and SUZUKI, Y. *Prostaglandins*, **20**, 655 (1980)
45. GIRARD, Y., LARUE, M., JONES, T.R. and ROKACH, J. *Tetrahedron Letters*, **23**, 1023 (1982)
46. JONES, T., MASSON, P., HAMEL, R., BRUNET, G., HOLME, G., GIRARD, Y. *et al. Prostaglandins*, **24**, 279–291 (1982)
47. SIROIS, P., ROY, S. and BORGEAT, P. *Prostaglandins and Medicine*, **5**, 429 (1981)
48. SAMHOUN, M.N. and PIPER, P.J. In *Leukotrienes and Other Lipoxygenase Products*, Ed. P.J. Piper. p. 161. Chichester: Research Studies Press, John Wiley and Sons (1983)
49. DRAZEN, J.M., AUSTEN, K.F., LEWIS, R.A., CLARK, D.A., GOTO, G., MARFAT, A. *et al. Proceedings of the National Academy of Sciences of the United States of America*, **77**, 4354 (1980)
50. KRELL, R.D., TSAI, B.S. and GILES, R.E. In *Leukotrienes and Other Lipoxygenase Products*. Ed. P.J. Piper. pp. 222–233. Chichester: Research Studies Press, John Wiley and Sons (1983)
51. PIPER, P.J., SAMHOUN, M.N., TIPPINS, J.R., WILLIAMS, T.J., PALMER, M.A. and PECK, M.J. In *SRS-A and Leukotrienes*. Ed. P.J. Piper. pp. 81–99. Chichester: Research Studies Press, John Wiley and Sons (1981)
52. PIPER, P.J. and SAMHOUN, M.N. *British Journal of Pharmacology*, **77**, 267 (1982)
53. YUSKO, P., HALL, R.A. and FORD-HUTCHINSON, A.W. *Prostaglandins*, **25**, 397 (1983)
54. DAHLÉN, S.E., HEDQVIST, P., HAMMARSTRÖM, S. and SAMUELSSON, B. *Nature*, **288**, 484 (1980)
55. PIPER, P.J. and SAMHOUN, M.N. *Prostaglandins*, **21**, 793 (1981)

56. SMEDGARD, G., HEDQVIST, P., DAHLÉN, S.E., REVENAS, B., HAMMARSTRÖM, S. and SAMUELS-
SON, B. *Nature*, **295**, 327 (1982)
57. KRELL, R.D., OSBORN, R., VICKERY, L., FALCONE, K., O'DONNELL, M., GLEASON, J. *et al. Prostaglandins*, **22**, 387 (1981)
58. HEDQVIST, P. AND DAHLÉN, S.E. In *Leukotrienes and Other Lipoxygenase Products*. Ed.
P.J. Piper. p. 134. Chichester: Research Studies Press, John Wiley and Sons (1983)
59. HAMEL, R., MASSON, P., FORD-HUTCHINSON, A.W., JONES, T.R., BRUNET, G. and PIECHUTA, H.
Prostaglandins, **24**, 419 (1982)
60. WEICHMAN, B.M., MUCCITELLI, R.M., OSBORN, R.R., HOLDEN, D.A., GLEASON, J.C. and WAS-
SERMAN, M.A. *Journal of Pharmacology and Experimental Therapeutics*, **222**, 202 (1982)
61. SIROIS, P., ROY, S., BORGEAT, P., PICARD, S. and VALLERAND, P. *Prostaglandins, Leukotrienes and Medicine*, **8**, 157 (1982)
62. HAMEL, R. and FORD-HUTCHINSON, A.W. *Prostaglandins*, in press (1983)
63. GOETZL, E.J., GOLDMAN, D.W., NACCACHE, P.H., SHA'AFI, R.I. and PICKETT, W.C. In *Advances in Prostaglandin, Thromboxane and Leukotriene Research: Leukotrienes and
Other Lipoxygenase Products*. Eds B. Samuelsson, R. Paoletti and P.W. Ramwell. Vol.
9. p. 273. New York: Raven Press (1982)
64. GRYGLEWSKI, R.J., DEMBINSKA-KIEC, A., GRODZINSKA, L. and PANCZENKO, B. In *Lung Cells
in Diseases*. Ed. A. Bouhuys. Amsterdam: North-Holland Biomedical Press (1976)
65. ADCOCK, J.J. and GARLAND, L.G. *British Journal of Pharmacology*, **69**, 167 (1980)
66. PIPER, P.J. and TIPPINS, J.R. In *Advances in Prostaglandin, Thromboxane and Leukotriene
Research: Leukotrienes and Other Lipoxygenase Products*. Eds B. Samuelsson, R.
Paoletti and P.W. Ramwell. Vol. 9. p. 183. New York: Raven Press (1982)
67. HOLROYDE, M.C., ALTOUNYAN, R.E.C., COLE, A.H., DIXON, M. and ELLIOT, E.V. *Lancet*, **ii**, 17
(1981)
68. WEISS, J.W., DRAZEN, J.M., COLES, N., McFADDEN, E.R., WELLER, P.W., COREY, E.J. *et al.*
Science, **216**, 196 (1982)
69. GRIFFIN, M., WEISS, J., LEITCH, A.G., McFADDEN, E.R., COREY, E.J., AUSTEN, K.F. *et al. New
England Journal of Medicine*, **308**, 436 (1983)
70. AHMED, T., GREENBLATT, D.W., BIRCH, S., MARCHETTE, B. and WANNER, A. *American
Review of Respiratory Diseases*, **124**, 110 (1981)
71. PEATFIELD, A.C., PIPER, P.J. and RICHARDSON, P.S. *Journal of Physiology*, **325**, 56 (1982)
72. RICHARDSON, P.S., PEATFIELD, A.C., JACKSON, D.M. and PIPER, P.J. In *Leukotrienes and
Other Lipoxygenase Products*. Ed. P.J. Piper. p. 178. Chichester: Research Studies
Press, John Wiley and Sons (1983)
73. MAROM, Z., SHELHAMER, J.H., BACH, M.K., MORTON, D.R. and KALINER, M. *American
Review of Respiratory Diseases*, **126**, 449 (1982)
74. COLES, S.H., NEILL, K.H., REID, L.M., AUSTEN, K.F., NII, Y., COREY, E.J. *et al. Prostaglandins*, **25**, 155 (1983)
75. LEWIS, R.A., DRAZEN, J.M., COREY, E.J. and AUSTEN, K.F. In *SRS-A and Leukotrienes*. Ed.
P.J. Piper. p. 101. Chichester: Research Studies Press, John Wiley and Sons (1981)
76. PECK, M.J., PIPER, P.J. and WILLIAMS, T.J. *Prostaglandins*, **21**, 315 (1981)
77. BISGAARD, H., KRISTENSEN, J. and SONDERGAARD, J. *Prostaglandins*, **23**, 797 (1982)
78. CAMP, R.D.R., COUTTS, A.A., GREAVES, M.W., KAY, A.B. and WALPORT, M.J. *Journal of Investigative Dermatology*, **78**, 329 (1982)
79. BRAY, M.A., CUNNINGHAM, F.M., FORD-HUTCHINSON, A.W. and SMITH, M.J.H. *British Journal
of Pharmacology*, **72**, 483 (1981)
80. WEDMORE, C.V. and WILLIAMS, T.J. *Nature*, **289**, 646 (1981)
81. DAHLÉN, S.E., BJORK, J., HEDQVIST, P., ARFORS, K.E., HAMMARSTRÖM, S., LINDGREN, N.A. *et
al. Proceedings of the National Academy of Sciences of the United States of America*, **78**,
3887 (1981)
82. FORD-HUTCHINSON, A.W., BRAY, M.A., DOIG, M.V., SHIPLEY, M.E. and SMITH, M.J.H. *Nature*,
286, 264 (1980)
83. GOETZL, E.J. and PICKETT, W.C. *Journal of Immunology*, **125**, 1789 (1980)
84. SMITH, M.J.H., FORD-HUTCHINSON, A.W. and BRAY, M.A. *Journal of Pharmacy and Pharmacology*, **32**, 517 (1980)
85. BJORK, J., HEDQVIST, P. and ARFORS, K.E. *Inflammation*, **6**, 189 (1982)
86. BRAY, M.A., FORD-HUTCHINSON, A.W. and SMITH, M.J.H. *Prostaglandins*, **22**, 213 (1981)
87. BATTACHERJEE, P., HAMMOND, B., SALMON, J.A., STEPNEY, R. and EAKINS, K.E. *European
Journal of Pharmacology*, **73**, 21 (1981)

88. FEUERSTEIN, G., ZUKOWSKA-GROJEC, Z. and KOPIN, I.J. *European Journal of Pharmacology*, **76,** 107 (1981)
89. CASEY, L., CLARKE, J., FLETCHER, J. and RAMWELL, P. In *Advances in Prostaglandin, Thromboxane and Leukotriene Research, Leukotrienes and Other Lipoxygenase Products.* Eds B. Samuelsson, R. Paoletti and P.W. Ramwell. Vol. 9. p. 201. New York: Raven Press (1982)
90. LUX, W.E., FEUERSTEIN, G., SMITH, G.P. and FADEN, A.I. *Advances in Prostaglandin, Thromboxane and Leukotriene Research*, **9,** 338 (1982)
91. FENIUK, L., KENNEDY, I. and WHELAN, C.J. In *Leukotrienes and Other Lipoxygenase Products.* Ed. P.J. Piper. p. 108. Chichester: Research Studies Press, John Wiley and Sons (1983)
92. YOKOCHI, K., OLLEY, P.M., SIDERIS, E., HAMILTON, F., HUHTANEN, D. and COCEI, F. In *Advances in Prostaglandin, Thromboxane and Leukotriene Research: Leukotrienes and Other Lipoxygenase Products.* Eds B. Samuelsson, R. Paoletti and P.W. Ramwell. Vol. 9. p. 211. New York: Raven Press (1982)
93. BURKE, J.A., LEWIS, R., GUO, A.G. and COREY, E.J. *Journal of Pharmacology and Experimental Therapeutics*, **221,** 235 (1982)
94. LETTS, L.G. and PIPER, P.J. *British Journal of Pharmacology*, **76,** 169 (1982)
95. LETTS, L.G. and PIPER, P.J. In *Advances in Prostaglandin, Thromboxane and Leukotriene Research.* Eds B. Samuelsson and R. Paoletti. Vol. 11. p. 391. New York: Raven Press (1983)
96. KENNEDY, I., WHELAN, C.J. and WRIGHT, G. *British Journal of Pharmacology*, in press (1983)
97. LETTS, L.G., PIPER, P.J. and NEWMAN, D.L. In *Leukotrienes and other Lipoxygenase Products.* Ed. P. J. Piper. p. 94. Chichester: Research Studies Press, John Wiley and Sons (1983)
98. MICHELASSI, F., LANDA, L., HILL, R.P., LOWENSTEIN, E., WATKINS, W.D., PETKAU, A.J. *et al. Science,* **217,** 841 (1982)
99. KITO, G., OKUDA, H., OHKAWA, S., TERAO, S. and KIKUCHI, L. *Life Sciences*, **29,** 1325 (1981)
100. PIPER, P.J., LETTS, L.G., TIPPINS, J.R. and BARRETT, K. In *Leukotrienes and Other Lipoxygenase Products.* Ed. P.J. Piper. p. 299. Chichester: Research Studies Press, John Wiley and Sons (1983)
101. PIPER, P.J., LETTS, L.G. and GALTON, S.A. *Prostaglandins*, **25,** 591–599 (1983)
102. MONCADA, S., HERMAN, A., HIGGS, E. and VANE, J. *Thrombosis Rsearch*, **11,** 323 (1977)
103. RAE, S.A., DAVIDSON, E.M. and SMITH, M.J.H. *Lancet*, **ii,** 1122 (1982)
104. BRAIN, S.D., CAMP, R.D.R., DOWD, P.M., KOBZA-BLACK, A., WOOLLARD, P.M., MALLET, A.I. *et al.* In *Leukotrienes and Other Lipoxygenase Products.* Ed. P.J. Piper. p. 248. Chichester: Research Studies Press, John Wiley and Sons (1983)
105. FELS, A.O.S., PAWLOWSKI, N.A., CRAMER, E.B., KING, T.K.C., COHN, A.Z. and SCOTT, W.A. *Proceedings of the National Academy of Sciences of the United States of America*, **79,** 7866 (1982)
106. RANKIN, J.A., HITCHCOCK, M., MERRILL, W., BACH, M.K., BRASHLER, J.R. and ASKENASE, P.W. *Nature*, **297,** 329 (1982)
107. DOIG, M.V. and FORD-HUTCHINSON, A.W. *Prostaglandins*, **20,** 1007 (1980)
108. BACH, M.K., BRASHLER, J.R., HAMMARSTRÖM, S. and SAMUELSSON, B. *Biochemical and Biophysical Research Communications*, **93,** 1121 (1980)
109. HONGLUM, J., PAI, J., ATRACHE, V., SOK, D. and SIH, C.J. *Proceedings of the National Academy of Sciences of the United States of America*, **77,** 5688 (1980)

Chapter 4

Platelet-activating factor

J.M. Lynch, G.S. Worthen and P.M. Henson

Introduction

Platelet-activating factor (PAF) is, at present, the only member of a novel class of lipid mediators. The full extent of its action is unknown. It has been implicated as a mediator of immediate hypersensitivity, inflammation, and cardiovascular and pulmonary homeostasis and may have a number of additional specific effects.

The name 'platelet-activating factor' was given to the soluble mediator of leucocyte-dependent histamine release from rabbit platelets. Initially, it was considered to be a basophil-derived mediator of anaphylaxis in the rabbit. However, it is now known that PAF has a variety of activities which involve neither platelets nor anaphylaxis and is produced by a number of cell types other than the basophil. Therefore the term 'platelet-activating factor' is somewhat misleading and inadequate. However, there is no generally acceptable replacement at this time. Based either wholly or partially on the chemical structure of PAF, various groups have proposed alkyl-glycerol-ether-phosphorylcholine (AGEPC), alkyl-acetyl-glyceryl-phosphorylcholine (AAGPC) or PAF-acether. Since structural conformation is lacking for PAF from a number of sources, we will use the term 'Platelet Activating Factor' for preparations of biological origin and AGEPC for synthetic or semisynthetic material of defined character.

Historical overview of platelet-activating factor

In 1966, Barbaro and Zvaifler[1] demonstrated that platelets from rabbits sensitized to produce reaginic antibody released vasoactive amines when presented with the appropriate antigen. While they felt that this response was a direct effect of antigen on platelet-bound reaginic antibody, it soon became apparent that it was due to the contaminating leucocytes[2,3]. Henson[4] suggested in 1969 that the leucocyte-dependent histamine release was mediated by a soluble factor not requiring direct contact between the leucocytes and the platelets, an observation that was later confirmed[5,6]. In 1971, Siraganian and Osler[7] proposed that the basophil was the source of

73

the soluble factor. This was confirmed by Benveniste *et al.*[8] who designated
the soluble factor as 'Platelet-activating Factor' (PAF).

Direct evidence that PAF was produced *in vivo* was not obtained until
1978[9,10] due to technical difficulties in the isolation of PAF from blood.
Prior to this, evidence for *in vivo* PAF production and its actions was
gained from the study of antigen-induced anaphylaxis in rabbits immunized
to produce only IgE antibody[11,12]. In this system, sublethal doses of
intravenous antigen induced shock with physical findings of systemic
hypotension, pulmonary hypertension, decreased dynamic compliance and
increased total pulmonary resistance[13]. Intravenous antigen also induced a
hypercoagulable state[12,14], as well as neutropenia[11], thrombocytopenia[12,15]
and a rapid decrease in metachromatically stainable basophils[11,16]. The
neutropenia and thrombocytopenia were transient, returning to prechal-
lenge levels within 60 minutes. During this thrombocytopenic period,
platelet aggregates could be found lodged within the microvasculature, in
particular the microvasculature of the lung. In the rabbit the platelet is the
major source not only of 5-hydroxytryptamine but of histamine and, in the
IgE rabbit model, platelets were shown to release histamine[15] and platelet
factor[17] upon antigen challenge. Depletion of platelets by anti-platelet
antibody prior to antigen challenge abrogated lethal effects and reduced
those pathophysiological aspects of anaphylaxis in the rabbit[16] which are
platelet dependent. That the recovery of platelet counts following antigen
challenge involved those platelets which had disappeared was shown by
experiments in which ^{51}Cr-labelled platelets were not lost but returned to
the circulation[12].

It had been shown that platelets exposed *in vitro* to PAF became specifically desensitized to PAF[18] and, when platelets isolated after anaphylaxis
were tested for responsiveness to PAF, they were found to be specifically
desensitized[19]. While these data were suggestive of *in vivo* PAF activity,
the isolation of PAF from blood was not accomplished until the presence of
a factor, found in serum and plasma, which inactivated PAF was discovered. This factor was acid labile while PAF was not and, using this differential, Pinckard *et al.*[9,10] were able to isolate PAF from rabbit blood
collected into acid during anaphylaxis.

While the rabbit basophil was demonstrated to be the source of PAF in
the IgE rabbit model by Siraganian and Osler[7] and Benveniste *et al.*[8],
demonstration of PAF in other species and cell types was long fraught with
controversy. PAF could be extracted from the mixture resulting from prolonged incubation of rabbit, human and porcine leucocytes at pH 10.5[20,21].
Reports of human basophil release of PAF suffered from lack of characterization of the activity[24] or from the presence of other leucocytes in the
preparation[22,23]. More recently, Betz *et al.*[24] and Sanchez-Crespo *et al.*[25]
have reported that human basophils fail to release PAF, while Camussi *et
al.*[26] obtained positive evidence. Another cell type involved in anaphylac-
toid responses is the mast cell, and human and rabbit mast cells were
initially reported to release PAF[23]. This was subsequently refuted[27], but
now it appears that mast cells derived from mouse bone marrow do release
PAF[28].

In 1970, Henson[29] reported the enhancement of histamine release from
opsonized zymosan-stimulated rabbit platelets by neutrophils. He was

unable to demonstrate a soluble mediator for this phenomenon and the mechanism of enhancement remained unexplained until 1979[30] when the problem was re-examined. At that time, it was found that rabbit neutrophils produced PAF when activated by phagocytic stimuli. The discrepancy between these two reports was due to the failure to use albumin (which stabilizes PAF activity[8]) in the reaction buffer in the initial experiments. It is now clear that PAF can be produced by neutrophils[25,26,31], platelets[32-34], monocytes[25,26] eosinophils[35] and macrophages[27,36-40], from humans, rabbits, rats and monkeys.

Concurrent with the association of PAF release with the inflammatory response, there appeared a report which brought together two widely divergent paths of inquiry. In recent years, it has been recognized that a polar lipid produced in the renal medulla had potent anti-hypertensive activity and this anti-hypertensive lipid has been the focus of intensive study[41]. Blank et al.[42] reported the synthesis of an ether lipid which fitted the known structural limits and had the activity of the previously described anti-hypertensive polar renomedullary lipid. Their ether lipid was identical to that proposed as the structure of PAF[43,44] and it has since been shown that isolated perfused rat kidney produces PAF[45].

Yet other sources of platelet-activating factors include saliva from humans[46], isolated perfused rat lungs[47] and endothelial cells[48]. The full significance of these findings is not yet known, and it is expected that this listing is still incomplete.

Structure and metabolism of PAF

In 1975, Benveniste et al.[49] reported data which suggested that PAF was a phospholipid. They demonstrated that PAF activity was extracted with ethanol and comigrated with a phospholipid in thin-layer chromatography.

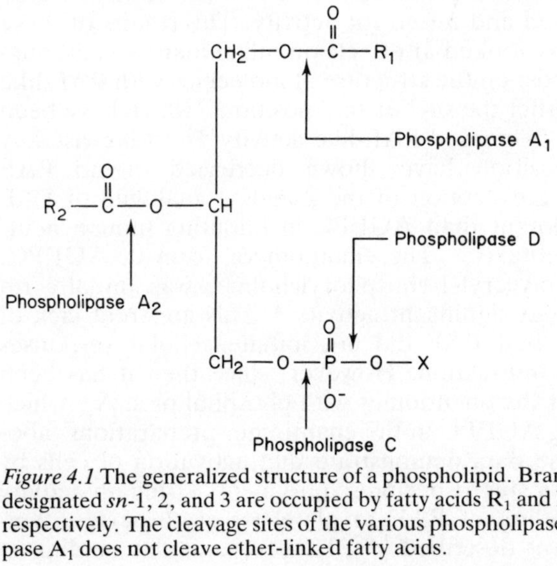

Figure 4.1 The generalized structure of a phospholipid. Branches from the glycerol backbone, designated sn-1, 2, and 3 are occupied by fatty acids R_1 and R_2 and the polar head group, respectively. The cleavage sites of the various phospholipases are noted by arrows. Phospholipase A_1 does not cleave ether-linked fatty acids.

Later, Benveniste *et al.*[21] showed that PAF activity was destroyed by incubation with phospholipases A_2, C or D, but not by phospholipase A_1 from *Rhizopus* nor by sphingomyelinase, suggesting that PAF was phospholipid in nature with a critical ester-linked moiety in the second position. The polar head group of PAF was resistant to methylation suggesting that it was a phosphatidylcholine species.

In 1979, Demopoulous *et al.*[43] and Benveniste *et al.*[44] suggested that 1-*0*-Alkyl-2-Acetyl-*sn*-Glyceryl-3-Phosphorylcholine (AGEPC), a lipid prepared semisynthetically by both groups, possessed the activity of PAF, fitted the known structural limitations and probably was PAF. The structure was identical to that proposed for the anti-hypertensive renomedullary lipid[42]. The AGEPC structure was confirmed by mass spectroscopy of highly purified PAF from rabbit basophils[50]. While the structure of PAF from other sources has not been confirmed, no differences have been demonstrated using standard chemical and physical methods[51,52].

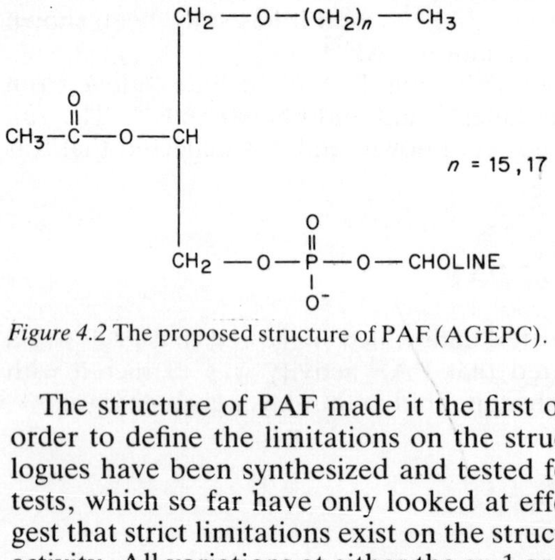

Figure 4.2 The proposed structure of PAF (AGEPC).

The structure of PAF made it the first of a novel class of mediators. In order to define the limitations on the structure of PAF, a variety of analogues have been synthesized and tested for activity. The results of these tests, which so far have only looked at effects on inflammatory cells, suggest that strict limitations exist on the structure of molecules with PAF-like activity. All variations at either the *sn*-1 or *sn*-3 positions, which have been tested at this time, display decreased PAF-like activity[53-56]. Likewise any variations at the *sn*-2 position have shown decreased or no PAF activity[43,53,54,57-59], with the exception of the 2-maleyl analogue of PAF which was slightly more potent than AGEPC in initiating human neutrophil and monocyte chemotaxis[57]. The enantiomeric form of AGEPC, 3-*O*-Hexadecyl-2-Acetyl-*sn*-Glyceryl-1-Phosphorylcholine, was initially reported to have depressed but significant activity[58]. This apparent lack of stereospecificity suggested that PAF did not initiate cellular responses through a receptor–ligand interaction. However, since then it has been shown that pretreatment of the enantiomer with phospholipase A_2, which destroys any contaminating AGEPC in the enantiomer preparations, abolishes all activity[59,60]. These data demonstrate that activation of cells by AGEPC does in fact have a stereospecific requirement. Using an activity subtraction technique, binding of PAF to platelets, erythrocytes, lymphocyes and neutrophils was described[61,62]. However, similar binding to liposomes can be shown and it therefore appears to be a physical partitioning of PAF to lipophilic sites[63]. More recently, Valone *et al.*[64] using ^{3}H-labelled PAF, have reported a saturable high-affinity binding site on human platelets, as well as an infinite capacity binding consistent with lipophilic partitioning. Ether analogues of phosphatidic acid have been synthesized which appear to have significant platelet-activiting activity but did not, on the basis of desensitization studies, appear to stimulate through the same 'receptor' as PAF[65,66]. Whether these or any analogues not yet isolated naturally will prove to mediate certain effects now ascribed to AGEPC is not known.

With the elucidation of the structure of PAF, it became feasible to look for the cellular machinery which synthesized this potent mediator. It seemed likely that PAF was released upon synthesis as it did not appear to be a constituent of human neutrophil granules[67], nor is it found in extracts of resting basophils or neutrophils[68,69]. Due to the rapid release of PAF upon stimulation, one potential pathway of synthesis was the acetylation of a lyso-alkylphosphorylcholine[70]. Analysis of the ether lipid of neutrophils and monocytes reveals that most of the alkylphosphorylcholines are potential PAF precursors[71,72]. Excess acetate, which would increase the rate of acetylation, increased the release of PAF from macrophages[73] and the presence of labelled acetate resulted in the release of labelled PAF[70], thus supporting the hypothesis. The enzyme which mediates this acetylation, an acetyltransferase, has been described for a variety of cells and tissues[74-78]. The demonstration of increased acetyltransferase activity in neutrophils and eosinophils stimulated to produce PAF also supports this hypothesis[75].

While the concentration of lyso-phospholipids in resting cells is quite low, those stimuli which induce PAF release are also know to stimulate phospholipase A_2 which would result in the production of the appropriate lyso-alkylphosphorylcholines. This suggested that the synthesis of PAF may be a two-step phenomenon[79]. Inhibition of phospholipase A_2 inhibited the release of PAF from rabbit platelets and this evidence coupled with the production of lyso-PAF by exogenous phospholipase A_2 using platelets as substrate supports that hypothesis[80].

Another potential pathway of PAF synthesis rests upon the activity of a cholinephosphotransferase which mediates the conversion of 1-alkyl-2-acetylglycerol to PAF[81]. It is not known whether the activity of this enzyme is increased upon stimulation of the cells, but production of PAF by both perfused kidney[45] and perfused lung[47] leads to the interesting possibility that this enzyme may be responsible for the base-line production of PAF by those organs.

All powerful mediators must be regulated tightly. At least one enzyme has been described which regulates PAF by enzymatically inactivating it. Pinckard *et al.*[9,10] demonstrated the presence of an acid-labile factor in rabbit serum which appeared to enzymatically inhibit PAF. Such a factor has been isolated from human serum[82] and has been shown to be an acetyl-hydrolase highly specific for the deacetylation of PAF[83]. The same or similar enzymes have been located in the cytosolic fraction from a number of tissues[84]. The product of this acetylhydrolase has been shown to be lyso-PAF which, therefore, has been proposed to be both precursor and metabolite for PAF. Increased acetylhydrolase activity has been shown in stimulated neutrophils and eosinophils in parallel to the increased activity of PAF synthetic enzymes[75]. Lyso-PAF can be further degraded to a glycerylphosphorylcholine by an alkylmono-oxygenase[85].

PAF production in inflammation

PAF release can be induced from inflammatory cells[30] and this release is synthesis dependent[67–69]. The control of PAF synthesis in the inflammatory environment is poorly understood, although this is an area of great interest. It has been shown that the synthesis of PAF was dependent on temperature, free Ca^{2+}, an energy source and phospholipase A_2 activity[18,24,80]. The release of PAF from neutrophils, monocytes and macrophages has been induced by phagocytic stimuli, immune complexes and Ca^{2+} ionophores[25,26,31]. Platelets have been stimulated to release PAF by thrombin, collagen and Ca^{2+} ionophores[32–34] and endothelial cells show enhanced release in the presence of Ca^{2+} ionophores[48].

PAF-induced platelet stimulation

PAF was named for its ability to induce rabbit platelet aggregation and the release of granule constituents, the first activity described for it[8]. Platelets can be activated by a wide variety of stimuli and, as the platelet-activating properties of PAF became better understood, Vargaftig et al.[86] proposed that only those activities which fit a specific set of criteria (copurification on thin-layer or high-performance liquid chromatography with hog leucocyte PAF, inactivation by phospholipase A_2 and the ability to stimulate platelets in the presence of indomethacin and ADP scavengers) be termed PAF. Most recently, the specificity of desensitization to PAF has been shown using analogues of AGEPC and this has been suggested as a test of identity with PAF[60]. As a result of the more specific definition of PAF, several factors termed 'platelet-activating factors' should not be confused with PAF. These include antigen-induced lung platelet activating factor[87], the antigen-induced rat platelet activating factors[88–90] and the platelet activating factor of thrombotic thrombocytopenia purpura[91].

Most of the early studies on the effects of PAF were done on rabbit platelets, because it was not until several years after the initial observations that PAF stimulation of platelets from other species was demonstrated[92]. The relative potency of PAF on platelets from different species has been shown to vary greatly, with guinea-pig platelets being the most sensitive, of those tested, to AGEPC, while rat platelets appear to be unresponsive to AGEPC in any concentration[86,93].

The difficulties in demonstrating PAF stimulation of human platelets seem to have stemmed from the relative insensitivity of human platelets to PAF, when compared to rabbit platelets, and the difficulty in retaining responsiveness through washing. Even when those problems were overcome, there appeared to be significant individual variation in the degree of human platelet response to PAF or AGEPC[31,94-97]. This variability has been overcome in part and the sensitivity to PAF increased by the synergistic effects of pretreatment of the platelets with substimulatory doses of ADP or adrenaline[33,94,98-100].

The activation of platelets *in vitro* is very rapid with the shape change being almost instantaneous, the release of 5-[^{3}H]hydroxytryptamine reaching completion in 90 seconds and aggregation reaching completion only slightly slower[18,101]. Stimulation by PAF shares the same dependencies on temperature, free Ca^{2+} and energy as such other platelet stimuli as thrombin[102].

Platelet activation by PAF *in vivo*, as demonstrated by thrombocytopenia, is also very rapid whether induced by antigen administration to allergic animals[12,15] or by intravenous infusion of PAF or AGEPC. PAF-induced thrombocytopenia is transient and does not involve platelet consumption with sequestration of the platelets occurring primarily in the lung[12,15]. The bronchoconstriction associated with anaphylaxis in the rabbit[16] or intravenous infusion of AGEPC appears to be dependent on platelets and is abrogated by prior platelet depletion.

Other inflammatory effects of PAF

While early reports of the effects of PAF on neutrophils were conflicting[66,103,104], it is now accepted that PAF or AGEPC possess neutrophil-stimulating capacity[105-110]. As opposed to the platelet, work with the PAF-mediated effects on neutrophils has been done with either well-characterized PAF or AGEPC avoiding confusion in the literature with other mediators. Human neutrophils were reported to be less sensitve to PAF than were rabbit neutrophils which was also the case with platelets.

PAF/AGEPC *in vitro* induces neutrophil shape change, aggregation, oxygen radical production, chemotaxis and degranulation[62,104-107,109-112]. AGEPC stimulates neutrophil adherence to monolayers of cultured endothelial cells[112], as well as activating lipoxygenase metabolism of arachidonic acid[113,114]. AGEPC also has been shown to induce a stimulus-specific desensitization of neutrophils, such as was seen with platelets[109,110]. In the rabbit, *in vivo*, intravenous infusions of PAF or AGEPC result in a transient neutropenia[115,116], while intradermal AGEPC induces neutrophil infiltrates[117]. However, it has not yet been established that these are direct effects. In addition to having an effect on platelets and neutrophils, AGEPC has been shown to be chemotactic for monocytes[57] and to induce wheal and flare[118], vascular leakage[119] and pain [118], when injected intradermally in man and to produce similar inflammatory effects in the rat paw[120].

PAF mediates virtually all of the *in vitro* cellular functions which are associated with inflammation. However, its relative importance in the inflammatory response is not yet known. Because PAF is quickly inactivated *in vivo*, it is likely that its role in mediating inflammation will prove to be that of an amplification mechanism or a short-term modulator of the response.

Physiology

Recent evidence suggests that PAF has potent effects on large-scale physiological events, some of which may be platelet independent. In particular, the vasoactive and bronchoconstrictive properties of PAF may be of considerable importance in a variety of disorders, including asthma. Although asthma is clinically and pathophysiologically characterized by airways obstruction, a considerable body of evidence suggests that bronchoconstriction may be a sequel of airways inflammation[122].

Thus, the ability of PAF, both to be produced by inflammatory cells and to magnify the inflammatory response, may be relevant to the pathophysiology of asthma. To date, however, PAF release has been linked tentatively only to IgE-mediated anaphylaxis in the rabbit[121].

The system that best illustrates the physiological effects of PAF remains the rabbit model of anaphylaxis of Pinckard and coworkers. In this system, within 30–60 seconds of antigen challenge, there was acute basopenia, neutropenia, and thrombocytopenia[13]. ^{51}Cr studies showed the platelets to be sequestered in the lungs. Within 60 seconds of antigen challenge, elevated levels of plasma thromboxane B_2 and platelet factor 4 were found. Release of PAF into blood was noted at 60 seconds reaching its peak at 4–5 minutes. A rapid rise (within 60 seconds) in measured pulmonary resistance and decrease in dynamic compliance suggestive of bronchoconstriction, increase in right ventricular pressure suggestive of pulmonary vasoconstriction and systemic hypotension, reinforce the similarities of this animal model to human anaphylaxis.

Infusion of AGEPC into rabbits produced remarkably similar effects[121,122]. Acute baso-, neutro-, and thrombocytopenia occurred in response to small doses of AGEPC. Bronchoconstriction, pulmonary vasoconstriction, and systemic hypotension were all similar in magnitude and timing to that seen in anaphylaxis. Despite the fact that platelet depletion abrogated bronchoconstriction after AGEPC infusion but not after antigen challenge, these data sugges that AGEPC may be an important mediator of the physiology of anaphylaxis in the rabbit. The massive release of PAF during anaphylaxis may well be restricted to the rabbit, since, as was noted previously, several investigators have failed to show release of AGEPC by human basophils, or by rat mast cells and basophils. Mouse mast cells have been recently reported to produce PAF[28]. In additon, there remain a wide variety of cells that are capable of PAF release following diverse stimuli.

Effects on smooth muscle

A variety of studies now suggest that AGEPC may affect smooth muscle. We have recently obtained results similar to those of Halonen et al.[123] utilizing direct measurements of pulmonary artery pressure in the rabbit which demonstrated marked increases in pulmonary artery pressure following AGEPC infusion[124]. We found no increase in left ventricular-end-diastolic pressure, suggesting that true pulmonary vasoconstriction had occurred. We found similar lung mechanical changes to those found by Halonen et al., suggesting bronchoconstriction and systemic hypotension with peripheral vasodilatation. Sanchez-Crespo and colleagues[125] have recently reported hypotension in rats, whose platelets are unresponsive to PAF.

A number of authors have demonstrated AGEPC-induced smooth muscle constriction *in vitro*. In the isolated perfused lung, Heffner and colleagues, utilizing rabbit lung perfused with human platelets[126], and Voelkel *et al.*, utilizing rat lung perfused cell free [127], have demonstrated pulmonary vasoconstriction in response to AGEPC. These two studies illustrate admirably the multiplicity of effects and the species specificity which may occur with AGEPC. In the rabbit study, large amounts of thromboxane B_2 (TxB_2) were released, and vasoconstriction was blocked by prostaglandin synthetase inhibitors, and was platelet dependent. In the rat study, platelets were essentially absent, prostaglandin synthetase inhibitors were without effect, and large amounts of leukotrines C_4 and D_4 were released. The use of the leukotriene synthesis blocker, diethylcarbamazine, inhibited AGEPC-induced vasoconstriction. In both studies severe lung oedema ensued, which will be discussed later.

Findlay *et al.* have demonstrated the ability of AGEPC, at fairly high concentration ($1 \times 10^{-7}M$) to cause guinea-pig ileum contraction[128]. This contraction, however, appeared independent of the release of histamine, prostaglandins, leukotrienes, or endogenous neurotransmitters. Recently, AGEPC has been shown to cause contraction of guinea-pig lung parenchyma strips[129] and suggested as constricting coronary arteries[130] and cutaneous vessels[118]. No studies have looked directly at the ability of AGEPC to constrict airways smooth muscle *in vitro*. However, the *in vivo* data which suggests bronchoconstriction, the ability of AGEPC to cause prostaglandin and leukotriene release, and the recent descriptions of the potent bronchoconstriction properties of these agents[131] make it possible that PAF may be an important mediator in the bronchoconstriction of asthma.

Peripheral vasodilation has also been observed. As noted previously, AGEPC appears to be identical to the anti-hypertensive polar renomedullary lipid[42]. In the systemic circulation, it has been shown to cause vasodilatation and decreased arterial pressure. When applied directly to the systemic microvasculature[132], it elicits vasodilator responses. Systemic vasodilator effects are not blocked by indomethacin, and vasodilatation was accompanied by TxB_2 but not 6-keto-$PGF_{1\alpha}$ release[133]. Although PAF may exert some of its actions directly, many of its effects appear to be mediated by a variety of other physiologically active compounds. A consensus of the mode of action of PAF has not yet been reached.

Effects on vascular permeability

Enhanced vascular permeability, allowing the formation of oedema, and the penetration of normally excluded substances, is an important component of inflammatory states, including those in the airways. To date there are no data on the ability of AGEPC to increase airways permeability. However, there is now information suggesting that AGEPC can increase permeability in a number of vascular beds. It is important to realize that

AGEPC, because of its multiplicity of effects, might increase vascular permeability directly or by causing the influx of inflammatory cells which may themselves alter vascular permeability.

Pinckard and coworkers[118] demonstrated a pronounced wheal and flare response in humans following cutaneous injection of as little as 0.1 pmol of AGEPC, which was estimated to be between 100 and 1000 times more active than histamine on a molar basis. Studies with H_1 blockers were equivocal in humans. Studies in guinea-pigs and rabbits, however, demonstrated that H_1 blockade had no effect on AGEPC-induced oedema in skin. The time course of oedema appears to *precede* that of neutrophil influx, suggesting that it may be a 'direct' effect (which does not imply that there may not be intervening compounds). Sanchez-Crespo and coworkers[125] have shown a marked fall in blood volume in the rat (where platelets are probably not involved) following AGEPC infusion, and accumulation of ^{125}I-labelled albumin in peritoneal fluid. Although the other site(s) of protein penetration are unclear, this suggests an increase in vascular permeability. A number of recent reports implicate AGEPC in lung oedema. It is important to recognize, however, that lung oedema may be due either to increased vascular permeability or to increased vascular hydrostatic pressure (or both). Particularly in the case of the lung, it is difficult to exclude hydrostatic oedema as a contributing cause. The isolated perfused lung has been used to elucidate mechanisms of action of AGEPC. Heffner and coworkers[126], as mentioned above, have demonstrated platelet-dependent vasoconstriction and marked lung oedema following AGEPC infusion in isolated rabbit lung perfused with human platelets. The oedema in this case was blocked by inhibitors of smooth muscle contraction (nitroglycerin) as well as cyclo-oxygenase inhibitors. It is unlikely that the oedema in this case represents pressure-trauma to the lung vasculature. Voelkel and coworkers[127], by contrast, showed platelet-independent lung oedema and vasoconstriction following AGEPC infusion in rat lung perfused cell free. The oedema and vasoconstriction in this case was not blocked by cyclo-oxygenase inhibitors, and was associated with production of leukotrienes C_4 and D4. These latter compounds have been shown recently to produce oedema themselves[134]. We have shown a modest increase in rabbit lung albumin penetration *in vivo* occurring at a time when vascular pressures had normalized, suggesting a real increase in vascular permeability occurring as early as 1 hour after infusion[124]. Mojorad and Said[135] have reported marked increases in lung water 4 hours following AGEPC infusion into dogs.

PAF is thus capable of causing bronchoconstriction, pulmonary vasoconstriction, and increased vascular permeability in a variety of systems. Because of these abilities, it is a reasonable candidate as an important mediator of asthma.

Pharmacological modulation of PAF

Inhibition of the production of PAF has not yet been achieved by specific inhibitors. Non-specific inhibitors of cellular activation will block the release of PAF from basophils, neutrophils, monocytes, macrophages and platelets but control of the release of PAF from kidney and lung has not yet been studied. Inhibition of release from inflammatory cells has been accomplished by metabolic inhibitors such as 2-deoxyglucose[8,67], drugs which increase intracellular cyclic AMP levels such as theophylline and PGI_2[136-138], Ca^{2+} blockers and chelators[8,67] and inhibitors of phospholipase A_2.

Attempts to specifically inhibit PAF-induced activity have generally been unsuccessful. Analogues of AGEPC that have been tested do not antagonize AGEPC or PAF activity[69]. Desensitization of platelets by analogues of AGEPC has been reported to be proportional to their agonistic properties[58,59]. The specific inhibition of PAF or AGEPC stimulation of rabbit platelets by Fab fragments of a monoclonal antibody to rabbit platelets has been reported, but the mechanism of this inhibition is unknown[139]. The antibody appears to recognize only the rabbit platelet, thus limiting its application to the investigation of the mechanism of platelet stimulation by PAF.

Non-specific inhibition of PAF-induced activation of platelets and neutrophils has been achieved by such non-specific blockers of cell function as membrane active drugs, serine protease inhibitors, metabolic inhibitors and colchicine[140-143]. Prevention of Ca^{2+} fluxes either by chelating external Ca^{2+} or blocking intracellular transport has been shown to inhibit PAF-induced activation[18,140,143]. Human platelet stimulation by AGEPC appeared to be partially dependent on thromboxane production[94,95,143], but the effect of inhibition of the cyclo-oxygenase pathway could be overcome by pretreatment of the platelets with substimulatory doses of adrenaline[99]. In the neutrophil, prevention of AGEPC-induced activation has been achieved by inhibitors of the lipoxygenase pathway of arachidonic acid metabolism, but not the cyclo-oxygenase pathway[105,111,113].

Increasing the intracellular level of cyclic AMP has proven to be effective in inhibiting PAF or AGEPC-induced activation of platelets and neutrophils. These increases in cyclic AMP (cAMP) having been achieved by treatment with theophylline, dibutyryl-cAMP and the prostanoids, PGI_2 and PGE_1[98,100,140,144,145]. It has also been reported that AGEPC has regulatory activity in respect to preventing rises in cyclic AMP levels in platelets[146,147].

The lack of a PAF antagonist or a specific inhibitor of the acetyltransferase enzyme allows only non-specific pharmacological modulation of PAF effects or synthesis. The non-specific modulation of PAF effects in immediate hypersenstivity and inflammatory responses has not been studied in depth and almost nothing is known about modulation of pulmonary hypertension, smooth muscle contraction and the other effects of PAF. At the same time the inter-relationships between PAF, other mediators of these phenomena and the cells involved are also poorly understood. Parallel advances in both areas must take place before clinical pathologies can be determined to contain a PAF-mediated component or an intelligent treatment can be designed.

Conclusion

PAF has been shown to be involved in immediate hypersensitivity responses, to induce vascular responses, particularly in the lung, and to modulate cardiac function. It has potent effects as a mediator of inflammation being both produced by and activating inflammatory cells, and indirectly to induce bronchospasms. Thus a large body of data exists which may implicate PAF as a mediator of asthma. Quite recently Grandel and coworkers[148] have found increased levels of PAF in the blood of adolescent asthmatics undergoing exercise-induced bronchospasm. The preliminary data are the most direct association between PAF and asthma to date. The relative importance of PAF as a mediator of asthma remains to be determined.

References

1. BARBARO, J.F. and ZVAIFLER, N.J. *Proceedings of the Society for Experimental Biology and Medicine*, **122**, 1245 (1966)
2. SCHOENBECHLER, M.J. and SADUN, E.H. *Proceedings of the Society for Experimental Biology and Medicine*, **127**, 601 (1968)
3. SIRAGANIAN, R.P. and OLIVEIRA, B. *Federation Proceedings*, **27**, 315 (1968)
4. HENSON, P.M. *Federation Proceedings*, **28**, 1721 (1969)
5. HENSON, P.M. *Journal of Experimental Medicine*, **131**, 287 (1970)
6. SIRAGANIAN, R.P. and OSLER, A.G. *Journal of Immunology*, **106**, 1244 (1971)
7. SIRAGANIAN, R.P. and OSLER, A.G. *Journal of Immunology*, **106**, 1251 (1971)
8. BENVENISTE, J., HENSON, P.M. and COCHRANE, C.G. *Journal of Experimental Medicine*, **136**, 1356 (1972)
9. PINCKARD, R.N., FARR, R.S. and HANAHAN, D.J. *Federation Proceedings*, **37**, 1667 (1978)
10. PINCKARD, R.N., FARR, R.S. and HANAHAN, D.J.*Journal of Immunology*, **123**, 1847 (1979)
11. PINCKARD, R.N., HALONEN, M. and MENG, A.L. *Journal of Allergy and Clinical Immunology*, **49**, 301 (1972)
12. HALONEN, M. and PINCKARD, R.N. *Journal of Immunology*, **115**, 519 (1975)
13. HALONEN, M., FISHER, H.K., BLAIR, C., BUTLER, C. II and PINCKARD, R.N. *American Review of Respiratory Disease*, **114**, 961 (1976)
14. PINCKARD, R.N., TANIGAWA, C. and HALONEN, M. *Journal of Immunolgoy*, **115**, 525 (1975)
15. HALONEN, M., PINCKARD R.N. and MENG, A.L. *Journal of Immunology*, **111**, 331 (1973)
16. PINCKARD, R.N., HALONEN, M., PALMER, J.D., BUTLER, C., SHAW, J.O., and HENSON, P.M. *Journal of Immunology*, **119**, 2185 (1977)
17. McMANUS, L.M., MORLEY, C.A., LEVINE, S.P. and PINCKARD, R.N. *Journal of Immunology*, **123**, 2835 (1979)
18. HENSON, P.M. *Journal of Experimental Medicine*, **143**, 937 (1976)
19. HENSON, P.M. and PINCKARD, R.N. *Journal of Immunology*, **119**, 2179 (1977)
20. BENVENISTE, J. *Nature*, **249**, 581 (1974)
21. BENVENISTE, J., LECOUEDIC, J.P., POLONSKY, J. and TENCE, M. *Nature*, **269**, 170 (1977)
22. LEWIS, R.A., GOETZL, E.J., WASSERMAN, S., VALONE, F.H., RUBIN, R.H. and AUSTEN, K.F. *Journal of Immunology*, **114**, 87 (1975)
23. CAMUSSI, G., MENCIA-HUERTA, J.M. and BENVENISTE, J. *Immunology*, **33**, 523 (1977)
24. BETZ, S.J., LOTNER, G.Z. and HENSON, P.M. *Journal of Immunology*, **125**, 2749 (1980)
25. SANCHEZ-CRESPO, M., ALONSO, F. and EGIDO, J. *Immunology*, **40**, 645 (1980)
26. CAMUSSI, G., AGLIETTA, M., CODA, R., BUSSOLINO, F., PIACIBELLO, N. and TETTA, C. *Immunology*, **42**, 191 (1981)
27. MENCIA-HUERTA, J.M. and BENVENISTE, J. *European Journal of Immunology*, **9**, 409 (1979)
28. MENCIA-HUERTA, J.M., RAZIN, F., LEWIS, R.A., COREY, C.J. and AUSTEN, K.F. *Federation Proceedings*, **42**, 1380 (1983)
29. HENSON, P.M. *Journal of Immunology*, **105**, 490 (1970)
30. LYNCH, J.M., LOTNER, G.Z., BETZ, S.J. and HENSON, P.M. *Journal of Immunology*, **123**, 1219 (1979)
31. LOTNER, G.Z., LYNCH, J.M., BETZ, S.J. and HENSON, P.M. *Journal of Immunology*, **124**, 676 (1980)
32. CHIGNARD, M., LECOUEDIC, J.P., TENCE, M., VARGAFTIG, B.B. and BENVENISTE, J. *Nature*, **279**, 799 (1979)
33. CHIGNARD, M., LECOUEDIC, J.P., VARGAFTIG, B.B. and BENVENISTE, J. *British Journal of Haematology*, **46**, 455 (1980)

34. NAMM, D.H. and HIGH, J.A. *Thrombosis Research*, **20**, 285 (1980)
35. LYNCH, J.M., DAVIES, J. and HENSON, P.M. Unpublished data
36. ARNOUX, B., DUVAL, D. and BENVENISTE, J. *European Journal of Clinical Investigation*, **10**, 437 (1980)
37. MENCIA-HUERTA, J.M. and BENVENISTE, J. *Cellular Immunology*, **57**, 281 (1981)
38. ARNOUX, B., DURAND, J., RIGAUD, M., VARGAFTIG, B.B. and BENVENISTE, J. *Agents and Actions*, **11**, 555 (1981)
39. CAMUSSI, G., BUSSOLINO, F., GHEZZO, F. and PEGORARO, L. *Blood*, **59**, 16 (1982)
40. ROUBIN, R., MENCIA-HUERTA, J.M. and BENVENISTE, J. *European Journal of Immunology*, **12**, 141 (1982)
41. MUIRHEAD, E.E., RIGHTSEL, W.A., LEACH, B.E., BYERS, L.W., PITCOOK, J.A. and BROOKS, B.B. *Annals of the Academy of Medicine (Singapore)*, **5**, 365 (1976)
42. BLANK, M.L., SYNDER, F., BYERS, L.W., BROOKS, B. and MUIRHEAD, E.E. *Biochemical and Biophysical Research Communications*, **90**, 1194 (1979)
43. DEMOPOULOS, C.A., PINCKARD, R.N. and HANAHAN, D.J. *Journal of Biological Chemistry*, **254**, 9355 (1979)
44. BENVENISTE, J., TENCE, M., VARENNE, P., BIDAULT, J., BOULLET, C. and POLONSKY, J. *Comptes Rendus de l'Academie des Sciences Naturelles Serie D (Paris)*, **289**, 1037 (1979)
45. PIROTSKY, E. and BENVENISTE, J. *International Archives of Allergy and Applied Immunology*, **66**, (Supplement 1), 176 (1981)
46. COX, C.P., WARDLOW, M.L., JORGENSON, R. and FARR, R.S. *Journal of Immunology*, **127**, 46 (1981)
47. WORTHEN, G.S., VOELKEL, N., LYNCH, J.M. and HENSON, P.M. Unpublished data
48. LYNCH, J.M., WORTHEN, G.S. and HENSON P.M. Unpublished data
49. BENVENISTE, J., KAMOUN, P. and POLONSKY, J. *Federation Proceedings*, **34**, 985 (1975)
50. HANAHAN, D.J., DEMOPOULOS, C.A., LIEHR, J. and PINCKARD, R.N. *Journal of Biological Chemistry*, **255**, 5514 (1980)
51. CLARK, P.O., HANAHAN D.J. and PINCKARD, R.N. *Biochemica et Biophysica Acta*, **628**, 69 (1980)
52. PINCKARD, R.N., McMANUS, L.M., DEMOPOULOS, C.A., HALONEN, M., CLARK, P.O., SHAW, J.O. et al. *Journal of the Reticuloendothelial Society*, **28**, 95s (1980)
53. TENCE, M., MICHEL, E., COFFIER, F., POLONSKY, J., GODFROID, J.J. and BENVENISTE, J. *Agents and Actions*, 11, **558**, (1980)
54. TENCE, M., COFFIER, F., HEYMANS, F., POLONSKY, J., GODFROID, J.J. and BENVENISTE, J. *Biochimie (Paris)*, **63**, 723 (1981)
55. SATOUCHI, K., PINCKARD, R.N., McMANUS, L.M. and HANAHAN, D.J. *Journal of Biological Chemistry*, **256**, 4425 (1981)
56. SATOUCHI, K., PINCKARD, R.N. and HANAHAN, D.J. *Archives of Biochemistry and Biophysics*, **211**, 683 (1981)
57. GOETZEL, E.J., DERIAN, C.K., TAUBER, A.I. and VALONE, F.H. *Biochemical and Biophysical Research Communications*, **94**, 881 (1980)
58. HANAHAN, D.J., MUNDER, P.G., SATOUCHI, K., McMANUS, L.M. and PINCKARD, R.N. *Biochemical and Biophysical Research Communications*, **99**, 183, (1981)
59. WYKLE, R.L., MILLER, C.H., LEWIS, J.C., SHMITT, J.D., SMITH, J.A. SURLES, J.R. et al. *Biochemical and Biophysical Research Communications*, **100**, 1651 (1981)
60. KERALY, C.L. and BENVENISTE, J. *British Journal of Haematology*, **51**, 313 (1982)
61. SHAW, J.O. and HENSON, P.M. *American Journal of Pathology*, **98**, 791 (1980)
62. CAMMUSSI, G., BUSSOLINO, F., TETTA, C., BRUSCA, R. and RAGNI, R. *Panminerva Medica-Europa Medica*, **22**, 1 (1980)
63. MARGOLIS, H., KRAMP, W., LUNCH J.M. and HENSON P.M. Unpublished data
64. VALONE, F.H., COLES, E., REINHOLD, U.R. and GOETZL, E.J. *Journal of Immunology*, **129**, 1637 (1982)
65. SIMON, M.F., CHAP, H. and DOUSTE-BLAZY, L. *Biochemical and Biophysical Research Communications*, **108**, 1743 (1982)
66. HUMPHREY, D.M., McMANUS, L.M., SATOUCHI, K., HANAHAN, D.J. and PINCKARD, R.N. *Laboratory Investigation*, **46**, 422 (1980)
67. BETZ, S.J. and HENSON, P.M. *Journal of Immunology*, **125**, 2756 (1980)
68. TENCE, M., POLONSKY, J., LECOUEDIC, J.P. and BENVENISTE, J. *Biochimie*, **62**, 251 (1980)
69. PINCKARD, R.N., McMANUS, L.M. and HANAHAN, D.J. *Advances in Inflammation Research*. Vol.4. New York: Raven Press, (1982)

70. CHAP, H., MAUCO, G., SIMON, M.F., BENVENISTE, J. and DOUSTE-BLAZY, L. *Nature*, **289**, 312 (1981)
71. MUELLER, H.W., O'FLAHERTY, J.T. and WYKLE, R.L. *Lipids*, **17**, 72 (1982)
72. SUGIURA, T., ONUMA, Y., SEKIGUCHI, N. and WAKU, K. *Biochimica et Biophysica Acta*, **712**, 515 (1982)
73. MENCIA-HUERTA, J.M., ROUBIN, R. and BENVENISTE, J. *International Archives of Allergy and Applied Immunology*, **66**, (Supplement 1), 178 (1981)
74. WYKLE, R.L., MALONE, B. and SNYDER, F. *Journal of Biological Chemistry*, **255**, 10256 (1980)
75. LEE, T.C., MALONE, B., WASSERMAN, S.I., FITZGERALD, V. and SNYDER, F. *Biochemical and Biophysical Research Communications*, **105**, 1303 (1982)
76. NINIO, E., MENCIA-HUERTA, J.M., HEYMANS, F. and BENVENISTE, J. *Biochimica et Biophysica Acta*, **710**, 23 (1982)
77. MENCIA-HUERTA, J.M., ROUBIN, R., MORGAT, J.L. and BENVENISTE, J. *Journal of Immunology*, **129**, 804 (1982)
78. ROUBIN, R., MENCIA-HUERTA, J.M., LANDES, A. and BENVENISTE, J. *Journal of Immunology*, **129**, 809 (1982)
79. MENCIA-HUERTA, J.M., NINIO, E., ROUBIN, R. and BENVENISTE, J. *Agents and Actions*, **11**, 556 (1981)
80. BENVENISTE, J., CHIGNARD M., LECOUEDIC, J.P. and VARGAFTIG, B.B. *Thrombosis Research*, **25**, 375 (1982)
81. RENOOIJ, W. and SNYDER, F. *Biochimica et Biophysica Acta*, **663**, 545 (1981)
82. FARR, R.S., COX, C.P., WARDLOW, M.L. and JORGENSEN, R. *Clinical Immunology and Immunopathology*, **15**, 318 (1980)
83. FARR, R.S. Personal Communication
84. BLANK, M.L., LEE, T.C., FITZGERALD, V. and SNYDER, F. *Journal of Biological Chemistry*, **256**, 179 (1981)
85. LEE, T.C., BLANK, M.L., FITZGERALD, V. and SNYDER, F. *Archives of Biochemistry and Biophysics*, **208**, 353 (1981)
86. VARGAFTIG, B.B., CHIGNARD, M., BENVENISTE, J., LEFORT, J. and WAL, F. *Annals of the New York Academy of Sciences*, **370**, 119 (1981)
87. KRAVIS, T.C. and HENSON, P.M. *Journal of Immunology*, **115**, 1677 (1975)
88. KATER, L.A., GOETZL, E.J. and AUSTEN, K.F. *Journal of Clinical Investigation*, **57**, 1173 (1976)
89. FESUS, L., CSABA, B. and MUSZBEK, L. *Clinical and Experimental Immunology*, **27**, 512 (1977)
90. VALONE, F.H., WHITMER, D.I., PICKETT, W.O., AUSTEN, K.F. and GOETZL, E.J. *Immunology*, **37**, 841 (1979)
91. LIAN, E., HARKNESS, D.R., BYRNES, J.J., WALLACH, H. and NUNEZ, R. *Blood*, **53**, 333 (1979)
92. BENVENISTE, J., LECOUEDIC, J.P. and KAMOUN, P. *Lancet*, **i**, 344 (1975)
93. NAMM, D.H., TADEPALLI, A.S. and HIGH, J.A. *Thrombosis Research*, **25**, 341 (1982)
94. O'DONNELL, M.C., HENSONS, P.M. and FIEDEL, B.A. *Immunology*, **35**, 953 (1979)
95. McMANUS, L.M., HANAHAN, D.J. and PINCKARD, R.N. *Journal of Clinical Investigation*, **67**, 903 (1981)
96. MARCUS, A.J., SAFIER, C.B., ULLMAN, H.L., WONG, K.T.H., BROEKMAN, M.J., WEKSLER, B.B. *et al. Blood*, **58**, 1027 (1981)
97. TSIEN, W.H., ASHLEY, C.J. and SHEPPARD, H. *Thrombosis Research*, **28**, 587 (1982)
98. RAO, G.H.R., SCHMID, H.H.O., REDDY, K.R. and WHITE, J.G. *Biochemica et Biophysica Acta*, **715**, 205 (1982)
99. VARGAFTIG, B.B., FOUQUE, F., BENVENISTE, J. and ODIOT, J. *Thrombosis Research*, **28**, 557 (1982)
100. RAO, G.H.R. and WHITE, J.G. *Prostaglandins, Leukotrienes and Medicine*, **9**, 459 (1982)
101. HENSON, P.M. *Journal of Clinical Investigation*, **60**, 481, (1977)
102. BECKER, E.L. and HENSON, P.M. *Advances in Immunology*, **17**, 93 (1973)
103. O'DONNELL, M.C., SIEGEL, J.N. and FIEDEL, B.A. *Clinical and Experimental Immunology*, **43**, 135 (1981)
104. CZARNETZKI, B.M. and BENVENISTE, J. *Agents and Actions*, **11**, 549 (1981)
105. CAMUSSI, G., TETTA, C., BUSSOLINO, F., CALIGARIS CAPPIO, F., CODA, R., MASERA, C. *et al. International Archives of Allergy and Applied Immunology*, **64**, 25 (1981)
106. O'FLAHERTY, J.T., MILLER, C.H., LEWIS, J.C., WYKLE, R.L., BASS, D.A., McCALL, C.E. *et al. Inflammation*, **5**, 193 (1981)

107. O'FLAHERTY, J.T., WYKLE, R.L., MILLER, C.H., LEWIS, J.C., WAITE, M., BASS, D.A. *et al.*
American Journal of Pathology, **103,** 70 (1981)
108. O'FLAHERTY, J.T., WYKLE, R.L., LEES, C.J., SHAEWMAKE, T., McCALL, C.E. and THOMAS, M.J.
American Journal of Pathology, **105,** 164 (1981)
109. O'FLAHERTY, J.T., LEES, C.J., MILLER, C.H., McCALL, C.E., LEWIS, J.C., LOVE, S.H. *et al. Journal of Immunology*, **127,** 731 (1981)
110. SHAW, J.O., PINCKARD, R.N., FERRIGNI, K.S., McMANUS, L.M. and HANAHAN, D.J. *Journal of Immunology*, **127,** 1250 (1981)
111. SMITH, R.J. and BOWMAN, B.J. *Biochemical and Biophysical Research Communications*, **104,** 1495 (1982)
112. INGRAHAM, L.M., COATES, T.D., ALLEN, J.M., HIGGINS, C.P., BAEHNER, R.L. and BOXER, L.A.
Blood, **59,** 1259 (1982)
113. CHILTON, F.H., O'FLAHERTY, J.T., WALSH, C.E., THOMAS, M.J., WYKLE, R.L., DECHATELET, L.R. *et al. Journal of Biological Chemistry*, **257,** 5402 (1982)
114. LIN, A.H., MORTON, D.R. and GORMAN, R.R. *Journal of Clinical Investigation*, **70,** 1058 (1982)
115. McMANUS, L.M., HANAHAN, D.J., DEMOPOULOS, C.A. and PINCKARD, R.N. *Journal of Immunology*, **124,** 2919 (1980)
116. McMANUS, L.M., PINCKARD, R.N., FITZPATRICK, F.A., O'ROURKE, R.A., CRAWFORD, M.H. and HANAHAN, D.J. *Laboratory Investigation*, **45,** 303 (1981)
117. HUMPHREY, D.M., PINCKARD, R.N., McMANUS, L.M. and HANAHAN, D.J. *Federation Proceedings*, **40,** 1003 (1981)
118. PINCKARD, R.N., KNIKER, W.T., LEE, L., HANAHAN, D.J. and McMANUS, L.M. *Journal of Allergy and Clinical Immunology*, **65,** 196 (1980)
119. STIMLER, N.P., BLOOR, C.M., HUGLI, T.E., WYKLE, R.L., McCALL, C.E. and O'FLAHERTY, J.T.
American Journal of Pathology, **105,** 64 (1981)
120. BONNET, J., LOISEAU, A.M., ORVOEN, M. and BESSIN, P. *Agents and Actions*, **11,** 559 (1981)
121. DUNNILL, M.S. *Journal of Clinical Pathology*, **13,** 27 (1960)
122. HALONEN, M., PALMER, J.D., LOHMAN, I.C., McMANUS, L.M. and PINCKARD, R.N. *American Review of Respiratory Disease*, **122,** 915 (1980)
123. HALONEN, M., PALMER, J.D., LOHMAN, I.C., McMANUS, L.M. and PINCKARD, R.N. *American Review of Respiratory Disease*, **124,** 416 (1981)
124. WORTHEN, G.S., GOINS, A.I., MITCHELL, B.C., LARSEN, G.L., REEVES, J.T. and HENSON, P.M.
Chest, in press, 1983.
125. SANCHEZ-CRESPO, M., ALONSO, F., INARRA, P., ALVAREZ, V. and EGIDO, J. *Immunopharmacology*, **4,** 173 (1982)
126. HEFFNER, J.E., SHOEMAKER, S.A., CANHAM, E.M., PATEL, M., McMURTRY, I.F., MORRIS, H.G. *et al. Journal of Clinical Investigation*, **71,** 351 (1983)
127. VOELKEL, N.F., WORTHEN, G.S., REEVES, J.T., HENSON, P.M. and MURPHY, R.C. *Science*, **218,** 286 (1982)
128. FINDLAY, S.R., LICHTENSTEIN, L.M., HANAHAN, D.J. and PINCKARD, R.N. *American Journal of Physiology*, **241,** C130 (1981)
129. O'FLAHERTY, J.T., LEES, C.J. and STIMLER, N.P. *Federation Proceedings*, **40,** 1015 (1981)
130. BURKE, J.A., LEVI, R., HANAHAN, D.J. and PINCKARD, R.N. *Federation Proceedings*, **41,** 823 (1982)
131. WEISS, J.W., DRAZEN, J.M., COLES, N., McFADDEN, E.R., WELLER, P.F., COROY, E.J. *et al. Science*, **216,** 196 (1982)
132. SMITH, K.A., PREWITT, R.L., BYERS, L.W. and MUIRHEAD, E.E. *Hypertension*, **3,** 460 (1981)
133. FEUERSTEIN, G., ZUKOWSKA GROJEC, Z., KRAUSZ, M.M., BLANK, M.L., SNYDER, F. and KOPN, I.J. *Clinical and Experimental Hypertension*, **4,** 1335 (1982)
134. DAHLEN, S.E., BJORK, J., HEDQUIST, P., ARFORS, K.E., HAMMARSTRÖM, S., LINDGREN, J.A. *et al. Proceedings of the National Academy of Sciences of the United States of America*, **78,** 3887 (1981)
135. MOJORAD, M. and SAID, S.I. *American Review of Respiratory Disease* (Supplement), **125,** 278 (1982)
136. BUSSOLINO, F. and BENVENISTE, J. *Immunology*, **40,** 367 (1980)
137. CAMUSSI, G., TETTA, C., SEGOLONI, G., DEREGIBUS, M.C. and BUSSOLINO, F. *Agents and Actions*, **11,** 550 (1981)
138. ALONSO, F., SANCHEZ-CRESPO, M. and MATO, J.M. *Immunology*, **49,** 493 (1982)
139. LYNCH, J.M., SPEARS, P. and HENSON, P.M. *Federation Proceedings*, **41,** 528 (1982)
140. HENSON, P.M. and OADES, Z.G. *Journal of Experimental Medicine*, **143,** 953 (1976)

141. SHAW, J., PRINTZ, M., HIRABAYASHI, K. and HENSON, P.M. *Journal of Immunology*, **121**, 1939 (1978)
142. CAZENAVE, J.P., BENVENISTE, J. and MUSTARD, J.F. *Laboratory Investigation*, **41**, 275 (1979)
143. CHESNEY, C.M., PIFER, D.D., BYERS, L.W. and MUIRHEAD, E.E. *Blood*, **59**, 582 (1982)
144. BUSSOLINO, F. and CAMUSSI, G. *Prostaglandins*, **20**, 781 (1980)
145. IEYASU, H., TAKAI, Y., KAIBUCHI, K., SAWAMURA, M. and NISHIZUKA, Y. *Biochemical and Biophysical Research Communications*, **108**, 1701 (1982)
146. MILLER, O.V., AYER, D.E. and GORMAN, R.R. *Biochimica et Biophysica Acta*, **711**, 445 (1982)
147. HASLAM, R.J. and VANDERWEL, M. *Journal of Biological Chemistry*, **257**, 6879 (1982)
148. GRANDEL, K.E., SCHWARTZ, E., GREENE, D., WARLOW, M.L., PINCKARD, R.N. and FARR, R.S. *Federation Proceedings*, **42**, 1026 (1983)

Chapter 5

Eosinophils and neutrophils

A.B. Kay

Introduction

Asthma covers a broad clinical spectrum, ranging from mild readily reversible bronchospasm to severe chronic intractable obstruction to airflow. The mechanisms which lead to airways narrowing in bronchial asthma are complex. There seems little doubt that in some instances mast-cell-derived agents which constrict bronchial smooth muscle play a direct role in the narrowing of the airways. However, the infiltration of inflammatory cells which follows mast cell activation might have more relevance to the underlying pathology. In this chapter, the role of eosinophils and neutrophils in pathogenesis will be considered in terms of (*a*) the mast-cell-derived chemical mediators which activate these granulocytes, and (*b*) the relationship between the 'allergic' and inflammatory aspects of asthma. First, some general biological properties of eosinophils and neutrophils are compared and contrasted.

General properties of eosinophils and neutrophils

In many respects, eosinophils and neutrophils are similar in that they are non-dividing granule-containing cells which arise in the bone marrow and have a limited lifespan in the circulation. Both cell types have secretory, as well as phagocytic, properties and possess similar membrane markers for immunoglobulin and complement.

It is generally believed that eosinophils have a specialized role in host defence against invading parasites, in much the same way that neutrophils destroy certain bacteria. However, in some diseases, of which bronchial asthma is an example, eosinophils seem to be inappropriately recruited and there is often considerable tissue damage which might result, at least in part, from eosinophil-derived products. Similarly, the secretory properties of neutrophils are likely to contribute to the events associated with narrowing of the airways.

89

Formation and fate

EOSINOPHILS

There is comparatively little information on eosinophil turnover in man. Most studies have been performed in the rat in which it has been shown that, before birth, eosinophil production occurs in the thymus and lymph nodes[1]. In adult animals, the majority of eosinophils are produced in the bone marrow[2], possibly under the influence of a T-lymphocyte-dependent low-molecular-weight (<1500) eosinophilopoietin[3]. It is unlikely that all cells of the granulocyte series originate from the same pluripotent stem cell, but rather that eosinophils and neutrophils (and possibly basophils) develop under separate genetic control from an, as yet, unidentified precursor cell which may, or may not, have a common cell of origin[4]. Nevertheless, eosinophil bone marrow precursors, such as metamyelocytes and band forms, are easily recognized and these, like other granulocyte precursors, proceed through several divisions before maturing and entering the bloodstream[5]. Protein synthesis is apparently very active in the eosinophil metamyelocyte, as shown by a highly developed endoplasmic reticulum and the presence of up to four nucleoli. With maturation and the appearance of granules, morphological signs of protein synthesis disappear[6]. Eosinophils are usually considered as 'end-stage' cells, although mitotic division is occasionally observed within tissues. The cells can remain viable for several days *in vitro*.

For every circulating eosinophil, there are approximately 200 mature cells in the bone marrow reserve and 500 in loose submucosal connective tissue. Therefore, there is a dynamic turnover of eosinophils, with production and maintenance of a reserve pool in the marrow, and transport via the blood to certain tissue sites. The eventual fate of the cell is not fully understood, although intact or ruptured eosinophils may be engulfed by macrophages or may pass through the intestinal and respiratory mucosae and be excreted. This is thought to be similar to the elimination of neutrophils where the bulk of cells are probably excreted intact or degraded in faeces and respiratory tract secretions, the remainder being removed by tissue macrophages.

NEUTROPHILS

Neutrophils also develop from undifferentiated stem cells in the bone marrow. Granule development is apparent at the promyelocyte stage, at which time primary (or azurophil) peroxidase-positive granules are recognizable. At the myelocyte stage the specific (or secondary) granules develop. Myelocyte formation, the mitotic phase, takes about 7.5 days, and the development of mature neutrophils, the postmitotic phase, is also approximately 7.5 days. The blood transit time (half-life) is 6 hours and the cell has up to 48 hours to perform its tissue function.

Morphology

EOSINOPHILS

In all species the eosinophil is characterized by the presence of large intracytoplasmic granules (*Figure 5.1*). Human eosinophils contain about

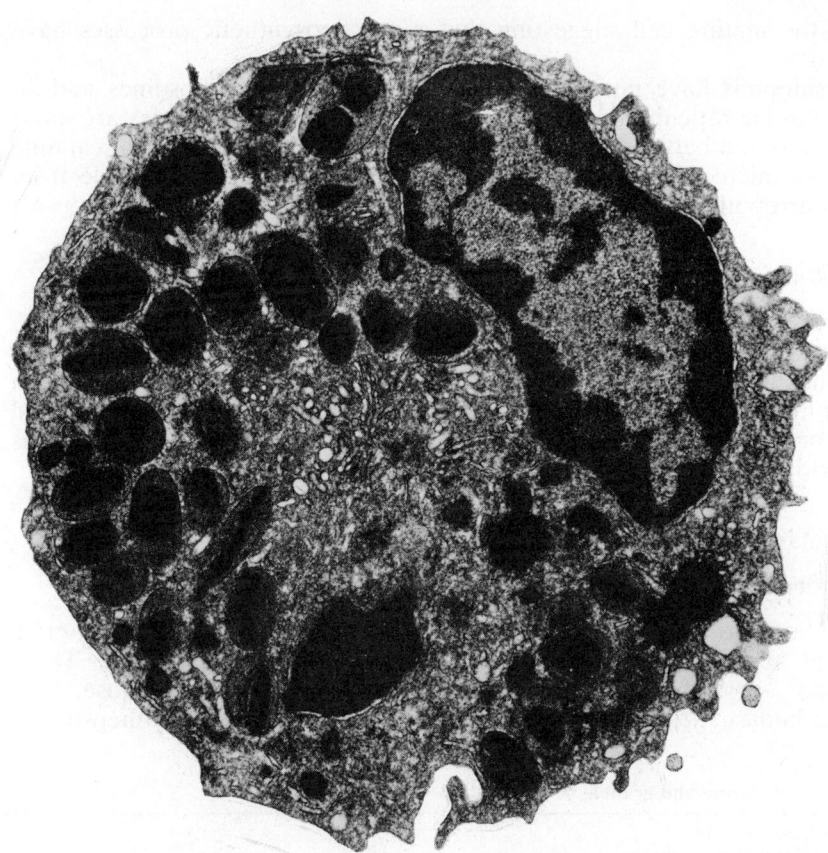

Figure 5.1 An electron micrograph of a human blood eosinophil. Magnification × 10 700. (Prepared by Miss Anne Dewar, Cardiothoracic Institute, London.)

20 refractile granules[7] which stain a yellow-pink colour with acid aniline dyes such as eosin or chromotrope 2R. The granules are often spherical or ovoid and about 0.5–1.0 μm in diameter. Ultrastructural studies indicate that the granules are bounded by a double-layered membrane, containing a rectangular or square crystalline-like core (or 'internum') surrounded by a less electron-dense matrix[8,9]. The granules contain a number of biological agents, many of which are also present in neutrophils. However, the high peroxidase content and the presence of arginine-rich cationic proteins are distinct features of the cell.

In addition to the large crystalloids, a smaller granule is present, but only in mature eosinophils[10]. These do not contain a crystalline core but stain intensely for acid phosphatase and arylsulphatase. These smaller granules are thought to be derived from the Golgi apparatus.

The eosinophil nucleus is similar in appearance to those of other mature granulocytes and contains clumps of condensed chromatin distributed against the nuclear membrane with filamentory connections between nuclear lobes. Nucleoli, the site of ribosomal RNA production, are absent from the mature cell suggesting that major biosynthetic processes have ceased[11].

Eosinophils have mitochondria, Golgi apparatus[12], ribosomes and an endoplasmic reticulum[13]. Many of these intracellular organelles are more numerous and better developed than those of the neutrophil. By scanning electron microscopy, the eosinophil membrane is indistinguishable from the neutrophil and shows surface villi, ruffles and ridge-like profiles[14].

NEUTROPHILS

The essential difference between eosinophils and neutrophils is in the structure of the intracellular granules. Primary and secondary neutrophil granules have a limiting unit membrane of about 7–9 nm in width with a trilaminar structure. Both types of granule are extremely pleomorphic and can only be successfully differentiated by cytochemical techniques, such as peroxidase staining. Secondary granules tend to be smaller.

Granular constituents

EOSINOPHILS

In addition to peroxidase and basic proteins, eosinophil granules contain several other hydrolytic and proteolytic enzymes[15] (*Table 5.1*). These include arylsulphatase, phospholipases, acid phosphatase, β-glucuronidase, acid β-glycerophosphatase, ribonuclease and cathepsin.

TABLE 5.1. Eosinophil granule proteins

Major basic protein
Eosinophil cationic protein
Eosinophil peroxidase
Eosinophil-derived neurotoxin
Arylsulphatase B
Phospholipase D
Charcot–Leyden crystal protein (lyso-phospholipase)
Histaminase

Approximately half the granule protein consists of the arginine-rich *major basic protein* (MBP)[16]. Human MBP has a molecular weight of approximately 9200 (*see* Ackerman *et al.*[17]). MBP is highly lethal for certain helminthic larvae *in vitro*[18], and appears to act as a ligand to facilitate adherence of eosinophils to the surface of certain parasites[19].

Another arginine-rich cationic protein associated with human eosinophil granules has also been described by Olsson and Venge[20]. This *eosinophil cationic protein* (ECP) has a molecular size of 21 000 and is immunochemically distinct from MBP[17]. ECP also damages schistosomula of *Schistosoma mansoni in vitro* in a similar fashion to that described for MBP and, on a molar basis, ECP appears to be more potent[21].

The matrix of the eosinophil granule is rich in a relatively cyanide-insensitive *peroxidase*[22] which differs from myeloperoxidase of the neutrophil both antigenically and biochemically[23]. Peroxidase has been shown to be discharged into phagosomes after phagocytosis[24] and onto the surface of certain helminthic worms following adherence[25].

Eosinophil peroxidase, in the presence of H_2O_2 and a halide, induced non-cytotoxic mast cell degranulation[26]. The *in vivo* significance of this observation is unknown but it may be an important amplification mechanism in the release of pharmacological mediators of hypersensitivity.

Human eosinophils contain about eight times more *arylsulphatase* than neutrophils[27]. Arylsulphatase can apparently interfere with the biological activities of leukotrienes C_4 and D_4[28] (which comprise most of the activity of the slow-reacting substance of anaphylaxis, SRS-A), even though these lipid mediators do not contain recognized substrates for this enzyme. It is often stated that this observation supports the view that eosinophils play an important role in inactivating mast cell products.

Phospholipase D, previously associated only with tissues of plant origin, was identified in human eosinophils (but not in any other blood leucocyte tested) and it could destroy the activity of 'platelet-activating factor' (PAF)[29]. The role of PAF (1-O-hexadecyl- and 1-O-octadecyl-2-acetyl-sn-glyceryl-3-phosphorylcholine) in immediate-type reactions, at least in man, is unclear. Phospholipase D may have important actions on other lipid substrates which might have more relevance to the physiological role of eosinophils.

Histaminase activity has been demonstrated in human eosinophils and neutrophils in comparable amounts[30]. The enzyme is not detected in mononuclear cells. Histaminase promotes oxidative deamination of histamine to imidazole acetic acid. The other major enzymatic pathway of histamine degradation is by *N*-methylation to 1-methylhistamine which is catalysed by histamine methyltransferase (HMT). HMT was not detected in neutrophils, eosinophils or lymphocytes and appears to reside mainly in the monocyte.

A role for the eosinophil in 'deactivating' histamine has been proposed by a number of workers[31]. However, histaminase is widely distributed in many organs and tissues and so it is unlikely that there is an absolute requirement for eosinophils in histamine catabolism through oxidative deamination. The product of histaminase action, imidazole acetic acid, has a number of eosinophil-related biological activities which include 'chemotaxis'[32] and eosinophil complement receptor enhancement[33].

Charcot–Leyden crystals (CLC) have been recognized for over a 100 years and are associated with a number of conditions characterized by a tissue or peripheral blood eosinophilia. For instance, the presence of CLC in sputa from asthmatic patients is indicative of an 'eosinophilic response'. It is now known that CLC is comprised almost solely of a single membrane-derived protein having a molecular size of approximately 13 000[34]. The protein has been shown to be lyso-phospholipase and may play a role in the inactivation of otherwise toxic lyso-phospholipids. It is now apparent that basophils are also a source of CLC, indicating that the presence of these refractile crystals might be indicative of a broader spectrum of inflammatory responses than was originally supposed[35].

Eosinophils also possess a *neurotoxin* of molecular weight 18 000[36]. The protein appears to act by damaging myelinated neurones in experimental animals (the 'Gordon phenomenon'). Its biological or pathological significance is unknown, although it may explain the neurological abnormalities observed in the hypereosinophilic syndrome and certain parasitic diseases.

NEUTROPHILS

Neutrophil granules also contain a wide range of enzymes. Secondary granules, which are more numerous in mature neutrophils, contain distinct markers such as lactoferrin and vitamin-B_{12}-binding protein. The recognized constituents derived from human neutrophil granules are shown in *Table 5.2*. When neutrophils engulf particles or come into contact with

TABLE 5.2. Neutrophil granule proteins

Primary (azurophil) granules	*Secondary (specific) granules*
Acid hydrolases	Lysozyme
Acid β-glycerophosphatase	Lactoferrin
β-Glucuronidase	Vitamin-B_{12}-binding protein (cobalophilin)
N-Acetyl-β-glucosaminidase	Collagenase
α-Mannosidase	Acidic proteins
Arylsulphatase	
β-Galactosidase	
5'-Nucleotidase	
α-Fucosidase	
Acid protease (cathepsin)	
Neutral proteases	
Chymotrypsin-like protease	
Elastase	
Collagenase	
Cationic proteins	
Myeloperoxidase	
Lysozyme	
Acid mucopolysaccharide	

Adapted from Klebanoff and Clark[37].

appropriately opsonized surfaces, there is a significant extracellular release of granular constituents. Thus, although degranulation is associated with phagocytosis, phagocytosis is not necessary for the extracellular release of granule-derived enzymes. Interestingly, secondary granule constituents seem more accessible for extracellular release than those derived from primary granules. It is clear that the array of enzymes of neutrophil origin has considerable potential for tissue damage.

Cell surface receptors for complement and immunoglobulins on eosinophils and neutrophils

There is general agreement that eosinophils do not have easily demonstrable receptors for IgA, IgM and IgD. Neutrophils express IgA$_1$ and IgA$_2$ receptors but the significance of this is unknown. There are conflicting data regarding the presence of IgE receptors on eosinophils and this controversy has yet to be resolved[38–40]. Using a modification of the rosette technique in which purified myeloma proteins are covalently linked to indicator red cells, it was shown that human eosinophils bear receptors for human IgG$_1$, IgG$_2$, IgG$_3$ and IgG$_4$ but not IgE.

Human peripheral blood eosinophils also express complement (C) receptors, namely CR1 (C3b/C4) and CR3 (C3b')[41,42]. There are also specific receptors for C5a. As with immunoglobulin, complement receptor expression, at least as shown by the rosette technique, appears to be about half that observed with neutrophils. Enhanced expression of immunoglobulin receptors is a useful marker of cell 'activation'. Measurement of complement and IgG receptors have been successfully employed in studies in bronchial asthma (*see below*).

Eosinophil and neutrophil chemotaxis

Eosinophils and neutrophils are motile cells which 'crawl' on glass and respond in chemotaxis (migration towards gradient) and/or chemokinesis (increased rate of random movement). A large number of eosinophil and neutrophil chemotactic agents have been recognized, but the biological significance of many of them is unclear. It is generally assumed that mast-cell-derived products might play a role in the recruitment of eosinophils and neutrophils to the site of allergic tissue reactions. Chemotactic agents for these cell types have been also recognized in association with the complement system, the coagulation cascade, bacteria (and other micro-organisms) as well as activated T lymphocytes.

Mast-cell-derived chemotactic factors can be divided into amines, acidic peptides and arachidonic acid metabolites. Amines, particularly histamine, and one of the major catabolites, imidazole acetic acid, are both chemotactic and chemokinetic for human eosinophils over the concentration range of 1×10^{-4} to 1×10^{-6} M[32,43].

The eosinophil chemotactic factor of anaphylaxis (ECF-A) is a family of closely related acidic peptides, in the molecular weight range 360–1000, which reside preformed within mast cell granules[44]. They possess a number of biological activities for eosinophils and (to a lesser extent) neutrophils. These properties include chemotaxis, chemokinesis, eosinophil accumulation *in vivo*[45], chemotactic deactivation and complement receptor enhancement[46] (*see below*). At the present time only two of these peptides (valine-glycine-serine-glutamic acid and alanine-glycine-serine-glutamic acid) have been identified[47]. There are a number of higher-molecular-weight ECF-A mast-cell peptides (i.e. 600–1000 daltons) which are more hydrophobic, appear to be more biologically active but are not as yet chemically characterized[48].

Various arachidonic acid metabolites possess eosinophil, as well as neutrophil, chemotactic properties. The most potent appears to be the leukotriene LTB_4 since it can attract neutrophils and eosinophils at concentrations of about 10^{-8} M[49]. 5-Hydroxyeicosatetraenoic acid (5-HETE) also attracts eosinophils as does the prostaglandin PGD_2.

There is also considerable interest in a high-molecular-weight neutrophil chemotactic factor also believed to be mast cell associated. Unlike many other mediators, it can be measured in the serum of asthmatic subjects following various challenge procedures (*see below*).

The potent chemotactic fragment, C5a, also promotes eosinophil locomotion[50], as do products of the coagulation cascade, such as fibrinopeptide B[51].

Bacterial products and material derived from metazoan parasites have eosinophil as well as neutrophil chemotactic properties. Several T-lymphocyte-derived eosinophil chemotactic factors have been described.

They may be relevant to the eosinophilia which sometimes accompanies delayed-type hypersensitivity reactions and parasitic granulomata (reviewed by Colley[52]).

The question as to whether the various mast cell products preferentially attract eosinophils from a mixed leucocyte population has given rise to some controversy. Since most of the studies have employed blood eosinophils from patients with eosinophilia, it is possible that these cells were already 'activated' and might have responded in a different fashion from normal eosinophils.

Allergy and the eosinophil

Association between the eosinophil and allergy

In general, the allergic diseases associated with eosinophilia are those in which an immediate-type hypersensitivity reaction is predominant, i.e. those reactions involving mast cells sensitized by IgE and triggered by specific allergen. Common examples are hay fever and other forms of allergic rhinitis, extrinsic bronchial asthma and general anaphylactic reactions, for example in subjects sensitive to certain drugs and stinging insects.

Present evidence suggests that the interaction of sensitized mast cells with specific antigen leads to the release of factors which are chemotactic for eosinophils, and that eosinophils migrate into the site of degranulated mast cells as a result of chemotaxis and/or chemokinesis.

Possible protective effects of the eosinophil

The precise role of the eosinophil, once it has arrived at the site of an immediate-type reaction, is still the subject of some speculation. There is some evidence for believing that, in these situations, eosinophils may have a regulatory role in dampening mast cell activity (*Figure 5.2*). As stated above, the eosinophil's content of histaminase might be relevant to its role in these reactions (although there are plenty of non-eosinophil sources of this enzyme). Similarly, the relatively high content of arylsulphatase in eosinophils might serve to inactivate leukotrienes C_4 and D_4 (potent constrictors of smooth muscle). This putative action of arylsulphatase needs clarification since it was first described when the chemical structure of the leukotrienes was unknown. When the activities of SRS-A became identified as those of LTC_4, LTD_4 and LTE_4, there was a need for re-examination of these putative actions of arylsulphatase, since these lipidopeptides do not contain a free sulphate or free sulphone group. Recently, it was shown that eosinophil peroxidase inactivated LTC_4, LTD_4 and LTE_4 in reactions dependent on H_2O_2 and a halide[53]. The mechanism of this inactivation is unknown. On the other hand, the leukotriene-*generating* capacity of eosinophils appears to be four to five times greater than that of neutrophils[54].

Eosinophils are also said to contain phospholipase D[29]. Phospholipase D can inactivate platelet-activating factor. These observations are sometimes used to strengthen the argument that eosinophils dampen down mast-cell-dependent allergic reactions.

Mast cell   Eosinophil

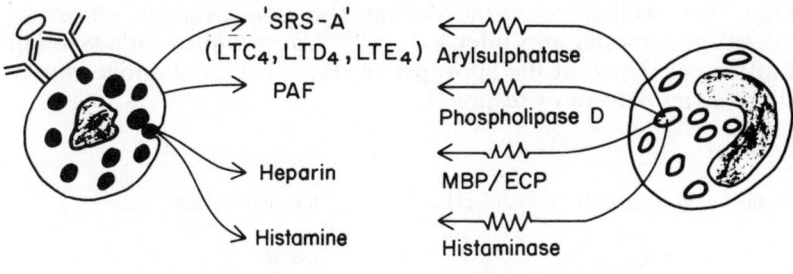

Figure 5.2 Inactivation of mast cell mediators by eosinophil-derived products. At one level of control, eosinophil-derived products neutralize or inactivate mast cell mediators. PAF—platelet-activating factor; MBP—major basic protein; ECP—eosinophil cationic protein.

The Charcot–Leyden crystal protein may also play a role in regulating mast cell events, since lyso-phospholipases are known to inactivate potentially toxic lyso-phospholipids formed as a result of the action of phospholipase A_2. Alternatively, or in addition, eosinophils might be serving in other ways in the allergic response. For instance, they may have a special role in phagocytosing mast cell granules or IgE allergen complexes.

Eosinophils, allergy and helminth immunity

It has been proposed that immediate-type (IgE-mediated) hypersensitivity might have been retained in phylogeny because of the benefit this mechanism confers in adaptive immunity to metazoan parasites (*Figure 5.3*)[55]. This raises the question as to whether allergies (immediate-type hypersensitivity) are the result of an inability to distinguish 'common allergens' from certain metazoan parasite antigens. It would not be surprising, because of their complexity, if pollen grains, animal danders and the house dust mite share antigenic determinants with helminths. Furthermore, since many enter the body by similar routes (i.e. the skin and gut), they may be expected to recruit similar immunological mechanisms. In global terms, the fight for survival against helminths has always been very severe and, therefore, the occasional inappropriate recruitment of defences by a non-parasitic signal would be relatively inconsequential. Hypereosinophilia, raised concentrations of IgE, and signs and symptoms of the release of mast cell mediators may represent, in common 'allergies', the same sequence of events which follows invasion by helminths, although the magnitude of the response is much smaller and, furthermore, poses no serious threat to the survival of the species since 'allergies', by themselves, are usually relatively trivial. The hypereosinophilia and signs of histamine release seen in certain drug reactions may be a consequence of a similar mechanism.

It could be argued that bacterial antigens might also be expected to evoke a similar response since many are likely to share the same antigens as helminths. However, the 'eosinopenic factor' characteristic of acute infections may 'mask' the recruitment of eosinophils. It is relevant that eosinophilia was well recognized during the convalescent phase of pneumococcal pneumonia and infections with *Haemophilus influenzae* in pre-antibiotic eras. Thus, at the appropriate stage, bacterial antigens may also elicit the same pattern of response.

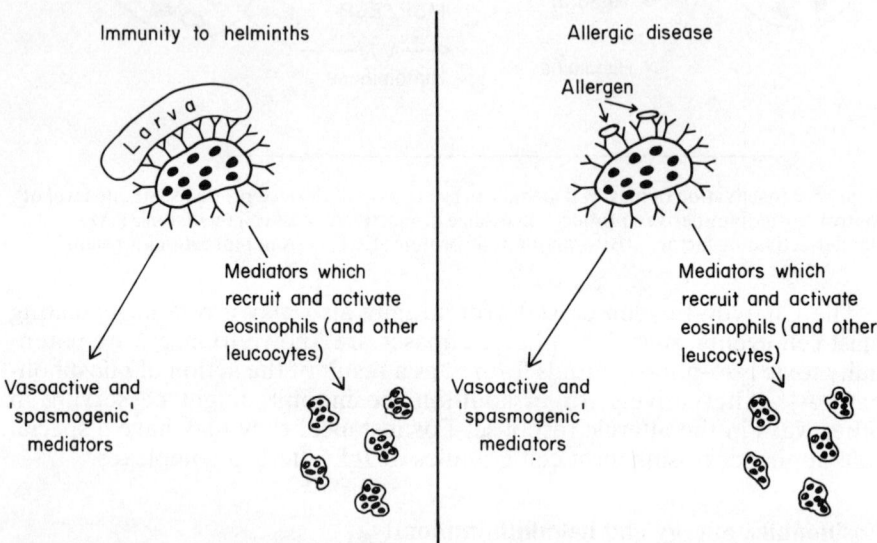

Figure 5.3 Similarities between the eosinophil/mast cell (basophil)/IgE interactions in immunity to helminths and allergic disease. In both situations there are mediators which have direct action on tissues (i.e. vasocactive and 'spasmogenic' mediators), as well as mediators which recruit and activate eosinophils (and other leucocytes). In immunity to helminths, vasoactive and spasmogenic mediators might increase local concentrations of complement and immunoglobulin whereas in allergic disease they are responsible for the immediate signs and symptoms, i.e. rhinorrhoea, bronchospasm, etc. Similarly the recruitment and activation of eosinophils and other leucocytes by mediators in the context of immunity to helminths might accelerate the killing of larvae, whereas in allergic disease this leads to the secretion of granule enzymes which contribute to tissue damage.

In evolutionary terms, the advantages of the mast cell/IgE/eosinophil interaction in limiting access of helminths probably greatly outweigh the disadvantages of the relatively trivial hypersensitivity reactions which occur when various antigens are 'mistakenly identified'. It seems unlikely that specialized cells and proteins, such as mast cells, eosinophils, and IgE, would have evolved primarily for their injurious effects.

Thus, the mast cell/IgE/eosinophil axis might be a distinct advantage in protecting against helminths since otherwise, unlike allergies, these worm infestations might endanger the species in its fight for survival. These ideas have been discussed in some detail elsewhere[55-57].

Allergy and the neutrophil

Comparatively little attention has been given to the neutrophil as a cell which participates actively in acute allergic reactions. It is well recognized, at least in the skin, that neutrophil infiltration is an early event following mast cell degranulation. For instance, when the 'skin window' technique was used to study cell infiltration following IgE-mediated skin 'prick' tests in man, there was marked neutrophil infiltration during the first 2–4 hours and this, in turn, was followed by the accumulation of large numbers of eosinophils[45]. Similar results have been observed in antigen-challenged guinea-pig skin passively sensitized by IgG_1[56] (IgG_1 is a tissue-sensitizing antibody comparable to human IgE). Neutrophil infiltration in these circumstances might be due to the release of high-molecular-weight neutrophil chemotactic factor which appears to be a selective chemoattractant for this cell type[58].

Neutrophils might play a special role in the elimination of certain inhalant allergens. For instance, it has recently been shown that a factor in normal human serum (granulocyte pollen-binding protein—GPBP) promotes the firm adherence of human neutrophils to intact pollen grains[59,60]. This has been shown for a number of grass, weed, tree and flower pollens. GPBP has been tentatively identified as transferrin. However, this neutrophil/pollen adherence reaction appears to be independent of the conventional transferrin receptor. The adherence reaction appears to require magnesium ions and may be unique to pollen, in that transferrin did not promote adherence of neutrophils to inert particles such as Sepharose and Sephadex beads.

Inflammatory cells and the progression of asthma

A blood and tissue eosinophilia are hallmarks of both allergic and non-allergic asthma[61–63]. One of the typical features of asthma deaths is plugging of the lumen of small and medium-sized bronchi by inspissated mucus, cells and cell debris[64]. The cells include epithelial cells shed off from the basement membrane together with varying numbers of eosinophils, macrophages and lymphocytes. Eosinophil infiltration, both in and around walls of the bronchi, is a very characteristic feature and this is often associated with the presence of Charcot–Leyden crystals and Curshmann's spirals in the sputum plugs. Neutrophils are not usually observed at autopsy of asthma deaths, but are often seen in the bronchi of asthmatics dying from non-asthmatic causes.

There is evidence that eosinophils and neutrophils migrate into bronchial tissues as a result of the release of mast-cell-derived chemotactic factors. These include histamine, ECF-A, high-molecular-weight NCF, LTB_4 and PAF. High-molecular-weight neutrophil chemotactic factor of anaphylaxis (variously referred to as NCF, NCF-A, or high-molecular-weight NCF has a molecular weight of approximately 600 000 daltons and an isoelectric point between 6.5 to 6.8[65]. It can be identified in the circulation of asthmatic subjects following the inhalation of specific antigen[58,66] during exercise-induced asthma[67] and in association with food-induced wheeze[68]. The time-course of release of NCF was similar to that of histamine and its appearance in the circulation was blocked by prior administration of disodium cromoglycate (DSCG)[68]. The *in vitro* release of NCF from lung fragments, has also been documented.[69].

Many of the features of bronchial asthma can be explained on the basis of the recognized biological activities of mast-cell-derived mediators. In *Figure 5.4*, an attempt has been made to link the various clinical manifestations of the disease with these pharmacological and pathological aspects. It has been suggested that the events associated with obstruction of the bronchi might be divided into three main phases. These have been termed (*a*) a rapid, spasmogenic phase, (*b*) a late, sustained phase and (*c*) a subacute/chronic inflammatory phase. The phases might act in sequence following the initial release of mast-cell-derived agents as a result of IgE/allergen interaction or non-immunological triggers such as exercise, infection or complement activation.

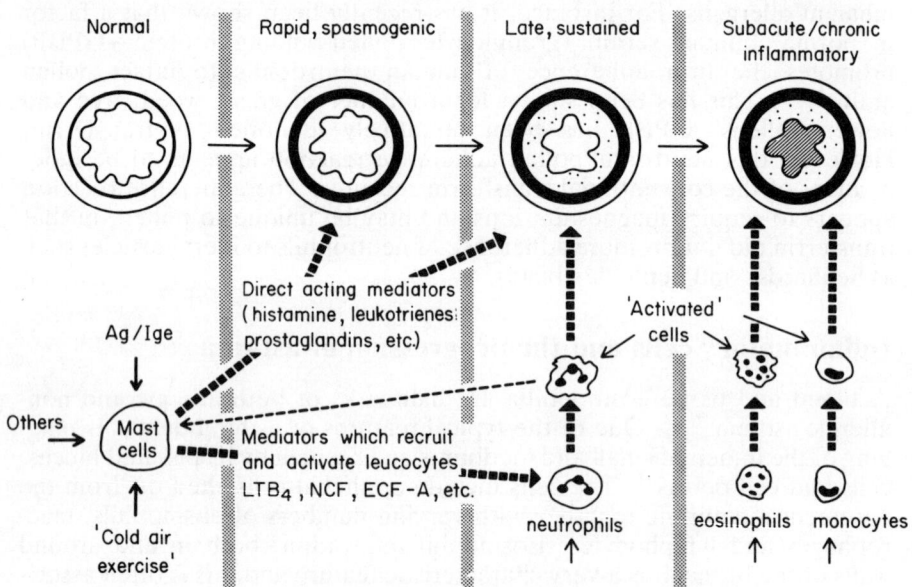

Figure 5.4 A diagrammatic representation of the progression of the asthmatic reaction (*see* text for explanation).

(*a*) *Rapid, spasmogenic phase:* when asthmatic subjects are subjected to allergen challenge, an exercise task or inhalation of a non-specific irritant such as sulphur dioxide, there is an increase in airways resistance which is rapid (10–15 min) in onset. Such reactions are readily reversible, either spontaneously or by bronchodilators such as β_2-specific sympathomimetics. As mentioned above, elevations in the concentrations of plasma histamine and NCF were demonstrated and the time-course of mediator release paralleled the fall in forced expiratory volume per second (FEV_1) or peak expiratory flow rate (PEFR). This rapid phase is probably mediated largely through histamine acting either directly on smooth muscle or via vagal reflexes. It can be inhibited by prior administration of disodium cromogly-cate (DSCG), or by histamine H_1-receptor antagonists. The rapid spasmogenic phase is not affected by corticosteroids given immediately prior to challenge. Mast-cell-associated chemotactic factors, such as NCF[70] and leukotriene B_4[49], activate leucocytes *in vitro* as shown by enhanced expression of membrane receptors for complement (C3b). Recent studies suggest that, in asthma, neutrophils and monocytes can be activated *in vivo*[72]. Using the rosette technique to measure C3b receptors, there was a time-dependent increase in the percentage of neutrophil and monocyte rosettes in asthmatic subjects who wheezed following either a treadmill exercise task or inhalation of specific allergen. NCF peaked at 15 min, whereas the increase in the percentage of C3b neutrophil and monocyte rosettes continued for up to 60 minutes. In contrast, asthmatic subjects who did not develop exercise-induced asthma (EIA) following the same exercise task, or who had bronchospasm induced by methacholine, had no significant increase in either rosette formation, elevation of NCF or fall in the peak expiratory flow rate. Enhancement of C3b rosettes following these manoeuvres was inhibited by prior administration of DSCG. These studies suggest that leucocytes are 'activated' following exercise-induced asthma or allergen challenge and that this may have particular relevance to the events which precede the development of late-phase asthmatic reactions.

(*b*) *Late, sustained phase:* following bronchial challenge with specific allergen many subjects have a second, usually more severe, rise in airways resistance which is maximal 6–8 hours following exposure. Compared to the rapid spasmogenic phase, the late-phase reaction is slower both in onset and disappearance, i.e. more sustained. Late-phase reactions are associated with more lung hyperinflation and sometimes take several days to resolve. They are often followed by greatly enhanced bronchial hyper-reactivity. The pathogenesis of late reactions is incompletely understood. There is probably some bronchial infiltration by neutrophils since, at least in human skin, IgE-dependent responses are associated with neutrophil accumulation 4–8 hours following antigen challenge. It was originally proposed that the late reaction was an example of a type III, or Arthus, response with neutrophil infiltration resulting from the generation of chemotactic factors following activation of complement by immune complexes. Recent evidence suggests that late reactions might be associated with reactivation of mast cells, since there was also a late sustained rise in the concentration of circulating serum NCF[71] and histamine[73]. There is evidence to suggest that eosinophilia is associated with late reactions. For instance, relatively large numbers of eosinophils were observed at lung lavage in individuals who developed allergen-induced late-phase reactions (J. de Monchy, personal communication). There is also a small but significant rise in blood eosinophil counts during late-phase reactions. Eosinophils may have particular relevance to the inflammatory events of asthma, as discussed below. It is also possible that leukotrienes, prostaglandins and thromboxanes play a role in the late reactions as these mediators tend to have sustained biological effects and might, for instance, cause prolonged contraction of bronchial smooth muscle, together with oedema of the sub-mucosa, as a result of their effects on the microvasculature[74]. Furthermore late reactions are inhibited by prior administration of corticosteroids[75]. Since one of the postulated actions of corticosteroids is to prevent (via lipo-modulin/macrocortin) the release of free arachidonic acid, it is reasonable to speculate that late reactions might, in part, be associated with arachido-nic acid metabolites.

(c) *Subacute/chronic inflammatory phase:* continuing asthma in the untreated or partially controlled patient is likely to be associated, to a greater or lesser degree, with a substantial inflammatory reaction in and around the bronchi. As stated above, infiltration of the bronchi with large numbers of eosinophils and mononuclear cells are characteristic findings at autopsy. Several studies of bronchoalveolar lavage (BAL) fluid in asthma indicated that the eosinophil is a prominent cell when compared to fluid obtained from normal individuals and from patients with diseases such as sarcoidosis and bronchial carcinoma[76]. In a placebo-controlled double-blind study, it was shown that DSCG suppressed the local accumulation of eosinophils in bronchial mucus and BAL fluid[77]. In addition, this compound also seemed to inhibit the local concentrations of house dust mite specific IgE whereas it had no effect on the levels of total IgE, IgG, IgA and IgM, C3 and C4. Eosinophils and mononuclear cells might be recruited by mast-cell-derived chemotactic factors, such as ECF-A and LTB_4. Eosinophils especially might contribute to tissue damage as a result of release of the basic proteins derived from their crystalloid granules. High levels of sputum major basic protein (MBP) have been reported in asthma[78] and MBP has been shown to damage cells that are diverse in origin, including ascites tumour cells, mononuclear phagocytes and, importantly, ciliated respiratory epithelial cells[79]. MBP is thought to play a special role in tissue damage associated with severe asthma, since it was detected in mucous plugs, damaged epithelial surfaces and also beneath the basement membrane from bronchi of patients dying from this disease[80]. Thus, it seems likely that in asthma the eosinophil damages respiratory tissue. Eosinophil cationic protein (ECP) concentrations in the serum also appear to be related to the asthmatic process, in that increased levels were detected following bronchial challenge[81]. The relatively high leukotriene-generating capacity of eosinophils has already been mentioned[54]. This has clear implications for the eosinophils as pro-inflammatory cells.

Corticosteroids, eosinophils, neutrophils and the asthmatic response

It has been known for many years that the administration of corticosteroids is associated with an abrupt fall in the blood eosinophil count. The beneficial effects of corticosteroids in a number of eosinophil-related disorders, including bronchial asthma, is undisputed, although it is uncertain whether, in these situations, corticosteroids are acting principally 'against the eosinophil' or exerting their major effects by other pathways.

The eosinopenic effects of adrenal corticosteroids seem to be due to a combination of rapid tissue sequestration of eosinophils[82] and inhibition of the egress of mature cells from the bone marrow[83]. There is also a dampening of the rate of eosinophil migration in the tissues following the administration of corticosteroids[84]. In many lung diseases, for instance cryptogenic pulmonary eosinophilia, treatment with corticosteroids leads to complete remission, with apparent reversal of eosinophil-mediated tissue damage. In other situations, e.g. chronic bronchial asthma, there is massive deposition of eosinophil-derived material even in the face of apparent prolonged corticosteroid therapy[80]. It is likely that corticosteroids also inhibit eosinophil and neutrophil locomotion, possibly through the generation of agents such as lipomodulin/macrocortin which inhibit the action of phospholipase A_2[85–87]. This might dampen the subsequent influx of neutrophils, eosinophils and monocytes which in turn minimize release of lysosomal enzymes and further tissue destruction.

On the other hand, it is well known that many asthmatics are resistant to the effects of corticosteroids and that these patients require much higher doses of oral prednisolone for prolonged periods of time[88]. In a recent study, it was shown that corticosteroid-resistant asthmatics have an apparent defect of leucocyte 'activation'[89]. Although these studies were undertaken with peripheral blood monocytes, rather than neutrophils or eosinophils, recent evidence suggests that the test of activation used in these studies (complement (C3b) receptor enhancement—CRE) is a property of all phagocytic cells. When asthmatic patients took a course of oral prednisolone (and subsequently responded clinically to this treatment), their peripheral blood monocytes underwent less CRE, after exposure to a chemotactic factor *in vitro*, than cells from normal untreated subjects. In contrast, corticosteroid-*resistant* asthmatics taking prednisolone had a similar degree of monocyte CRE to that of normal individuals. This suggests that, in these resistant patients, corticosteroids had less anti-inflammatory effect. It is yet to be determined whether this defect is related to lipomodulin generation.

Summary

Various properties of eosinophils and neutrophils are compared and contrasted. The putative role for these cells in acute allergic reactions is discussed with particular relevance to the biological advantages of IgE/mast-cell/eosinophil interactions. The possible contributions of eosinophils and neutrophils to the progression of asthma are considered. Present evidence suggests that mast-cell mediators recruit and activate inflammatory cells and that these infiltrating leucocytes, particularly eosinophils, damage respiratory tissues. The anti-inflammatory actions of corticosteroids in bronchial asthma are also discussed.

References

1. RYTÖMMA, T. *Acta Pathologica et Microbiologica Scandinavica*, **50,** Supplementum 140, 1 (1960)
2. RINGOEN, A.R. *Handbook of Haematology*. p. 181. London: Hamish Hamilton (1938)

3. MAHMOUD, A.A.F., STONE, M.K. and KELLERMEYER, R.W. *Journal of Clinical Investigation*, **60**, 675 (1977)
4. CURRY, J.L. and TRENTIN, J.J. *Developmental Biology*, **15**, 395 (1967)
5. CARTWRIGHT, G.E., ATHENS, J.W., HAAB, O.P., RAAB, S.O., BOGGS, D.R. and WINTROBE, M.M. *Annals of the New York Academy of Sciences*, **113**, 963 (1964)
6. BRYANT, B.J. and KELLEY, L.S. *Proceedings of the Society for Experimental Biology and Medicine*, **99**, 681 (1958)
7. LASZLO, J. and RUNDLES, R.W. In *Hematology*. Ed. W.J. Williams. Chap. 75. New York: McGraw-Hill (1972)
8. BESSIS, M. and THIERY, H. *International Review of Cytology*, **12**, 199 (1961)
9. FALLER, A. *Zeitschrift für Zellforschung und mikroskopische Anatomie*, **69**, 551 (1966)
10. PARMLEY, R.T. and SPICER, S.S. *Laboratory Investigation*, **30**, 557 (1974)
11. ZUCKER-FRANKLIN, D. *Seminars in Hematology*, **5**, 209 (1968)
12. GOODMAN, J.R., REILLY, E.B. and MOORE, R.E. *Blood*, **12**, 428 (1957)
13. HIRSCH, J.G. In *The Inflammatory Process*. Ed. B.W. Zweifach. p. 245. New York: Academic Press (1965)
14. POLLIACK, A. and DOUGLAS, S.C. *British Journal of Haematology*, **30**, 303 (1975)
15. ARCHER, G.T. and HIRSCH, J.G. *Journal of Experimental Medicine*, **118**, 287 (1963)
16. BEHRENS, M. and MARTI, H.R. *Biochimica et Biophysica Acta*, **65**, 551 (1962)
17. ACKERMAN, S.J., DURACK, D.T. and GLEICH, G.J. *Advances in Host Defense Mechanisms*, **1**, 269 (1982)
18. BUTTERWORTH, A.E., WASSOM, D.L., GLEICH, G.J., LOEGERING, D.A. and DAVID, J.R. *Journal of Immunology*, **122**, 221 (1979)
19. BUTTERWORTH, A.E., VADAS, M.A., WASSOM, D.L., DESSEIN, A., HOGAN, M., SHERRY, B. *et al.* *Journal of Experimental Medicine*, **150**, 1456 (1979)
20. OLSSON, I. and VENGE, P. *Blood*, **44**, 235 (1974)
21. McLAREN, D. J., McKEAN, J.R., OLSSON, I., VENGE, P. and KAY, A.B. *Parasite Immunology*, **3**, 359 (1981)
22. ARCHER, R.K. and BROOME, J. *Acta Haematologica*, **29**, 147 (1963)
23. SALMON, S.E., CLINE, M.J., SCHULTZ, J. and LEHRER, R.I. *New England Journal of Medicine*, **282**, 250 (1970)
24. COTTRAN, R.S. and LITT, M. *Journal of Experimental Medicine*, **129**, 1291 (1969)
25. McLAREN, D.J., MacKENZIE, C.D. and RAMALHO-PINTO, F.J. *Clinical and Experimental Immunology*, **30**, 105 (1977)
26. HENDERSON, W.R., CHI, E.Y. and KLEBANOFF, S.J. *Journal of Experimental Medicine*, **152**, 265 (1980)
27. TANAKA, K.R., VALENTINE, W.N. and FREDRICKS, R.E. *British Journal of Haematology*, **8**, 86 (1962)
28. WASSERMAN, S.I., GOETZL, E.J. and AUSTEN, K.F. *Journal of Immunology*, **114**, 645 (1975)
29. KATER, L.A., GOETZL, E.J. and AUSTEN, K.F. *Journal of Clinical Investigation*, **57**, 1173 (1976)
30. ZEIGER, R.S., YURDIN, D.L. and COLTEN, H.R. *Journal of Allergy and Clinical Immunology*, **58**, 172 (1976)
31. ARCHER, R.K. *The Eosinophil Leucocytes*. Oxford: Blackwell Scientific Publications (1963)
32. TURNBULL, L.W. and KAY, A.B. *Immunology*, **31**, 797 (1976)
33. ANWAR, A.R.E. and KAY, A.B. *Journal of Immunology*, **121**, 1245 (1978)
34. WELLER, P.F., GOETZL, E.J. and AUSTEN, K.F. *Proceedings of the National Academy of Sciences of the United States of America*, **77**, 7440 (1980)
35. ACKERMAN, S.J., WEIL, G.J. and GLEICH, G.J. *Journal of Experimental Medicine*, **155**, 1597 (1982)
36. DURACK, D.T., ACKERMAN, S.J., LOEGERING, D.A. and GLEICH, G.J. *Proceedings of the National Academy of Sciences of the United States of America*, **78**, 5165 (1981)
37. KLEBANOFF, S.J. and CLARK, R.A. In *The Neutrophil: Function and Clinical Disorders*. p. 489. Amsterdam: North-Holland (1978)
38. ISHIZAKA, K., TOMIOKA, H. and ISHIZAKA, T. *Journal of Immunology*, **105**, 1459 (1970)
39. CAPRON, M., CAPRON, A., GOETZL, E.J. and AUSTEN, K.F. *Nature*, **289**, 71 (1981)
40. KAY, A.B. In *Proceedings of the XIth International Congress of Allergology and Clinical Immunology*. Eds J.W. Kerr and M.A. Ganderton. p. 245. Basingstoke: Macmillan (1983)
41. ANWAR, A.R.E. and KAY, A.B. *Journal of Immunology*, **119**, 976 (1977)
42. DIERICH, M.P., MUSSEL, H.H., SCHEINER, O., EHLEN, T., BURGER, R., PETERS, H. *et al.* *Immunology*, **45**, 85 (1982)

43. CLARK, R.A.F., GALLIN, J.I. and KAPLAN, A.P. *Journal of Experimental Medicine*, **142,** 1462 (1975)
44. KAY, A.B. and AUSTEN, K.F. *Journal of Immunology*, **107,** 988 (1971)
45. BRYANT, D.H. and KAY, A.B. *Clinical Allergy*, **7,** 211 (1977)
46. ANWAR, A.R.E. and KAY, A.B. *Nature*, **269,** 522 (1977)
47. GOETZL, E.J. and AUSTEN, K.F. *Proceedings of the National Academy of Sciences of the United States of America*, **72,** 4123 (1975)
48. GOETZL, E.J. and AUSTEN, K.F. In *The Eosinophil in Health and Disease*. p. 149. New York: Grune & Stratton (1980)
49. NAGY, L., LEE, T.H., GOETZL, E.J., PICKETT, W.C. and KAY, A.B. *Clinical and Experimental Immunology*, **47,** 541 (1982)
50. KAY, A.B. *Clinical and Experimental Immunology*, **6,** 75 (1970)
51. KAY, A.B., PEPPER, D.S. and McKENZIE, R. *British Journal of Haematology*, **27,** 669 (1974)
52. COLLEY, D.G. In *The Eosinophil in Health and Disease*. p. 293. New York: Grune & Stratton (1980)
53. HENDERSON, W.R., JORG, A. and KLEBANOFF, S.J. *Journal of Immunology*, **128,** 2609 (1982)
54. JORG, A., HENDERSON, W.R., MURPHY, R.C. and KLEBANOFF, S.J. *Jounal of Experimental Medicine*, **155,** 390 (1982)
55. KAY, A.B. *Journal of Allergy and Clinical Immunology*, **64,** 90 (1979)
56. KAY, A.B. In *Recent Advances in Clinical Immunology*. p. 113. Edinburgh: Churchill Livingstone (1980)
57. GROVE, D.I. *Allergy*, **37,** 139 (1982)
58. ATKINS, P.C., NORMAN, M., WEINER, H. and ZEIMAN, B. *Annals of Internal Medicine*, **86,** 415 (1977)
59. SASS-KUHN, S.P., MOQBEL, R., MacKAY, J.A., CROMWELL, O. and KAY, A.B. *Journal of Clinical Investigation*, **73,** 202 (1984)
60. KAY, A.B., SASS-KUHN, S.P., MOQBEL, R. and MacKAY, J. Unpublished observations
61. LOWELL, F.C. *Journal of the American Medical Association*, **202,** 875 (1967)
62. FRANKLIN, W. *New England Journal of Medicine*, **290,** 1469 (1974)
63. HORN, B.R., ROBIN, E.D., THEODORE, J. and VAN KESSEL, A. *New England Journal of Medicine*, **292,** 1152 (1975)
64. DUNNILL, M.S. In *Allergy: Principles and Practices*. p. 678. St Louis: C.V. Mosby Co. (1978)
65. LEE, T.H., NAGAKURA, T., PAPAGEORGIOU, N., IIKURA, Y. and KAY, A.B. *New England Journal of Medicine*, **308,** 1502 (1983)
66. BROWN, M.J., IND, P.W., CAUSON, R. and LEE, T.H. *Journal of Allergy and Clinical Immunology*, **69,** 20 (1982)
67. LEE, T.H., NAGY, L., NAGAKURA, T., WALPORT, M.J. and KAY, A.B. *Journal of Clinical Investigation*, **69,** 889 (1982)
68. PAPAGEORGIOU, N., LEE, T.H., NAGAKURA, R., CROMWELL, O., WRAITH, D.G. and KAY, A.B. *Journal of Allergy and Clinical Immunology*, **72,** 75 (1983)
69. O'DRISCOLL, B.R., CROMWELL, O. and KAY, A.B. *Journal of Allergy and Clinical Immunology*, **72,** 695 (1983)
70. LEE, T.H., NAGY, L., NAGAKURA, T., WALPORT, M.J. and KAY, A.B. *Federation Proceedings*, **41,** 734 (Abstract) (1982)
71. KAY, A.B., PAPAGEORGIOU, N., LEE, T.H., CARROLL, M. and DURHAM, S.R. *Journal of Allergy and Clinical Immunology*, **71,** 146, 230 (Abstract) (1983)
72. NAGY, L., LEE, T.H. and KAY, A.B. *New England Journal of Medicine*, **306,** 497 (1982)
73. DURHAM, S.R., LEE, T.H., MERRETT, T.G., MERRETT, J., BROWN, M.J., CAUSON, R. et al. *Journal of Allergy and Clinical Immunology*, **71,** 146, 231 (Abstract) (1983)
74. CAMP, R.D.R., COUTTS, A.A., GREAVES, M.W., KAY, A.B. and WALPORT, M.J. *British Journal of Pharmacology*, **75,** 168P (1982)
75. BOOIJ-NORD, H., ORIE, N.G.M. and DE VRIES, K. *Journal of Allergy and Clinical Immunology*, **48,** 344 (1971)
76. MICHEL, F.B., GODARD, P., AUBAS, P., MARIA Y., DUJOL, P., CALVAYRAC, P. et al. *Respiration*, **42,** Suppl. 1, 7 (1981)
77. DIAZ, P., GALLEGUILLOS, F.R., GONZALEZ, M.C. and KAY, A.B. Unpublished observations
78. FRIGAS, E., LOEGERING, D.A. and GLEICH, G.J. *Laboratory Investigation*, **42,** 35 (1980)
79. GLEICH, G.J., FRIGAS, E., LOEGERING, D.A., WASSOM, D.L. and STEINMULLER, D. *Journal of Immunology*, **123,** 2925 (1979)
80. FILLEY, W.V., HOLLEY, K.E., KEPHART, G.M. and GLEICH, G.J. *Lancet*, **ii,** 11 (1982)

81. DAHL, R., VENGE, P. and OLSSON, I. *Allergy*, **33,** 211 (1978)
82. ANDERSEN, V. and BRO-RASMUSSEN, F. Presented at *XIIth Congress of the International Society of Hematology*. September, New York (1968)
83. HUDSON, G. *Bone Marrow Reactions*. London: Edward Arnold (1966)
84. ZWEIMAN, B., SLOTT, R.J. and ATKINS, P.C. *Journal of Allergy and Clinical Immunology*, **58,** 657 (1976)
85. BLACKWELL, G.J. and FLOWER, R.J. *Nature*, **278,** 456 (1979)
86. HIRATA, F., SCHIFFMAN, E., VENKATASUBRAMANIAN, K., SALOMAN, D. and AXELROD, J. *Proceedings of the National Academy of Sciences of the United States of America*, **77,** 2533 (1980)
87. HIRATA, F. *Journal of Biological Chemistry*, **256,** 7730 (1981)
88. CARMICHAEL, J., PATERSON, I.C., DIAZ, P., CROMPTON, G.K., KAY, A.B. and GRANT, I.W.B. *British Medical Journal*, **282,** 1419 (1981)
89. KAY, A.B., DIAZ, P., CARMICHAEL, J. and GRANT, I.W.B. *Clinical and Experimental Immunology*, **44,** 576 (1981)

Chapter 6

Acetylcholine

Laurie J. Smith

Introduction

Asthma has been defined as a disease characterized by increased responsiveness of the airways to a variety of stimuli, manifested by slowing of forced expiration with the ability to change either spontaneously or with treatment[1]. This increased responsiveness of the airways has been extensively studied. Virtually all asthmatics develop bronchoconstriction when exposed to aerosols of cholinomimetic agents in concentrations not producing any changes in non-asthmatic subjects[1]. This property of heightened airways reactivity to cholinergic agents has focused attention on the role of the parasympathetic nervous system in asthma. This chapter will review acetylcholine, the parasympathetic nervous system and its role in asthma relating to antigenic and non-specific stimuli.

Acetylcholine as a neurotransmitter

Acetylcholine is a major neurotransmitter in the human body. It is stored in vesicles in highly concentrated ionic form in nerve endings (axons). When an action potential travels down a nerve, a complex sequence of events occurs resulting in the explosive release of hundreds of quanta of acetylcholine. The acetylcholine diffuses across a synaptic or junctional cleft to combine with specialized macromolecular receptors on the postjunctional membrane. Located in the region of this neuroeffector junction is a high concentration of acetylcholinesterase. This enzyme is capable of hydrolysing, and thus inactivating, acetylcholine with tremendous rapidity allowing the axon to recover within milliseconds.

Acetylcholine receptors

The type of response to the action potential depends upon the nature of the postjunctional receptor area. Although acetylcholine is always the neurotransmitter, there are four different receptor types distinguished by their location and response to agonists and antagonists. All postganglionic

107

parasympathetic fibres and a few postganglionic sympathetic fibres (sweat glands and sympathetic vasodilator fibres) stimulate the type I cholinergic receptors. These receptors are referred to as muscarinic, because of the preferential stimulating action that muscarinic alkaloids have on these receptors. They are blocked by atropine. Type II cholinergic receptors respond to acetylcholine from all preganglionic fibres of both the parasympathetic and sympathetic systems, i.e. the receptor is on the ganglion cell. These sites are inhibited by hexamethonium and stimulated by dimethylphenylpiperazinium. Type III receptors are found in striated muscle as acetylcholine is also the neurotransmitter from the motor nerves to skeletal muscle. This receptor is blocked by decamethonium and stimulated by phenyltrimethylammonium. Type II and type III receptors are stimulated at low doses and blocked at high doses by nicotine and are referred to as nicotinic receptors. They are both inhibited by d-tubocurarine. Cholinoceptive neurones of the central nervous system have either nicotinic or muscarinic receptors; type IV. They are blocked by either d-tubocurarine or atropine, respectively[2] (*Table 6.1* and *Figure 6.1*). In this chapter we are interested in acetylcholine as it functions as a neurotransmitter for parasympathetic postsynaptic fibres.

TABLE 6.1. Acetylcholine receptors

Type	Situation	Specific agonist	Specific antagonist
I	Postganglionic parasympathetic (and some sympathetic) nerve fibre terminals to effector cells	Muscarine	Atropine
II	Preganglionic sympathetic and parasympathetic nerve fibre terminals to ganglia cells	Dimethylphenyl-piperazinium Nicotine, low concentrations	Hexamethonium d-Tubocurarine Nicotine, high concentrations
III	Somatic motor nerve to striated muscle	Phenyltrimethyl-ammonium Nicotine, low concentrations	Decamethonium d-Tubocurarine Nicotine, high concentrations
IV Muscarinic	CNS nerve junctions	Muscarine Oxotremorine	Atropine
IV Nicotinic	CNS nerve junctions	Nicotine, low concentrations	Nicotine, high concentrations d-Tubocurarine

Parasympathetic nervous system and the vagal reflex

The autonomic nervous system is a part of the central nervous system, acting as an efferent outflow of motor neurones innervating tissues and organs chiefly involved in maintaining tonic activity, homeostasis and stress adaptation. Sensory fibres travel with many of the effector nerves and can be considered as part of the system. The autonomic nervous system can be

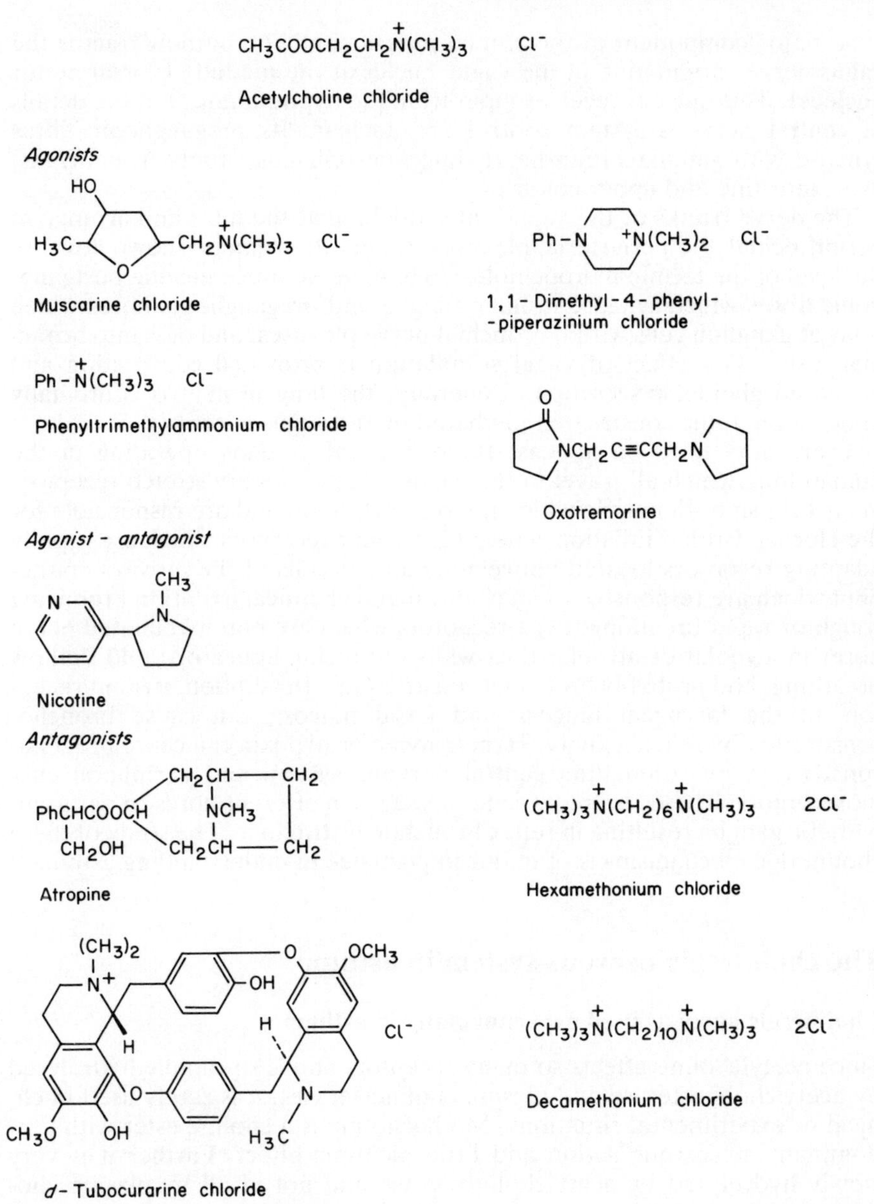

$$CH_3COOCH_2CH_2\overset{+}{N}(CH_3)_3 \quad Cl^-$$

Acetylcholine chloride

Agonists

Muscarine chloride

$$Ph-\overset{+}{N}(CH_3)_3 \quad Cl^-$$

Phenyltrimethylammonium chloride

1,1 - Dimethyl - 4 - phenyl - -piperazinium chloride

Oxotremorine

Agonist - antagonist

Nicotine

Antagonists

Atropine

$$(CH_3)_3\overset{+}{N}(CH_2)_6\overset{+}{N}(CH_3)_3 \quad 2Cl^-$$

Hexamethonium chloride

$$(CH_3)_3\overset{+}{N}(CH_2)_{10}\overset{+}{N}(CH_3)_3 \quad 2Cl^-$$

Decamethonium chloride

d- Tubocurarine chloride

Figure 6.1 Acetylcholine receptors. Structures of specific agonists and antagonists.

divided into two main systems, the sympathetic (thoracolumbar) outflow and parasympathetic (cranial and sacral) outflow. The sympathetic system is distributed to effectors throughout the body and may discharge overall as a unit for the 'fight and flight' reaction. The parasympathetic system does not innervate all smooth muscle and visceral organs, and each part often acts independently rather than in concert.

A major component of the cranial parasympathetic outflow tract is the vagus nerve, originating in the vagus nuclei of the medulla (dorsal motor nucleus). This nucleus receives input from the hypothalmus, but the details of central nervous system control are unclear. Its preganglionic fibres synapse with ganglia within heart, lung, oesophagus, stomach, pancreas, liver, intestine and upper colon[3].

The nerve trunks of the vagus enter the lung at the hilus and arrange in peribronchial and periarterial plexuses. Innervation can be shown down to the level of the terminal bronchioles[4]. These nerve fibres include postganglionic fibres which synapse in hilar ganglia and preganglionic fibres which relay at ganglion cells within bronchial nerve plexuses, and pass into bronchial walls. The effect of vagal stimulation is bronchial constriction and increased glandular secretion. Generally, the lung in man is continually under some tonic constriction mediated by the vagus nerve[5].

There appear to be at least three afferent systems operating in the human lung which all travel in the vagus: (1) pulmonary stretch receptors in airways smooth muscle which inhibit inspiration and are responsible for the Hering–Breuer inflation reflex; (2) irritant receptors which are rapidly adapting receptors located between columnar cells of the airways epithelium which are responsive to mechanical and chemical irritation producing cough or rapid breathing; (3) J receptors which are non-myelinated nerve fibres in alveolar or alveolar duct walls producing apnea or rapid shallow breathing, and probably bronchial constriction[6]. In addition, irritant receptors in the laryngeal mucosa and nasal mucosa can cause bronchoconstriction by reflex activity. Hypercapnea or hypoxia can cause bronchoconstriction by stimulating central nervous system and peripheral chemoreceptors. These receptors send messages in afferent fibres to parasympathetic ganglia resulting in reflex bronchoconstriction[7]. The study of these cholinergic mechanisms is of major importance in understanding asthma.

The cholinergic nervous system in asthma

Cholinergic agonists used experimentally in asthma

Since acetylcholine affects so many receptors and is so rapidly hydrolysed by acetylcholinesterase and plasma cholinesterases, it is rarely used in clinical or experimental situations. Methacholine is a choline ester with predominant muscarinic action and little nicotinic effect. Further it is very slowly hydrolysed by acetylcholinesterase and not at all by plasma cholinesterases. Methacholine is frequently used in experimental situations to investigate aspects of the cholinergic nervous system. Another choline ester, carbachol, is even more resistant to hydrolysis by acetylcholinesterase and non-specific cholinesterases. However, carbachol has more nicotinic effects than methacholine, especially on autonomic ganglia. It appears to act both directly on receptors and to stimulate the release of endogenous acetylcholine from terminals of cholinergic fibres. Pilocarpine, a naturally occurring alkaloid, is occasionally used to study cholinergic effects. It has dominant muscarinic effects but sweat glands are particularly sensitive to this drug[8] (*Figure 6.2*).

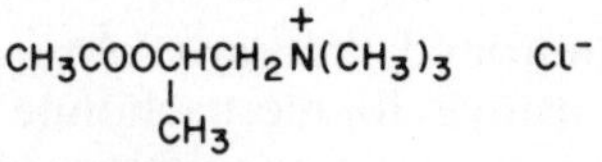

$$CH_3COOCHCH_2 \overset{+}{N}(CH_3)_3 \quad Cl^-$$
$$\underset{CH_3}{|}$$

$$NH_2 COOCH_2 CH_2 \overset{+}{N}(CH_3)_3 \quad Cl^-$$

Metacholine chloride

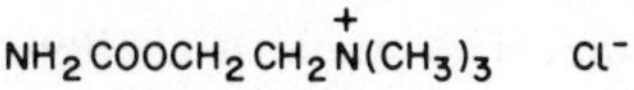

Carbachol chloride

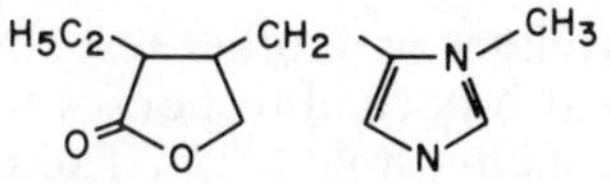

Pilocarpine

Figure 6.2 Cholinergic agonists used in man.

Cholinergic hypersensitivity

Asthmatic subjects demonstrate increased bronchial responsiveness to cholinergic stimuli when compared to normal subjects[9]. In fact, a recent textbook[1] states 'all asthmatic patients are exquisitely sensitive to methacholine aerosol.' This phenomenon has been known for many years. John Curry, in 1947[10], citing references dating back to 1912, reviewed the literature concerning response to cholinergic stimulation, using methacholine, pilocarpine or carbachol given subcutaneously, orally or by aerosol. He reports that the early investigators showed repeatedly that cholinergic stimulation had the potential to trigger symptoms of asthma in many asthmatic subjects, but few normal individuals. Curry himself demonstrated that intravenous, subcutaneous, and aerosolized methacholine could provoke symptoms of asthma and decrease vital capacity in asthmatic subjects, and some allergic rhinitis subjects (during their pollen season). He also found that this sensitivity correlated with histamine provocation but was more sensitive. The more severe asthmatics were, the more sensitive to methacholine they were. These early studies generally employed a single dose of cholinergic agent to provoke symptoms.

In 1965, Townley et al.[11] described a provocation technique which used a fixed concentration of methacholine delivered by aerosol. He administered increasing numbers of inhalations of methacholine until a 20% drop in FEV_1 from base-line was reached. He found current asthmatics to be more sensitive to cholinergic stimulation than former asthmatics. Hay fever patients were less responsive, with approximately one-half of these subjects having a bronchoconstrictor response to the higher doses of methacholine. Parker et al.[12] at that time recommended using inhalation of methacholine as a test for bronchial asthma.

Since then, the methacholine inhalation test has been used frequently in studying asthmatic subjects. The technique of giving an increasing number of inhalations of a fixed concentration of methacholine has been replaced by an approach using a fixed number of breaths of increasing concentrations of methacholine. In 1975, a committee of the American Academy of Allergy and Immunology published suggested guidelines for standardizing bronchial inhalation challenges[13]. These guidelines have been further refined by other investigators[14]. These refinements have allowed reproducible observations to be made about the nature of the bronchial responsiveness in asthma. The modern challenge tests have confirmed the early observation that most, if not all, asthmatics are sensitive to methacholine. Furthermore, as suggested by Curry[10], this sensitivity to inhalation of methacholine correlates directly with the severity of the asthma. Asthmatics requiring continual medication respond to lower doses of methacholine than asthmatics requiring little or no medication[15].

Bronchial responsiveness to methacholine correlates with other tests of bronchial lability. Several studies have shown that bronchial responses to inhaled histamine correlate closely with those of methacholine[16,17]. These responses are not exactly similar, however, as the methacholine effect can be completely abolished by atropine while the histamine response may be unaffected or only slightly altered[18,19]. Bronchial sensitivity to methacholine correlates with the ability of exercise to induce asthma[20], although methacholine challenge is positive in more subjects than is exercise[21]. The mechanisms producing asthma via exercise have been claimed to be related to respiratory heat loss[22]. When asthma produced by isocapnic hyperventilation in cold air is compared to bronchial responsiveness to methacholine, there is a close positive correlation between the two tests[23].

Methacholine sensitivity can be found in other diseases besides asthma. Subjects with allergic rhinitis may have increased bronchial sensitivity to methacholine[11]. Although the incidence of a positive methacholine test varies among studies[9], there is a tendency towards a higher incidence among allergic rhinitis subjects who experience any lower respiratory symptoms[24]. The response in hay fever subjects generally requires doses higher than needed in asthma for a comparable response[11].

Methacholine sensitivity has also been found in some patients with chronic obstructive pulmonary disease[25,26]. This relationship may reflect pre-existing bronchoconstriction, rendering a bronchus more likely to respond to a constricting stimulus. However, many of these subjects with marked constriction do not respond to methacholine. It is possible that pre-existing methacholine reactivity may predispose to the development of chronic obstructive pulmonary disease. Some patients with cystic fibrosis also show an increased reactivity to methacholine[27] or histamine[28]. Recently, 50% of patients in one series with sarcoid were shown to be methacholine responsive[29]. The significance of methacholine sensitivity in other populations besides asthma is unclear.

Cholinergic hypersensitivity and non-specific bronchial responsiveness

The basis for the increased bronchial reactivity seen in asthma is not clear. Methacholine, when delivered by aerosol, acts directly on bronchial smooth muscle via acetylcholine receptors to produce bronchoconstriction. This effect is not significantly altered when given following aerosolized hexamethonium (a ganglionic blocker) in a dose which does significantly alter the response to aerosolized histamine in the same human volunteers[30]. This suggests that methacholine is acting at a site distal to the ganglion, presumably the muscarinic receptor, and that reflex mechanisms are not important. The increased bronchomotor responses may be due to changes in number of receptors, or binding affinity, or increase in smooth muscle responsiveness to the neurotransmitter. That the response to inhaled methacholine or acetylcholine does not involve an exaggerated reflex response is further supported by studies in animals showing that cooling of the vagus nerve in dogs did not alter the bronchial response to aerosolized acetylcholine[31], and acetylcholine aerosol, while causing bronchoconstriction, cannot be shown to stimulate rapidly adapting receptors in dog lung under conditions where histamine clearly does[32]. It is possible that changes in bronchial smooth muscle account for some of this increased response; however, this is currently under investigation[9].

In addition to the postganglionic hyper-responsiveness, there is also evidence for bronchospasm in asthma to be mediated via reflex activity. Simonsson showed that aerosols of citric acid, histamine phosphate and carbon dust caused bronchoconstriction in patients with asthma and bronchitis, and that this could be abolished with intravenous atropine[33]. The mechanism responsible for this was thought to involve the stimulation of cough and irritant receptors in the airways, initiating reflex parasympathetic activity resulting in bronchoconstriction. Conditions in which the airways epithelium is damaged, therefore leading to increased sensitivity of vagal sensory nerve endings, have been associated with increased bronchial responsiveness. Viral upper respiratory infections are frequently associated with increased bronchial sensitivity, not only in asthmatic subjects, but in normals as well[12]. This increase in bronchial reactivity can be blocked by atropine and may be due to sensitization of rapidly adapting sensory receptors[34]. Ozone, in a concentration which does not alter baseline lung function, can cause increased responsiveness to aerosols of histamine and methacholine in both non-atopic and atopic individuals. This effect can be blocked by atropine[35]. Sulphur dioxide, in concentrations that do not affect normal subjects, can cause bronchospasm in asthmatic subjects. Sulphur dioxide directly stimulates afferent nerve endings in the larynx and tracheobronchial tree resulting in reflex bronchospasm[36]. Insults to bronchial mucosa, like ozone and upper respiratory infections, which may produce bronchial hyper-reactivity in non-asthmatic subjects cause transient effects lasting from 24 hours up to 8 weeks and the change in bronchial responsiveness is generally of a smaller magnitude than that produced in asthmatic subjects[9].

In addition to increased receptor sensitivity and increased sensitivity of sensory nerve endings, there is evidence of other mechanisms contributing to bronchial hyper-reactivity. In dogs, 5-hydroxytryptamine, in doses too low to cause direct constriction, may enhance efferent vagal activity in airways[31]. Other evidence suggests that histamine may act similarly in some dogs in a synergistic fashion with vagal stimulation[32]. Therefore, histamine may not only exert its effect directly on smooth muscle and via reflex stimulation, but also via a direct enhancing effect on efferent vagal activity.

The central nervous system may modulate bronchial hyper-reactivity. There are connections between the dorsal motor nucleus of the vagus and the hypothalamus, but their nature requires further investigation. Studies have shown that some asthmatics can respond to suggestion with bronchoconstriction. Those who exhibit this response tend to have greater airways sensitivity to methacholine and histamine and have a greater tendency to react to suggestion with emotional responses measured as changes in blood pressure, pulse amplitude and electromyogram[38]. Further, this response can be blocked by atropine[39]. Some asthmatics have been demonstrated to respond to hypnotic suggestions with bronchoconstriction or bronchodilatation[40]. A few asthmatics can increase their threshold response to methacholine or even transiently abolish it with hypnotic suggestion[41]. These studies provide evidence that there may be a connection between the central nervous system and regulation of bronchial hyper-reactivity, presumably via modulating the parasympathetic nervous system.

There have been suggestions that bronchial hyper-responsiveness may be, in part, due to blockade of the β-adrenergic nervous system. This topic has recently been reviewed in detail[9]. β-Adrenergic dysfunction does not appear to be a major cause of bronchial hyper-reactivity although it may modify it[42]. It has been shown, however, that the degree of β blockade, as measured by blood pressure responses to increasing doses of isoproterenol, is directly related to the degree of bronchial reactivity as measured by methacholine bronchial challenge[43].

There has also been some suggestion that α-adrenergic sensitivity may contribute to bronchial hyper-reactivity. Simonsson showed that an α-receptor agonist could cause a decrease in airways conductance in the presence of cholinergic and β-adrenergic antagonists[44]. Overall, it is difficult to demonstrate a significant α-adrenergic effect producing bronchial hyper-reactivity[9]. It has been shown, however, that α-adrenergic sensitivity, as measured by pupillary responses to an α stimulator, correlates directly with bronchial methacholine sensitivity[43]. Therefore, cholinergic hypersensitivity accompanies and correlates directly with the degree of β-adrenergic blockade and α-adrenergic sensitivity. There is no direct evidence of a cause-and-effect relationship.

Cholinergic hypersensitivity and response to antigen and histamine

Allergen-provoked asthma requires the cooperation of IgE fixed to mast cells responding to the presence of specific antigen with the release of mast cell mediators. Although histamine, slow-reacting substance of anaphylaxis (SRS-A) and other mast cell mediators are capable of causing bronchoconstriction by a direct mechanism[45], there is evidence that parasympathetic reflex mechanisms may also be important in antigen-provoked asthma. In 1972, Gold et al.[46] performed antigen challenges on naturally sensitized dogs and measured respiratory resistance. They showed that vagal blockade abolished increased respiratory resistance to antigen challenge. Further, unilateral bronchial exposure to antigen produced bilateral bronchoconstriction and this response could be prevented by vagal cooling on the side of the exposure. In the same year, Yu et al.[47] reported the results of antigen challenge in humans. Airways resistance change in response to inhaled antigen was blocked by intravenous atropine in five of seven subjects. The other two subjects, not blocked by intravenous atropine, demonstrated complete obliteration of antigen response with aerosolized atropine. These studies were interpreted as showing that a major aspect of antigen-induced bronchoconstriction was based on cholinergic stimulation.

Later, Krell et al.[48] found that atropine did not attenuate antigen response in most allergic dogs they studied. Rosenthal et al.[49] could not show an alteration in antigen response in humans when using aerosolized atropine to block ragweed antigen-induced bronchospasm. Another study by Orehek[50], using allergen-induced bronchoconstriction in 10 allergic asthmatics, found ipratropium bromide (an atropine-like drug described in Chapter 9) completely blocked the response in five subjects, had no effect in three and intermediate effects in two others. Results of more detailed studies in animals suggest that differences in site of bronchoconstrictive response may be one cause of these conflicting reports. Constriction in airways down to 1.0 mm in diameter in the dog, due to antigen challenge, may be due largely to vagal reflex mechanisms although, overall, there is a substantial component of direct airways constriction which is atropine resistant[51].

Several explanations can be invoked to explain the differences reported from different studies. Doses of antigen, methods of delivery, degree of vagal blockade and intersubject variation may be quite important. Gold used a single antigen dose which had been determined on a previous day to be a provocative concentration. Rosenthal et al. performed a dose–response curve on each study day. This resulted in much longer time of antigen exposure in Rosenthal's study than in Gold's, for example. It appears that, although cholinergic mechanisms do participate in antigen-induced asthma, the direct effects of mast-cell-derived mediators predominate.

As stated previously, histamine exerts its effect by both direct and reflex mechanisms. Histamine has been shown to directly stimulate the rapidly adapting receptors in dog lung[32]. Yanta et al.[37] showed that the pulmonary response to inhaled histamine can vary in different dogs. They all have a direct constrictor response to histamine. However, some showed evidence of constant vagal tone modulating, i.e. enhancing, a histamine response and others showed evidence of a reflex response to histamine. This suggests that interaction between histamine and the cholinergic nervous system may be quite variable from subject to subject.

Since histamine and antigen cause bronchospasm via both a direct effect on smooth muscle and an interaction with the cholinergic nervous system, one might expect degrees of bronchial reactivity to antigen to correlate with degree of non-specific bronchial sensitivity to methacholine or histamine. Makino[52] did find that bronchial sensitivity to inhaled antigen correlated with bronchial sensitivity to acetylcholine. Others have found similar relationships[53]. Further, bronchial response to inhaled histamine has been found to correlate quite well to response to inhaled antigen[54].

Recurrent antigen exposure has the potential to increase bronchial responses to methacholine and histamine. This requires a delayed bronchial response to allergen inhalation and does not generally follow a simple immediate bronchospastic response to antigen[55]. A possible mechanism for this is that the inflammatory reaction from the late antigen response sensitizes the rapidly adapting receptors to be more responsive to non-specific stimuli.

There is evidence that, although acetylcholine per se or cholinergic stimulation cannot trigger mast cells to release mediators directly, acetylcholine may be able to exert an enhancing effect in the presence of antigen-induced mediator release. Kaliner[56] has shown that acetylcholine can enhance antigen-induced mediator release from mast cells in human lung, presumably by increasing levels of cyclic GMP (guanosine cyclic 3′:5′-monophosphate). Therefore, cholinergic stimulation has the potential to augment bronchial response to inhaled antigen.

Mucus

Cholinergic efferent nerves can be shown to terminate near mucous glands which contain both serous and mucous cells and are the main source of tracheal secretion. Goblet cells contribute only a small amount of mucus and there is little evidence of significant innervation. Cholinergic stimulation increases the volume of mucus secreted and the output of mucus glycoproteins, as well as stimulating ciliary activity and mucociliary transport[57]. Aerosols of both histamine and acetylcholine, at concentrations which can cause bronchoconstriction, have been demonstrated to increase tracheal mucus velocity[58]. Atropine has been demonstrated to inhibit the production of tracheal secretion and volume of sputum, although another study has suggested that atropine might also stimulate mucociliary clearance[59]. Another inhibitor of cholinergic activity, ipratropium bromide, did not slow mucus transport or mucociliary clearance[58].

Summary

Increased responsiveness of airways is a hallmark of asthma. Cholinergic mechanisms account for a significant proportion of this hyper-reactivity. Asthmatics have increased responsiveness to inhaled methacholine pointing to a sensitivity in the postganglionic area, either receptor sensitivity or increased end-organ response. They also show evidence of heightened reflex activity. The affector side of the parasympathetic reflex arc is spontaneously more sensitive to a variety of non-specific stimuli, like histamine, and can be rendered even more sensitive in the presence of some viral infections or irritants like ozone and sulphur dioxide. Reacting in an extremely sensitive manner, the affector system sends stimuli into the vagus triggering an effector response greater than normal because of the heightened postganglionic responsiveness. In addition, in some undefined manner, other mediators, such as 5-hydroxytryptamine and histamine, may augment naturally occurring parasympathetic tone. Parasympathetic tone and reactivity may also be modified by psychological factors, including suggestion and hypnosis. Disequilibrium of the sympathetic nervous system accompanies and may amplify this hyper-reactivity of the cholinergic nervous system. All of these mechanisms may combine to produce the pathophysiology seen in asthma: constriction of bronchial smooth muscle and increased mucus production.

References

1. MIDDLETON, E. Jr, REED, C.E. and ELLIS, E.F. *Allergy Principles and Practice*. Chap. 36. St Louis: C.V. Mosby Co. (1978)
2. GILMAN, A.G., GOODMAN, L.S. and GILMAN, A. *The Pharmacological Basis of Therapeutics*. Chap. 4. New York: Macmillan Publishing Co. (1980)

3. MOUNTCASTLE, V.B. *Medical Physiology*. Chap. 33. St Louis: C.V. Mosby Co (1980)
4. RICHARDSON, J.B. *American Review of Respiratory Disease*, **119**, 785 (1979)
5. WIDDICOMBE, J.G. and STERLING, G.M. *Archives of International Medicine*, **126**, 311 (1970)
6. WIDDICOMBE, J.G. *American Review of Respiratory Disease*, **115**, 99 (1977)
7. WIDDICOMBE, J.G. *Postgraduate Medical Journal*, **51** (Suppl.) 36 (1975)
8. GILMAN, A.G., GOODMAN, L.S. and GILMAN, A. *The Pharmacological Basis of Therapeutics*. Chap. 2. New York: Macmillan Publishing Co. (1980)
9. BOUSHEY, H.A., HOLTZMAN, M.J., SHELLER, J.R. and NADEL, J.A. *American Review of Respiratory Disease*, **121**, 389 (1980)
10. CURRY, J. *Journal of Clinical Investigation*, **26**, 430 (1947)
11. TOWNLEY, R.G., DENNIS, M. and ITKIN, I.H. *Journal of Allergy*, **36**, 121 (1965)
12. PARKER, C.D., BILBO, R.E. and REED, C.E. *Archives of Internal Medicine*, **115**, 452 (1965)
13. CHAI, H., FARR, R.S., FROELICH, L.A., MATHISON, D.A. *et al. Journal of Allergy and Clinical Immunology*, **56**, 323 (1975)
14. RYAN, G., DOLOVITCH, M.B., ROBERTS, R.S., FRITH, P.A. and JUNIPER, E.F. *American Review of Respiratory Disease*, **123**, 195 (1981)
15. JUNIPER, E.F., FRITH, P.A. and HARGREAVE, F.E. *Thorax*, **36**, 575 (1981)
16. JUNIPER, E.F., FRITH, P.A., DUNNETT, C., COCKEROFT, D.W. and HARGREAVE, F.E. *Thorax*, **33**, 705 (1978)
17. SALOME, C.M., SCHOEFFEL, R.C. and WOOLCOCK, A.J. *Clinical Allergy*, **10**, 541 (1980)
18. ITKIN, I.H. and ANAND, S.C. *Journal of Allergy*, **45**, 1978 (1970)
19. CASTERLINE, C.L., EVANS III, R. and WARD, G.W. *Journal of Allergy and Clinical Immunology*, **58**, 607 (1976)
20. KIVILOOG, J. *Scandinavian Journal of Respiratory Diseases*, **54**, 347 (1973)
21. CATHAM, M., BLEECKER, E.R., SMITH, P.L., ROSENTHAL, R.R., MASON, P. and NORMAN, P.S. *American Review of Respiratory Disease*, **126**, 235 (1982)
22. DEAL, E.C., McFADDEN, E.R. Jr, INGRAM, R.H. Jr, BRESLIN, F.J. and JAEGAR, J.J. *American Review of Respiratory Disease*, **121**, 621 (1980)
23. O'BYRNE, P.M., RYAN, G., MORRIS, M., McCORMACK, D., JONES, N.L., and MORSE, J.L.C. *et al. American Review of Respiratory Disease*, **125**, 281 (1982)
24. COCKCROFT, D.W., KILLIAN, D.N., MELLON, J.J.A. and HARGREAVE, F.E. *Clinical Allergy*, **7**, 235 (1977)
25. SIMONSSON, B.G. *Acta Allergologica*, **20**, 325 (1965)
26. KLEIN, R.C. and SALVAGGIO, J.E. *Journal of Allergy*, **37**, 258 (1966)
27. BURDON, J.G.W., CADE, J.F., SUTHERLAND, P.W. and PAIN, M.C.F. *Medical Journal of Australia*, **2**, 77 (1980)
28. MELLIS, C.M. and LEVISON, H. *Paediatrics*, **61**, 446 (1978)
29. BECHTEL, J.J., STARR, T. III, DANTZKER, D.R. and BOWER, J.J. *American Review of Respiratory Disease*, **124**, 759 (1981)
30. HOLTZMAN, M.J., SHELLER, J.R., DIMEO, M., NADEL, J.A. and BOUSHEY, H.A. *American Review of Respiratory Disease*, **122**, 17 (1980)
31. HAHN, H.L., WILSON, A.G., GRAF, P.D., FISCHER, S.P. and NADEL, J.A. *Journal of Applied Physiology*, **44**, 144 (1978)
32. VIDRUK, E.H., HAHN, H.L., NADEL, J.A. and SAMPSON, S.R. *Journal of Applied Physiology*, **43**, 397 (1977)
33. SIMONSSON, B.G., JACOBS, F.M. and NADEL, J.A. *Journal of Clinical Investigation*, **46**, 1812 (1967)
34. EMPEY, W., LAITINEN, L.A., JACOBS, L., GOLD, W.M. and NADEL, J.A. *American Review of Respiratory Disease*, **113**, 131 (1976)
35. HOLTZMAN, M.J., CUNNINGHAM, J.H., SHELLER, J.R., IRSIGLER, G.B., NADEL, J.A. and BOUSHEY, H.A. *American Review of Respiratory Disease*, **120**, 1059 (1979)
36. SHEPPARD, D., WONG, W.S., UEHARA, C.B., NADEL, J.A. and BOUSHEY, H.A. *American Review of Respiratory Disease*, **122**, 873 (1980)
37. YANTA, M.A., LORING, S.H., INGRAM, R.H. Jr and DRAZEN, J.M. *Journal of Applied Physiology*, **50**, 869 (1981)
38. HORTON, D.J., SUDA, W.L., KINSMAN, R.A., SOUHRADA, J. and SPECTOR, S. *American Review of Respiratory Disease*, **117**, 1029 (1978)
39. McFADDEN, E.R. Jr, LUPARELLO, T., LYONS, H.A. and BLEECKER, E. *Psychosomatic Medicine*, **31**, 134 (1969)
40. SMITH, M.M., COLEBATCH, J.H.J. and CLARKE, P.S. *American Review of Respiratory Disease*, **102**, 236 (1970)

118   Acetylcholine

41. SMITH, L.J., WAIN, H.J. and EVANS, R. III, *Journal of Allergy and Clinical Immunology*, **67** (Suppl.), 44 (1980)
42. MORLEY, J. *Bronchial Hyperreactivity*. p. 31. London: Academic Press (1982)
43. KALINER, M., SHELHAMER, J.H., DAVIS, P.B., SMITH, L.J. and VENTER, J.C. *Annals of Internal Medicine*, **96**, 349 (1982)
44. SIMONSSON, B.G., SVEDMYER, N., ANDERSON, R. and BORGH, N.P. *Scandinavian Journal of Respiratory Disease*, **53**, 227 (1972)
45. LICHTENSTEIN, L.M. and AUSTEN, K.F. *Asthma: Physiology, Immunopharmacology, and Treatment*. Chaps 7, 10. New York: Academic Press (1977)
46. GOLD, W.M., KESSLER, G.F. and YU, D.Y. *Journal of Applied Physiology*, **33**, 719 (1972)
47. YU, D.Y., GALANT, S.P. and GOLD, W.M. *Journal of Applied Physiology*, **32**, 823 (1972)
48. KRELL, R.D., CHAKRIN, L.W., WARDELL, J.R., McCOY, J. and GIANNONE, E. *Journal of Allergy and Clinical Immunology*, **58**, 19 (1979)
49. ROSENTHAL, R.R., NORMAN, P.S., SUMMER, W.R. and PERMUTT, S. *Journal of Applied Physiology*, **42**, 600 (1977)
50. LICHTENSTEIN, L.M. and AUSTEN, K.F. *Asthma: Physiology, Immunopharmacology and Treatment*. Chap. 16. New York: Academic Press (1977)
51. PATTERSON, R., SUSKO, I.M. and HARRIS, K.E. *Journal of Clinical Investigation*, **62**, 519 (1978)
52. MAKINO, A. *Japanese Journal of Allergology*, **13**, 127 (1964)
53. FELARCA, A.B. and ITKIN, I.H. *Journal of Allergy*, **37**, 223 (1966)
54. COCKCROFT, D.W., RUFFIN, D.E., FRITH, P.A., CARTIER, A., JUNIPER, E.F., DOLOVICH, J. et al. *American Review of Respiratory Disease*, **120**, 1053 (1979)
55. COCKCROFT, D.W., RUFFIN, R.E., DOLOVICH, J. and HARGREAVE, F.E. *Clinical Allergy*, **7**, 503 (1977)
56. KALINER, M. *Journal of Allergy and Clinical Immunology*, **60**, 204 (1977)
57. LICHTENSTEIN, L.M. and AUSTEN, K.F. *Asthma: Physiology, Immunopharmacology and Treatment*. Chap. 16. New York: Academic Press (1977)
58. WANNER, A. *American Review of Respiratory Disease*, **116**, 100 (1977)
59. CHOPRA, S.K. *American Review of Respiratory Disease*, **118**, 367 (1978)

Part 3

Pharmacological approaches

Section 1 Competitive antagonists

Chapter 7

H$_1$ antihistamines

Noemi Eiser

Introduction

In 1910, Dale and Laidlow[1,2] implicated histamine in the pathogenesis of asthma and other allergic disorders when they reported that intravenous histamine produced anaphylactic shock, associated with respiratory distress in certain laboratory animals. This prompted the search for agents which, in combating the effects of histamine, might be useful in the treatment of allergic diseases. The first successes in this search came from France. By 1933, Fourneau and Bovet[3] had reported that certain phenolic ethers could inhibit some of the actions of histamine. Four years later, Staub and Bovet[4] showed that one of these ethers, thymoxyethyl-diethylamine(1), had antianaphylactic properties. These original agents, because of their toxicity, were unsuitable for clinical use. However, clinically effective and relatively non-toxic 'antihistamines', such as phenbenzamine(2), mepyramine(3), diphenhydramine(4) and tripelennamine(5) were described shortly afterwards[5-8].

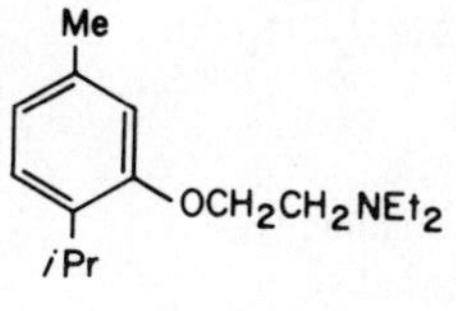

121

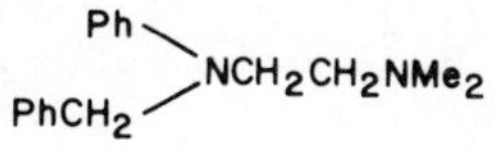

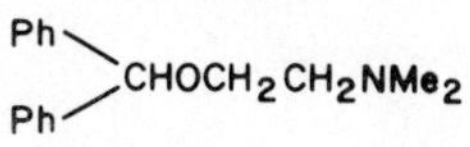

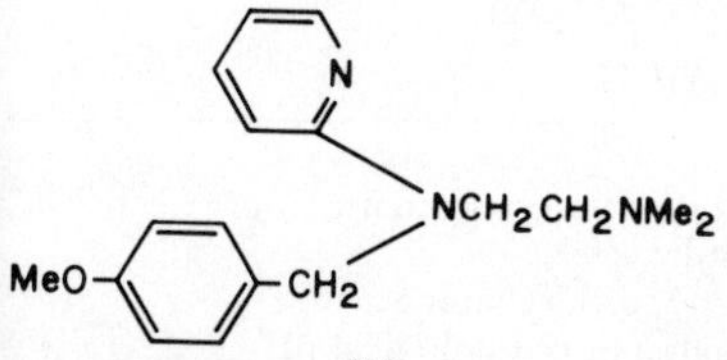

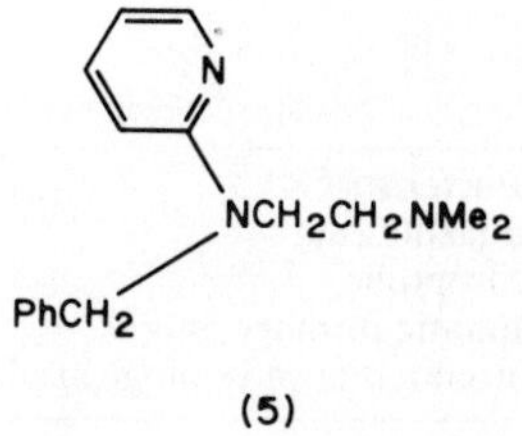

The observation that these 'classical antihistamines' failed to inhibit his-tamine-induced gastric acid secretion[9] led to the suggestion that there were two types of histamine receptor[10]: the H_1-receptor, whose actions were prevented by mepyramine, a 'classical antihistamine' and the non-H_1- or H_2-receptor, whose actions were refractory to mepyramine antagonism. Black and colleagues[11] gave substance to this concept when they developed specific agonists and antagonists of this H_2-receptor. H_1-receptors pre-dominate in the tracheobronchial tree of most animal species, including man and mediate bronchoconstriction. When H_2-receptors are present they seem to mediate bronchodilatation[12,13]. There is some controversy regarding the existence of H_2-receptors in human airways, but, if present, their role appears to be trivial and without clinical significance[14-19].

The 'classical antihistamines' are competitive inhibitors of the histamine H_1-receptor. There is a marked similarity between the structures of hista-mine and most of the H_1-receptor antagonists, in that an ethylamine chain, either straight or as part of a ring, usually forms an integral part of the molecule (*Table 7.1*). Several classes of H_1-receptor antagonists are recog-nized. Drugs of the ethanolamine, alkylamine and ethylenediamine types epitomize the group as a whole and are illustrated in *Table 7.1* together

TABLE 7.1. Comparison between histamine and H_1-receptor antagonists

Histamine	*H_1-receptor antagonist*
(1) *Structures*	
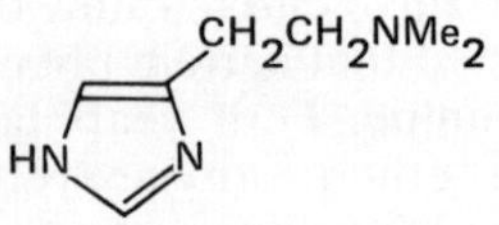 $CH_2CH_2NMe_2$ imidazole ring, HN N	(*a*) Ethanolamine type: 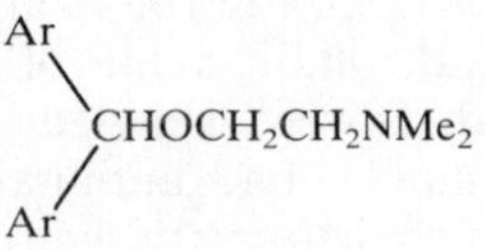 Ar — CHOCH$_2$CH$_2$NMe$_2$ — Ar
	(*b*) Alkylamine type: 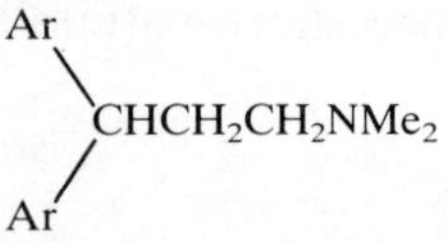 Ar — CHCH$_2$CH$_2$NMe$_2$ — Ar
	(*c*) Ethylenediamine type: 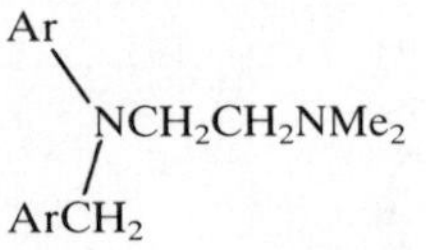 Ar — NCH$_2$CH$_2$NMe$_2$ — ArCH$_2$
(2) *Characteristics*	
(i) Imidazole ring	Aryl and/or heteroaromatic ring
(ii) Hydrophilic	Lipophilic
(iii) Aliphatic primary amine	Aliphatic tertiary amine
(iv) Protonated at physiological pH	Protonated at physiological pH

with a comparison between some of their characteristics and those of histamine.

The similarity between the structure of a number of biogenic amines, including histamine, 5-hydroxytryptamine, acetylcholine and adrenaline, is probably responsible for the relative non-specificity of their respective competitive antagonists[20]. For instance, most H_1-receptor antagonists have significant anti-cholinergic and tranquilizing properties, while some are also inhibitors of α-adrenergic receptors or 5-hydroxytryptamine[7,21–24]. Due to this lack of specificity, most produce central nervous system effects and some of these drugs have anti-parkinsonian activity[25], while others have anti-emetic[26], local anaesthetic[27] or quinidine-like activity[28]. The specificity of these individual H_1-receptor antagonists varies considerably.

Early estimates of the potency of the H_1-receptor antagonists compared their effect on either the lethal dose of histamine or on the size of histamine-induced intradermal wheals in guinea-pigs. However, it is known now that these were inappropriate models, since both H_1- and H_2-receptors mediate the cardiovascular and inflammatory responses to histamine in most species[29–32]. Other, more specific, methods of estimating potency have been used, such as recording the effects on histamine-induced contractions of isolated guinea-pig ileum or tracheal strip. In one such study, Cheng and Woodward[33] compared the potency of a number of antagonists of the H_1-receptor by estimating their pA_2 values—the negative logarithm of the molar concentration of antagonist producing a two-fold shift to the right of the histamine dose–response curve in isolated guinea-pig ileum. Part of their results are shown in *Table 7.2*. Considerable differences in potency were demonstrated. For instance, terfenadine(6) was one-sixth as potent at the H_1-receptor as chlorpheniramine(7) in this model.

Unfortunately, there seems to be little correlation between the potency of H_1-receptor antagonists established *in vitro* and their clinical efficacy in

TABLE 7.2. Antihistaminic effects of drugs on histamine response of isolated guinea-pig ileum

Drugs	pA_2 Value	
	Mean	Range
(1) Ethanolamines		
Diphenhydramine	7.93	7.71 – 8.20
(2) Ethylenediamines		
Mepyramine	9.03	8.84 – 9.34
Tripelennamine	8.70	8.30 – 9.65
(3) Alkylamines		
Chlorpheniramine	9.01	8.76 – 9.37
(4) Piperazines		
Buclizine	5.53	5.31 – 5.75
(5) Phenothiazines		
Chlorpromazine	8.60	8.31 – 9.06
Promethazine	8.87	8.32 – 10.78
(6) Piperidines		
Terfenadine	8.23	7.91 – 8.55

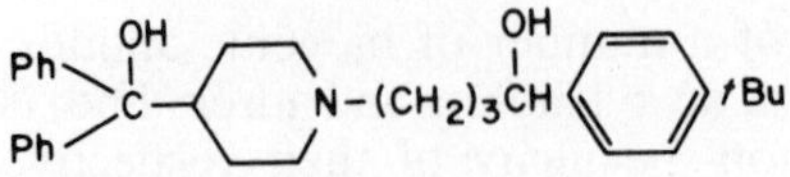

(6) 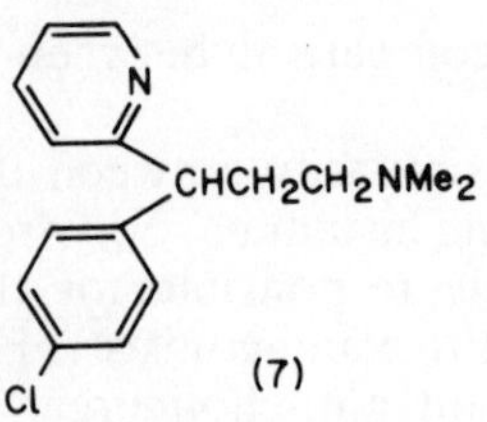   (7)

allergic diseases. It is probable that a combination of factors are responsible, including inadequate local concentrations of the drugs, the contribution of the H$_2$-receptor to the vascular response to histamine in the nose or skin, the modulation of the autonomic nervous system and the contribution of other mediators of the allergic responses.

Effects of H$_1$-receptor antagonists when given to asthmatics by various routes

Oral

Several pieces of evidence pointed to the important aetiological role of histamine in the asthmatic attack. For instance, Weiss and colleagues[34] had demonstrated that intravenous histamine caused dyspnoea, wheeze and a fall in vital capacity in asthmatic subjects, while antigen-induced histamine release had been observed, both *in vitro* and *in vivo*, in sensitized guinea-pigs by Bartosche and coworker[35] and by Code[36]. These data stimulated a plethora of clinical trials directed towards establishing the role of H$_1$-receptor antagonists in the treatment of asthma. Unfortunately, the validity of many of these trials is open to doubt, since they were, in the main, uncontrolled, open trials, reporting changes in symptoms rather than objective changes in airways function. The differences in potency and specificity of the H$_1$-receptor antagonists, already mentioned, as well as differences in the type and severity of asthma studied, makes the interpretation and comparison of these trials difficult.

In 1948, Vallery-Radot and coworkers[37] claimed that diphenhydramine was the most effective H$_1$-receptor antagonist in the treatment of asthma, while, in contrast, Arbesman[38] found that it was frequently less useful than tripelennamine. It was reported that diphenhydramine was a better treatment for atopic rather than non-atopic asthmatics[39], for seasonal rather than perennial asthma[40], for mild rather than severe asthma[41], was particularly helpful in suppressing cough[42] especially in infantile asthma[37], but was unhelpful in asthma precipitated by respiratory infection[43]. However, with conventional oral doses of diphenhydramine, the improvements in asthma varied between 12 to 65% of cases in the different trials[40-44], and in one series[45] no objective changes in spirometric measurements were obtained despite improvements in symptoms. Trials with another H$_1$-receptor antagonist, phenindamine(8), produced improvements in asthma ranging from 15 to 75%[46-49]. Again the best results were in the children[46] and, in one trial, 27% of patients had symptomatic improvement without concomitant improvements in vital capacity[48]. Results with tripelennamine were no more encouraging. Arbesman and colleagues[50] reported improvements in 46% of seasonal asthmatics, but only 37% of perennial asthmatics, whereas Feinberg[51] found that a mere 28% of his asthmatics improved. Similarly, oral chlorpheniramine up to 4 mg four times daily, improved the symptoms of only 25% of asthmatics in one series[52], but when compared with placebo in a double-blind trial, chlorpheniramine 12 mg twice daily did not change asthma scores[53]. Karlin[54] found no consistent change in peak expiratory flow rate (PEFR) in a group of asthmatic children with either diphenhydramine, promethazine(9), or tripelennamine in the usual dose or in double the usual dose.

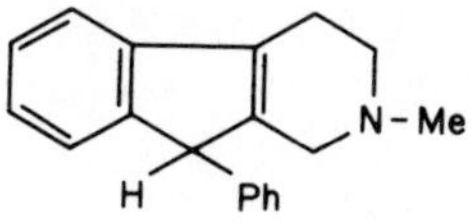

(8)

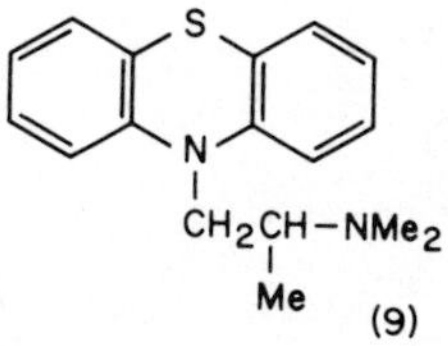

(9)

In general, therefore, the results with oral H_1-receptor antagonists in the treatment of asthma have been disappointing and many have concluded, on the basis of these and other similar trials, that the earlier oral H_1-receptor antagonists had a very limited place in the management of asthma[53-59]. Nevertheless, there is some evidence that H_1-receptor antagonists, given in adequate dosage, can produce bronchodilatation when given parenterally.

Parenteral

ON BRONCHIAL TONE

In 1949, Herxheimer[60] showed that intravenous mepyramine 50–100 mg and promethazine 25 mg increased the vital capacity in mild, though not in severe, asthma. Similarly, intramuscular thiazinamium(10) 25 mg was shown to increase the maximum forced expiratory volume in 1 second (FEV_1) of asthmatics by 25% while 50 mg was more effective than 2 puffs of a conventional isoprenaline aerosol[61,62]. Furthermore, Popa[63] has observed a similar degree of bronchodilatation following chlorpheniramine 10 mg i.v. and aminophylline 5.5 mg/kg i.v. It appears that the extent of bronchodilatation achieved with intravenous chlorpheniramine varies between asthmatics and is dependent on the degree of pre-existing bronchial tone[18]. It is also dose dependent over a range of 2.5–10 mg (personal observation). Since intravenous chlorpheniramine has no effect on the basal bronchial tone of normal subjects[14,17,18], it is possible that, in some asthmatics, there is a continuous release of histamine from pulmonary mast cells into the bronchi in the resting state which is partially responsible for their initial bronchomotor tone, and that H_1-receptor antagonists relieve this tone by competitive inhibition of the bronchial H_1-receptors. Another possibility is that the basal bronchial tone is mediated via the cholinergic nervous system and that H_1-receptor antagonists relieve this tone by their non-specific anti-cholinergic activity. This seems unlikely since chlorpheniramine 20 mg i.v. does not prevent the bronchial response to inhaled methacholine[17,18]. Nevertheless, in one study[64], intravenous clemastine(11), which is said to be a more specific H₁-receptor antagonist without anti-cholinergic properties[65,66], did not alter bronchial tone. The explanation for this single observation could be that the dose of clemastine 1 mg was insufficient to inhibit the H₁-receptor or that since these were seasonal asthmatics, studied outside the season when their lung function was normal, there was little histamine to inhibit.

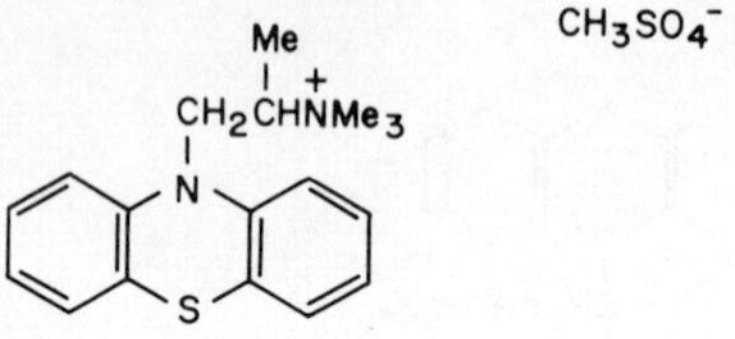

(10)

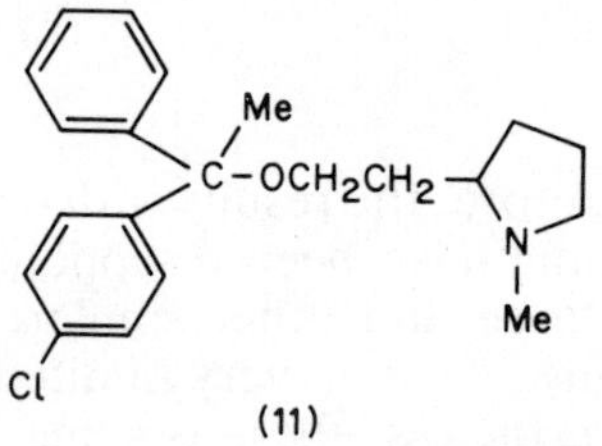

(11)

ON INDUCED BRONCHOCONSTRICTION

In 1946, Curry[67] first demonstrated that intravenous diphenhydramine could prevent histamine-induced bronchospasm in asthmatics. Similar results were obtained with inhaled diphenhydramine some years later[68] and, since then, it has been established that chlorpheniramine and clemastine can protect against histamine-induced bronchoconstriction, both in normal and in asthmatic subjects, whether given orally, intravenously or by inhalation[14–18,64,66,69–71].

Histamine is only one of the many mediators released during the immediate allergic response. It is perhaps not too surprising, therefore, that Schild and coworkers[72] found that, in excised human asthmatic bronchi, mepyramine was 10^4 times more potent in protecting against histamine than against antigen-induced bronchoconstriction and that, in early *in vivo* studies, tripelennamine and diphenhydramine had little effect on antigen-induced bronchospasm[73,74]. Oral chlorpheniramine 12 mg has been found recently to be similarly ineffective[75]. Nevertheless, once more H₁-receptor antagonists have proved to be more useful when given parenterally, rather than orally. Both Popa and Eiser have demonstrated that, when given in adequate dosage, 10–20 mg intravenously (i.v.), chlorpheniramine can prevent the early response to inhaled antigen[16,18,71]. Chlorpheniramine 20 mg i.v. provided protection against antigen-induced bronchospasm equivalent to that produced by the inhalation of disodium cromoglycate 20 mg (personal observation). Others have found that thiazinamium 25 mg intramuscularly (i.m.) and inhaled disodium cromoglycate 6 mg were equally effective[61].

The role of histamine as a mediator of exercise-induced asthma remains controversial. To date, the few reports concerning the protective effect of H_1-receptor antagonists on exercise-induced asthma have been somewhat inconclusive. No attentuation of the response to exercise was reported following mepyramine 50 mg i.m.[76], nor following oral chlorpheniramine 4 mg[77], whereas a decrease in expected bronchoconstriction was demonstrated after premedication with thiazinamium 50 mg i.m.[78], inhaled clemastine, 1 ml of 0.05% solution[79], and chlorpheniramine 10 mg and 20 mg i.v. (personal observation) and, again, the effect of the chlorpheniramine was comparable with that produced by disodium cromoglycate. Further work is needed to clarify the role of mediators in the production of exercise-induced asthma and the role of H_1-receptor antagonists in prophylaxis for this condition.

Why were the results of the early clinical trials so disappointing? The answer may be related to the relative non-specificity of these drugs and the facility with which they cross the blood-brain barrier. Similar peak blood levels of chlorpheniramine are achieved after administration of 4 mg i.v. and 12 mg p.o.[80]. However, as previously mentioned, after intravenous chlorpheniramine, bronchodilatation is dose dependent over a range of 2.5–10 mg and so, in order to achieve useful bronchodilatation with oral H_1-receptor antagonists, very large doses would be required. The associated sedation, also dose related, produced by most H_1-receptor antagonists makes the use of such doses unacceptable, except perhaps at night. Many years ago, Herxheimer[60] suggested that H_1-receptor antagonists might find a useful role in combating nocturnal asthma. This would appear reasonable, since histamine sensitivity and plasma histamine levels are greater by night than by day[81,82].

INHALED

It was Herxheimer[60] who recognized the potential advantage of giving H_1-receptor antagonists by inhalation rather than by mouth, in order to achieve higher local concentrations of the drug in the bronchi without the concomitant systemic effects. Unfortunately, with some of the H_1-receptor antagonists, relief of bronchial tone may be opposed and, therefore, reduced and even reversed, by either local irritation[83] or local histamine release. Church and Gradidge[84] observed histamine release in human lung *in vitro* in the presence of chlorpheniramine, diphenhydramine and other H_1-receptor antagonists and the concentrations of histamine obtained were within the range of those known to produce bronchial muscle constriction[85]. Furthermore, in clinical practice, some H_1-receptor antagonists, when given to patients by inhalation, have produced bronchospasm[86,87].

Apparently conflicting results have emerged from the studies of the effects of inhaled clemastine on the bronchial tone of asthmatics. Nogrady and colleagues[83] reported that inhaled clemastine 0.5 mg increased basal FEV_1 by 21%, as compared with 29% produced by salbutamol 5 mg. Their patients were in-patients recovering from acute asthma and so were in an unstable clinical state, with increased initial bronchomotor tone. The dose of the clemastine chosen was the maximum which did not produce throat irritation. The asthmatics in the subsequent studies were in a more stable condition with more normal initial lung function. Thus, Thomson and Kerr[15] reported only a 12% improvement in FEV_1 following inhaled clemastine, while Hartmann and colleagues[64] and Partridge and Saunders[88] observed no significant change. These results would be expected if the mechanism of action of the clemastine was to relieve the bronchial tone induced by continuous histamine release, since Nogrady's patients had increased initial bronchial tone, whereas the others did not. In particular, Hartmann's patients, pollen-sensitive asthmatics, were studied outside the pollen season when their lung function was normal and so their response to H_1-receptor antagonists might be expected to be the same as that of normal subjects. Furthermore, Partridge and Saunders gave their patients twice the dose of clemastine given by the others, which may have produced some local irritation.

The study in which inhaled clemastine was shown to protect against exercise-induced asthma[79] was mentioned previously.

Conclusions

H_1-receptor antagonists, when given in adequate dosage, can not only protect significantly against antigen- and exercise-induced asthma, but also produce bronchodilatation comparable with that seen after inhaled isoprenaline and salbutamol or after intravenous aminophylline. However, many factors govern the degree of bronchodilatation achieved with these drugs. These factors include marked individual variation in the response between asthmatic patients, the degree of pre-existing bronchial tone in the airways, the potency and specificity of the histamine antagonist and the dose and route by which the drug is given. What then is the role of the H_1-receptor antagonists in naturally occurring asthma?

At present the role of this class of drug appears limited. Most H_1-receptor antagonists are unsuitable for use during the day because of the marked sedation produced when they are given in adequate dosage. Nevertheless, they may find a place in the treatment of nocturnal asthma and the 'early morning dip'. In the future it is likely that new H_1-receptor antagonists will be developed which are more specific than those currently available. One promising, new, selective H_1-receptor antagonist is terfenadine(6). This drug exhibits no detectable antagonism against the H_2-receptor nor against α- and β-adrenergic receptors and has no demonstrable anti-cholinergic and anti-5-hydroxytryptamine activity[33]. Furthermore, terfenadine does not cross the blood–brain barrier[89,90]. Since this drug produces no significant sedation in doses up to 200 mg three times daily, it should be possible for the first time to carry out adequate dose–response studies to establish the efficacy of an oral H_1-receptor antagonist in asthma.

It is still unclear as to whether inhaled H_1-receptor antagonists have a place in the therapeutic armamentarium against asthma or not. Most of the known drugs are unsuitable because they are local irritants. The least irritant drug investigated so far, clemastine, produced tantalizing initial results in unstable asthmatics. These results require confirmation with careful dose–response studies in asthmatic patients with varying degrees of bronchoconstriction before any firm conclusions can be reached.

H_1-receptor antagonists have been with us for half a century. Yet, despite a wealth of experimental data, their role in the treatment of asthma remains nebulous. It is highly unlikely that even the more specific H_1-receptor antagonists will ever rival mast cell stabilizers, selective β_2-adrenergic stimulants and steroids as the mainstay of treatment for asthma.

Nevertheless, they may yet prove a useful adjunct to the treatment of difficult cases, particularly of nocturnal asthma.

References

1. DALE, H.H. and LAIDLOW, P.P. *Journal of Physiology*, **41,** 318 (1910)
2. DALE, H.H. and LAIDLOW, P.P. *Journal of Physiology*, **52,** 355 (1919)
3. FOURNEAU, E. and BOVET, D. *Archives Internationales de Pharmacodynamie et de Thérapie*, **46,** 178 (1933)
4. STAUB, A.-M. and BOVET, D. *Comptes Rendus des Seances de la Société Biologie et de ses Filiales*, **125,** 818 (1937)
5. HALPERN, B.N. *Archives Internationales de Pharmacodynamie et de Thérapie*, **68,** 339 (1942)
6. BOVET, D., HORCLOIS, R. and WALTHERT, F. *Comptes Rendus des Seances de la Société de Biologie et de ses Filiales*, **138,** 99 (1944)
7. LOEW, E.R., MacMILLAN, R. and KATSER, M.E. *Journal of Pharmacology and Experimental Therapeutics*, **86,** 229 (1946)
8. YONKMAN, F.F., CHESS, D., MATHIESON, D. and HANSEN, N. *Journal of Pharmacology and Experimental Therapeutics*, **87,** 256 (1946)
9. LOEW, E.R. and CHICKERING, O. *Proceedings of the Society for Experimental Biology and Medicine*, **48,** 65 (1941)
10. ASH, A.S.F. and SCHILD, H.O. *British Journal of Pharmacology*, **27,** 427 (1966)
11. BLACK, J.W., DUNCAN, W.A.M., DURANT, G.J., GANELLIN, C.R. and PARSONS, M.E. *Nature*, **236,** 385 (1972)
12. CHAKRIN, L.W. and KRELL, R.D. *H_2-antagonists in Peptic Ulcer Disease and Progress in Histamine Research*. Eds A. Torsoli, P.E. Lucchelli and R.W. Brimblecombe. p. 338. Amsterdam: Excerpta Medica (1980)
13. CHAND, N. *Advances in Pharmacology and Chemotherapy*, **17,** 103 (1980)
14. MACONOCHIE, J.G., WOODINGS, E.P. and RICHARDS, D.A. *British Journal of Clinical Pharmacology*, **7,** 231 (1979)
15. THOMSON, N.C. and KERR, J.W. *Thorax*, **35,** 428 (1980)
16. EISER, N.M., McRAE, K.D., SNASHALL, P.D. and GUZ, A. In *The Mast Cell: Its role in health and disease*. Eds J. Pepys and A.M. Edwards. p. 261. London: Pitman Medical (1979)
17. EISER, N.M., MILLS, J.M., McRAE, K.D., SNASHALL, P.D. and GUZ, A. *Clinical Science*, **58,** 537 (1980)
18. EISER, N.M., MILLS, J.M., SNASHALL, P.D. and GUZ, A. *Clinical Science*, **60,** 363 (1981)
19. NOGRADY, S.G. and BEVAN, C. *Thorax*, **36,** 268 (1981)
20. PEARLMAN, D.S. *Drugs*, **12,** 258 (1976)
21. WINDER, C.V., KAISER, M.E., ANDERSON, M.M. and GLASSCO, E.M. *Journal of Pharmacology and Experimental Therapeutics*, **87,** 121 (1946)
22. STONE, C.A., WENGER, H.C., LUDDEN, C.T., STAVORSKI, J.M. and ROSS, C.S. *Journal of Pharmacology and Experimental Therapeutics*, **131,** 73 (1961)
23. LEGGE, D.A., TIEDE, J.J., PETERS, G.A. and GEDGE, S.W. *Annals of Allergy*, **27,** 23 (1969)
24. NICKERSON, M. and COLLIER, B. In *The Pharmaceutical Basis of Therapeutics*. Eds L.S. Goodman and A. Gilman. p. 533. New York: Macmillan Publishing Company (1975)
25. FRANZ, D.N. In *The Pharmacological Basis of Therapeutics*. Eds L.S. Goodman and A. Gilman. p. 227. New York: Macmillan Publishing Company (1975)

26. CHINN, H.I. and SMITH, P.K. *Pharmacological Reviews*, **7**, 33 (1965)
27. LEAVITT, M.D. and CODE, C.F. *Journal of Laboratory and Clinical Medicine*, **32**, 334 (1947)
28. DOUGLAS, W.W. In *The Pharmacological Basis of Therapeutics*. Eds L.S. Goodman and A. Gilman. p. 590. New York: Macmillan Publishing Company (1975)
29. PARSONS, M.E. and OWEN, D.A.A. *International Symposium on Histamine H$_2$-Receptor Antagonists*. Eds C.J. Wood and M. Alison-Simpkins. p. 127. Welwyn: SK&F Labs (1973)
30. POWELL, J.R. and BRODY, M.J. *International Symposium on Histamine H$_2$-Receptor Antagonists*. Eds C.J. Wood and M. Alison-Simpkins. p. 137. Welwyn: SK&F Labs (1973)
31. LEVI, R. and CAPURRO, V. *International Symposium on Histamine H$_2$-Receptor Antagonists*. Eds C.J. Wood and M. Alison-Simpkins. p. 175. Welwyn: SK&F Labs (1973)
32. OWEN, D.A.A., FLYNN, S.B., GRISTWOOD, R.W., HARVEY, C.A. and WOODWARD, D.F. *Further Experience with H$_2$-receptor Antagonists in Peptic Ulcer Disease and Progress in Histamine Research*. Eds A. Torsoli, P.E. Luccheli and R.W. Brimblecome. p. 271. Amsterdam: Excerpta Medica (1980)
33. CHENG, H.C. and WOODWARD, J.K. *Drug Development Research*, **2**, 181 (1982)
34. WEISS, S., ROBB, G.P. and BLUMGART, H.L. *American Heart Journal*, **4**, 664 (1928)
35. BARTOSCHE, R., FELDBERG, W. and NAGEL, E. *Pflügers Archiv für die gesamte Physiologie des Menschen und der Tiere*, **230**, 129 (1932)
36. CODE, C.F. *American Journal of Physiology*, **127**, 78 (1939)
37. VALLERY-RADOT, P., HAMBURGER, J. and HALPERN, B. *Semaine des Hôpitaux Paris*, **24**, 655 (1948)
38. ARBESMAN, C.E. *New York State Journal of Medicine*, **47**, 1775 (1947)
39. HALPERN, B.N. and HAMBURGER, J. *Canadian Medical Association Journal*, **59**, 322 (1948)
40. KOELSCHE, G.A., PRICKMAN, L.E. and CARRYER, H.M. *Proceedings of Staff Meeting Mayo Clinic*, **20**, 432 (1945)
41. EYERMAN, C.H. *Journal of Allergy*, **17**, 210 (1946)
42. BERNSTEIN, T.B., ROSE, J.M. and FEINBERG, S.M. *Illinois Medical Journal*, **92**, 90 (1947)
43. LEVIN, S.L. *Journal of Allergy*, **17**, 145 (1946)
44. WALDBOTT, G.L. *Journal of Allergy*, **17**, 142 (1946)
45. LEVY, L. and SEABURY, J.H. *Journal of Allergy*, **18**, 244 (1947)
46. LEVIN, S.J. and MOSS, S.S. *Journal of Pediatrics*, **34**, 616 (1949)
47. COHEN, E.B., DAVIS, H.P. and MOWRY, W.A. *American Journal of Medicine*, **5**, 44 (1948)
48. CRIEP, L.H. and AARON, T.H. *Journal of Allergy*, **19**, 304 (1948)
49. STEINBERG, L. and GOTTESMAN, J. *Annals of Allergy*, **6**, 569 (1948)
50. ARBESMAN, C.E., KOEPF, G.F. and LENZNER, A.R. *Journal of Allergy*, **17**, 275 (1946)
51. FEINBERG, S.M. *Journal of the American Medical Association*, **132**, 702 (1946)
52. AMERICAN ACADEMY OF ALLERGY COMMITTEE ON THERAPY REPORT *Journal of Allergy*, **21**, 255 (1950)
53. DRUG COMMITTEE OF THE AMERICAN COLLEGE OF ALLERGISTS (CASEBOLT, J.; HOWARD, L.A.; MILLER, J.; LANOFF, G. and ROHR, J.H.) *Annals of Allergy*, **30**, 95 (1972)
54. KARLIN, J.M. *Annals of Allergy*, **30**, 342 (1972)
55. ENGLISHER, D.L. *New York State Journal of Medicine*, **47**, 1696 (1947)
56. EDITORIAL. *Lancet*, **ii**, 1182 (1955)
57. FEINBERG, S.M. *Annals of the New York Academy of Sciences*, **50**, 1186 (1950)
58. CHAI, H. *Chest*, **78**, 420 (1980)
59. CIRILLO, V.J. and TEMPERO, K.F. *American Journal of Hospital Pharmacy*, **33**, 1200 (1976)
60. HERXHEIMER, H. *British Medical Journal*, **ii**, 901 (1949)
61. BOOIJ-NOORD, H.O., ORIE, N.G.M., BERG, W. and DE VRIES, K. *Journal of Allergy*, **46**, 1 (1970)
62. SIMONSSON, B.G., *Acta Allergologica*, **19**, 305 (1964)
63. POPA, V.T. *Journal of Allergy and Clinical Immunology*, **59**, 54 (1977)
64. HARTMAN, N.V., MAGNUSSEN, H., HOLLE, J.P. and SCHÜLER, E. *Thorax*, **36**, 737 (1981)
65. KALLOS, P. *Clinical Trials Journal*, **8**, 23 (1971)
66. NOGRADY, S.G. and BEVAN, C. *Thorax*, **33**, 700 (1978)
67. CURRY, J.J. *Journal of Clinical Investigation*, **25**, 792 (1946)
68. CASTERLINE, C. and EVANS, R. *Journal of Allergy and Clinical Immunology*, **59**, 420 (1977)
69. SCHACHTER, E.N., BROWN, S., LACH, E. and GERSTEN HABER, B. *Chest*, **82**, 143 (1982)
70. WOENNE, R., KATTAN, M., ORANGE, R.P. and LEVISON, H. *Journal of Allergy and Clinical Immunology*, **62**, 119 (1978)
71. POPA, V.T. *Chest*, **78**, 442 (1980)
72. SCHILD, H.O., HAWKINS, D.F., MONGAR, J.L. and HERXHEIMER, H. *Lancet*, **ii**, 376 (1951)

73. SCHILLER, I.W. and LOWELL, F.C. *Annals of Allergy*, **5**, 564 (1947)
74. CURRY, J.J. and LOWELL, F.C. *Journal of Allergy*, **19**, 9 (1948)
75. LOWHAGEN, O. and LINDHOLM, N.B. *The Mast Cell: Its Role in Health and Disease*. Eds J. Pepys and A.M. Edwards. p. 332. London: Pitman Medical (1979)
76. McNEILL, R.S., NAIRN, J.R., MILLAR, J.S. and INGRAM, C.G. *Quarterly Journal of Medicine*, **35**, 55 (1966)
77. LEOPOLD, J.D., HARTLEY, J.P.R. and SMITH, A.P. *British Journal of Clinical Pharmacology*, **8**, 249 (1979)
78. ZIELINSKI, J. and CHODOSOWSKI, E. *Respiration*, **34**, 31 (1977)
79. HARTLEY, J.P.R. and NOGRADY, S.G. *Thorax*, **35**, 675 (1980)
80. PEETS, E.A., JACKSON, M. and SYMCHOWICZ, S. *Journal of Pharmacology and Experimental Therapeutics*, **180**, 364 (1972)
81. DE VRIES, K., GOEI, J.T., BOOIJ-NOORD, H. and ORIE, N.G.M. *Internal Archives of Allergy*, **20**, 93 (1962)
82. BARNES, P., FITZGERALD, G., BROWN, M. and DOLLERY, C. *New England Journal of Medicine*, **303**, 263 (1980)
83. NOGRADY, S.G., HARTLEY, J.P.R., HANDSLIP, P.D.J. and HURST, N.P. *Thorax*, **33**, 479 (1978)
84. CHURCH, M.K. and GRADIDGE, C.F. *British Journal of Pharmacology*, **66**, 68P (1979)
85. HAWKINS, D.F. *British Journal of Pharmacology*, **10**, 230 (1955)
86. CHARLIER, R. and PHILPPOT, E. *Archives Internationales de Pharmacodynamie et de Thérapie*, **78**, 559 (1949)
87. HERXHEIMER, H. *Management of Bronchial Asthma*. p. 52. London: Butterworths (1952)
88. PARTRIDGE, M.R. and SAUNDERS, K.B. *Thorax*, **34**, 771 (1979)
89. CHENG, H.C. and WOODWARD, J.K. *Arzneimittel-Forschung*, **32**, 1160 (1982)
90. WEICH, N.L. and MARTIN, J.S. *Arzneimittel-Forschung*, **32**, 1167 (1982)

Chapter 8

SRS-A antagonists

P. Sheard, M.C. Holroyde, J.R. Bantick and T.B. Lee

Development of FPL 55712

Slow-reacting substance of anaphylaxis (SRS-A, now known to consist primarily of a mixture of leukotrienes LTC_4 and LTD_4)[1] has long been considered to be an important mediator of anaphylactic/allergic reactions. The development of the Fisons compound FPL 55712, the first selective antagonist of SRS-A to be reported[2], followed directly on from work in our laboratories which had led to the introduction of the anti-asthma drug, sodium cromoglycate (1)[3].

A variety of tests were used at that time in attempting to evaluate potential anti-allergy/asthma activity of compounds which were synthesized in our laboratories. One such test was antagonism of SRS-A-induced contractions of isolated guinea-pig ileum preparations.

Although sodium cromoglycate, the disodium salt of a bischromone-2-carboxylic acid, inhibits mediator release during certain immediate hypersensitivity reactions in whole animals, and in animal and human tissues *in vitro*, it does not antagonize SRS-A (or indeed other putative mediators of such immediate hypersensitivity reactions). However, on testing a series of monochromone-2-carboxylic acids, one compound (2) showed weak but selective antagonist activity against SRS-A (with concentration producing 50% inhibition or $IC_{50} = 1.9 \times 10^{-4}M$)*.

Encouraged to continue routine screening for anti-SRS-A activity, our attention was drawn to compound (3), an analogue of sodium cromoglycate. The original batch of this compound showed relatively potent and selective SRS-A antagonist activity on the guinea-pig ileum [$IC_{50} = 1.3 \times 10^{-6}M$, based on the molecular weight of (3)].

Compound (3) was selected for further development and a large scale batch was synthesized. However, this newly synthesized material was found to have no activity as an antagonist of SRS-A at a concentration of $2 \times 10^{-4}M$. Analysis by thin-layer chromatography revealed that the large-scale batch was pure, but the original batch contained a trace of impurity

---

* Throughout this chapter drug activities are expressed in molar terms, and have been converted from other published units where necessary.

which was isolated, and its structure (4) was derived by proton magnetic resonance spectroscopy and mass spectrometry. Compound (4) proved to be a selective antagonist of SRS-A ($IC_{50} = 1 \times 10^{-7}$M) and it was confirmed that (4) had been responsible for all the apparent anti-SRS-A activity observed in the original batch of (3).

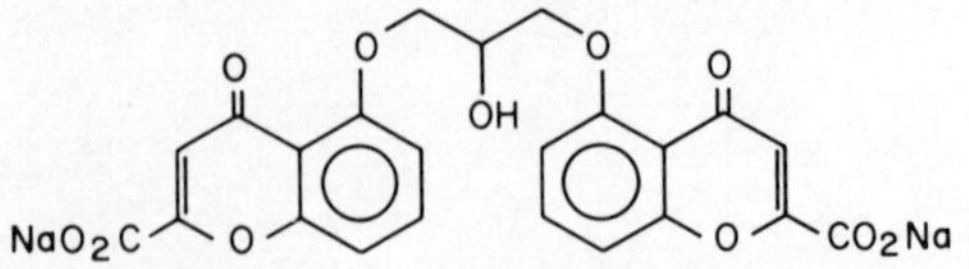

(1) 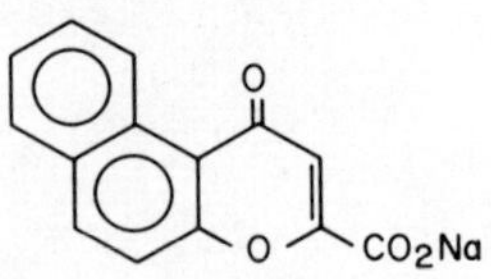   (2)

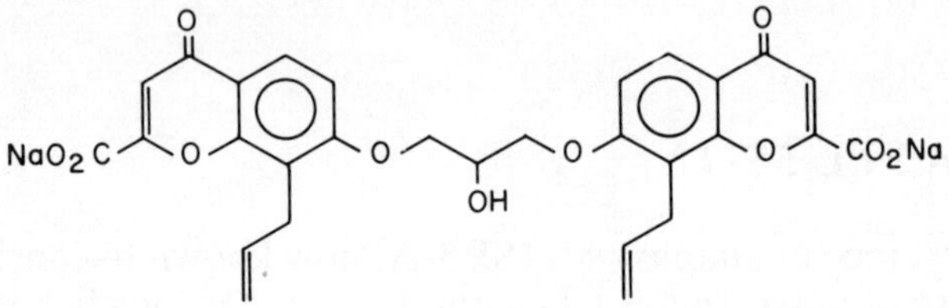

(3)

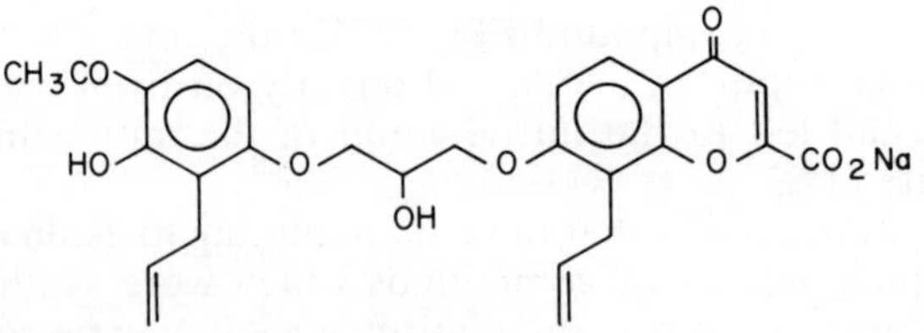

(4)

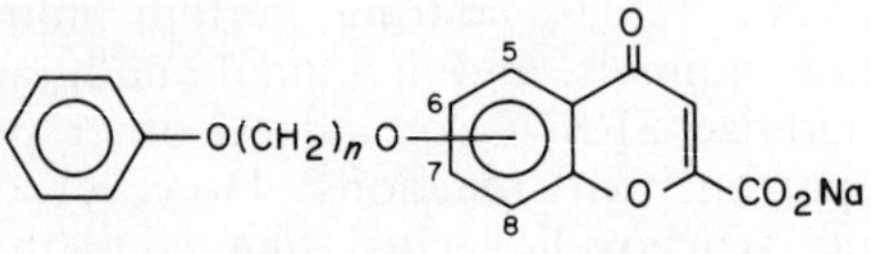

(5)

It was considered that a compound with similar or greater potency against SRS-A, a potentially important mediator of asthma and possibly other allergic reactions, might be a useful therapeutic substance. Thus, a specific structure–activity study based on (4) was initiated.

As a starting point for such work, compound (4) posed something of a problem in terms of the number of substituents present in the molecule. In order to simplify identification of the features contributing to activity, it was decided to take the basic skeleton of (4), an ω-phenoxyalkoxy-chromone-2-carboxylic acid, to optimize the activity of such a parent structure, and then reintroduce the substituent groups in a planned sequence to assess their relative importance.

From the parent structures, with varying chain lengths and substitution positions on the chromone ring (5), it was established that for substitution positions 5 and 7 there was a definite optimum, but at different chain lengths[4]. Chain elongation at substituent positions 6 and 8 was not proceeded with far enough to reach a peak of potency, but both series seemed intrinsically less active.

The most active compound (6) (*Table 8.1*) uncovered in these studies was linked in the 7-position, as in (4), but its five-carbon linking chain conferred much greater activity ($IC_{50} = 1 \times 10^{-6}M$) than was observed with (7) ($IC_{50} = 1.85 \times 10^{-5}M$), which contained the original hydroxyl-substituted three-carbon chain present in (4).

TABLE 8.1. Antagonist activities of compounds on guinea-pig ileum *in vitro*

Number	Compound	IC_{50} (μM)
6	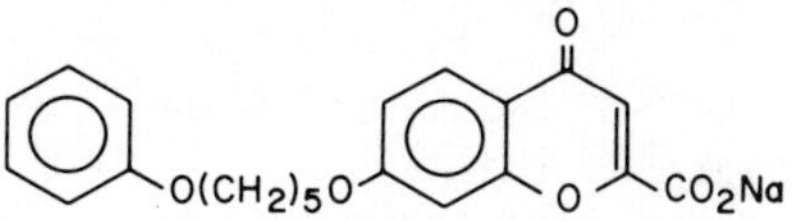 O(CH$_2$)$_5$O ... CO$_2$Na	1.0
7	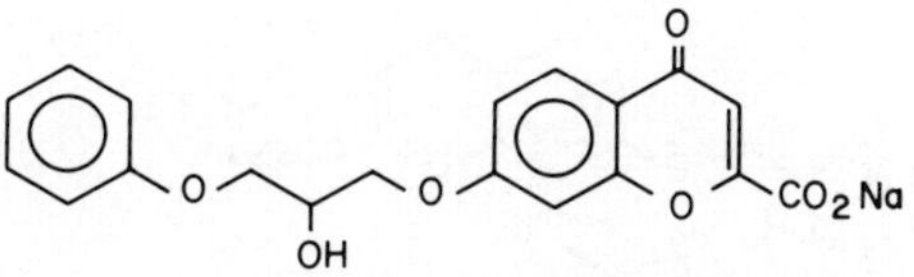 O ... OH ... O ... CO$_2$Na	18.5
8	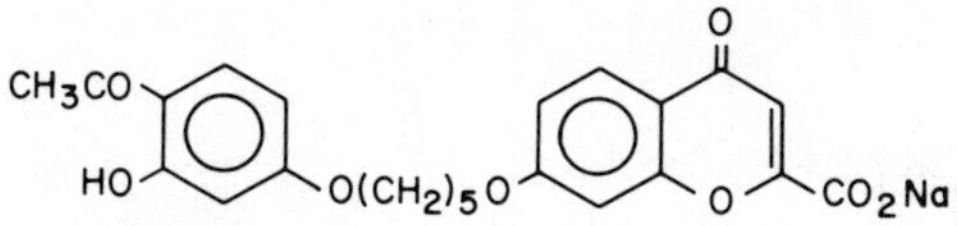 CH$_3$CO, HO ... O(CH$_2$)$_5$O ... CO$_2$Na	15
9	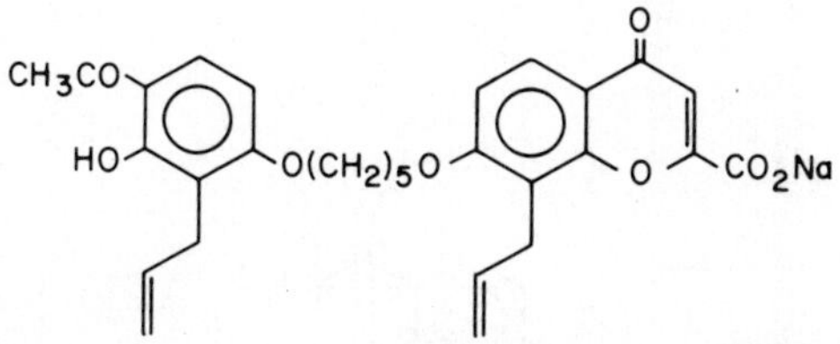 CH$_3$CO, HO ... O(CH$_2$)$_5$O ... CO$_2$Na	2.3

Surprisingly, addition of the acetyl, hydroxyl and allyl groups present in (4) to the optimum compound (6), led to a decrease in activity (compounds (8) and (9), *Table 8.1*). This approach was therefore abandoned, and attention was turned again to the original lead structure (4). Comparison of (8) with (9) indicated the contribution the allyl groups might be making to the activity of (4). Hence the allyl groups of (4) were chosen as a target for modification, the first being a simple reduction to propyl, which gave a compound (10) (FPL 55712) with increased potency (*Table 8.2*).

Many analogues of FPL 55712 were synthesized, but without further improvement in activity. However, the results served to reveal just how fortuitous the substitution pattern 2-alkyl-3-hydroxy-4-acetyl on the phenyl ring had been in the lead compound (4). Only when the 2-alkyl substituent

136

TABLE 8.2. Antagonist activities of compounds on guinea-pig ileum *in vitro*

Number	Compound	IC_{50} (μM)
10	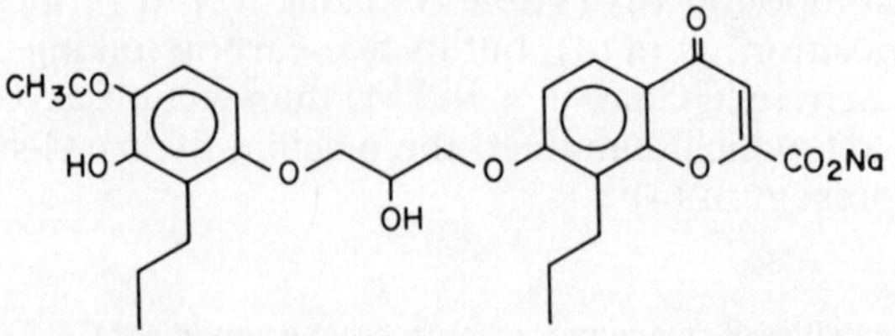 FPL 55712	0.01*
11	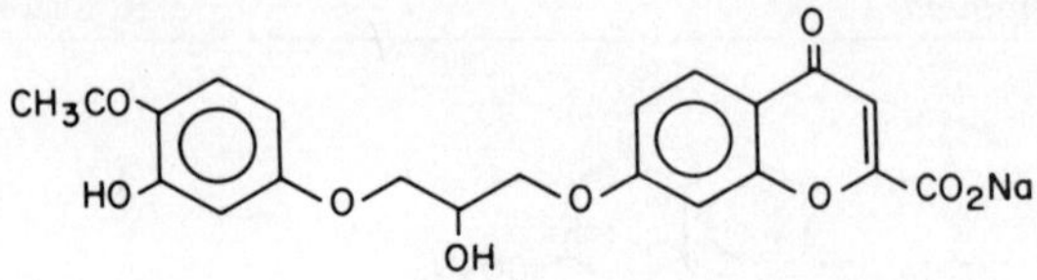	64
12	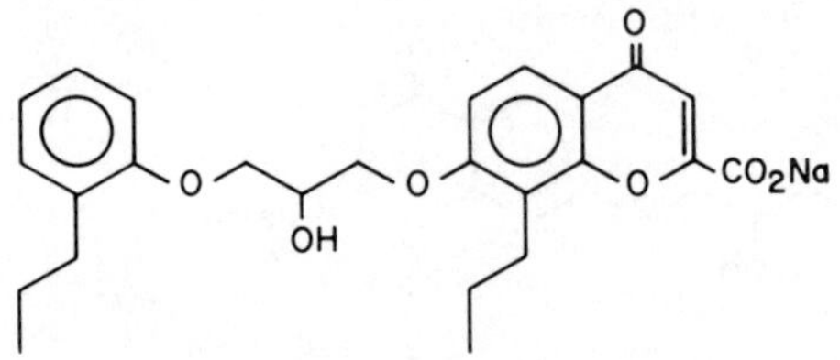	0.095
13	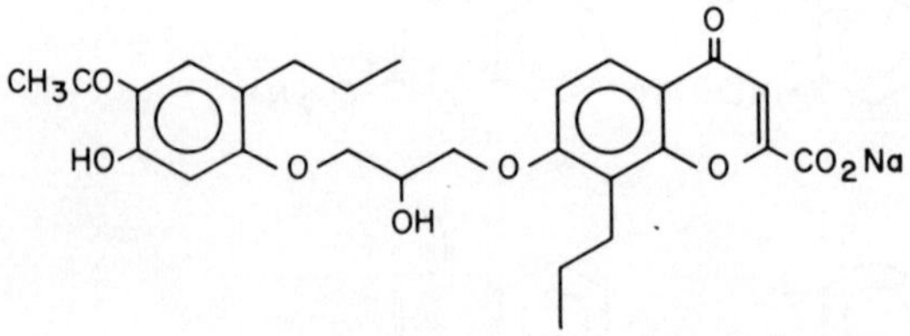	6.0
14	(a) R = H (b) R = nBu	0.23 3.6
15	(a) R_2 = Me, R_1 = OH (b) R_2 = H, R_1 = H	84 0.093

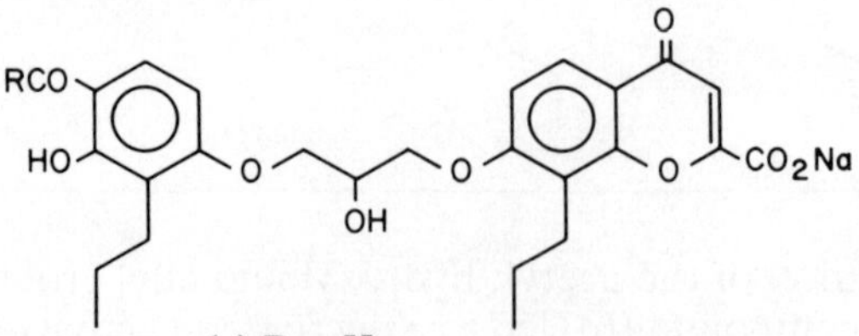

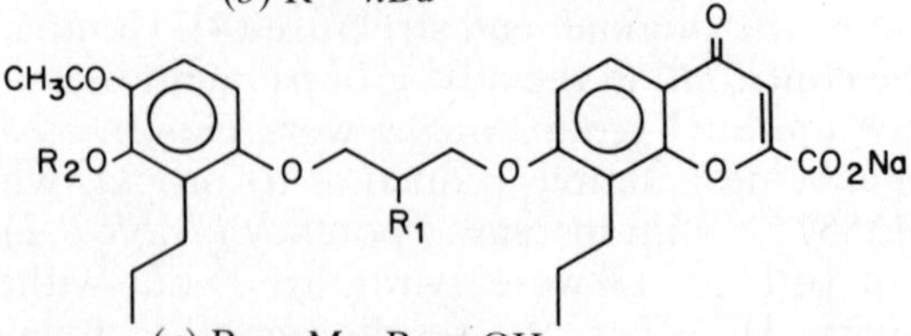

* Original result; *see* footnote to *Table 8.3*.

was also present on the phenyl ring did the vicinal-hydroxyacetyl combination confer enhanced activity. Illustrative of this are the compounds in *Table 8.2* where the vicinal-hydroxyacetyl grouping when alone had a marked detrimental effect [(11) compared with (7)], but in (10) the grouping further improved the already potent 2-alkylphenoxy compound (12).

Some indication of the optimum nature of the substituents and their positions is provided by (13) where the groups have an isomeric substitution pattern, by (14a) and (14b) with differing acyl groups, and by (15a) where the strong hydrogen bonding present in FPL 55712 between the hydroxyl and the adjacent carbonyl of the acetyl has been abolished.

An earlier observation[4] that removal of the chain hydroxyl from FPL 55712 increased potency was not borne out by subsequent retesting, which showed that the compound (15b) was less active.

Thus, in spite of the synthesis of a large number of analogues of (4), the most potent compound to emerge from the series, (10) (FPL 55712), only differed from (4) by a trivial chemical transformation.

Initial work showed that FPL 55712 was a very selective antagonist of the then uncharacterized slow-reacting substance of anaphylaxis in its action on the guinea-pig ileum (*Table 8.3*).

TABLE 8.3. Antagonist activity of FPL 55712 on guinea-pig ileum *in vitro*

Agonist	IC_{50} (μM) as mean $\pm$ s.e.m. of (n) observations		
SRS-A^{gp}	0.038 $\pm$	0.006*	(28)
LTD$_4$	0.064 $\pm$	0.008	(9)
Prostaglandin E$_1$	9.0 $\pm$	2.7	(5)
Prostaglandin F$_{2\alpha}$	9.4 $\pm$	5	(5)
Bradykinin	19 $\pm$	10	(5)
Acetylcholine	38 $\pm$	11	(5)
Histamine	41 $\pm$	11	(5)
5-Hydroxytryptamine	55 $\pm$	24	(5)

* Values from recent experiments. Over a number of years we have observed a slight decrease in the measured potency from that first quoted[2]; *see Table 8.2*.

The widely used sodium salt of FPL 55712 has maximum solubility in water at ambient temperatures of about 10^{-2}M and, for some applications, the several-fold more soluble lysine salt is advantageous[5]. In practice, the solubilization of the compound is often complicated by the presence of trace quantities of calcium and magnesium ions. The salts formed with these ions are extremely insoluble, and can cause problems with precipitation or cloudiness of the solution.

FPL 55712 is only minimally absorbed after oral dosing. An earlier communication[6] quoted the plasma half-life in guinea-pigs as 0.6 minutes after i.v. administration. Recently an improved method of analysis[7] of the distribution of radiolabelled FPL 55712 in the rat and the dog, following i.v. administration, revealed that the plasma concentration data were consonant with a two-compartment model with α and β phases of 5 minutes and 115 minutes for the dog, and 6 minutes and 99 minutes for the rat. In both species, FPL 55712 was excreted almost entirely via the bile, and there was no detectable metabolism of the compound. This rapid biliary clearance is consistent with the relatively high molecular weight of the compound and its high acidity (pK_a about 1.8) coupled with moderate lipophilicity (distribution coefficient between octanol and aqueous buffer at pH 7.4, log D = 1.92 ± 0.01).

Biological effects of FPL 55712

In vitro

GASTROINTESTINAL AND UTERINE PREPARATIONS

In the years since the first publication on FPL 55712, this compound has been extensively used by numerous groups as a pharmacological tool to identify the presence of SRS-A or peptidoleukotrienes. Consequently, the activity of FPL 55712 as a leukotriene antagonist has been examined on a number of tissues, particularly guinea-pig ileum, but also on rat gastrointestinal tissues and guinea-pig uterus. The data have been expressed in a variety of ways, and are summarized in *Table 8.4*. In some of these studies the type of antagonism, as indicated by analysis of Schild plots[23], was shown to be competitive[11,12,15,16].

TABLE 8.4. Antagonism of SRS-A or leukotriene-induced responses of gastrointestinal and uterine preparations *in vitro*

Agonist	$10^8 \times IC_{50}$ (M)	pA_2	$10^8 \times K_B$ (M)	Ref.
Guinea-pig ileum				
SRS-A^{gp}	1.0 ± 0.2 (5)			2
SRS-A^{gp}	3.8 ± 0.6 (28)			8
SRS-A^{dog}	circa 10.0			9
SRS-A^{monkey}			16.6 ± 8.2 (5)	10
SRS-A^{rat}		7.25 (5)		11
SRS-A^{rat}		7.5 (12)		12
SRS-A^{gp}			2.4 (7)	13
SRS-A^{rat}	1.1 ± 0.09 (4)			14
LTD$_4$	6.4 ± 0.8 (9)	7.33 ± 0.1 (12)	3.0 ± 0.3 (5)	8, 15
LTD$_4$		7.25 (7)	8.2 ± 0.7 (16)	16
LTD$_4$		7.1 ± 0.1		17
LTD$_4$	5.9			18
LTC$_4$		7.1 (2)		8
LTC$_4$		6.4 ± 0.1		19
LTE$_4$	3.5			20
LTE$_4$	4.0			18
Rat stomach				
SRS-A^{rat}		5.74 ± 6.90 (time dependent)		11
LTC$_4$		6.41*		21
LTD$_4$		6.67*		21
Rat colon				
LTC$_4$		6.61*		21
LTD$_4$		6.23*		21
Guinea-pig uterus				
LTD$_4$	960†			22

Results are expressed as mean ± s.e.m. of (*n*) observations where possible.
* Derived from data provided in publication.
† Significant inhibition produced by this dose, but not quantified.

AIRWAYS PREPARATIONS

The belief that leukotrienes may be important in the pathogenesis of asthma has focused attention on the activity of leukotrienes and FPL 55712 on isolated airways preparations from animals and man. The data obtained from such experiments are often difficult to compare due to the diverse experimental designs, but the results from experiments using guinea-pig tissues are summarized in *Table 8.5*. Once again, it should be noted that, in at least one of the investigations using guinea-pig trachea, the antagonist activity of FPL 55712 was shown to be competitive[16] and was stated to be 'apparently competitive' in a second[25].

TABLE 8.5. Antagonism of SRS-A or leukotriene-induced responses of guinea-pig isolated airways preparations

Agonist	$10^7 \times IC_{50}$ (M)	pA_2	$10^7 \times K_B(M)$	Ref.
Lung parenchymal strip				
SRS-A^{gp}	1.74 ± 0.38 (7)			8
SRS-A^{rat}		7.04 (6)		12
SRS-A^{gp}			11 (5)	13
SRS-A^{gp}	$< 20^a$			24
LTD$_4$	$< 20^a$			24
LTD$_4$	15.6 ± 2.2 (4)			8
LTD$_4$		6.03 (5)	10.01 ± 1.67 (13)	16
LTD$_4$		6.93 (6)	3.95 ± 1.72 (6)	25
LTD$_4$		6.96^b		26
LTC$_4$	$-^c$			25
LTC$_4$	$-^c$			26
Trachea				
LTD$_4$		6.51 (8)	5.79 ± 0.78 (13)	16
LTD$_4$			3.7 (3)	25
LTD$_4$		circa 5.6^b		27
LTC$_4$	9.6 (6)^d			25
LTC$_4$		6.9 ± 0.1 (5)		19

Results are expressed as mean ± s.e.m. of (*n*) observations where possible.
[a] Response abolished by this concentration.
[b] Derived from data provided in publication.
[c] Responses not antagonized by FPL 55712.
[d] Significant inhibition produced by this concentration; higher concentrations enhanced response.

Human tissue has been used less frequently. Using preparations of human bronchus, Sheard *et al.*[8] obtained an IC$_{50}$ of $(4.4 \pm 0.6) \times 10^{-7}$M (mean ± s.e.m., $n = 3$) against SRS-A derived from guinea-pig lungs. Dahlen *et al.*[28] showed that contractions induced by both LTC$_4$ and LTD$_4$ were reversed by $(1-10) \times 10^{-6}$M FPL 55712, and identical findings were obtained by Jones *et al.*[29]. Hanna *et al.*[30] obtained qualitatively similar results, although reportedly requiring a high concentration of 2.6×10^{-4}M for complete reversal of the response. Lung parenchymal strips were also used by Sheard *et al.*[8], who obtained an IC$_{50}$ of $(6.6 \pm 1.0) \times 10^{-7}$M ($n = 5$) against SRS-A^{gp} and 1.2×10^{-6}M in a single experiment using LTD$_4$. Jones *et al.*[29] also employed human trachea, and found that responses to both LTC$_4$ and LTD$_4$ could be partially inhibited by pretreatment of the tissue with $(2-4) \times 10^{-6}$M FPL 55712, and that established responses could be partially reversed by concentrations of $(0.5-10) \times 10^{-6}$M. Concentrations greater than 2×10^{-5}M were required for complete reversal.

CARDIOVASCULAR PREPARATIONS

Although SRS-A has traditionally been viewed in terms of its pulmonary activity, increasing attention is being paid to its actions on the cardiovascular system. In isolated perfused guinea-pig hearts, the reduction in contractility and coronary flow produced by both LTC_4 and LTD_4 is antagonized by FPL 55712, although only single concentrations have been used to date. In one study, a concentration of $4.8 \times 10^{-7}M$ antagonized LTD_4 more effectively than LTC_4[31], whereas in another study using $3.8 \times 10^{-6}M$ the reverse order of activity was obtained[32]. Kito et al.[33] showed that contractile responses of isolated rabbit coronary arteries to LTD_4 were inhibited dose dependently by FPL 55712 and, using the data in their publication, an approximate pA_2 of 7.3 can be calculated (as described by Van den Brink and Lien[34]). Guinea-pig pulmonary arteries are also contracted by LTC_4 and LTD_4; a single concentration of $1 \times 10^{-5}M$ FPL 55712 was shown to inhibit the response to LTC_4 [$K_B = (5-10) \times 10^{-7}M$] but not that to LTD_4[35]. Although human intracranial arteries have been shown to contract to LTD_4, any effect of FPL 55712 on this response is complicated by the reported direct relaxant effect of the antagonist at a concentration of $1 \times 10^{-6}M$[36]. This response appears to be unique and requires confirmation.

ENZYME INHIBITION

A number of studies have been carried out on the ability of FPL 55712 to inhibit a variety of enzymes as summarized in *Table 8.6*. It should not be assumed automatically that such activity occurs *in vivo*, since in only one of

TABLE 8.6. Inhibition of enzyme activity

Enzyme	Arachidonic acid metabolite assayed	Source	IC_{50} (μM)	Ref.
Cyclic-AMP phospho-diesterase		Rat brain	3	37
Cyclic-GMP phospho-diesterase		Rat brain	13	37
PG synthetase	PGD_2	Cell-free homogenate from RBL-1 cells	No effect at 100	38
PG synthetase	PGD_2	Guinea-pig pulmonary anaphylaxis	No effect at 10	39
PG synthetase	PGE_2	Bull seminal vesicle microsomes	10	40
PG synthetase	PGE_2	Bull seminal vesicle microsomes	circa 6	41
Thromboxane synthetase	TxB_2	Human platelet microsomes	6.5	42
5-Lipoxygenase	5-HETE	Cell-free homogenate from RBL-1 cells	21	38
5-Lipoxygenase	5-HETE	Intact human neutrophil—ionophore stimulated	70 (no effect at 10–20)	41
12-Lipoxygenase	12-HETE	Human platelet microsomes	100	43

the studies in which enzyme inhibition was reported was an intact cell preparation used and in this study FPL 55712 was only weakly active[41].

It is interesting that FPL 55712 appears to have an inhibitory effect on the generation of PGE_2 and thromboxanes, but not on the production of PGD_2. These results need verification but imply that FPL 55712 has a selective inhibitory effect on certain of the specific terminal enzymes associated with the cyclo-oxygenase pathway.

The pharmacological relevance of these enzyme inhibitory studies is not known.

In vivo

RESPIRATORY

The contraction of airways smooth muscle produced by leukotrienes is inhibited by FPL 55712, not only *in vitro*, but also *in vivo*. The compound is not absorbed orally and so has to be given intravenously or by aerosol. Furthermore, due to its short plasma half-life (*see above*), the compound must be administered shortly before the agonist. The respiratory actions of FPL 55712 have been studied primarily in the guinea-pig and are summarized in *Table 8.7*.

Although most groups agree that FPL 55712 has a short duration of action when given intravenously (e.g. 5.5 min at 1.9×10^{-6} mol/kg[20]), substantial inhibition was reported by Feniuk *et al.*[46] 30 min after a dose of 1.9

TABLE 8.7. Inhibition of SRS-A or leukotriene-induced bronchoconstriction in anaesthetized guinea-pigs by FPL 55712

Agonist and route of administration	FPL 55712: route of administration	Time interval[a]	ID_{50} ($\mu mol/kg$)	Ref.
SRS-A[gp] i.v.	i.v.	30 s	9.6[b]	44
SRS-A[gp] aerosol	i.v.	I	25.6 ± 5.0[c]	8
LTD_4 i.v.	i.v.	?	1–3[d]	45
LTD_4 i.v.	i.v.	30 s	1.9–19[e]	46
LTD_4 i.v.	i.v.	?	3.5	18
LTD_4 i.v.	i.v.	?	3.8	47
LTD_4 i.v.	aerosol[f]	?	9.6 mM	48
LTD_4 aerosol[g]	i.v.	I	24	15
LTD_4 aerosol[g]	aerosol[h]	5 min	35 s nebulization[i]	15
LTC_4 i.v.	i.v.	2 min	< 1.9[j]	49
LTC_4 i.v.	i.v.	?	11.5	47
LTE_4 i.v.	i.v.	30 s	0.38	20
LTE_4 i.v.	i.v.	?	2.1	18
LTE_4 i.v.	i.v.	?	1.9	47
LTE_4 i.v.	aerosol[f]	?	15 mM	48

ID_{50} given in $\mu mol/kg$ unless otherwise stated.
[a] Interval between administration of antagonist and leukotriene; I = immediate.
[b] This dose produced significant but unquantified inhibition.
[c] Mean ± s.e.m., $n = 5$.
[d] Animals pretreated with 0.28 mmol/kg indomethacin.
[e] Dose-dependent inhibition seen over this dose range. Animals pretreated with indomethacin 14 $\mu mol/kg$ and propranolol 1.2 $\mu mol/kg$ i.v.
[f] Duration of nebulization or dose delivered not specified.
[g] 1.6 μM solution nebulized ultrasonically for 2 min.
[h] 8 mM solution nebulized for various times.
[i] Corresponds to dose of 98 nmol/kg delivered to trachea.
[j] 1.9 $\mu mol/kg$ inhibited response to LTC_4 by 66% ($n = 3$).

$\times\ 10^{-5}$ mol/kg. Similarly, when given by aerosol, FPL 55712 was reported to have a surprisingly long half-life of 120 min against LTD_4[48], whereas our own studies[15] indicate a half-life (against nebulized LTD_4) of 10–15 min. In general the balance of the evidence suggests that FPL 55712 has a short duration of action.

CARDIOVASCULAR

The potent action of LTD_4 in producing coronary vasoconstriction (previously demonstrated *in vitro*) has also been shown *in vivo* in anaesthetized sheep[50]. Injection of LTD_4 into the left circumflex coronary artery produced profound coronary vasoconstriction and impaired regional ventricular contraction. These responses were not affected by pretreatment with ibuprofen, but FPL 55712 $1.9\ \times\ 10^{-6}$ mol/kg i.v. administered 2–5 min before LTD_4 abolished the coronary vasoconstriction and partially inhibited the impairment of contractility[50].

Similar results were obtained in anaesthetized pigs by Boyd *et al.*[51], who showed that bolus intracoronary injections of FPL 55712 $(0.19–1.9)\ \times\ 10^{-6}$ mol inhibited dose dependently the coronary vasoconstrictor action of LTD_4.

Several groups have described increased cutaneous vascular permeability in response to intradermal injections of leukotrienes, either alone or admixed with a vasodilator such as prostaglandin E_2. Patterson *et al.*[52] produced wheals on the skin of anaesthetized monkeys with SRS-A derived from rats, and demonstrated dose-dependent inhibition of the response by FPL 55712, using doses of $(1.9–192)\ \times\ 10^{-12}$ mol admixed with the SRS-A. Morley *et al.*[53] showed similar inhibition in conscious guinea-pigs using FPL 55712 $(0.19–192)\ \times\ 10^{-10}$ mol to antagonize responses to $LTC_4 \times PGE_2$, $LTD_4 + PGE_2$, and SRS-A^{rat}. Peck *et al.*[54] also demonstrated inhibition by FPL 55712 $(2 \times 10^{-8}$ mol in 0.1 ml) of the cutaneous response in guinea-pigs to LTD_4 $(2 \times 10^{-10}$ mol in 0.1 ml), mixed with PGE_2 $(8.5 \times 10^{-10}$ mol in 0.1 ml).

FPL 55712 also inhibits cutaneous responses to leukotrienes when given intravenously. In guinea-pigs, ID_{50} (the dose producing 50% inhibition) doses of 1.6×10^{-5} mol/kg versus LTD_4 and 2.1×10^{-5} mol/kg versus LTE_4 were reported by Crowley *et al.*[18]. In rats, the same authors reported values of 1.2×10^{-5} mol/kg versus LTD_4 and 7.3×10^{-6} mol/kg versus LTE_4. The latter value contrasts with the value of 2.3×10^{-6} mol/kg reported earlier by the same group[20].

NEURAL

The possible interaction of leukotrienes with nerve function has so far received little attention. However, Palmer *et al.*[55] revealed that LTC_4 produces a unique prolonged excitation of cerebellar Purkinje neurones in the rat following local administration by pressure ejection from a micropipette. This response could be prevented or reversed by local application of a $2 \times 10^{-5}M$ solution of FPL 55712. Subsequently, the same group showed that LTD_4, but not LTB_4, produces a similar response, which is also inhibited by FPL 55712[56]. The physiological relevance of these observations is unknown but clearly deserves further study.

Mucociliary function

Inhalation of allergens by sensitized dogs[57] and asthmatic humans[58] produces a reduction in tracheal mucus velocity which can be prevented by inhalation of FPL 55712. These studies provided the first indirect evidence that SRS-A may be involved in mucus production and/or transport.

Subsequently, Peatfield et al.[59] demonstrated a dose-dependent stimulation by LTC_4 of mucin output in the tracheas of anaesthetized cats. FPL 55712 was tested at a single concentration of $9.5 \times 10^{-6}M$ and was found to inhibit only the response to the highest dose of LTC_4 used ($6 \times 10^{-5}M$). LTC_4 had no effect in vitro on isolated pieces of cat trachea. In contrast, both LTC_4 and LTD_4 have been reported to produce dose-dependent increases in mucous glycoprotein secretion from cultured human airways in vitro[60]. Responses to both leukotrienes were substantially reduced in the presence of FPL 55712 at $1.9 \times 10^{-7}M$. Furthermore, Johnson et al.[61] have shown that FPL 55712 1.9×10^{-6} mol/kg significantly inhibits the stimulation of tracheal mucus secretion produced by local arterial injection of LTC_4 in anaesthetized dogs.

Mast-cell-stabilizing activity

IN VITRO

FPL 55712 has been shown to inhibit the release of histamine induced by dextran plus phosphatidylserine from rat peritoneal mast cells (IC_{50} circa $1 \times 10^{-7}M$)[62] and the antigen-induced release of histamine from passively sensitized rat peritoneal mast cells (IC_{50} $3.5 \times 10^{-7}M$)[48]. In both of these studies, FPL 55712 was in fact more active than sodium cromoglycate. FPL 55712 also inhibited the antigen-induced release of histamine from fragmented rat, dog and monkey lung[63] and fragmented guinea-pig lung[42]. In the experiments with rat lung, FPL 55712 produced a flat concentration–response curve with approximately 40% inhibition of histamine release over the concentration range $(0.1–100) \times 10^{-6}M$. With dog lung, a bell-shaped concentration–response curve was obtained with maximum inhibition of 50% at $1 \times 10^{-6}M$, while with monkey and guinea-pig lung, normal concentration–response curves were obtained but maximum inhibition of only 29 and 34%, respectively, was obtained at $1 \times 10^{-4}M$.

Like sodium cromoglycate, FPL 55712 did not inhibit anti-IgE-induced histamine release from human leucocytes at concentrations up to $1 \times 10^{-3}M$[62].

IN VIVO

When tested in rat passive cutaneous anaphylaxis (PCA), FPL 55712 was shown to possess weak anti-allergic activity (the dose producing 50% inhibition or $ED_{50} = 1.1 \times 10^{-5}$ mol/kg i.v.)[64]. By comparison, in the same experiment, sodium cromoglycate was about ten times more active. In rat passive lung anaphylaxis (PLA), FPL 55712 at a dose of 2×10^{-5} mol/kg i.v. was shown to produce 49% inhibition of antigen-induced bronchoconstriction, compared with an ED_{50} for sodium cromoglycate of 2.4×10^{-6} mol/kg i.v.[65]. When given by aerosol the ED_{50} values of FPL

55712 and sodium cromoglycate as inhibitors of IgE-mediated bronchoconstriction in rats were 3.8×10^{-2}M and 1.9×10^{-4}M, respectively[66].

It has also been shown in our laboratories that, when inhaled as an aqueous aerosol from a 10^{-2}M solution 10 minutes before antigen, FPL 55712 inhibited the antigen-induced fall in FEV_1 in an asthmatic volunteer by 60%.

The activity of FPL 55712 in each of these *in vivo* models could be claimed to have been due to its property of antagonizing SRS-A at receptor sites in the skin and lung. However, in another *in vivo* model, that of rat passive peritoneal anaphylaxis, FPL 55712 was shown to possess genuine mast-cell-stabilizing activity albeit weaker than that of sodium cromoglycate: ED_{50} values (inhibition of histamine release) $= 3.2 \times 10^{-8}$ mol per rat i.p. for FPL 55712 and 5.2×10^{-9} mol per rat i.p. for sodium cromoglycate[67].

It is perhaps not surprising that FPL 55712 should retain some of the mast-cell-stabilizing activity associated with other chromone derivatives such as sodium cromoglycate. This activity is most pronounced in rat peritoneal mast cells. It is less marked in whole tissues particularly those of the guinea-pig and monkey. However, this intrinsic mast-cell-stabilizing activity which FPL 55712 possesses must be taken into account when the compound is used as an investigative tool in experimental models of anaphylaxis.

Toxicology

In acute toxicity studies in mice and rats, the approximate intravenous median lethal dose of FPL 55712 was $(3.8–5.8) \times 10^{-4}$ mol/kg. There were no deaths at 2×10^{-4} mol/kg or less. Following oral administration there were no deaths at the maximum dose tested of 3.8×10^{-3} mol/kg. In a variety of pharmacological studies, the compound had no specific or potent effect on the major physiological systems of the body.

Administration of $(0.08–1.9) \times 10^{-5}$ mol/kg per day for 28 days to rats (s.c.) or dogs (i.v.) produced no systemic toxicity, although the rats displayed dose-dependent irritant or necrotic lesions at the site of injection.

Single and multiple (52 days) dose-inhalation studies in rats gave no evidence of irritation or cytotoxic potential on the respiratory tract or of systemic toxicity.

Inhalation of the compound as an aqueous aerosol of solutions of the lysine salt of up to 6.2×10^{-2}M for 5 minutes, by normal volunteers, gave no evidence of irritation of either the upper or lower respiratory tract.

Characterization of leukotriene receptors

The extreme potency of the leukotrienes, the unequal distribution of responsive tissues throughout the body (some smooth muscles are completely unresponsive to leukotrienes), and the discovery that minor alterations of some parts of the leukotriene molecule lead to drastic changes in activity, have led to the belief that leukotrienes act on discrete receptors. Although such receptors have not been rigorously characterized, nor their existence proven, it is convenient to assume their existence when considering the action of leukotrienes. Many synthetic analogues of LTD_4 and LTC_4 have been examined[68–70] and have allowed some of the requirements for optimal receptor fit to be established.

In the light of these findings, it is interesting to consider the activity of FPL 55712 and its influence on the characterization of putative leukotriene receptor subtypes.

FPL 55712 displays antagonism on various tissues of not only LTC_4, LTD_4 and LTE_4 but also a variety of leukotriene analogues which vary considerably in agonist potency. These analogues include the sulphones of LTC_4, LTD_4 and LTE_4[71]; LTC_5[72]; LTC_3, and 11-$trans$-LTC_3[73], $(5R,6S)$-LTD_4, $(5R,6R)$-LTD_4, 11-$trans$-LTD_4 and $(5R,6S)$-11-$trans$-LTD_4[27]. These results are consistent with the concept that FPL 55712 acts at a single receptor which is stimulated by several leukotriene analogues, each of which has a different affinity for the receptor. However, there is mounting evidence that there may be more than one receptor type activated by these peptidoleukotrienes. For instance, responses of airways preparations to SRS-A or LTD_4 in $vitro$ appear to be significantly less sensitive than ileum to inhibition by FPL 55712[12,16,74]. The receptor in rat fundus also appears to be less sensitive to inhibition than that in guinea-pig ileum[11].

In the guinea-pig lung parenchymal strip, Drazen et $al.$[26] reported that LTD_4 produced a biphasic dose–response curve of which only the initial phase was inhibited dose dependently by FPL 55712, while LTC_4-induced responses were not antagonized. This led to the suggestion that there may be two receptors in this tissue with only one being sensitive to FPL 55712. These results have been essentially confirmed by Krell et $al.$[25]. However, it should be noted that, in contrast to these findings, inhibition of LTC_4-induced responses of guinea-pig lung parenchymal strips has been reported with FPL 55712 at concentrations of $2 \times 10^{-6} M$[75] and higher (up to 2×10^{-5} M)[76].

Using guinea-pig tracheal preparations, Krell et $al.$[25] found that LTC_4 produced a biphasic dose–response curve with only the initial phase being antagonized by FPL 55712. LTD_4-induced responses in this tissue were inhibited in an apparently competitive manner by FPL 55712.

It is worth noting that the chemoattractant leukotriene LTB_4, which is present in impure preparations of SRS-A[77], also contracts guinea-pig lung parenchymal strips, but by a thromboxane-dependent mechanism[78] which is not inhibited by FPL 55712[75,79]. The chemokinetic effect of LTB_4 on human neutrophils is also not inhibited by FPL 55712[80]. These data suggest that the LTB_4 receptor (if such a discrete receptor exists) is probably distinct from other leukotriene receptors.

Amongst vascular tissues, FPL 55712 is reported to antagonize contractile responses of guinea-pig pulmonary artery to LTC_4 but not to LTD_4[35]. Intriguingly, dog coronary arteries have been reported to relax in response to LTC_4 and LTD_4, but neither response was inhibited by up to $5 \times 10^{-7} M$ FPL 55712[31]. This deserves investigation with higher concentrations of antagonist.

The process of identifying and classifying leukotriene receptors is only just beginning, but clearly there is already suggestive evidence that multiple receptors or receptor subtypes may exist, with differing affinities for both agonists and antagonists. This has important implications for the therapeutic applications of SRS-A antagonists, as the development of more selective antagonists may allow more selective treatment of disorders in which leukotrienes are shown to play a role. In particular, FPL 55712 may not represent the optimal configuration for activity at airways leukotriene receptors.

Other antagonists of SRS-A

Since the intial publication[2] on FPL 55712, several groups of workers have used the structure as a basis for further modification to improve the range of activity or bioavailability profile. The iodo-substituted derivative (16) was found to be a slightly less potent SRS-A antagonist on the guinea-pig trachea, but to possess a different selectivity profile against other agonists (*Table 8.8*)[81]. In an inbred asthmatic rat assay *in vivo*, the iodo compound ($ED_{50} = 4.6 \times 10^{-6}$ mol/kg i.v.) was over three times as active as FPL 55712 at inhibiting antigen-induced bronchoconstriction[82].

TABLE 8.8. Antagonist activity of FPL 55712 and compound 16 on guinea-pig trachea *in vitro*

Agonist	ED_{50} (μM)	
	FPL 55712	(16)
SRS-A	0.33	1.46
$PGF_{2\alpha}$	14.6	234
Histamine	455	35
5-Hydroxytryptamine	39	31
Acetylcholine	> 800	> 600

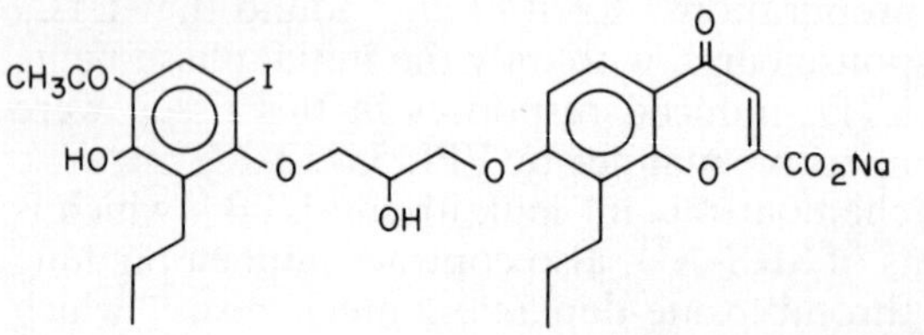

Other workers have sought to develop SRS-A antagonists with greater mast-cell-stablizing activity than FPL 55712, by adding the ω-phenoxyalkoxy chain of FPL 55712 and its attendant substituents onto structures possessing high levels of activity as inhibitors of mediator release.

Several structures which incorporate cyclic 1,3-dicarbonyl-2-nitro or -2-cyano systems, and are potentially capable of conferring mast-cell-stabilizing activity have been utilized in this way. Representative compounds are shown in *Table 8.9*. For compounds in the 3-nitrocoumarin series represented by (17), an extensive structure–activity study of antagonism on the guinea-pig ileum has been reported[67]. The conclusions concerning the features important for activity were remarkably similar to those

TABLE 8.9. Antagonist activity of compounds on guinea-pig ileum *in vitro*

No.	Compound	$10^8 \times IC_{50}$ (M)
17	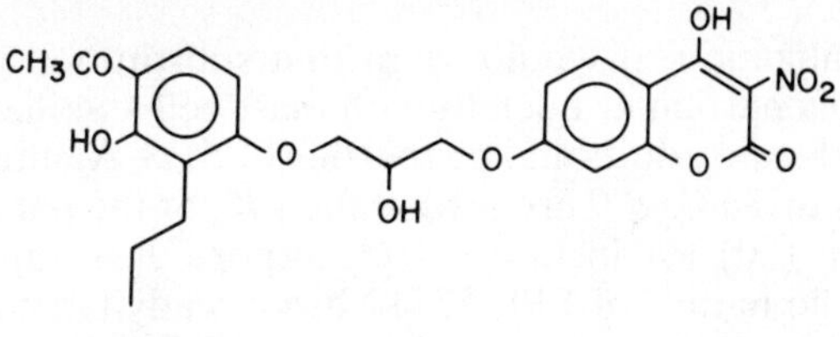	8
18	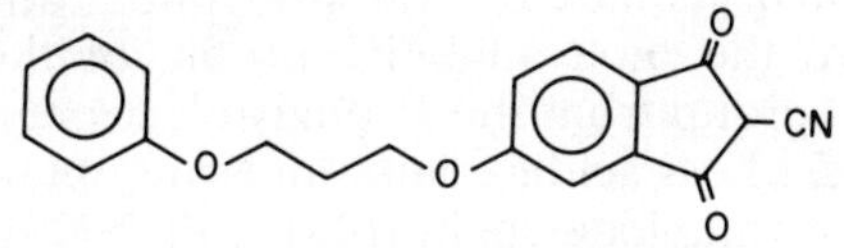	90
19	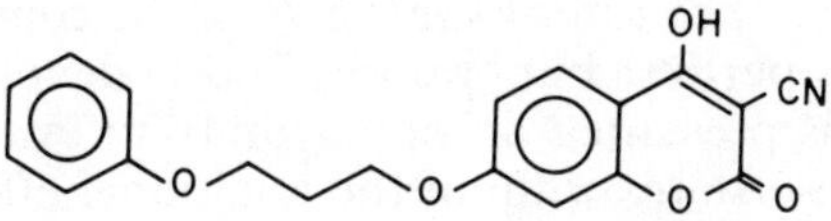	200
20	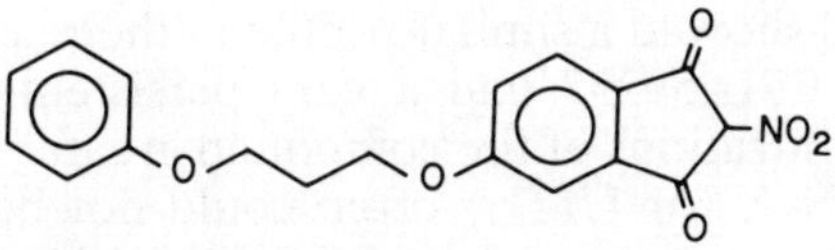	10
21	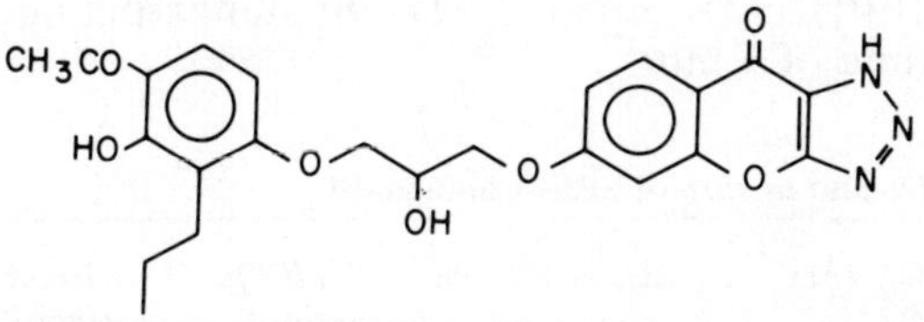	6.3

for the chromone-2-carboxylic acid series[4]. Optimum activity was associated with the same linking chain and substituent pattern around the phenyl ring as in FPL 55712.

SRS-A antagonist activity was further maximized (three-fold enhancement over (17)) by the addition of an 8-methyl substituent to the nitrocoumarin nucleus. Selected compounds of the series possessed high levels of mast-cell-stabilizing activity as evidenced by the rat passive peritoneal anaphylaxis test, where (17) for instance, with an ED_{50} of 6.5×10^{-10} mol per rat, was over eight times more potent than sodium cromoglycate (*see* p. 144).

Compounds containing the FPL 55712 side-chain were not described in the series represented by (18) and (19)[83] and, in the series represented by (20)[84], the activity for the FPL 55712 analogue was not reported. However, it seems reasonable to expect from the examples given in *Table 8.9* that such compounds would be potent antagonists. The benzopyrano[2,3-*d*]-*v*-triazoles represented by (21)[85] also appear to combine SRS-A antagonism with the mast-cell-stabilizing properties of the parent heterocyclic nucleus[86], although the latter activity is rather weak for (21) and the other examples quoted.

Hence, as a generalization, it would seem that substitution of the FPL 55712 side-chain onto a particular nucleus with mast-cell-stabilizing activity will confer on the molecule additional properties of SRS-A antagonism.

All the compounds in *Table 8.9* are acidic, the pK_a of the parent nitroin-dandione of structure (20) for instance being reported as approximately 1[87]. The strongly acidic nature of FPL 55712 has already been referred to as a contributory factor in its lack of oral absorption, and attempts have been made to improve the bioavailability profile of the compound by separating the carboxyl group from the strongly electronegative chromone ring to give weaker acids. Less acidic compounds are obtained on insertion of a phenyl ring (22)[88] or alkylene chain [(23) (FPL 57231) and (24) (FPL 59257)][8], but, in each case, there was only minimal improvement as indicated by the plasma clearance rates (*Table 8.10*). The compounds retained SRS-A antagonist properties but were almost devoid of mast-cell-stabilizing activity. This presented an opportunity to evaluate the role of SRS-A in allergic disease states without the additional effect of cromogly-cate-like activity which might complicate clinical assessment. The two propionic acid analogues, (23) and (24), were as selective on the guinea-pig ileum as FPL 55712 and showed a similar profile in their activities on other tissues[8]. Interestingly, FPL 59257 had a very persistent action *in vitro*. After exposure to concentrations of the compound greater than 2×10^{-6}M, tissue responses to SRS-A (or LTD$_4$) often could not be fully restored. Using lower concentrations, a pA_2 value of 7.75 ± 0.18 (mean $\pm$ s.e.m., $n = 8$) was obtained for FPL 59257 versus LTD$_4$ on guinea-pig ileum, after an antagonist contact time of 5 min[15].

TABLE 8.10. Activities *in vivo* and *in vitro* of SRS-A antagonists

Compound no.	$10^8 \times IC_{50}$ (M)	pK_a	Plasma half-life i.v. (min)	$10^7 \times ED_{50}$ (mol/kg i.v.)[a]
10 (FPL 55712)	3.8	1.8[b]	c	2.0 ± 0.4
22	40	3.3[b]	$\leqslant 10$ (guinea-pig)	—
23 (FPL 57231)	5.5	4.1–4.2[b]	$\leqslant 10$ (dog)	2.7 ± 0.6
24 (FPL 59257)	40[d]	4.1–4.2[b]	20 (rat)	e

[a] Antagonism of bronchoconstriction induced by inhalation of nebulized SRS-A in the anaesthetized guinea-pig.
[b] Value from closely related analogue.
[c] See p. 137.
[d] At time of maximum inhibition, i.e. on response immediately following that in presence of compound.
[e] In individual animals, 1×10^{-5} mol/kg inhibited by 51%, 2×10^{-5} mol/kg by 52 and 53%, and 3×10^{-5} mol/kg by 77%.

In an *in vivo* model of bronchoconstriction in guinea-pigs using an aerosol of partially purified SRS-A and intravenous administration of compound immediately prior to exposure to the agonist, both propionic acids were approximately equipotent with FPL 55712, but FPL 59257 showed a persistence of effect which attenuated subsequent control responses and prevented the determination of an accurate ED$_{50}$ value (*Table 8.10*). Such duration of action should be an advantageous feature for SRS-A antagonists employed in clinical therapy.

In studies to investigate the role of SRS-A in hypoxic pulmonary vaso-constriction in conscious sheep, intravenous pretreatment with FPL 57231 3.6×10^{-6} mol/kg per min prevented the pulmonary vasoconstriction induced by hypoxia, and infusion of the compound after the induction of vasoconstriction reversed the response[89], implicating SRS-A as a direct or indirect mediator of hypoxic pulmonary vasoconstriction.

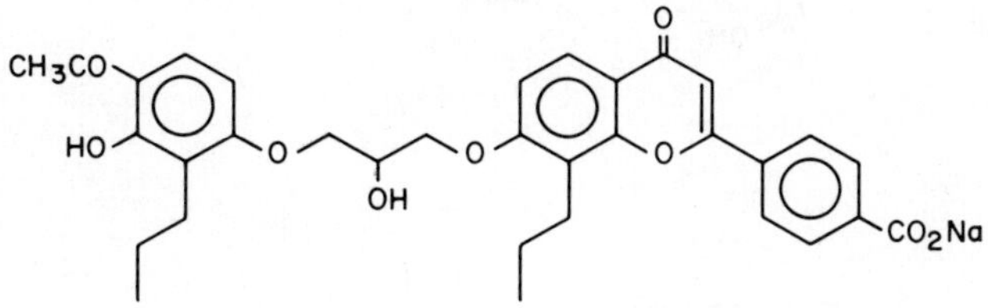

(22)

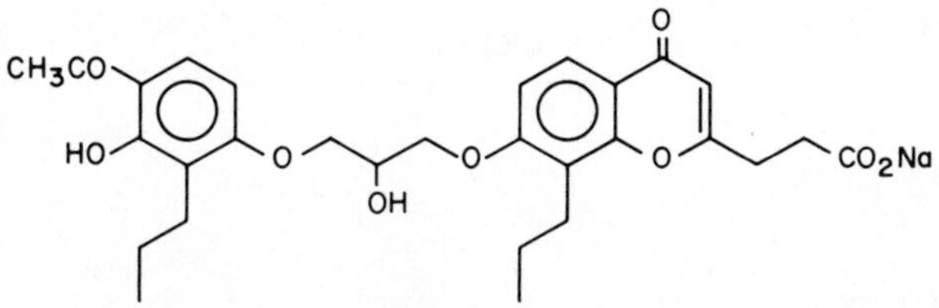

(23)

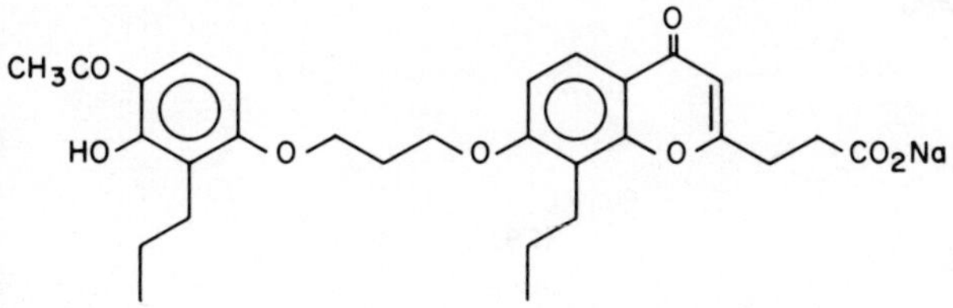

(24)

Airway mucus plugging is an important component of severe asthma, and of relevance to this is the finding that antigen challenge of trachea from allergic sheep *in vitro* increased glycoprotein secretion and absorption of ions (and consequently water)[90]. The mucus thus produced might be expected to be physically abnormal and difficult to clear from the airways. FPL 57231 blocked the increase in glycoprotein secretion[90], suggesting SRS-A as a mediator of the alteration in the physical properties of airways secretions. This, then, may be at least in part the mechanism of the anti-gen-induced decrease in tracheal mucus velocity referred to earlier in this chapter, p. 143). Ciliary dysfunction appears unlikely to be involved in the latter since slight ciliostimulation of tracheal epithelial cells in sheep has been observed after antigen challenge in both *in vitro* and *in vivo* experiments[91]. This increase in beat frequency *in vitro* was blocked by FPL 57231 (1.8×10^{-5}M), but not by antihistamines[91], suggesting that SRS-A may also be involved in the mediation of this observed ciliostimulation.

Examples of the variety of acidic moieties which demonstrate antagonist activity to SRS-A when substituted by the side-chain of FPL 55712, or a closely related structure, have been extended still further by claims that activity is associated with, for instance, benzoic acids, cinnamic acids, phenylacetic acids, phenoxyacetic acids, and salicylic acids (selected example (25))[92], and phenylthioacetic acids (selected example (26))[93].

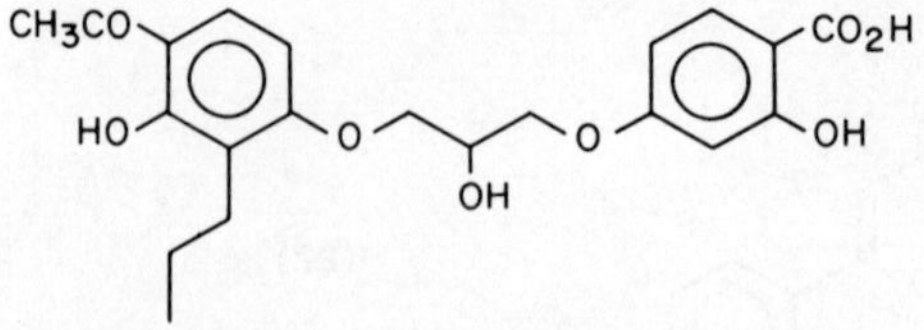

(25)

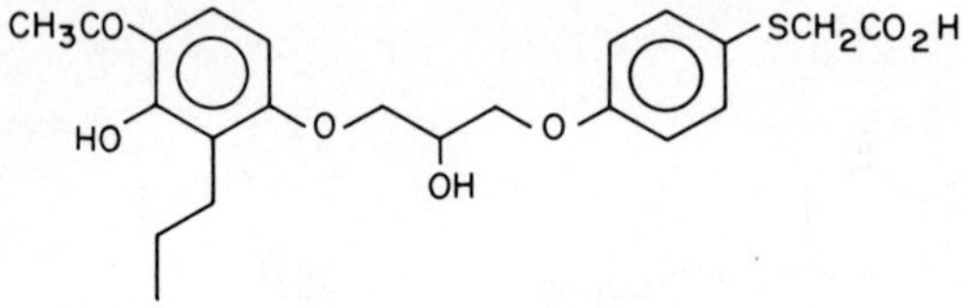

(26)

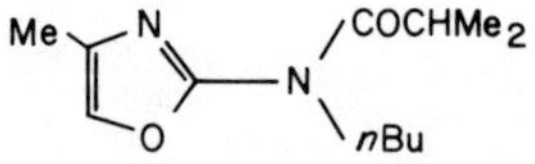

(27)

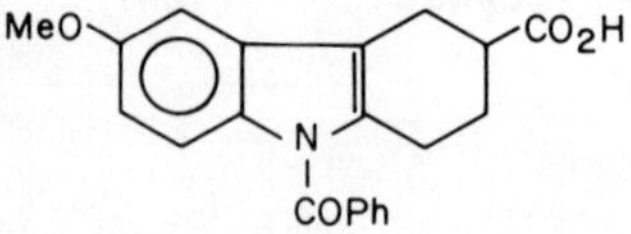

(28)

Amongst a series of anti-allergic 2-(acylamino)oxazoles[94], one compound (27) (isamoxole) has been claimed to be a moderately potent (pA_2 versus SRS-A^{gp} = 5.3) and fairly selective antagonist of SRS-A, being at least 10 times less potent against other agonists on guinea-pig ileum[95]. It should be noted that this compound is, in fact, a much weaker and less selective antagonist than FPL 55712.

A tetrahydrocarbazole derivative (28) (oxarbazole) has been reported to inhibit, in a dose-related manner, bronchoconstrictor responses induced by crude SRS-A^{rat} or by bradykinin in anaesthetized guinea-pigs[96]. This compound was ineffective against bronchoconstriction induced by histamine, carbachol, 5-hydroxytryptamine and PGF$_{2\alpha}$, and has been loosely referred to as an SRS-A antagonist. However, the activity which oxarbazole demonstrates in vivo is similar to that of non-steroidal anti-inflammatory drugs (its structure is similar to that of indomethacin), and its activity as an antagonist of SRS-A^{gp} in vitro (IC$_{50}$ = 4.6 × 10^{-5}M) is much weaker than that of FPL 55712[15]. The selectivity of oxarbazole in vitro has not been reported.

Recently, several series of imidodisulphamides have been described as antagonists of SRS-A on the guinea-pig ileum. In the case where the sulphonamide nitrogens were in an acyclic chain (29)[97], substituent schemes were utilized to explore the influence of lipophilic and electronic factors on activity. Halogen analogues [(29) X = Cl or Br, $n = 2$)] were identified as being moderately potent and selective antagonists, though closely related compounds additionally inhibited potassium chloride-induced contractions of the ileum (at 2×10^{-6}M, FPL 55712 did not significantly inhibit such contractions).

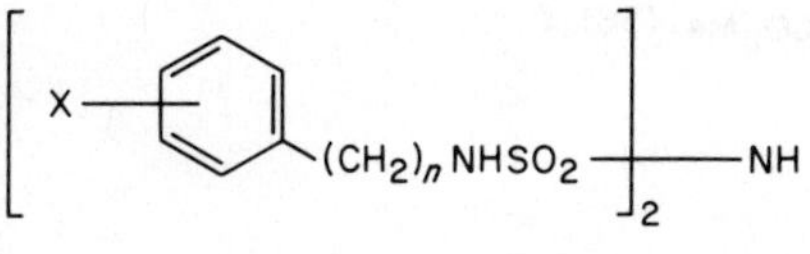

(29)

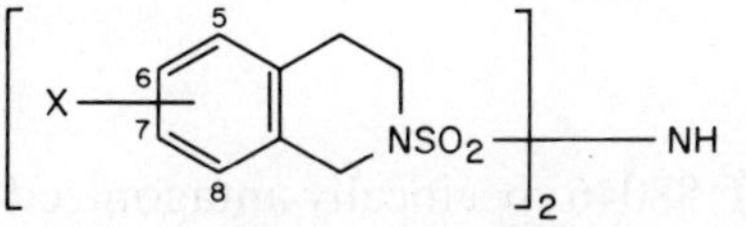

(30)

Greater potency was exhibited by compounds of the tetrahydro-isoquinoline series (30)[98] where in most cases X represents electron-withdrawing substituents. Inhibition of SRS-A responses was reported for single doses of compounds only, rendering true comparisons of potency difficult, but the activities recorded were remarkably tolerant of structural variation of X. Selected examples (*Table 8.11*) are the dihalogen isomers

TABLE 8.11. Inhibition of SRS-A-induced contraction of guinea-pig ileum by compounds at 5 μM

No.	X in compound (30)	Inhibition (%)
31	$7,8-Cl_2$	42
32	$5,8-Br_2$	50
33	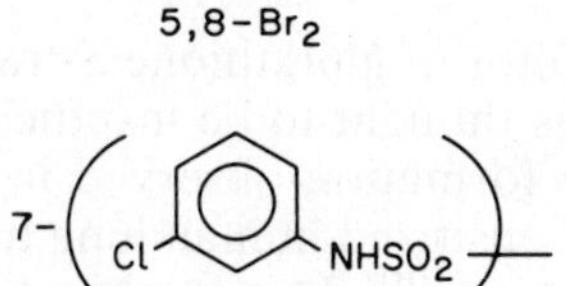 7- (Cl—⬡—NHSO$_2$)	67.5
34	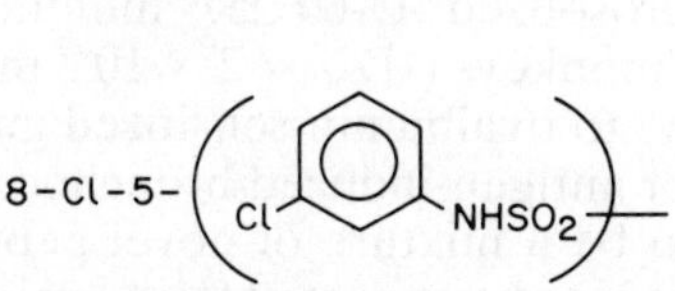 8-Cl-5- (Cl—⬡—NHSO$_2$)	63

(31) and (32), differing little in activity from the much more sterically demanding phenylaminosulphonyl substituents (33) and (34)[99]. Compound (33) (SK&F 88046) is stated to be equipotent with FPL 55712 against contractions of the guinea-pig ileum induced by partially purified SRS-A[100].

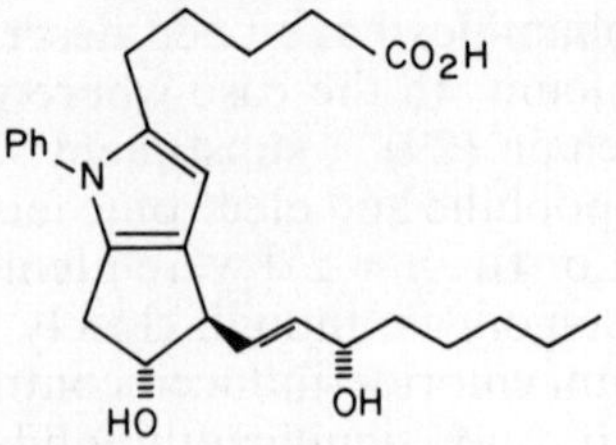

At concentrations of $(1-50) \times 10^{-6}$M, SK&F 88046 specifically antagonized LTD_4 in a dose-related manner on guinea-pig parenchymal strips, but like FPL 55712 was inactive against LTC_4 on this tissue, providing further support for the existence of more than one leukotriene receptor. In spontaneously breathing guinea-pigs, SK&F 88046 6.4×10^{-6} mol/kg i.v. significantly inhibited the changes in pulmonary resistance and dynamic lung compliance induced by intravenous administration of LTD_4.

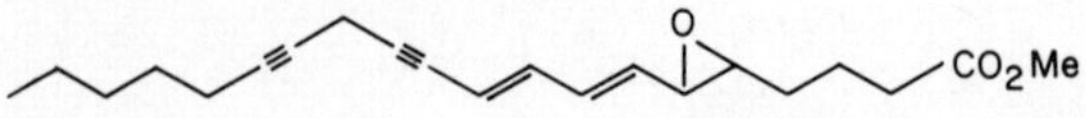

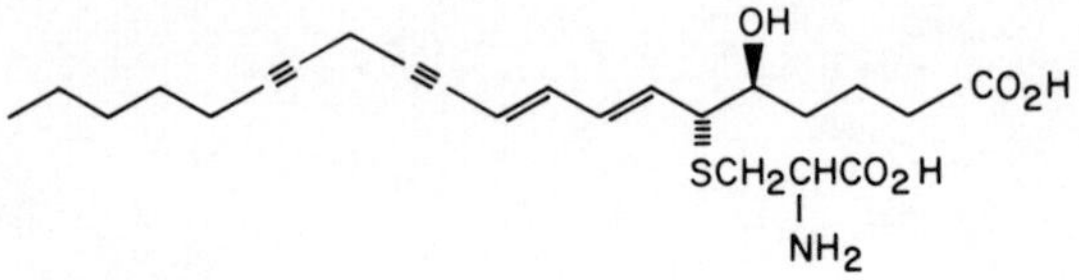

The N-phenylpyrrole analogue (35) (U-60,257) of prostacyclin has the dual mode of action of inhibiting the formation of leukotrienes as well as of being an apparently competitive antagonist of LTD_4 on guinea-pig ileum, as determined by a superfusion technique[101]. In the isolated organ bath, U-60,257 markedly affected the subsequent ability of the tissue to recover responsiveness to LTD_4, an effect perhaps similar to that shown by (24) (FPL 59257).

U-60,257 was found to be an inhibitor of glutathione S-transferase (ID_{50} = 8.2×10^{-5}M), but this activity was thought to be insufficient to account for all the inhibition of leukotriene formation observed in rat peritoneal cells ($ID_{50} = 1 \times 10^{-5}$M), or in IgE-sensitized human lung fragments (ID_{50} = 8.5×10^{-6}M) on challenge with antigen[101]. This combination of activities is reflected *in vivo* where aerosolized U-60,257 inhibited pulmonary anaphylaxis in *Ascaris*-sensitive monkeys ($ID_{50} = 2 \times 10^{-7}$ mol), and administration of 2×10^{-7} mol/kg i.v. to ovalbumin-sensitized guinea-pigs produced half-maximal inhibition of antigen-induced bronchoconstriction[102].

Now that SRS-A is known to be a mixture of novel peptidolipids, primarily leukotrienes C_4 and D_4, it is to be expected from precedents of close structural relationships between agonists and antagonists that systematic modification of the leukotriene molecular architecture will lead to the discovery of new antagonists of SRS-A. An early example of this is the claim that diacetylene epoxide (36) antagonized ($IC_{50} = 1 \times 10^{-5}$M) the contraction of guinea-pig ileum induced by (37), a diacetylene analogue of LTE_4

approximately 20 times less potent than LTE_4 itself[103]. Also many unnatural isomers of LTC_4, LTD_4 and LTE_4, differing in the geometry, or in the positions of their double bonds, or additionally, in some cases, with their substituents being diastereotopic in the unnatural configuration, (5R,6S), are claimed[104] to be partial agonists/antagonists of SRS-A on the guinea-pig ileum at concentrations between 2×10^{-10} and 2×10^{-6}M. It is further claimed that the compounds display this combination of activities in their effects on pulmonary mechanics in anaesthetized guinea-pigs (dose range 2×10^{-7} mol/kg to 2×10^{-4} mol/kg i.v.).

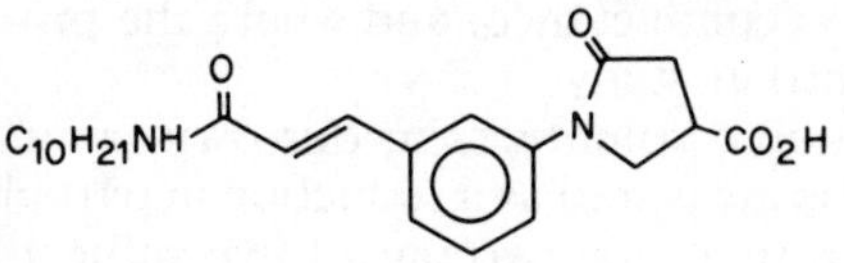

(38)

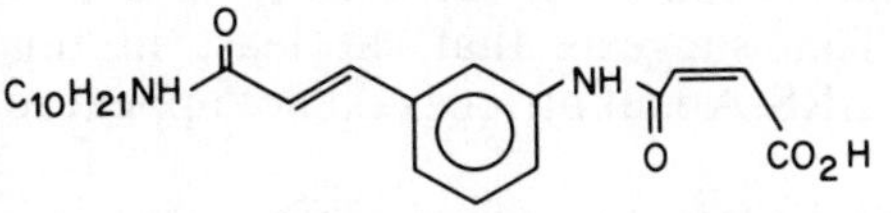

(39)

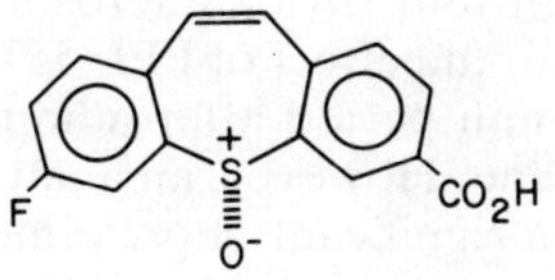

(40)

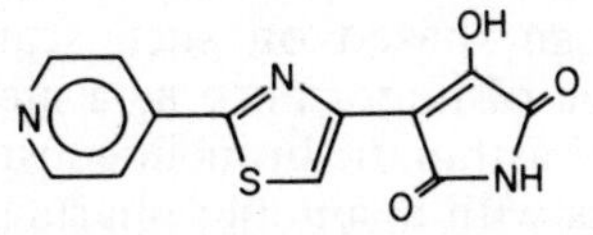

(41)

In addition to the foregoing compounds, SRS-A antagonist activity has been claimed for a number of diverse structural types, for which biological data are not available. Selected representative examples of these structures are oxopyrrolidino-carboxylic acids (38)[105], phenylaminocarbonyl-propenoic acids (39)[106], dibenzothiepin acids (40) (which are also claimed as prostaglandin antagonists)[107], and hydroxypyrroline-2,5-diones (41) (which also inhibit glycolic acid oxidase)[108].

Clinical evaluation of antagonists of SRS-A

Only limited studies have been carried out to date with SRS-A antagonists in man.

In a preliminary open study, inhalation of aerosols from 5×10^{-3}M solutions of both FPL 55712 and FPL 59257 substantially inhibited the bronchoconstrictor response and abolished the cough response induced by inhalation of nebulized LTC_4 in two non-atopic volunteers[109].

In a study by Ahmed *et al.*[58] in six ragweed-sensitive patients, referred to earlier in this chapter, inhalation of FPL 55712 as an aerosol from a $2 \times 10^{-2}M$ solution prevented the antigen-induced fall in tracheal mucus velocity (TMV), but was said not to protect against the airways effects of antigen challenge as measured by specific airways conductance (SGaw). This study, though, was specifically designed to investigate changes in TMV. At each time of antigen challenge a provocation dose which would produce a 35% fall in SGaw was administered (PD$_{35}$). The PD$_{35}$ was higher after drug treatment than after placebo, but the difference was reported not to be significant. The effect of FPL 55712 in similar patients with the emphasis on changes in airways conductance, and where the provocation dose is not varied, deserves further study.

In antigen provocation studies on atopic volunteers in our own laboratories, in which airways obstruction was measured as a reduction in partial expiratory flow rate, it has been shown that only two out of five subjects were partially protected following inhalation of an aerosol from a $5 \times 10^{-3}M$ solution of FPL 59257[110]. This suggests that, at least in this experimental model of acute asthma, SRS-A/leukotrienes do not appear to play a dominant role.

Finally, FPL 55712 has been administered to four chronic asthmatics who had proved difficult to stabilize with conventional therapy[111]. FPL 55712 2.5×10^{-4} mol was given daily in four divided aerosol doses via a Wright nebulizer for seven days. Overall, the effect of FPL 55712 on FEV$_1$ (the highest recorded value over a 30-min period after administration of saline or drug) was no different from saline. However, an analysis of covariance of individual responses revealed a significant improvement in FEV$_1$ after FPL 55712 in two of the patients.

It is difficult to draw firm conclusions on the possible benefits to be derived from SRS-A antagonists in man, based on such scanty data. However, it appears that SRS-A may be of importance as a mediator of mucociliary dysfunction in asthma and of asthmatic bronchoconstriction in some patients. Thus, SRS-A antagonists with a suitable pharmacokinetic profile may yet prove to be potentially useful therapeutic agents in the treatment of asthma and possibly other immunological and inflammatory diseases.

Prospects

Although the SRS-A antagonist, FPL 55712, has been known for about 10 years, the true potential of this type of compound in various disease states in man is still not clear. The few clinical studies with FPL 55712 itself suggest that some allergic asthmatic patients might derive benefit from it. Although SRS-A has primarily been considered in the past as a potentially important mediator of asthmatic bronchoconstriction, more recently evidence has emerged to suggest the involvement of SRS-A in disturbance of mucociliary and cardiovascular function.

The implications of the studies on mucociliary transport are that SRS-A may contribute to impairment of ventilatory function in allergic asthma, not only by contraction of bronchial smooth muscle, but also by impairing mucus clearance leading to mucus plugging of the airways, which is one of the characteristic pathological features of severe asthma. SRS-A may also contribute to the bronchial hyper-reactivity seen in subjects with asthma, since it is known to potentiate the smooth muscle contracting effects of other agonists such as histamine. The full potential of an antagonist of SRS-A in asthma may be revealed only after long-term administration of the drug in order to establish its beneficial effect on these more chronic aspects of this disease.

Further, the observation that FPL 57231 prevents the pulmonary vasoconstriction induced by hypoxia in sheep suggests that SRS-A may play a role in the pathogenesis of diseases in which pulmonary hypertension is a feature, for example cor pulmonale, chronic bronchitis and emphysema[112]. Again, an assessment of the clinical value of antagonists of SRS-A in the treatment of such diseases would require long-term studies.

That leukotrienes have potent effects on the cardiovascular system, including negative inotropism, coronary vasoconstriction, and increased vascular permeability, suggests that antagonists of SRS-A may also prove to be useful in alleviating cardiovascular disorders which are associated with the formation of leukotrienes.

The verification or otherwise of these suppositions is for the future and will require more concerted efforts to examine those presently known antagonists of SRS-A and also antagonists with a more suitable pharmacokinetic profile, e.g. improved biological half-life, good oral absorption.

The elucidation of the structure of the leukotrienes has revitalized interest in SRS-A and synthetic analogues of the leukotrienes with antagonist activity have started, and will continue, to emerge. It is to be confidently expected that the next 10 years will reveal a clearer picture of the potential therapeutic role of antagonists of of SRS-A.

References

1. LEWIS, R.A., DRAZEN, J.M., AUSTEN, K.F., CLARK, D.A., and COREY, E.J. *Biochemical and Biophysical Research Communications*, **96**, 271 (1980)
2. AUGSTEIN, J., FARMER, J.B., LEE, T.B., SHEARD, P. and TATTERSALL, M.L. *Nature New Biology*, **248**, 215 (1973)
3. COX, J.S.G. *Nature*, **216**, 1328 (1967)
4. APPLETON, R.A., BANTICK, J.R., CHAMBERLAIN, T.R., HARDERN, D.N., LEE, T.B. and PRATT, A.D. *Journal of Medicinal Chemistry*, **20**, 371 (1977)
5. BANTICK, J.R., HARDERN, D.N., LEE, T.B. and TAYLOR, J.E. (Fisons) German Patent 2803230 (1978)
6. SHEARD, P., LEE, T.B. and TATTERSALL, M.L. *Monographs in Allergy*, **12**, 245 (1977)
7. MEAD, B., PATTERSON, L.H. and SMITH, D.A. *Journal of Pharmacy and Pharmacology*, **33**, 682 (1981)
8. SHEARD, P., HOLROYDE, M.C., GHELANI, A.M., BANTICK, J.R. and LEE, T.B. In *Advances in Prostaglandin, Thromboxane and Leukotriene Research*. Eds. B. Samuelsson and R. Paoletti, Vol. 9. p. 229. New York: Raven Press (1982)
9. KRELL, R.D. and CHAKRIN, L.W. *International Archives of Allergy and Applied Immunology*, **56**, 39 (1978)
10. WEICHMAN, B.M., HOSTELLEY, L.S., BOSTICK, S.P., MUCCITELLI, R.M., KRELL, R.D. and GLEASON, J.G. *Journal of Pharmacology and Experimental Therapeutics*, **221**, 295 (1982)
11. FENIUK, L., KENNEDY, I. and WHELAN, C.J. *Journal of Pharmacy and Pharmacology*, **34**, 586 (1982)

12. COLEMAN, R.A., KENNEDY, I. and WHELAN, C.J. *British Journal of Pharmacology*, **66**, 83P (1979)
13. FLEISCH, J.H., HAISCH, K.D. and SPAETHE, S.M. *Journal of Pharmacology and Experimental Therapeutics*, **221**, 146 (1982)
14. JAKSCHIK, B.A., KULCZYCKI, A., MacDONALD, H.H. and PARKER, C.W. *Journal of Immunology*, **119**, 618 (1977)
15. HOLROYDE, M.C. and GHELANI, A.M. (Fisons unpublished results)
16. FLEISCH, J.H., RINKEMA, L.E. and BAKER, S.R. *Life Sciences*, **31**, 577 (1982)
17. HOLME, G. Personal communication
18. CROWLEY, H.J., O'DONNELL, M., YAREMKO, B. and WELTON, A.F. *Federation Proceedings*, **41**, 823 (1982)
19. HOLME, G., BRUNET, G., PIECHUTA, H., MASSON, P., GIRARD, Y. and ROKACH, J. *Prostaglandins*, **20**, 717 (1980)
20. WELTON, A.F., CROWLEY, H.J., MILLER, D.A. and YAREMKO, B. *Prostaglandins*, **21**, 287 (1981)
21. GOLDENBERG, M.M. and SUBERS, E.M. *European Journal of Pharmacology*, **78**, 463 (1982)
22. WEICHMAN, B.M. and TUCKER, S.S. *Prostaglandins*, **24**, 245 (1982)
23. ARUNLAKSHANA, O. and SCHILD, H.O. *British Journal of Pharmacology*, **14**, 48 (1959)
24. PIPER, P.J. and SAMHOUN, M.N. *Prostaglandins*, **21**, 793 (1981)
25. KRELL, R.D., OSBORN, R., VICKERY, L., FALCONE, K., O'DONNELL, M., GLEASON, J. *et al. Prostaglandins*, **22**, 387 (1981)
26. DRAZEN, J.M., AUSTEN, K.F., LEWIS, R.A., CLARK, D.A., GOTO, G., MARFAT, A. *et al. Proceedings of the National Academy of Sciences of the United States of America*, **77**, 4354 (1980)
27. TSAI, B.S., BERNSTEIN, P., MACIA, R.A., CONATY, J. and KRELL, R.D. *Prostaglandins*, **23**, 489 (1982)
28. DAHLEN, S.E., HEDQVIST, P., HAMMARSTRÖM, S. and SAMUELSSON, B. *Nature*, **288**, 484 (1980)
29. JONES, T.R., DAVIS, C. and DANIEL, E.E. *Canadian Journal of Physiology and Pharmacology*, **60**, 638 (1982)
30. HANNA, C.J., BACH, M.K., PARE, P.D. and SCHELLENBERG, R.R. *Nature*, **290**, 343 (1981)
31. BURKE, J.A., LEVI, R., GUO, Z.G. and COREY, E.J. *Journal of Pharmacology and Experimental Therapeutics*, **221**, 235 (1982)
32. LETTS, L.G. and PIPER, P.J. *British Journal of Pharmacology*, **76**, 169 (1982)
33. KITO, G., OKUDA, H., OHKAWA, S., TERAO, S. and KIKUCHI, K. *Life Sciences*, **29**, 1325 (1981)
34. VAN DEN BRINK, F.G. and LIEN, E.J. *European Journal of Pharmacology*, **44**, 251 (1977)
35. HAND, J.M., WILL, J.A. and BUCKNER, C.K. *European Journal of Pharmacology*, **76**, 439 (1981)
36. AITKEN, V., BOULLIN, D.J. and TAGARI, P. *Vth International Conference on Prostaglandins*, Abstract 258. Florence (1982)
37. CHASIN, M. and SCOTT, C. *Biochemical Pharmacology*, **27**, 2065 (1978)
38. CASEY, F.B., APPLEBY, B.J. and BUCK, D.C. *Federation Proceedings*, **41**, 820 (1982)
39. BLAIR, I.A., DOLLERY, C.T., ENNIS, M., HOULT, J.R.S., ROBINSON, C. and WADDELL, K.A. *British Journal of Pharmacology*, **78**, 49 p (1983)
40. MIELENS, Z.E., FERGUSON, E.W. and FERRARI, R.A. *Agents and Actions*, **11**, 673 (1981)
41. HALLAM, C. and MITCHELL, P.D. (Fisons unpublished results)
42. WELTON, A.F., HOPE, W.C., TOBIAS, L.D. and HAMILTON, J.G. *Biochemical Pharmacology*, **30**, 1378 (1981)
43. HAWORTH, D., FISHER, R.W. and CAREY, F. *Biochemical Society Transactions*, **10**, 239 (1982)
44. O'DONNELL, M., FALCONE, K. and KRELL, R.D. *Federation Proceedings*, **40**, 721 (1981)
45. ASPINALL, R.L. *Federation Proceedings*, **41**, 820 (1982)
46. FENIUK, L., KENNEDY, I. and WHELAN, C.J. In *Leukotrienes and other Lipoxygenase Products*. Ed. P.J. Piper. Chichester: John Wiley and Sons, in press (1983)
47. WELTON, A.F., O'DONNELL, M., CROWLEY, H., MEDFORD, A. and YAREMKO, B. *Vth International Conference on Prostaglandins*, Abstract 484. Florence (1982)
48. WELTON, A.F., O'DONNELL, M., HOPE, W.C., TOBIAS, L.D. and CROWLEY, H. *Vth International Conference on Prostaglandins*, Abstract 334. Florence (1982)
49. SCHIANTARELLI, P., BONGRANI, S. and FOLCO, G. *European Journal of Pharmacology*, **73**, 363 (1981)
50. MICHELASSI, F., LANDA, L., HILL, R.D., LOWENSTEIN, E., WATKINS, W.D., PETKAU, A.J. *et al. Science*, **217**, 841 (1982)

51. BOYD, L.M., EZRA, D., FEUERSTEIN, G. and GOLDSTEIN, R.E. *European Journal of Pharmacology*, **89**, 307 (1983)
52. PATTERSON, R., ORANGE, R.P. and HARRIS, K.E. *Journal of Allergy and Clinical Immunology*, **62**, 371 (1978)
53. MORLEY, J., PAGE, C. and PAUL, W. *Agents and Actions*, **11**, 585 (1981)
54. PECK, M.J., PIPER, P.J. and WILLIAMS, T.J. *Prostaglandins*, **21**, 315 (1981)
55. PALMER, M.R., MATHEWS, R., MURPHY, R.C. and HOFFER, B.J. *Neuroscience Letters*, **18**, 173 (1980)
56. PALMER, M.R., MATHEWS, R., HOFFER, B.J. and MURPHY, R.C. *Journal of Pharmacology and Experimental Therapeutics*, **219**, 91 (1981)
57. WANNER, A., ZARZECKI, S., HIRSCH, J. and EPSTEIN, S. *Journal of Applied Physiology*, **39**, 950 (1975)
58. AHMED, T., GREENBLATT, W., BIRCH, S., MARCHETTE, B. and WANNER, A. *American Review of Respiratory Disease*, **124**, 110 (1981)
59. PEATFIELD, A.C., PIPER, P.J. and RICHARDSON, P.S. *British Journal of Pharmacology*, **77**, 391 (1982)
60. MAROM, Z., SHELHAMER, J.H., BACH, M.K., MORTON, D.R. and KALINER, M. *American Review of Respiratory Disease*, **126**, 449 (1982)
61. JOHNSON, H.G., CHINN, R.A., CHOW, A.W., BACH, M.K., MORTON, D.R. and NADEL, J.A. *XIth International Congress of Allergology and Clinical Immunology*. Abstract 146P. London (1982)
62. CONROY, M.C. and BLANCUZZI, V. *Monographs in Allergy*, **14**, 307 (1979)
63. KRELL, R.D., McCOY, J., OSBORN, R. and CHAKRIN, L.W. *International Journal of Immunopharmacology*, **2**, 55 (1980)
64. SHEARD, P. In *SRS-A and Leukotrienes*. Ed. P.J. Piper. p. 209. Chichester: Wiley (1981)
65. FARMER, J.B., RICHARDS, I.M., SHEARD, P. and WOODS, A.M. *British Journal of Pharmacology*, **55**, 57 (1975)
66. O'DONNELL, M. and WELTON, A.F. *Federation Proceedings*, **41**, 821 (1982)
67. BUCKLE, D.R., OUTRED, D.J., ROSS, J.W., SMITH, H., SMITH, R.J., SPICER, B.A. *et al. Journal of Medicinal Chemistry*, **22**, 158 (1979)
68. DRAZEN, J.M., LEWIS, R.A., AUSTEN, K.F., TODA, M., BRION, F., MARFAT, A. *et al. Proceedings of the National Academy of Sciences of the United States of America*, **78**, 3195 (1981)
69. LEWIS, R.A., DRAZEN, J.M., AUSTEN, K.F., TODA, M., BRION, F., MARFAT, A. *et al. Proceedings of the National Academy of Sciences of the United States of America*, **78**, 4579 (1981)
70. BAKER, S.R., BOOT, J.R., JAMIESON, W.B., OSBORNE, D.J. and SWEATMAN, W.J.F. *Biochemical and Biophysical Research Communications*, **103**, 1258 (1981)
71. JONES, T., MASSON, P., HAMEL, R., BRUNET, G., HOLME, G., GIRARD, Y. *et al. Prostaglandins*, **24**, 279 (1982)
72. HAMMERSTRÖM, S. *Journal of Biological Chemistry*, **255**, 7093 (1980)
73. HAMMERSTRÖM, S. *Journal of Biological Chemistry*, **256**, 2275 (1981)
74. GHELANI, A.M., HOLROYDE, M.C. and SHEARD, P. *British Journal of Pharmacology*, **71**, 107 (1980)
75. PIPER, P.J. and SAMHOUN, M.N. *British Journal of Pharmacology*, **77**, 267 (1982)
76. SIROIS, P., ROY, S. and BORGEAT, P. *International Journal of Immunopharmacology*, **4**, 293 (1982)
77. MORRIS, H.R., TAYLOR, G.W., PIPER, P.J. and TIPPINS, J.R. *Agents and Actions*, Suppl. **6**, 27 (1979)
78. SIROIS, P., ROY, S., BORGEAT, P., PICARD, S. and VALLERAND, P. *Prostaglandins, Leukotrienes and Medicine*, **8**, 157 (1982)
79. SIROIS, P., BORGEAT, P., JEANSON, A., ROY, S. and GIRARD, G. *Prostaglandins and Medicine*, **5**, 429 (1980)
80. ELLIOTT, E.V. (Fisons unpublished results)
81. ROKACH, J., HAMEL, P.A. and HIRSCHMANN, R.F. (Merck) United States Patent 4252818 (1981)
82. HOLME, G., PIECHUTA, H. and SHARE, N.N. *International Journal of Immunopharmacology*, **2**, 263 (1980)
83. BUCKLE, D.R. and SMITH, H. (Beecham) British Patent 1555753 (1979)
84. BUCKLE, D.R. and SMITH, H. (Beecham) German Patent 2722039 (1977)
85. BUCKLE, D.R. and SMITH, H. (Beecham) European Patent 54398 (1982)
86. BUCKLE, D.R. and SMITH, H. (Beecham) European Patent 7727 (1980)

158   SRS-A antagonists

87. BUCKLE, D.R., CANTELLO, B.C.C., SMITH, H. and SPICER, B.A. *Journal of Medicinal Chemistry*, **18**, 726 (1975)
88. LEE, T.B., HARDERN, D.N. and BANTICK, J.R. (Fisons) United States Patent 4042708 (1977)
89. AHMED, T., OLIVER, W., FRANK, B.L., ROBINSON, M.J. and WANNER, A. *American Review of Respiratory Disease*, **125** (Suppl.), 271 (1982)
90. PHIPPS, R., DENAS, S. and WANNER, A. *Federation Proceedings*, **41**, 1509 (1982)
91. MAURER, D.R., SCHOR, J., SIELCZAK, M., WANNER, A. and ABRAHAM, W.M. *Cell Motility*, Suppl. **1**, 67 (1982)
92. OXFORD, A.W. and ELLIS, F. (Glaxo) British Patent 2058785 (1981)
93. HARDERN, D.N., LEE, T.B. and BANTICK, J.R. (Fisons) European Patent 56172 (1982)
94. ROSS, W.J., HARRISON, R.G., JOLLEY, M.R.J., NEVILLE, M.C., TODD, A., VERGE, J.P. *et al. Journal of Medicinal Chemistry*, **22**, 412 (1979)
95. DAWSON, W. and SWEATMAN, W.J.F. *British Journal of Pharmacology*, **71**, 387 (1980)
96. MIELENS, Z.E. *Pharmacology*, **17**, 323 (1978)
97. ALI, F.E., DANDRIDGE, P.A., GLEASON, J.G., KRELL, R.D., KRUSE, C.H., LAVANCHY, P.G. *et al. Journal of Medicinal Chemistry*, **25**, 947 (1982)
98. ALI, F.E., GLEASON, J.G., HILL, D.T., KRELL, R.D., KRUSE, C.H., LAVANCHY, P.G. *et al. Journal of Medicinal Chemistry*, **25**, 1235 (1982)
99. ALI, F.E. (SK&F) European Patent 38177 (1981)
100. GLEASON, J.G., KRELL, R.D., WEICHMAN, B.M., ALI, F.E. and BERKOWITZ, B. In *Advances in Prostaglandin, Thromboxane and Leukotriene Research*. Eds B. Samuelsson and R. Paoletti. Vol. 9. p. 243. New York: Raven Press (1982)
101. BACH, M.K., BRASHLER, J.R., SMITH, H.W., FITZPATRICK, F.A., SUN. F.F. and McGUIRE, J.C. *Prostaglandins*, **23**, 759 (1982)
102. SMITH, H.W., BACH, M.K., HARRISON, A.W., JOHNSON, H.G., MAJOR, N.J. and WASSERMAN, M.A. *Prostaglandins*, **24**, 543 (1982)
103. ROSENBERGER, M. (Roche) European Patent 36663 (1981)
104. JAMIESON, W.B., BAKER, S.R. and ROSS, W.J. (Lilly) British Patent 2094301 (1982)
105. KADIN, S.B. (Pfizer) European Patent 47119 (1982)
106. KADIN, S.B. (Pfizer) United States Patent 4296129 (1981)
107. ROKACH, J., ROONEY, C.S. and CRAGOE, E.J. (Merck) European Patent 52912 (1982)
108. CRAGOE, E.J. and ROONEY, C.S. (Merck) United States Patent 4296237 (1981)
109. HOLROYDE, M.C., ALTOUNYAN, R.E.C., COLE, M., DIXON, M. and ELLIOTT, E.V., *Lancet*, **i**, 17 (1981)
110. ALTOUNYAN, R.E.C. and COLE, M. *Proceedings of the XIth International Congress of Allergology and Clinical Immunology*. Ed. J.W. Kerr. p. 271. London: Macmillan (1983)
111. LEE, T.H., WALPORT, M.J., WILKINSON, A.H., TURNER-WARWICK, M. and KAY, A.B. *Lancet*, **ii**, 304 (1981)
112. CROFTON, J. and DOUGLAS, A. *Respiratory Diseases*, 3rd ed. Oxford: Blackwell Scientific Publications (1981)

Chapter 9

Anti-cholinergic drugs

G.E. Pakes

Over the last few decades, the value of anti-cholinergic drugs (*Figure 9.1*) in the treatment of asthma has often gone unrecognized by clinicians in the wake of the greater popularity of β-adrenoceptor agents and the methyl-xanthine derivatives. Nevertheless, a reawakening of interest in anti-cholinergic drugs has occurred in view of the recently clarified patho-physiological role of the parasympathetic nervous system in asthma. It is

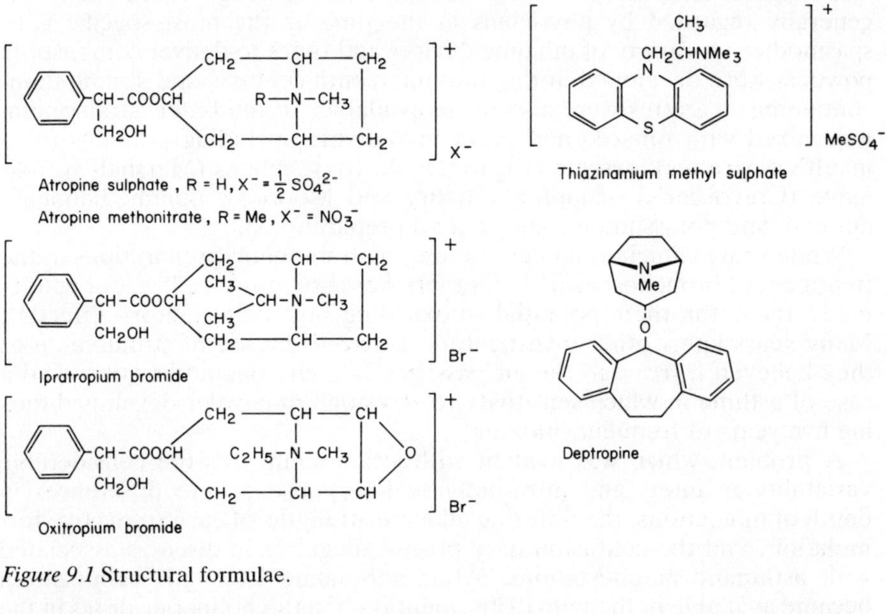

Figure 9.1 Structural formulae.

the purpose of this chapter to show how anti-asthmatic anti-cholinergic drugs have evolved from primordial herbal remedies to the highly effective and relatively safe quaternary compounds ipratropium bromide and oxitro-pium bromide. Lastly, a discussion is presented of the importance of anti-cholinergic agents in patients with bronchospastic diseases who fail to respond adequately to sympathomimetic drugs and theophylline.

159

The history of anti-cholinergic drugs in asthma

Anti-cholinergic drugs are probably the oldest single class of pharmacological agents to be used in the treatment of asthma. Inhalational therapy for respiratory diseases was practiced in India as early as 4000 years ago[1], and one commonly used herbal remedy made from the plant *Nardostachys jatamansi* contains an anti-cholinergic alkaloid, which has since been shown to counteract histamine-induced bronchospasm[2]. Sanskrit accounts in Indian Ayurvedic medicine mention toxicity from over-indulgence in smoking (dry mouth and throat, elevated skin temperatures, and rapid pulse), suggesting overdose of an atropine-like substance[1]. The first specific mention of *Datura* species (*D. stramonium, D. innoxa*, and *D. metel*) in the treatment of asthma was in the *Yogaratrakara* in the seventeenth century[3]. According to this source, the root of the *Datura* plant was ground into a powder with dry ginger, long pepper, black pepper and red arsenic, prepared into a paste with a base of ghee, dried, and finally smoked in a pipe.

Datura was introduced to England in 1802 by General Gent, who in India had observed the smoking of this plant for respiratory conditions[4,5]. Preparations of the shredded leaves (often of questionable origin) were available from apothecaries and street vendors in England in the early 1800s[6]. By the 1850s, lobelia, belladonna leaves and hyoscyamine were commonly used as home remedies for asthma, although stramonium was generally regarded by physicians at the time as the most specific anti-spasmodic[7]. A variety of inhaling devices and tubes to deliver combustible powders were developed in the mid-nineteenth century, and stramonium-containing cigarettes were also made available. In the latter, stramonium was mixed with tobacco and other ingredients, including cannabis (Grimault's cigarettes), arsenic (Cigarettes de Joy), cubebs (Marshall's), foxglove (Crevoisier's), camphor (Savory and Moore's), opium, henbane, aniseed, and potassium nitrate (several preparations).

While some clinicians lauded the use of stramonium preparations in the treatment of bronchospasm[5,8–11], others were not impressed[12,13], or condemned them for their potential intoxicating and hallucinatory effects[14]. Many years later, other investigators criticized the use of stramonium as they believed it irritated the air passages[15,16], and one author observed a case of asthma in which sensitivity to stramonium powder developed during five years of frequent smoking[17].

A problem which was evident with stramonium was the considerable variability in inter- and intra-individual response due to differences in depth of inhalations, the differing alkaloid strengths of each respective formulation, and the confusion over precise diagnosis in diseases associated with asthmatic manifestations. After adrenaline 1:100 for nebulization became available in the mid-1930s, mention of anti-cholinergic drugs in the treatment of respiratory diseases became rare.

There was little critical assessment of the value of anti-cholinergic drugs in asthma until spirometry allowed objective evaluation. In 1941, Dautrebande[18] demonstrated that atropine had a bronchodilatating effect, and he thought the drug was particularly useful in asthmatic patients with excessive bronchial mucus. In 1959, Herxheimer[19] showed that the smoking of cigarettes containing atropine sulphate 1.45 mg or 0.5 mg resulted in mean increases in vital capacity of 17% and 12%, respectively, in six asthmatic patients. Bronchodilatation with stramonium cigarettes was similar, with vital capacity increasing by a mean of 19%.

The respiratory effects of comparable aerosol doses of 17 different tropine derivatives (not all specifically named) were assessed in 96 asthmatic patients[20]. Four-hour monitoring of the magnitude and duration of increases in forced expiratory volume in one second (FEV_1) indicated that analogous atropine and hyoscine derivatives were almost equi-active, and homatropine was less active (quantitative data not given). The anti-muscarine agent, benzhexol (trihexyphenidyl), showed some transient bronchodilatory action.

Increasing the N-alkyl chain from methyl to ethyl in the atropine series resulted in a marked loss of bronchodilatating activity. N-Methylhyoscine was more active than N-butylhyoscine. The duration of action was significantly lengthened by quaternization. Atropine methonitrate was observed to have both potent and sustained activity, and further investigation was proposed.

In another study, several anti-cholinergic drugs were compared in antigen provocation tests utilizing vital capacity measurements[21]. Intravenous atropine sulphate 0.6 mg and L-hyoscyamine 0.5 mg both offered almost complete protection (80% and 99% for 2 to 3.5 hours, respectively) against subsequent doses of intravenous methacholine, as would be expected of anti-cholinergic agents against an acetylcholine derivative. However, both afforded little protection against intravenous histamine provocation (18% and 10% maximal protection at 30 minutes).

L-Hyoscyamine 0.5 mg orally and 0.05% by aerosol were similarly effective against methacholine provocation (70% protection), as were L-hyoscine (scopolamine) 0.3 mg subcutaneously (95% protection at 30 minutes), 0.6 mg orally (65% at 3 hours), and 0.06% aerosol (50% at 30 minutes). Each offered no significant protection against histamine challenge. Although the investigators concluded that L-hyoscyamine and L-hyoscine were as effective as bronchodilators as atropine sulphate, they felt that the pronounced sedative side-effects of the former agents would preclude their use in asthma therapy.

Mode and site of action

All anti-cholinergic drugs exert a bronchodilatating action mainly in large airways, in contrast to β-adrenoceptor agonists, which are usually thought to have a greater effect on small airways[22-24]. The anti-cholinergics probably produce bronchodilatation by competitive inhibition of cholinergic receptors on bronchial smooth muscle, antagonizing the action of acetylcholine at its membrane-bound receptor site. They thereby block the bronchoconstrictor action of vagal efferent impulses. Lung irritant receptors provide the chief afferent input for this vagal reflex[25].

Atropine and the other anti-cholinergic agents decrease the elevation of intracellular guanosine cyclic 3':5'-monophosphate (cyclic GMP) occurring during cholinergic stimulation. The direct role of cyclic GMP in altering bronchial muscle is uncertain. An increase in cyclic GMP levels in mast cells may enhance immunological release of mediators[26] and anti-cholinergic agents may prevent this by blocking cholinergic receptors on the mast cell surfaces[27]. For a more complete description of the role of cholinergic influences in asthma, the reader is directed to Chapter 6.

Most early clinical work suggested that atropine affected only the large airways[28,29]. However, Cooper *et al.*[30] demonstrated that inhaled or intravenous atropine exerts significant effects on elastic recoil pressure and upstream resistance, as well as total lung resistance, suggesting that the agent has significant effects on small, as well as large, airways function.

Atropine sulphate and methonitrate

Dose–response studies

A wide range of inhaled doses of atropine have been examined in single dose–response studies. Thus, while very low doses of 0.005–0.05 mg were suggested as being optimal for maximum bronchodilatation[20], a dose of up to 6 mg has been said to be preferable by other authors[31]. Results from different laboratories are difficult to compare because of wide variation in the amounts of drug administered, different size of aerosol particles delivered (affecting depth of airways penetration[32]), and the diversity of methods of drug delivery (nebulization, metered dose aerosol).

Although some bronchodilatation occurs with atropine within 15 minutes after inhalation, maximal effects are usually observed between 30 and 120 minutes. In one of the earliest dose–response studies in 20 asthmatic children (ages 8 to 14 years)[31], nebulized atropine sulphate 0.05–0.1 mg/kg (1–6 mg) provided optimal bronchodilatation, and this was soon recommended in the literature as appropriate[33]. However, this dose range was reported to be poorly tolerated by some adult patients[34,35]. In a double-blind placebo-controlled crossover study, 0.005, 0.01, 0.025 and 0.05 mg/kg doses (mean, 0.4–4 mg) were administered by nebulization to 10 male patients with chronic bronchitis, and resulted in maximum increases in forced expiratory volume in one second (FEV_1) of 18% (at 60 minutes), 24% (at 30–60 minutes), 27% (at 60 minutes) and 35% (at 60 minutes), respectively[35]. Although the 0.05 mg/kg dose afforded marginally greater and longer-lasting (4 versus 3 hours) bronchodilatation than 0.025 mg/kg, the smaller dose was associated with fewer adverse reactions (dry mouth and increase in pulse rate). Effective bronchodilatation (increase in FEV_1 ⩾15%) lasted 1 hour with the 0.005 mg/kg dose and 2 hours with the 0.01 mg/kg dose. Thus, the most optimal, yet least discomforting, dose of inhaled atropine sulphate in adult patients was considered to be 0.025 mg/kg, or about 2 mg.

A single nebulized dose of atropine sulphate 0.05 mg/kg (average 3.7 mg) resulted in highly variable maximum serum atropine concentrations (1.3–5.8 ng/ml) in six male patients with chronic bronchitis[34]. Maximum increases in FEV_1 (37%) and specific airways conductance (SGaw 33%) occurred at 1.5 hours. The maximum concentrations of 4.8 and 5.8 ng/ml attained in two patients are slightly in excess of those reported from a 0.32 mg intravenous dose of atropine sulphate in healthy volunteers[36]. Measurable concentrations were present for 15 minutes to at least 4 hours, indicating that significant systemic absorption occurs after inhalation of atropine sulphate. There was no correlation between improvement in spirometric and plethysmographic parameters and serum concentration achieved.

In one comparative study, the milligram-for-milligram potency of atropine sulphate was found to be about one-half that of atropine methonitrate in 13 stable asthmatics[37]. Although both atropine sulphate 4 mg and atropine methonitrate 2 mg produced similar maximum increases in FEV_1 (46% at 60 minutes and 48% at 120 minutes, respectively), the duration of action was significantly longer with the methonitrate salt (6 versus 4 hours). The greater bronchodilatory potency of atropine methonitrate over atropine sulphate was also demonstrated by other authors[20,38,39], and is to be expected as the former is a quaternary salt.

Oral atropine, at single doses of up to 1 mg, was shown to have no effect in bronchial asthma[10]. Higher doses were productive of uncomfortable side-effects.

Effects in antigen-induced bronchospasm

Considerable variation has been observed in the ability of atropine sulphate to prevent bronchoconstriction induced by inhalation antigen challenges. Inhaled atropine was most effective in preventing bronchospasm provoked by methacholine[32,41–43], carbachol[20,44], charcoal dust[29], and cold air[29], showed some effect against citric acid[29] and house dust[43,45], and had little or no effect against ragweed or mixed pollens[20,43,46] and histamine[20,29,42]. In comparative trials with β-adrenoceptor stimulants, atropine proved to have a lesser protective effect against histamine-induced bronchospasm than salbutamol[42] and isoprenaline[20]. In 6 extrinsic asthmatic patients, atropine sulphate 1.2 mg was more effective than sodium cromoglycate 40 mg or thymoxamine 15 mg in the prevention of bronchospasm provoked by prostaglandin $F_{2\alpha}$[47].

Effect in exercise-induced bronchospasm

Studies of the effect of inhaled atropine on exercise-induced bronchospasm (EIB) have produced mixed results. In studies in which little or no protection against EIB was reported[41,48–52], atropine was administered less than 20 minutes before the exercise challenge. However, in trials where atropine markedly prevented EIB[53,54], a longer time was allowed for atropine to attain its maximal bronchodilatory effect.

Thus, in 20 asthmatic children (ages 8 to 16 years) given atropine sulphate 1 mg 45 minutes before a cycloergometer exercise challenge, FEV_1 values decreased by a mean of 10%, as compared with 22% with placebo[53]. A similar degree of protection was provided by ipratropium bromide 0.04 mg (a 13% decrease), while more protection occurred with ipratropium bromide 0.08 mg (a 1% decrease).

In another trial, 6 asthmatic children (ages 12 to 16 years) were given atropine sulphate 60 minutes before a treadmill test[54]. Postexercise specific airways conductance (SGaw) values were 34% higher than placebo with a nebulized dose of 0.03–0.04 mg/kg, 36% higher with double this dose, 25% higher with a 0.35 mg intramuscular dose, and 58% higher with a combination of the usual nebulized dose and the intramuscular dose. Thus, parenteral atropine appears to add to the bronchoprotective effect against EIB, as well as the bronchodilatation produced by inhaled drug, presumably by reaching the smaller airways.

Tinkelman et al.[55] have reported that atropine sulphate in high inhaled doses specifically blocked the effect of exercise in 17 of 18 asthmatic children. However, this group did not control for the pre-exercise bronchodilator effect of atropine.

Single dose comparative trials in asthma and bronchitis

Most of the trials in which atropine was assessed in single dose studies involved small treatment groups (less than 20 patients). The degree of bronchodilatation was measured primarily by spirometry (especially FEV_1), although a few trials also included plethysmographic measurements. In some trials, respiratory measurements were not performed after 3.5 hours[38,62,63] and, thus, a complete assessment of the bronchodilatory effects of atropine vis-à-vis comparative agents could not be made.

In most of the comparative trials reviewed, the patient populations were strictly defined as either asthmatic or bronchitic. However, in a few trials, patients with asthma also had chronic bronchitis[37,58,65]. Significant bronchodilatation ($FEV_1 \geqslant 15\%$ above base-line) was achieved in most patients after receiving atropine. However, a few patients showed no improvement in any respiratory parameter, suggesting that the vagal component in asthmatic conditions may vary considerably between individuals. Atropine was very useful in asthmatic patients who achieved insignificant bronchodilatation with isoprenaline[67] or salbutamol[57]. Possible reasons for the lack of response to the β-adrenoceptor agents (e.g. tachyphylaxis) were not explained in these trials.

The onset of bronchodilatation with inhaled atropine methonitrate was more delayed than with the β-adrenoceptor agents, but was of longer duration. Thus, while effective bronchodilatation was maintained for up to 7 hours or more with atropine methonitrate, it lasted only 0.5–2 hours with isoprenaline[31,38,58,63], 1–2 hours with fenoterol[37,69], and 2 hours with salbutamol[65]. As would be expected, atropine sulphate produced bronchodilatation of lesser magnitude and of shorter duration than atropine methonitrate in asthmatic patients. It was equal to or marginally better than isoprenaline[56,61,66].

The response to atropine tended to be better in patients with chronic bronchitis and asthma with a bronchitic component than in those with uncomplicated asthma[20,59,60,71], possibly due to greater vagal influence in the former two conditions. Thus, Crompton[60] found that, in 18 bronchitic patients, the maximum FEV_1 attained with subcutaneous atropine sulphate 0.6 mg was double that occurring in 18 asthmatics, whereas the response to isoprenaline was the same in both types of patients. Similar results were noted by Chick and Jenne[59]. In still another trial, aerosolized atropine methonitrate treatment resulted in a more rapid response in patients with chronic bronchitis than in those with asthma[71].

Atropine responsiveness was increased in atopic asthmatics by the addition of corticosteroids[20,72]. Thus, in 8 atopic asthmatic patients, a 16-week course of inhaled beclomethasone dipropionate 0.1 mg four times daily improved the maximum FEV_1 response to nebulized atropine methonitrate 1.9 mg by 14%, but not the response to salbutamol 4.2 mg[72]. In 3 of 6 adult status asthmaticus patients treated aggressively with intravenous corticosteroids, theophylline and β_2-adrenoceptor agents, atropine sulphate 5 mg by intermittent positive-pressure breathing improved spirometric values by greater than 15%[73]. However, as atropine takes so long to act, its use in status asthmaticus would be expected to be limited without a concurrent high-dose corticosteroid regimen. Some patients have actually been found to be 'atropine resistant' until the allergic component of their acute asthmatic condition is remedied by corticosteroids and sodium cromoglycate[20,72]. Corticosteroids did not improve response in patients with chronic bronchitis[20,60].

The combination of atropine with a β-adrenoceptor agent generally resulted in an increase in duration of action over that attained with either agent alone. In some trials, an increase in maximum bronchodilatation was also apparent, although this could be negligible[31]. Additive effects would be expected with the combination, as the two types of agents produce bronchodilatation by complementary mechanisms (β-adrenoceptor agents increasing cyclic AMP and atropine decreasing cyclic GMP) and affect different parts of the airways.

Comparative trials in obstructive airways disease

In several trials, atropine was evaluated in patients with a diagnosis of chronic obstructive airways disease. Thus, in 24 of such patients, subcutaneous atropine sulphate 0.5 mg was shown to produce a smaller overall decrease in total airways resistance (29%) than subcutaneous doses of adrenaline 1 mg (55%), orciprenaline 0.5 mg (44%) and terbutaline 0.5 mg (53%)[74]. Conversely, in 10 children (ages 9 to 16 years) with respiratory disease associated with cystic fibrosis, nebulized atropine sulphate 0.1 mg/kg produced a greater decrease in residual volume than nebulized isoprenaline 0.05 mg/kg (25% versus 16%)[75].

Long-term studies

Very few long-term studies have been reported comparing atropine with other bronchodilators, or even with placebo. In asthma patients, long-term treatment with atropine sulphate proved to be no better than placebo in two trials[64,76]. Thus, during an 8-week double-blind crossover trial in 6 adult asthmatics, the mean FEV_1 increased by 18% with oral atropine sulphate 0.5 mg four times daily and by 14% with placebo. Similarly, in 12 asthmatic children (ages 7 to 17 years) on oral atropine sulphate 0.02 mg/kg (mean 0.67 mg) three times daily for 4 weeks, mean morning and evening peak flow rates were no different from those which occurred during a 4-week placebo period[76]. A higher dosage only led to uncomfortable anticholinergic side-effects.

Although one author found no differences between nebulized atropine sulphate 0.02 mg/kg three times daily and placebo in an 8-week double-blind crossover trial, spirometric measurements were made only 20 minutes post inhalation and, thus, at a time when atropine would just be starting to produce a bronchodilatory effect[76]. As the 'placebo' used here was a sympathomimetic plus a propylene glycol diluent, the validity of this study in assessing long-term atropine response in asthma is questionable.

In a 1-week double-blind crossover study in 7 asthma patients, atropine sulphate 0.25 mg inhaled 4-hourly was significantly more effective than 0.3 ml of the α-blocker thymoxamine 1.5% inhaled 4-hourly[77]. The three patients who responded best to atropine had previously had marked bronchorrhoea.

Finally, in 15 patients with chronic bronchitis, the maximal responses of nebulized atropine sulphate 1 mg, isoprenaline 1 mg and placebo, each given four times daily for 3 weeks did not change weekly base-line lung function studies (taken 10 hours after the last drug inhalation)[78].

Side-effects

A disadvantage of atropine is that it produces notable anti-cholinergic side-effects in many patients, and these have been found to be dose related[31,61,79], and more frequent with oral and parenteral drug. Nevertheless, the incidence of dry mouth after single therapeutic doses of inhaled atropine sulphate or methonitrate has been reported as 8–10%[56,62], 33%[78], 38%[37], and even nearly 100%[31,38,57,67,68,75]. Although oral dryness with atropine is bothersome, it is generally mild. Dry mouth was more common and longer lasting with inhaled atropine sulphate 2 mg than with ipratropium 0.04 and 0.08 mg[80].

In single dose studies of inhaled atropine, flushing occurred in less than 10% of patients[31], lightheadedness in 25–33%[67,68], and giddiness in 38%[37], whereas blurred vision and urinary retention were rarely reported. Side-effects were fewer in patients on a combination of atropine methonitrate or sulphate with fenoterol than with each agent alone[37]. Unlike inhaled isoprenaline[38,56,67,78] and salbutamol[79], inhaled atropine did not produce tremors, significant increases in pulse rate or blood pressure, or palpitations even at doses of 6 mg. Very few patients have had to stop therapy because of side-effects, as the benefits usually outweigh the discomfort.

Of 15 patients who received nebulized atropine sulphate 1 mg four times daily for 3 weeks, one-third reported mild urinary hesitancy, dry mouth and blurred vision[78]. In another multiple-dose study[64], 3 of 6 asthmatics on oral atropine sulphate 0.5 mg four times daily complained of dry mouth, while 3 noticed no differences from placebo.

Reports of serious adverse reactions to atropine are rare. Nevertheless, in the study of Larsen et al.[75] in patients with cystic fibrosis, one 16-year-old girl with a history of meconium ileus developed partial bowel obstruction 12 hours after one inhalation of atropine sulphate 0.1 mg/kg. This resolved after cessation of treatment. A case report has also been published involving a 59-year-old man who developed an acute organic brain syndrome (pressured speech, flight of ideas, visual hallucinations) 7 days after starting inhaled atropine sulphate 1.2 mg every 6 hours[81]. After physostigmine 1 mg was administered intravenously, the patient's mental status returned to normal within five minutes. The patient, who had no previous psychiatric history, remained well when taken off all atropine subsequent to this episode.

Thiazinamium

Thiazinamium methylsulphate is an anti-cholinergic phenothiazine derivative, which also has antihistaminic properties (*Figure 9.1*). Although it has been available for the treatment of asthma since the early 1960s, studies on its pharmacokinetics in man have been reported mainly during the last 10 years[82–85]. Intramuscular injection of thiazinamium induces considerable bronchodilatation[86,87], but inconsistent results have been obtained after oral administration[84,85]. As thiazinamium is a quaternary ammonium compound, the latter is to be expected. The bioavailability of oral thiazinamium is only 2–3% of that occurring after an intramuscular injection[85]. Intrarectal thiazinamium is slightly better absorbed (3–9%)[83]. The elimination half-life of parenteral drug is short, being about 20 minutes in most patients[82].

In 17 patients with obstructive lung disease, intramuscular thiazinamium and inhaled sodium cromoglycate both afforded a marked protective effect in bronchial allergen tests, although only thiazinamium produced significant bronchodilatation[88]. In 18 patients with chronic bronchitis and emphysema, the bronchodilatating activity of intramuscular thiazinamium 50 mg was almost identical to that of inhaled ipratropium 0.02 mg (airways flow resistance falling maximally by 49% at 30 minutes), but greater than that occurring with intramuscular atropine sulphate 0.5 mg (maximal R_t decrease, 33% at 15 minutes)[70].

In an 8-week crossover comparative trial in 15 patients with chronic bronchitis, oral thiazinamium 300 mg three times daily proved less effective in spirometric measurements and subjective assessments than inhaled ipratropium 0.04 mg three times daily[89].

Compared with inhaled ipratropium bromide, intramuscular thiazinamium and intramuscular atropine were associated with 'extremely frequent side-effects' in the study by Vastag *et al.*[70]. Notable tachycardia occurred shortly after intramuscular injection of thiazinamium in two trials, and this was thought to be related to the high plasma concentrations rapidly achieved by this highly water-soluble drug[84,86]. Dry mouth was reported as 'frequent' with oral thiazinamium, and micturition problems of moderate severity affected 13% of patients[89].

Deptropine

Deptropine (dibenzheptropine) citrate is a tropinylether anti-cholinergic agent, which also has anti-5-hydroxytryptamine and antihistamine properties (*Figure 9.1*)[90]. Like atropine, deptropine can be administered parenterally, orally or by inhalation, and has a slow onset of action relative to β-adrenoceptor agents.

Response to deptropine has been found to differ considerably among asthmatic patients. Nevertheless, optimum bronchodilatation in most patients appears to occur with daily doses of 2–3 mg intramuscularly[91,92] and 0.2 mg by inhalation[93–95]. Although Schmidt[96] reported an average increase in maximum voluntary ventilation volume of 56% in asthmatic patients during a 6-week regimen of oral deptropine 2 mg daily, three other authors did not find 1.5–2 mg daily of oral drug to be significantly better than placebo in up to 3 months of treatment[97–99].

The bronchodilatory effect and duration of action of deptropine appear to be dose dependent. Thus, in 10 patients with asthma and 20 with chronic bronchitis, a low (0.1 mg) aerosolized dose of deptropine citrate resulted in no greater bronchodilatation than was observed with placebo, FEV_1 values rising only to a maximum of 5.3% above base-line[100]. Conversely, a high aerosolized dose (2 mg) resulted in a mean maximum FEV_1 increase of 64% at 2 hours in a similar group of patients[101]. Even at 5 hours, the FEV_1 was 54% above base-line.

In a double-blind crossover trial in 8 asthmatic patients and 8 chronic bronchitics, aerosolized deptropine 0.2 mg produced a lower degree of bronchodilatation than ipratropium 0.04 mg (maximum FEV_1, 29% versus 48%)[93]. The onset of action of the two drugs was similar, FEV_1 values for both being 18% above base-line at five hours. No significant differences have been noted in the bronchodilatory response between asthmatic and bronchitic patients in this trial, as well as in another[100].

Although the addition of aerosolized isoprenaline 0.3 mg to a dose of deptropine citrate 0.2 mg did not increase the maximal indirect breathing capacity (iMBC) more than that which occurred with deptropine alone (27% versus 26%), it hastened the onset of bronchodilatation (iMBC) increase at 30 minutes, 24% versus 5% above baseline)[95].

Dry mouth and throat were reported in 10–50% of patients treated with oral deptropine, difficulty with micturition in 31%, difficulty in coughing in 19%, and blurred vision in 12%[97,99,102]. Aerosolized deptropine 0.2 mg daily was associated with fewer anti-cholinergic side-effects, dry throat occurring in fewer than 7% of patients[95].

Ipratropium bromide

Ipratropium bromide (*Figure 9.1*) is a quaternary derivative of *N*-isopropylatropine[103]. In dogs, the milligram-for-milligram ratio of bronchodilatation to inhibition of salivation was found to be 1:220 with inhaled ipratropium, compared with 1:93 with inhaled atropine sulphate[104]. Bronchodilatation:tachycardia ratios were 1:550 and 1:300, respectively. In *in vitro* studies on isolated animal airways preparations, ipratropium demonstrated no important effects on ciliary beat frequency, while the same doses of atropine decreased ciliary activity by up to 30%[105,106]. Thus, inhaled ipratropium appeared to be more bronchoselective and possibly less productive of systemic anti-cholinergic side-effects than atropine. This subsequently led to considerable research of this drug in patients with asthma and chronic bronchitis.

Effect in antigen-induced bronchospasm

The protective effect of ipratropium bromide against experimental bronchoconstriction has been variable. As was the case with atropine, the type and concentration of antigen used, the dose of ipratropium, and the timing of ipratropium administration relative to antigen challenge have been largely responsible for this. Some studies did not allow enough time for ipratropium to act before measuring any protective response against antigen or exercise challenge.

In studies where the protective effect was monitored for 30 minutes or more, ipratropium gave variable or limited protection against bronchospasm induced by 5-hydroxytryptamine[107,108] and histamine[70,107,109–112], moderate protection against propranolol-induced bronchospasm[107], and greater and more consistent protection against bronchospasm induced by grass pollen[113,114], moulds, animal hair and house dust[113], cigarette smoke[108,115], prostaglandin $F_{2\alpha}$[116], and cold air[108]. The most marked protection was against acetylcholine and methacholine-induced bronchoconstriction[70,107–109,112,117,118], as would be expected for an anti-cholinergic agent.

When 10 asthmatics inhaled ipratropium 0.04 mg about 30 minutes prior to an inhalation challenge with acetylcholine 0.25 mg, the usual 4-fold rise in total respiratory resistance was prevented[70]. Similarly, inhalation of ipratropium 0.04 mg 20–120 minutes before a challenge with aerosolized acetylcholine 3% over 2 minutes reduced the fall in FEV_1 to 20–30%, in contrast to 50–60% without ipratropium ($p < 0.005$)[117].

In comparative trials, ipratropium was more active than the β_2-adrenoceptor stimulant orciprenaline (metaproterenol) against cholinergic challenge[119,120], and equally as effective as fenoterol in preventing methacholine-induced bronchospasm[110]. However, ipratropium has been generally less active than β_2-adrenoceptor agents against bronchospasm induced by histamine, ragweed, grass and animal extract allergens[111,119,121,122].

Effect in exercise-induced bronchospasm

Although some asthmatic patients are apparently well protected against exercise-induced bronchospasm (EIB) with ipratropium bromide, in other patients no response at all seems to occur. As β_2-adrenoceptor agents[123] or sodium cromoglycate[124,125] are effective in patients who fail to respond to ipratropium, the vagal reflex may not be important in some cases of EIB.

In contrast to studies in which the protective response was monitored less than 20 minutes post exercise[126–129], studies where the effect was monitored over at least 1 hour showed total or partial protection[53,130–132]. However, like atropine[41], ipratropium did not prevent the potentiation of EIB produced by breathing cold winter air[132].

Dose–response studies

Most investigators assessing the dose–response effects of ipratropium in asthmatic and bronchitic patients have not shown any significant increases in response at inhaled doses higher than 0.02–0.04 mg[133–137]. However, a few authors did report a better bronchodilatory response with doses of 0.08–0.28 mg of ipratropium[138–141].

The onset of maximum effect with inhaled ipratropium is slower than with isoprenaline, although some bronchodilator response occurs very rapidly (within 30 seconds)[142,143]. Fifty per cent of the eventual maximum response occurs by 3 minutes, 80% within 30 minutes, and the peak effect at 1–2 hours[134,136].

The duration of a significant bronchodilator response to a 0.02–0.04 mg dose is about 6 hours[136,144]. With higher doses (0.06 or 0.08 mg), a greater response is usually observed after the first several hours[133,141,145].

Pharmacokinetics

As with other inhaled drugs, about 90% of ipratropium bromide precipitates in the mouth and upper airways, and is swallowed[146,147]. Systemic absorption of an inhaled dose is limited, and only very low blood concentrations are likely to occur with the usual inhaled doses.

Two minutes after 5 healthy volunteers inhaled a very high dose (0.555 mg), ipratropium appeared in the plasma. A peak plasma concentration of 0.06 ng/ml was recorded at 3 hours, representing 0.03% of the inhaled dose. Based on urinary excretion, less than 5% of the inhaled dose was absorbed[148].

Plasma concentrations after ipratropium 0.04 mg by inhalation are 1000 times lower than those occurring after 0.15 mg intravenously and 15 mg orally, even though each of these routes results in equivalent bronchodilatation. Thus, it appears that ipratropium's bronchodilatory effect after inhalation is due to a local effect at the alveolar space, rather than a systemic effect.

Of the 0.555 mg inhaled dose 2.8% was eliminated in the urine after 24 hours, with only 0.4% of the dose being eliminated by this route over the next 5 days[148]. Faecal excretion of ipratropium bromide in these volunteers was 48% at 24 hours after dosing, and 69% by the end of 6–7 days. The elimination half-life of ipratropium bromide in healthy volunteers was 3.2–3.8 hours by all routes of elimination[148], which is considerably shorter than that reported for atropine (12.5–38 hours)[149].

Short-term comparisons with placebo and with β-adrenoceptor stimulants in airways disease

In short-term studies specifically designed to compare ipratropium with a placebo in patients with asthma or bronchitis, inhaled ipratropium usually resulted in a significantly greater improvement in respiratory function than a placebo[69,129,150–153]. Airways resistance decreased by 15–30% following doses of 0.04–0.08 mg in these trials. Similarly, in studies comparing ipratropium with other inhaled bronchodilators in patients with chronic obstructive airways diseases, utilizing placebo administration as part of the study design, ipratropium and the comparison drugs were superior to placebo.

Asthmatic patients in double-blind short-term comparative trials achieved similar maximum improvement in airways function with ipratropium 0.04 or 0.08 mg as they did with isoprenaline 0.075 to 0.2 mg[141,154–

[159]. However, the timing of the bronchodilator effect differed markedly. Ipratropium usually exerted its maximum effect at 1–2 hours, with a duration of effect of about 4–6 hours or more. Conversely, isoprenaline reached its maximum effect more rapidly (at about 15 minutes or less), but acted for a shorter duration (1–2 hours in most studies).

The few studies which have compared usual doses of ipratropium and orciprenaline in asthmatic patients demonstrated similar improvement in airways function with both agents[137,160,161].

Single dose studies comparing metered doses of ipratropium 0.04 or 0.08 mg with usual doses of salbutamol demonstrated that the maximum improvement achieved in airways function was less with ipratropium. There was about a 25–50% increase in FEV_1 with ipratropium, as compared with 35–75% with salbutamol. As with isoprenaline, the onset of maximum effect was slower with ipratropium (about 90–180 minutes versus 30–60 minutes). However, the overall duration of effect of ipratropium and salbutamol appeared to be similar, although some studies showed no significant differences after the first few hours due to the previously greater effect of salbutamol beginning to decline[122,162]. In one trial in which 22 patients with acute asthma received ipratropium 0.5 mg or salbutamol 10 mg by nebulization, the drugs were equally effective[163].

In contrast to short-term studies, multiple-dose studies, comparing usual doses of ipratropium and salbutamol over a few days to a few weeks, usually demonstrated no significant differences in regard to respiratory function indices, patient preference, or symptom scoring[164,165]. Nevertheless, salbutamol tended to be more effective[165]. The numbers of patients in such studies (16 and 11, respectively) may well have been too small to detect statistically significant differences.

In one study in which ipratropium and salbutamol response was assessed according to age in 29 asthmatic patients, ipratropium appeared to be more effective in patients over 40 years old (who may have lost their β-adrenergic responsiveness), while salbutamol was more effective in younger patients[166].

Usual doses of inhaled ipratropium, as well as very high doses (in one cumulative dose study) also fared less well than fenoterol in single dose studies in asthmatic patients. The maximum improvement in respiratory function was less with ipratropium (about a 25–50% increase in FEV_1, compared with 35–50% with fenoterol in most studies). However, unlike salbutamol, fenoterol has a relatively slow onset of maximum effect (1–2 hours[167]). Thus, ipratropium and fenoterol demonstrated a similar time course to maximal effects.

A multiple-dose study in a small number of asthmatic patients (13) detected no significant differences between ipratropium 0.04 mg five times daily for 4 days or fenoterol 0.4 mg five times daily[168]. Increasing the ipratropium dose to 0.08 mg did not improve the magnitude of response. In fact, 0.08 mg appeared to be less effective than 0.04 mg, possibly due to an increase in coughing with the higher dose.

Usual doses of inhaled ipratropium have been reported as less effective[169], equally effective[170], and more effective[171] than inhaled terbutaline. An explanation for the variable results is that, in the trial of Linehan et al.[170], low doses of terbutaline 0.05 mg were tested. In the two other trials, one measured effectiveness using peak expiratory flow (PEF) values[171] and the other utilized FEV_1 and specific airways conductance values[169]. Thus, more trials are necessary to compare the efficacy of ipratropium with that of terbutaline.

Comparisons with other anti-cholinergic drugs

In small groups of asthmatic patients, ipratropium 0.04 or 0.08 mg was as effective as inhaled atropine 2 mg in one single dose trial[80], but not another[169]. However, in the latter trial, most of the patients had a bronchitic component to their asthma. Ipratropium was shown to be superior to inhaled deptropine 0.1 mg[93].

Response in atopic versus non-atopic asthma

Four studies[122,166,172,173] compared the differential bronchodilatating response to inhaled ipratropium in atopic versus non-atopic asthmatics. Patients were defined as atopic if they had immediate hypersensitivity reactions to one or more allergens, seasonal variation related to allergen exposure, and onset of asthma early in life. Non-atopic patients were those with no immediate hypersensitivity reaction to allergens, no personal history of allergic rhinitis or eczema, and onset of asthma in adult life. Each of the studies reported no significant differences in ipratropium response between the two groups of patients. This is in contrast to the more prolonged and significantly greater increase ($p < 0.05$) in FEV_1 noted with salbutamol in atopic versus non-atopic asthmatics[122].

Studies in bronchitis

In several single dose studies in bronchitis patients, inhaled ipratropium 0.04 mg was as effective as orciprenaline 1.5 mg[161,174,175]. Both drugs produced about a 30% improvement in total airways resistance in patients with bronchitis secondary to mitral stenosis[175]. In one study, ipratropium 0.04 mg and orciprenaline 1.5 mg were equally effective in terminating bronchospasm in patients with an acute exacerbation of chronic bronchitis[176], which is surprising considering the relatively slow onset of maximum effect of the former drug.

Unlike the findings in asthmatic patients, in a few single dose studies in small groups of patients with chronic bronchitis, ipratropium and salbutamol were usually equally effective. In some studies, ipratropium was even more effective according to some evaluation parameters[177-180], or was longer acting[181]. Ipratropium was shown in two reports to be at least as rapid in onset of maximum effect as salbutamol[162,180], in contrast to the findings of its slower onset in patients with asthma.

As with comparisons with salbutamol, ipratropium and fenoterol were of similar effectiveness in most studies in bronchitis patients. Usual doses of both drugs increased the airways conductance by about 60–70% and the FEV_1 by about 20–30%. The time course of response was also similar, the maximum effect occurring at 30–60 minutes. At least a 15% increase in FEV_1 above base-line was maintained for about 2 to 4 or 5 hours.

Response in asthma versus bronchitis

As occurs with other bronchodilator drugs, the absolute effect of ipratropium was often somewhat less in bronchitis than in asthma in most studies in which data on the two respiratory conditions were distinguished[93,162,164,182,183]. However, with ipratropium, the decrease in effectiveness in bronchitis was comparatively small, and the relative effect of ipratropium compared with β_2-adrenoceptor agonist drugs was greater in bronchitis. Thus, in comparative studies, ipratropium was generally less effective than the β_2-adrenoceptor agonist drugs in asthma, but at least as effective in bronchitis. According to Verstraeten[184], this may be due partly to a more important vagal component to bronchitis than to asthma.

Studies in undifferentiated chronic obstructive airways disease

In studies which did not differentiate asthmatics from bronchitis patients, or did not report results separately, usual inhaled doses of ipratropium 0.04 or 0.08 mg were more effective than inhaled isoprenaline[150,185] or orally administered ephedrine 48 mg[186]. Such doses of ipratropium were usually equally effective as standard inhaled doses of fenoterol[187-190], orciprenaline[176,191], terbutaline[192] and salbutamol[193].

In all long-term studies of inhaled ipratropium bromide, the drug was well tolerated, and tachyphylaxis did not occur. In several small open studies, usually in patients with chronic bronchitis treated for up to 12 months[194-200], and in a large series (187 patients) in patients with undifferentiated chronic obstructive lung disease treated for up to 4 years[201], daily ipratropium therapy continued to be effective. FEV_1 values were maintained at about 15–30% above baseline throughout the treatment period. In some studies, the response was apparently even greater after 4–6 months than initially[197,199]. The doses used were usually about 0.04 mg three to four times daily, although occasionally doses as high as 0.8 mg daily were used[194].

In a 6-month study in 60 patients with moderate-to-severe chronic bronchitis, ipratropium 0.04 mg three times daily produced significant additional bronchodilatation and improved exercise performance when added to previous β_2-adrenoceptor and theophylline regimens[232].

In a 2-month comparative crossover study in 60 patients with chronic bronchitis, ipratropium aerosol 0.04 mg or salbutamol 4 mg tablets, each given three times daily, produced similar changes in peak expiratory flow rate (PEFR), but subjective clinical assessment was significantly in favour of ipratropium[202].

Combined use with other bronchodilator drugs

As with atropine, ipratropium has been combined with β_2-adrenoceptor agents, methylxanthine derivatives, and sodium cromoglycate, usually with improved spirometric results. Addition of a systemic corticosteroid to a combined aerosol regimen increased the response still further in patients with asthma, but not in chronic bronchitis[165].

Several single dose or short-term studies in small groups of patients with chronic obstructive lung disease indicated that the combined use of ipratropium (usually 0.04 mg) with β_2-adrenoceptor agonist drugs such as inhaled salbutamol (usually 0.2 mg)[165,172,179,183,203–205] or fenoterol (usually 0.4 mg)[188,189,206–211], or inhaled[212] or orally administered orciprenaline[213], has often produced a greater or more prolonged response than occurred with the individual drugs. However, the increase in response was not always statistically significant. Occasionally, combined treatment was superior in patients with asthmatic bronchitis but not in patients with bronchitis and emphysema[209], or was statistically better than ipratropium alone, but not a β_2-adrenoceptor agonist alone[172,203], or vice versa[188,189]. The small numbers of patients in some of these trials may have been insufficient to definitely establish at a significant level any improvement which occurred with combined treatment.

A combination of a high dose of ipratropium 0.5–2 mg with a usual dose of sodium cromoglycate 20 mg, administered by ventilator, was more effective than either drug alone in preventing exercise-induced bronchospasm in asthmatic patients[214,215]. However, such combined treatment was less effective than a large dose of fenoterol 2 mg given alone[214].

When oral theophylline was combined with inhaled orciprenaline 1.5 mg or orciprenaline plus ipratropium 0.04 mg in 13 asthmatic patients with severe reversible bronchoconstriction, combined treatments produced the greatest improvements in respiratory function[212]. Thus, maximum increases in FEV_1 were 27%, 34% and 54% for orciprenaline, orciprenaline plus theophylline, and all three drugs, respectively. Similarly, in a placebo-controlled 2-week study in 12 patients with asthma[216], the combination of inhaled ipratropium 0.04 mg four times daily and theophylline (at a dosage sufficient to maintain therapeutic serum concentrations of 10–20 μg/ml) resulted in a significantly greater increase in respiratory function indices than occurred with ipratropium alone.

Studies in children

Although most studies of ipratropium use in children have involved single doses, a few have reported continued effectiveness of the drug over several weeks of treatment in small groups of patients[217–219]. In 12 children with bronchospasm, 0.02 mg appeared to be the optimum inhaled dose and no differences over base-line values were noted between doses of 0.01 and 0.04 mg[218].

In a trial in which children 3–5 years old received all drugs via nebulization, ipratropium 0.25 mg and salbutamol 5 mg produced very similar increases in peak expiratory flow rate between 10 and 30 minutes[220]. Both agents were significantly more effective than clemastine 1 mg or placebo. In another trial in which 32 very young asthmatic children (3 months to 2 years old) received ipratropium 0.25 mg by nebulization, 40% experienced an improvement in airways resistance and thoracic gas volume[221]. None of the children under 18 months old responded to salbutamol.

In a few children with exercise-induced bronchospasm, ipratropium appeared to be less effective than salbutamol in preventing the bronchospastic response to exercise challenge[222], although ipratropium 0.06 mg was markedly more effective than placebo in another trial[130]. In uncontrolled single dose studies in children with bronchospastic disease, ipratropium aerosol, usually at a dose of 0.04 mg was reportedly an effective broncho-dilator, increasing FEV_1 values by about 35%[213] and decreasing airways resistance and total resistance by 25 and 40%, respectively[223,224]. In other comparative studies in such patients, ipratropium 0.02 or 0.04 mg often had a similar effect as usual doses of salbutamol[217], fenoterol[225], or orciprenaline[226].

Steroid-sparing effect

In a placebo-controlled study, the effect of ipratropium on systemic corti-costeroid requirements was evaluated in 32 chronic obstructive lung dis-ease patients who had received prednisone 10–20 mg or triamcinolone 4–10 mg orally, daily for at least 3 years[227]. Inhaled ipratropium 0.04 mg four times daily allowed the steroid dosage to be reduced over 2 months to one-half the initial dose in 34% of the patients, and to one-third in 19%. In the placebo group, the corticosteroid dosage could not be maintained below base-line levels.

Side-effects

Unlike the other anti-cholinergic drugs which have been used in asthma therapy, ipratropium aerosol has been well tolerated in all studies. Syste-mic side-effects are unlikely owing to the very low blood concentrations attained when the drug is given via a metered dose aerosol device. Thus, intra-ocular pressure was not altered in volunteers or glaucoma patients receiving up to 0.8 mg[228,229], although occasional patients have com-plained of vision disturbances, usually after inadvertently spraying part of the dose into the eyes[229]. Mucus production was unchanged even with very high doses, but such studies have not been performed during long-term use of ipratropium.

A bad taste in the mouth has been noted in 20–30% of patients in some studies[164,230], and transient dryness of the mouth and scratching in the trachea have occurred in up to 25% of patients receiving aerosolized solu-tions of the drug given over several minutes[231].

In 1982, a nebulizer solution of ipratropium bromide became available in some countries, the recommended dosage for adults being 0.1–0.5 mg up to four times daily[233]. The long-term tolerance of this preparation, and its effects on sputum viscosity, have yet to be established.

Oxitropium bromide

The latest anti-cholinergic agent to be studied in the treatment of asthma and other respiratory diseases is oxitropium bromide [(−)-N-ethyl-norhyoscine methobromide or Ba 253; Boehringer Ingelheim] (*Figure 9.1*). This compound has qualitative effects similar to those of ipratropium bro-mide. The absorption of oxitropium is also very low, as would be expected for a quaternary ammonium compound[234].

In a dose–response study in 11 patients with chronic bronchitis and one with asthma, oxitropium 0.02 and 0.2 mg and placebo reduced the mean total airways resistance maximally by 45% (at 30 minutes), 53% (at 2 hours) and 15% (at 4 hours), respectively[235]. At 8 hours, oxitropium 0.02 and 0.2 mg remained significantly ($p<0.05$) more effective than placebo, with respective decreases in total resistance of 28% and 40%, compared with a 7% increase with placebo. In another dose–response study, the bronchodilatory effects of the 0.2 mg dose seemed to last longer than the 0.02 mg dose[236].

Metered dose inhalation and powder inhalation of oxitropium bromide 0.2 mg both provided a marked protective effect (approximately 30% with each) in acetylcholine provocation tests in 24 asthmatics[237]. However, in another 24 asthmatic patients, these preparations offered very little protective effect (13%) in histamine challenge tests[237].

When bronchodilatation with inhaled oxitropium 0.2 mg and fenoterol 0.4 mg were compared in 12 asthmatic patients, 15 minutes after crude allergen extract provocation tests, specific airways resistance was observed to return to base-line faster with fenoterol (15 minutes versus 30 minutes)[238]. Capillary Po_2 increased significantly after fenoterol inhalation, but not following oxitropium inhalation. When oxitropium 0.2 mg, fenoterol 0.4 mg or sodium cromoglycate 20 mg were administered by inhalation 30 minutes before a crude allergen extract provocation test, only fenoterol provided almost complete protection. The mean protective effect of oxitropium was somewhat less than that of sodium cromoglycate, but the difference was not statistically significant ($p<0.05$)[238].

In exercise-sensitive asthmatic patients, oxitropium 0.1 mg, ipratropium 0.04 mg, fenoterol 0.4 mg and placebo were compared with regard to their protective effect against EIB[239]. Patients exercised on a cycloergometer when peak effects of the bronchodilators would have been apparent (60 minutes for oxitropium and ipratropium, and 10 minutes for fenoterol). Fenoterol exerted a good protective effect in all patients, whereas the anticholinergic agents differed very little from placebo. One patient benefited from oxitropium, 4 from ipratropium, and 2 from placebo.

Similarly, in another EIB trial in 13 asthmatic children (9 to 15 years old), a larger dose of oxitropium 0.2 mg was compared with fenoterol 0.4 mg and sodium cromoglycate 20 mg[240]. In this study, only 20 minutes was allowed between drug inhalation and exercise testing, and thus oxitropium would not have been evaluated at its peak effect. Nevertheless, oxitropium was significantly ($p<0.001$) more effective than placebo against EIB, but not as effective as fenoterol or sodium cromoglycate. The degree of protection (defined as the difference between the decrease in FEV_1 with and without agents), was 16.6%, 32.5% and 25.8%, respectively.

Oxitropium bromide has been compared with fenoterol in two controlled trials[236,238] and ipratropium bromide in one trial[139]. Thus, in a double-blind crossover study in 10 patients with asthma and 14 with chronic bronchitis, fenoterol 0.4 mg produced a more rapid rise in FEV_1 (within 5 minutes) than oxitropium 0.2 mg, although FEV_1 values were equivalent by 30 minutes[236]. The maximum FEV_1 increase was similar with both oxitropium (22%) and fenoterol (20%), and occurred at about the same time (0.5–2 hours). However, at 6 hours, significant bronchodilatation was apparent only with oxitropium, FEV_1 being 16% above base-line versus 8% with fenoterol.

In initial preclinical tests, it was suggested that oxitropium bromide possessed a greated bronchodilatating effect and a longer duration of action than ipratropium[241]. Preliminary clinical studies seem to affirm the latter, but not the former. The onset of action of oxitropium and ipratropium are similar, but not identical[139,242]. Where oxitropium 0.2 mg was compared with ipratropium 0.04 mg in 30 patients with chronic obstructive pulmonary disease, FEV_1 increased by about the same percentage at 15 minutes (16.4% and 17%, respectively)[139]. However, during the first 3 minutes, pulmonary resistance did not fall to as great a degree with oxitropium as with ipratropium (6% versus 15%). The author suggests that, because of its slow effect on pulmonary resistance, oxitropium bromide would be an unlikely candidate for the treatment of an acute bronchospastic attack.

One author[236] suggested that, as with atropine and ipratropium, bronchodilatation with oxitropium may be similar to that of β_2-adrenoceptor agents in patients with chronic bronchitis, but inferior to the latter agents in asthmatic patients[236]. However, careful assessment of the author's data reveals that oxitropium 0.2 mg actually produced similar maximum FEV_1 increases in 6 asthmatic patients and 6 bronchitic patients (28% and 26%, respectively), whereas fenoterol 0.4 mg produced a poorer response in the bronchitic group (39% versus 32%). Thus, oxitropium only tended to look better in these bronchitic patients by comparison. While FEV_1 values with oxitropium and fenoterol were equivalent at 6 hours in asthmatic patients, they remained slightly higher (by 6%) with oxitropium in the bronchitic group. A larger number of patients will be required for a proper study of the differential bronchodilatating effects of oxitropium and a β_2-adrenoceptor agent in asthma and bronchitis.

Like ipratropium, oxitropium by inhalation has not caused any important side-effects. However, it is too early to say whether one compound has advantages over the other.

Conclusions

Anti-cholinergic drugs have a long history of use in the treatment of asthma. The object of research over the past quarter of a century has been to synthesize a compound which produces optimal bronchodilatation with few side-effects. Ipratropium and oxitropium were to become the 'Holy Grail' for this crusade.

Like all of their predecessors, ipratropium and oxitropium, when given by inhalation, are slower acting than β_2-adrenoceptor agents and they have a longer duration of action. Bronchodilatation with these anti-cholinergic drugs may not be as great as that with some β-adrenoceptor agents in asthmatic patients. However, the effects of the two classes of drugs are often similar in patients with chronic bronchitis. The tachyphylaxis, tremor and cardiovascular side-effects produced by the β-adrenoceptor stimulants do not seem to occur with inhaled doses of anti-cholinergic drugs. It is somewhat disconcerting, though, that a few patients may not respond to these drugs, presumably because they have little or no vagal component to their bronchospasm.

The anti-cholinergic drugs would appear to be indicated primarily as an alternative to the β_2-adrenoceptor aerosols for the treatment of patients with asthma and chronic bronchitis who fail to respond adequately to sympathomimetic agents. In conclusion, the combination of anti-cholinergic drugs with β_2-adrenoceptor agents may well prove an important area of use in those patients not responding adequately to a single drug regimen, and possibly help to minimize corticosteroid requirements in such patients.

References

1. GANDEVIA, B. *Postgraduate Medical Journal*, **51** (Suppl. 7), 13 (1975)
2. GUPTA, S.S., PATEL, C.B. and MATHUR, V.S. *Journal of the Indian Medical Association*, **37**, 223 (1961)
3. KASHIKAR, C.G. *Chowkhamba Sanskrit Series*, **351**, 1 (1955)
4. CHRISTIE, T. *Edinburgh Medical and Surgical Journal*, **7**, 153 (1811)
5. SIGMOND, G.G. *Lancet*, **ii**, 392 (1836)
6. ENGLISH, W. *Edinburgh Medical Journal*, **7**, 153 (1811)
7. WILLIAMS, C.J.B. *The Pathology and Diagnosis of Disease of the Chest*, 4th ed. p. 328. London: Smith Elder (1840)
8. BEVERLEY, W.H. *British Medical Journal*, **2**, 465 (1884)
9. FOTHERGILL, J.M., *Chronic Bronchitis: Its Form and Treatment*. London: Baillière Tindal & Cox (1882)
10. FULLER, W.H. *On Diseases of the Chest* London: Churchill (1862)
11. NEALE, R. *The Medical Digest*, 3rd ed. London: Ledger Smith (1891)
12. GERHARDT, W.W. *The Diagnosis, Pathology and Treatment of Diseases of the Chest*, 4th ed. p. 183. Philadelphia: Lippincott (1860)
13. WOOD, G.B. *A Treatise on the Practice of Medicine*, 5th ed. Vol. 1. p. 887. Philadelphia: Lippincott (1858)
14. TURNER, D. *The Treatment of Asthma*. Transactions of the Intercolonial Medical Congress Australasia, 3rd Session. p. 117. Sydney: Government Printer (1893)
15. CARRYER, H.M., PRICKMAN, L.E., MAYTUM, C.K. and KOELSCHE, G.A. *Journal of the American Medical Association*, **131**, 21 (1946)
16. ALEXANDER, H.L. *Synopsis of Allergy*, 2nd ed. St Louis: Mosby (1947)
17. SWINEFORD, O. *Journal of Allergy*, **8**, 607 (1937)
18. DAUTREBANDE, L. *Archives Internationales de Pharmacodynamie et de Thérapie*, **66**, 379 (1941)
19. HERXHEIMER, H. *British Medical Journal*, **2**, 167 (1959)
20. ALTOUNYAN, R.E.C. *Thorax*, **19**, 406 (1964)
21. BEAKEY, J.F., BRESNICK, E., LEVINSON, L. and SEGAL, M.S. *Annals of Allergy*, **7**, 113 (1949)
22. HENSLEY, M.J., O'CAIN, C.F., McFADDEN, E.R. and INGRAM, R.H. *American Journal of Physiology*, **45**, 778 (1978)
23. INGRAM, R.H. and McFADDEN, E.R. *New England Journal of Medicine*, **297**, 596 (1977)
24. THOMSON, N.C., PATEL, K.R. and KERR, J.W. *Thorax*, **33**, 694 (1978)
25. SU, C. and BEVAN, J.A. *Pharmacology and Therapeutics* (B), **2**, 275 (1976)
26. KALINER, M. *Journal of Allergy and Clinical Immunology*, **60**, 204 (1977)
27. ENGELHARDT, A. *Scandinavian Journal of Respiratory Diseases, Supplementum*, **103**, 110 (1979)
28. GOLD, W.M., KESSLER, G.F. and YU, D.Y.C. *Journal of Applied Physiology*, **33**, 719 (1972)
29. SIMONSSON, B.G., JACOBS, F.M. and NADEL, J. *Journal of Clinical Investigation*, **46**, 1812 (1967)
30. COOPER, D.M., BRYAN, A.C. and LEVISON, H. *Federation Proceedings*, **33**, 439 (1974)
31. CAVANAUGH, M.J. and COOPER, D.M. *American Review of Respiratory Disease*, **114**, 517 (1976)
32. MUITTARI, A. *Annales Medicinae Internae Fenniae*, **57**, 193 (1968)
33. ZIMENT, I. *Respiratory Pharmacology*. p. 125. Philadelphia: W.B. Saunders Co. (1978)
34. KRADJAN, W.A., LAKSHMINARAYAN, S., HAYDEN, P.W., LARSON, S.W. and MARINI, J.J. *American Review of Respiratory Disease*, **123**, 471 (1981)
35. PAK, C.C.F., KRADJAN, W.A., LAKSHMINARAYAN, S. and MARINI, J.J. *American Review of Respiratory Disease*, **125**, 331 (1982)

36. HAYDEN, P.W., LARSON, S.M. and LAKSHMINARAYAN, S. *Journal of Nuclear Medicine*, **20**, 366 (1979)
37. ALLEN, C.J. and CAMPBELL, A.H. *Thorax*, **35**, 932 (1980)
38. CHAMBERLAIN, D.A., MUIR, D.C.F. and KENNEDY, K.P. *Lancet*, **ii**, 1019 (1962)
39. MALPASS, G.N. *American Journal of Pharmacy*, **123**, 5 (1951)
40. CULLUMBINE, H., McKEE, W.H.E. and CREASY, N.H. *Quarterly Journal of Experimental Physiology*, **40**, 309 (1955)
41. DEAL, E.C. Jr, McFADDEN, E.R. Jr, INGRAM, R.H. Jr and JAEGER, J.J. *Journal of Applied Physiology*, **45**, 238 (1978)
42. CASTERLINE, C.L., EVANS, R. III and WARD, G.W. Jr *Journal of Allergy and Clinical Immunology*, **58**, 607 (1976)
43. ROSENTHAL, R.R., NORMAL, P.S., SUMMER, W.R. and PERMUTT, S. *Journal of Applied Physiology*, **42**, 600 (1977)
44. DAUTREBANDE, L., LOVEJOY, F.W. and McCREDIE, R.M. *Archives Internationales de Pharmacodynamie et de Thérapie*, **139**, 198 (1962)
45. YU, D.Y.C., GALANT, S.P. and GOLD, W.M. *Journal of Applied Physiology*, **32**, 823 (1972)
46. FISH, J.E., ROSENTHAL, R.R., SUMMER, W.R., MENKES, H., NORMAN, P.S. and PERMUTT, S. *American Review of Respiratory Disease*, **115**, 371 (1977)
47. PATEL, K.R. *British Medical Journal*, **2**, 360 (1975)
48. KIVILOOG, J. *Pediatrics*, **56** (Suppl.), **940** (1975)
49. SLY, R.M., HEIMLICH, E.M., BUSSER, R.J. and STRICK, L. *Journal of Allergy*, **40**, 93 (1967)
50. TASHKIN, D.P., KATZ, R.M., KERSCHNAR, H., RACHELEFSKY, G.S. and SIEGEL, S.C. *Annals of Allergy*, **39**, 311 (1977)
51. RACHELEFSKY, G.S., TASHKIN, D.P., KATZ, R.M. KERSCHNAR, H. and SIEGEL, S.C. *Chest*, **73** (Suppl.), 1017 (1978)
52. GODFREY, S. and KONIG, P. *Pediatrics*, **56** (Suppl.), 930 (1975)
53. BORUT, T.C., TASHKIN, D.P., FISCHER, T.J., KATZ, R., RACHELEFSKY, G., SIEGEL, S.C. *et al. Journal of Allergy and Clinical Immunology*, **60**, 127 (1977)
54. CHEN, W.Y., BRENNER, A.M., WEISER, P.C. and CHAI, H. *Chest*, **79**, 651 (1981)
55. TINKELMAN, D.G., CAVANAUGH, M.J. and COOPER, D.M. *American Review of Respiratory Disease*, **114**, 87 (1976)
56. BRADY, R.E. and EASTON, J.G. *Annals of Allergy*, **42**, 211 (1979)
57. BURGE, P.S., HARRIES, M.G. and I'ANSON, E. *British Journal of Diseases of the Chest*, **74**, 259 (1980)
58. CAPEL, L.H. and FLETCHER, E.C. *British Journal of Diseases of the Chest*, **58**, 174 (1964)
59. CHICK, J.W. and JENNE, J.W. *Chest*, **72**, 719 (1977)
60. CROMPTON, G.K. *Thorax*, **23**, 46 (1968)
61. CROPP, G.J.A. *American Review of Respiratory Disease*, **112**, 599 (1975)
62. HEMSTREET, M.P.B. *Annals of Allergy*, **44**, 138 (1980)
63. KENNEDY, M.C.S. and THURSBY-PELHAM, D.C. *British Medical Journal*, **1**, 1018 (1964)
64. LIGHT, R.W. and GEORGE, R.B. *Annals of Allergy*, **38**, 58 (1977)
65. PIERCE, R.J., ALLEN, C.J. and CAMPBELL, A.H. *Thorax*, **34**, 45 (1979)
66. SNOW, R.M., MILLER, W.C., BLAIR, H.T. and RICE, D.L. *Annals of Allergy*, **42**, 286 (1979)
67. MARINI, J.J. and LAKSHMINARAYAN, S. *Chest*, **77**, 591 (1980)
68. MARINI, J.J., LAKSHMINARAYAN, S. and KRADJAN, W.A. *Chest*, **80**, 285 (1981)
69. MINETTE, A. and MARCQ, M. *Scandinavian Journal of Respiratory Diseases Supplementum*, **103**, 192 (1979)
70. VASTAG, E., NAGY, L. and MISKOVITZ, G. *European Journal of Clinical Pharmacology*, **10**, 201 (1976)
71. GANDEVIA, B.H. The reversibility of airways obstruction in asthma. In *Transactions of the World Asthma Conference*, Eastborne. Chest and Heart Association, London (1965)
72. JOLOBE, O.M.P. and LANE, D.J. *British Journal of Diseases of the Chest*, **75**, 413 (1981)
73. GREEN, A.W., STOKLOSA, J. and MIDDLETON, E. Jr *Journal of Allergy and Clinical Immunology*, **61**, 149 (1978)
74. KAIK, G., BONELLI, J. and MAGOMETSCHNIGG, D. *International Journal of Clinical Pharmacology*, **16**, 1 (1978)
75. LARSEN, G.L., BARRON, R.J., COTTON, E.K. and BROOKS, J.G. *American Review of Respiratory Disease*, **119**, 399 (1979)
76. HUTCHISON, A.A., OLINSKY, A. and LANDAU, L.I. *Australian Paediatric Journal*, **16**, 267 (1980)
77. WARDLE, E.N. *British Medical Journal*, **1**, 1085 (1977)

78. KLOCK, L.E., MILLER, T.D., MORRIS, A.H., WATANABE, S. and DICKMAN, M. *American Review of Respiratory Disease*, **112**, 371 (1975)
79. STARKE, I.D., PARKER, R.A. and TURNER-WARWICK, M. *Respiration*, **43**, 51 (1982)
80. SPECTOR, S. and BALL, R.E. JR *Chest*, **68**, 426 (1975)
81. BERGMAN, K.R., PEARSON, C., WALTZ, G.W. and EVANS III, R. *Chest*, **78**, 891 (1980)
82. JONKMAN, J.H.G., VAN BORK, L.E., DE ZEEUW, R.A. and ORIE, N.G.M. *Lancet*, **i**, 693 (1976)
83. JONKMAN, J.H.G., VAN BORK, L.E., WIJSBEEK, J., BOLHUIS-DE VRIES, A.S., DE ZEEUW, R.A., ORIE, N.G.M. *et al. Journal of Pharmaceutical Sciences*, **68**, 69 (1979)
84. JONKMAN, J.H.G., WIJSBEEK, J., HOLLENBEEK-BROUWER, S. and DE ZEEUW, R.A. *Journal of Pharmacy and Pharmacology*, **26** (Suppl.), 63P (1974)
85. VAN BORK, L.E. *Tubercle*, **56**, 244 (1975)
86. BOOIJ-NOORD, H., ORIE, N.G.M., TEN CATE, H.J. SLOOTS, S. and BOLT, D. *International Archives of Allergy*, **10**, 321 (1957)
87. VAN GEUNS, H.A. and SCHERRER, M. *International Archives of Allergy*, **7**, 111 (1955)
88. BOOIJ-NOORD, H., ORIE, N.G.M., BERG, W.C. and DE VRIES, K. *Journal of Allergy*, **46**, 1 (1970)
89. OTTO, A.J. *Scandinavian Journal of Respiratory Diseases Supplementum*, **103**, 151 (1979)
90. FUNCKE, A.B.H., DE JONGE, M.C., TERSTEEGE, H.M., MULDER, D., HARMS, A.F. and NAUTA, W. TH. *Acta Physiologica et Pharmacologica Neerlandica*, **11**, 104 (1962)
91. GRAY, W. and LECKIE, W.J.H. *British Journal of Diseases of the Chest*, **61**, 208 (1967)
92. SCHERRER, M. *Mededelingen Stichting Experimenteel Onderzoek Allergologie*, No. VII (1962)
93. BARBER, P.V., CHATTERJEE, S.S. and SCOTT, R. *British Journal of Diseases of the Chest*, **71**, 101 (1977)
94. COHEN, B.M. *Diseases of the Chest*, **48**, 471 (1965)
95. KENNEDY, M.C.S. *British Medical Journal*, **2**, 916 (1965)
96. SCHMIDT, F. The frequency and diagnosis of chronic asthmatic bronchitis and some clinical experiences with a new spasmolytic drug. Lecture given at the Antwerp Therapeutic Congress (1962)
97. GENERAL PRACTITIONER RESEARCH GROUP, *Practitioner*, **192**, 682 (1964)
98. LECKIE, W.J.H. and HORNE, N.W. *Thorax*, **20**, 317 (1965)
99. McNICOL, M.W. and BRUYNS, C. *British Journal of Diseases of the Chest*, **58**, 135 (1964)
100. RIPE, E. *Allergie und Asthma Band*, **16**, 41 (1970)
101. PRIME, F.J. *British Journal of Diseases of the Chest*, **62**, 81 (1968)
102. GIORDANO, S. and BEZANTE, T. *Minerva Pediatrica*, **21**, 1552 (1969)
103. PAKES, G.E., BROGDEN, R.N., HEEL, R.C., SPEIGHT, T.M. and AVERY, G.S. *Drugs*, **20**, 237 (1980)
104. BAUER, R., PUSCHMANN, S. and WICK, H. *Arzneimittel-Forschung*, **26**, 981 (1976)
105. IRAVANI, J. *International Journal of Clinical Pharmacology and Biopharmacy*, Suppl. 4, 20 (1972)
106. IRAVANI, J. and MORRIS-MELVILLE, G. *Postgraduate Medical Journal*, **51** (Suppl. 7), 108 (1975)
107. DE VRIES, K. *Postgraduate Medical Journal*, **51** (Suppl. 7), 106 (1975)
108. NOLTE, D. *Postgraduate Medical Journal*, **51** (Suppl. 7), 103 (1975)
109. CLARKE, P.S., JARRETT, R.G. and HALL, G.J.L. *Annals of Allergy*, **48**, 180 (1982)
110. FRITH, P.A., RUFFIN, R.E., COCKCROFT, D.W. and HARGREAVE, F.E. *Journal of Allergy and Clinical Immunology*, **61**, 175 (1978)
111. KILLIAM, D., MELLON, A. and HARGREAVE, F.E. *Journal of Allergy and Clinical Immunology*, **57**, 263 (1976)
112. WONNE, R., KATTAN, M., ORANGE, R.P. and LEVISON, H. *Journal of Allergy and Clinical Immunology*, **62**, 119 (1978)
113. KERSTEN, W. *Wiener Medizinische Wochenschrift*, **124** (Suppl. 21), 19 (1974)
114. OREHEK, J., GAYRARD, P., GRIMAUD, CH. and CHARPIN, J. *Postgraduate Medical Journal*, **51** (Suppl. 7), 105 (1975)
115. GAYRARD, P., OREHEK, J., GRIMAUD, CH. and CHARPIN, J. *Bulletin de Physio-Pathologie Respiratoire*, **10**, 451 (1974)
116. ALANKO, K. and POPPIUS, H. *Postgraduate Medical Journal*, **51** (Suppl. 7), 101 (1975)
117. BEUMER, H.M. *Postgraduate Medical Journal*, **51** (Suppl. 7), 101 (1975)
118. GAMAIN, B. *Postgraduate Medical Journal*, **51** (Suppl. 7), 102 (1975)
119. BEWTRA, A., NAIN, N. and TOWNLEY, R.G. *Clinical Pharmacology and Therapeutics*, **21**, 98 (1977)

120. NAIR, N.S., BEWTRA, A.K., WATT, G.D., BURKE, K.M. and TOWNLEY, R.G. *American Review of Respiratory Disease*, **115**, 68 (1977)
121. HARNETT, J. and SPECTOR, S.L. *Journal of Allergy and Clinical Immunology*, **57**, 261 (1976)
122. RUFFIN, R.E., FITZGERALD, J.D. and REBUCK, A.S. *Journal of Allergy and Clinical Immunology*, **59**, 136 (1977)
123. ANDERSON, S.D., SEALE, J.P., FERRIS, L., SCHOEFFEL, R. and LINDSAY, D.A. *Journal of Allergy and Immunology*, **64**, 612 (1979)
124. CHAN-YEUNG, M. *Chest*, **71**, 320 (1977)
125. HAYNES, R.L., INGRAM, R.H. Jr and McFADDEN, E.R. Jr *American Review of Respiratory Disease*, **113** (Part 2), 252 (1976)
126. DRY, J., PRADALIER, A., LEYNADIER, F. and HERMAN, D. *Therapie*, **32**, 181 (1977)
127. NOLTE, D. *Wiener Medizinische Wochenschrift*, **124** (Suppl. 21), 22 (1974)
128. STEMMAN, E.A. and KOSCHE, F. *Postgraduate Medical Journal*, **51** (Suppl. 7), 105 (1975)
129. POPPIUS, H., SALORINNE, Y. and VILJANEN, A.A. *Bulletin de Physio-Pathologie Respiratoire*, **8**, 643 (1972)
130. WEINBERG, E.G. *Postgraduate Medical Journal*, **51** (Suppl. 7), 128 (1975)
131. WOLKOVE, N., KREISMAN, H., FRANK, H. and GENT, M. *Journal of Allergy and Clinical Immunology*, **63**, 153 (1979)
132. WOLKOVE, N., KREISMAN, H., FRANK. H. and GENT, M. *Annals of Allergy*, **47**, 311 (1981)
133. GROSS, N.J. *Postgraduate Medical Journal*, **51** (Suppl. 7), 95 (1975)
134. LODDENKEMPER, R. *Postgraduate Medical Journal*, **51** (Suppl. 7), 97 (1975)
135. LODDENKEMPER, R. *Arzneimittel-Forschung*, **26**, 1017 (1976)
136. MAESEN, F. and BUYTENDIJK, H.J. *Postgraduate Medical Journal*, **51** (Suppl. 7), 97 (1975)
137. WOOD, M.J. and PATERSON, J.W. *Postgraduate Medical Journal*, **51** (Suppl. 7), 100 (1975)
138. IRSIGLER, G. *Postgraduate Medical Journal*, **51** (Suppl. 7), 96 (1975)
139. LULLING, J., DELWICHE, J.P. and PRIGNOT, J. *Respiration*, **42**, 188 (1981)
140. SIMONSSON, B.G., JONSON, B. and STROM, B. *Scandinavian Journal of Respiratory Disease*, **56**, 138 (1975)
141. STORMS, W.W., DE PICO, G.A. and REED, C.E. *American Review of Respiratory Disease*, **111**, 419 (1975)
142. BOHNING, W. and FABEL, H. *Postgraduate Medical Journal*, **51** (Suppl. 7), 95 (1975)
143. EMIRGIL, C., DWYER, K., BASKETTE, P. and SOBOL, B.J. *Current Therapeutic Research*, **17**, 215 (1975)
144. MAESEN, F.P.V. *Postgraduate Medical Journal*, **51** (Suppl. 7), 116 (1975)
145. RUFFIN, R.E. and NEWHOUSE, M.T. *Lung*, **155**, 141 (1978)
146. DAVIES, D.S. *Postgraduate Medical Journal*, **51** (Suppl. 7), 69 (1975)
147. ROMINGER, K.L. *Scandinavian Journal of Respiratory Diseases Supplementum*, **103**, 116 (1979)
148. ADLUNG, J., GOHLE, K.D., ZEREN, S. and WAHL, D. *Arzneimittel-Forschung*, **26**, 1005 (1976)
149. KALSER, S.C. and McLAIN, P.L. *Clinical Pharmacology and Therapeutics*, **11**, 214 (1970)
150. BAUER, R. and KUMMER, F. *International Journal of Clinical Pharmacology*, **8**, 135 (1973)
151. CHERVINSKY, P. *Journal of Allergy and Clinical Immunology*, **59**, 22 (1977)
152. HELLER, K.F. *Postgraduate Medical Journal*, **51** (Suppl. 7), 96 (1975)
153. LULLING, J., DELWICHE, J.P., LEDENT, C. and PRIGNOT, J. *British Journal of Diseases of the Chest*, **74**, 135 (1980)
154. BAIGELMAN, W. and CHODOSH, S. *Chest*, **71**, 324 (1977)
155. GROSS, N.J. *American Review of Respiratory Disease*, **112**, 823 (1975)
156. SCHLUETER, D.P. and NEUMANN, J.L. *Chest*, **73** (Suppl.), 982 (1978)
157. STRESEMANN, E. *Arzneimittel-Forschung*, **26**, 1015 (1976)
158. VLAGOPOULOS, T., TOWNLEY, R.G., GHAZANSHAHI, S., BEWTRA, A. and BURKE, K. *Annals of Allergy*, **36**, 223 (1976)
159. YEAGER, H. Jr, WEINBERG, R.H., KAUFMAN, L.V. and KATZ, S. *Journal of Clinical Pharmacology*, **16**, 198 (1976)
160. GAYRARD, P., OREHEK, J. and CHARPIN, J. *Revue Française des Maladies Respiratoires*, **1**, 481 (1973)
161. YERNAULT, J.C., DEJONGHE, M., DENAUT, M., ENGLERT, M. and DE COSTER, A. *Acta Tuberculosea et Pneumologica Belgica*, **66**, 421 (1975)
162. THIESSEN, B. and PEDERSEN, O.F. *Scandinavian Journal of Respiratory Diseases Supplementum*, **103**, 170 (1979)

163. WARD, M.J., FENTEM, P.H., RODERICK-SMITH, W.H. and DAVIES, D. *British Medical Journal*, **282**, 598 (1981)
164. LAITINEN, L.A., POPPIUS, H. and HAAHTELA, T. *Scandinavian Journal of Respiratory Diseases Supplementum*, **103**, 163 (1979)
165. LIGHTBODY, I.M., INGRAM, C.G., LEGGE, J.S. and JOHNSTON, R.N. *British Journal of Diseases of the Chest*, **72**, 181 (1978)
166. ULLAH, M., NEWMAN, G.B. and SAUNDERS, K.B. *Thorax*, **36**, 523 (1981)
167. HEEL, R.C., BROGDEN, R.N., SPEIGHT, T.M. and AVERY, G.S. *Drugs*, **15**, 3 (1978)
168. AHONEN, A., ALANKO, K. and MATTSON, K. *Current Therapeutic Research*, **24**, 65 (1978)
169. PIERCE, R.J., HOLMES, P.W. and CAMPBELL, A.H. *Australian and New Zealand Journal of Medicine*, **12**, 38 (1982)
170. LINEHAN, W.D. *Postgraduate Medical Journal*, **51** (Suppl. 7), 116 (1975)
171. JINDAL, S.K. and MALIK, S.K. *Indian Journal of Chest Diseases and Allied Sciences*, **21**, 130 (1979)
172. REBUCK, A.S. and MARCUS, H.I. *Scandinavian Journal of Respiratory Diseases Supplementum*, **103**, 186 (1979)
173. RUFFIN, R.E., McINTYRE, E., CROCKETT, A.J., ZIELONKA, K. and ALPERS, J.H. *Journal of Allergy and Clinical Immunology*, **69**, 60 (1982)
174. GUNTHER, W. and KAMBUROFF, P.L. *Current Medical Research and Opinion*, **2**, 281 (1974)
175. WETTENGEL, R. *Postgraduate Medical Journal*, **51** (Suppl. 7), 125 (1975)
176. KRIEGER, E. *Postgraduate Medical Journal*, **51** (Suppl. 7), 115 (1975)
177. JENKINS, C.R., CHOW, C.M., FISHER, B.L. and MARLIN, G.E. *Australian and New Zealand Journal of Medicine*, **11**, 513 (1981)
178. LEES, A.W., ALLAN, G.W. and SMITH, J. *British Journal of Clinical Practice*, **34**, 340 (1980)
179. DOUGLAS, N.J., DAVIDSON, I., SUDLOW, M.F. and FLENLEY, D.C. *Thorax*, **34**, 51 (1979)
180. POPPIUS, H. and SALORINNE, Y. *British Medical Journal*, **4**, 134 (1973)
181. CHAPMAN, T.T. *Postgraduate Medical Journal*, **51** (Suppl. 7), 112 (1975)
182. MARLIN, G.E., BUSH, D.E. and BEREND, N. *British Journal of Ckinical Pharmacology*, **6**, 547 (1978)
183. PETRIE, G.R. and PALMER, K.N.V. *Postgraduate Medical Journal*, **51** (Suppl. 7), 117 (1975
184. VERSTRAETEN, J.M. *Postgraduate Medical Journal*, **51** (Suppl. 7), 120 (1975)
185. KUMMER, F. *Postgraduate Medical Journal*, **51** (Suppl. 7), 115 (1975)
186. SILL, V., VOELKEL, N., LANSER, K. and MANVEDE, S. *Muenchener Medizinische Wochenschrift*, **118**, 177 (1976)
187. KAIK, G. *Therapiewoche*, **23**, 3260 (1973)
188. KAIK, G. *Wiener Klinische Wochenschrift*, **87**, 653 (1975)
189. KAIK, G. *Therapiewoche*, **25**, 2428 (1975)
190. STRIETZEL, G. *Praxis der Pneumologie*, **28**, 681 (1974)
191. ANASTASUTU, C. and DUTU, S. *Ftiziologie*, **23**, 305 (1974)
192. PETERSEN, B.N. and WEEKE, E. *Scandinavian Journal of Respiratory Diseases Supplementum*, **103**, 178 (1979)
193. SCHINDL, R. *Postgraduate Medical Journal*, **51** (Suppl. 7), 119 (1975)
194. BRINKMANN, O. *Postgraduate Medical Journal*, **51** (Suppl. 7), 130 (1975)
195. CUMMISKEY, J. and KEELAN, P. *Postgraduate Medical Journal*, **51** (Suppl. 7), 130 (1975)
196. CUMMISKEY, J., KEELAN, P., GRAY, P. and COX, G.A. *Journal of the Irish Medical Association*, **70**, 445 (1977)
197. HASLREITER, E. *Postgraduate Medical Journal*, **51** (Suppl. 7), 130 (1975)
198. JILG, J. *Postgraduate Medical Journal*, **51** (Suppl. 7), 131 (1975)
199. MINETTE, A. *Postgraduate Medical Journal*, **51** (Suppl. 7), 131 (1975)
200. ZEREN, S. *Postgraduate Medical Journal*, **51** (Suppl. 7), 133 (1975)
201. ULMER, W.T. *Postgraduate Medical Journal*, **51** (Suppl. 7), 133 (1975)
202. JAFFE, G.V., GRIMSHAW, J.J. and COX, G.A. *Practitioner*, **224**, 443 (1980)
203. CASALI, L., GRASSI, C., RAMPULLA, C. and ROSSI, A. *International Journal of Clinical Pharmacology and Biopharmacy*, **7**, 277 (1979)
204. KOK-JENSEN, A. *Ugeskrift For Laeger*, **141**, 2039 (1979)
205. LEITCH, A.G., HOPKIN, J.M.M., ELLISS, D.A., MERCHANT, S. and McHARDY, G.J.R. *Thorax*, **33**, 711 (1978)
206. ADDIS, C.J., BARCLAY, J. and CHANG, E.M. *European Journal of Clinical Pharmacology*, **16**, 97 (1979)
207. GUTERSOHN, J., JOOS, H. and HERZOG, H. *Postgraduate Medical Journal*, **51** (Suppl. 7), 113 (1975)

208. MARLIN, G.E., BEREND, N. and HARRISON, A.C. *Australian and New Zealand Journal of Medicine*, **9**, 511 (1979)
209. SERGYSELS, R., SCHANDEVYL, W., YERNAULT, J.C. and HENNEBERT, A. *Acta Tuberculosea et Pneumologica Belgica*, **67**, 163 (1976)
210. ULMER, W.T. *Medizinische Klinik*, **74**, 1548 (1979)
211. VERSTRAETEN, J.M. *Acta Tuberculosea et Pneumologica Belgica*, **65**, 395 (1974)
212. WILDBOLZ, U., KYD, K. and SCHERRER, M. *Lung*, **154**, 141 (1977)
213. LIN, M.T., LEE-HONG, E. and COLLINS-WILLIAMS, C. *Annals of Allergy*, **40**, 326 (1978)
214. RASMUSSEN, F.V., MADSEN, L. and BUNDGAARD, A. *Scandinavian Journal of Respiratory Diseases Supplementum*, **103**, 159 (1979)
215. THOMSON, N.C., PATEL, K.R. and KERR, J.W. *Thorax*, **33**, 694 (1978)
216. KREISMAN, H., FRANK, H., WOLKOVE, N. and GENT, M. *Thorax*, **36**, 387 (1981)
217. KOSCHE, F. and STEMMAN, E.A. *Postgraduate Medical Journal*, **51** (Suppl. 7), 127 (1975)
218. KUNKEL, G., RUDOLPH, R. and STOCK, U. *Postgraduate Medical Journal*, **51** (Suppl. 7), 127 (1975)
219. MANN, N.P. and HILLER, E.J. *Thorax*, **37**, 72 (1982)
220. GROGGINS, R.C., MILNER, A.D. and STOKES, G.M. *Archives of Disease in Childhood*, **56**, 342 (1981)
221. HODGES, I.G.C., GROGGINS, R.C., MILNER, A.D. and STOKES, G.M. *Archives of Disease in Childhood*, **56**, 729 (1981)
222. STEMMAN, E.A., WULLER, K., KOSCHE, F., BOTH, A. and BRAUN, S.H. *Praxis der Pneumologie*, **29**, 83 (1975)
223. HOFFMANN, D. and WONNE, R. *Postgraduate Medical Journal*, **51** (Suppl. 7), 126 (1975)
224. LOGVINOFF-POIDATZ, M. and GEUBELLE, G. *Postgraduate Medical Journal*, **51** (Suppl. 7), 127 (1975)
225. YEUNG, R., NOLAN, G.M. and LEVINSON, H. *Pediatrics*, **66**, 109 (1980)
226. HUTHER, W. *Postgraduate Medical Journal*, **51** (Suppl. 7), 126 (1975)
227. AJEWSKI, Z. and POPIAK, B. *Scandinavian Journal of Respiratory Diseases Supplementum*, **103**, 205 (1979)
228. SCHLEUFLER, G. *Postgraduate Medical Journal*, **51** (Suppl. 7), 132 (1975)
229. THUMM, H.W. *Therapie der Gegenwart*, **115**, 1244 (1976)
230. LAHDENSUO, A., VILJANEN, A.A. and MUITTARI, A. *Postgraduate Medical Journal*, **51** (Suppl. 7), 116 (1975)
231. ULMER, W.T. *Medizinische Klinik*, **66**, 326 (1971)
232. DYSON, A.J. Unpublished observations
233. CROMPTON, G.K. *Lancet*, **i**, 1243 (1982)
234. WAHL, D. *Ba253 Bericht Biochemie (Rat, Dog, Human)*, Boehringer Sohn, Abt. Biochemie (1977)
235. FLOHR, E. and BISCHOFF, K.O. *Respiration*, **38**, 98 (1979)
236. NOLTE, D. *Respiration*, **36**, 32 (1978)
237. BEUMER, H.M., GRIEBEN, CH., SCHUIJT, C. and SIEBELINK, J. *International Journal of Clinical Pharmacology, Therapy and Toxicology*, **19**, 168 (1981)
238. SCHULTZE-WERNINGHAUS, G. *Respiration*, **41**, 239 (1981)
239. LARSSON, K. *Respiration*, **43**, 57 (1982)
240. NEIJENS, H.J., WESSELIUS, T. and KERREBIJN, K.F. *Thorax*, **36**, 517 (1981)
241. SHELLEY, J.H. *Ba 253. Investigational Brochure*. Boehringer (1975)
242. MINETTE, A. and MARCQ, M. *Revue de l'Intstitut d'Hygiene des Mines*, **34**, 115 (1979)

Section 2   Functional antagonists

Chapter 10

Drugs acting at adrenoceptors

I.F. Skidmore

Introduction

Drugs that cause bronchodilatation by acting at adrenoceptors, particularly β_2-adrenoceptors, are the most common treatments for asthma in the United Kingdom. A similar situation exists in those countries where drugs of this type have been available for a considerable time. Elsewhere in the world, β_2-stimulant bronchodilators are increasingly competing with the old established bronchodilators such as theophylline. In recent years, β_2 stimulants have also been prescribed as prophylactic drugs, based on their ability to inhibit the release of spasmogens and inflammagens from human mast cells.

This chapter will review the origins and development of this highly effective group of drugs, the advances in pharmacology and medicinal chemistry that accompanied this development and the biochemical basis for their actions as bronchodilators and prophylactic agents. No attempt will be made to discuss quantitative structure–activity relationships in detail, for these have been adequately dealt with by others. Nor will much space be devoted to newer compounds still in the preclinical or early clinical phase unless they appear to represent a significant advance over established drugs. Finally, as in recent years there have been reports on the clinical activity of α-antagonists in asthma, the status of this class of drugs will be reviewed.

The development of β_2-adrenoceptor stimulants

As in many other therapeutic fields, herbal remedies containing an active principle structurally and pharmacologically related to todays drugs were in use in the ancient far East. Preparations of *Ephedra sinica* containing ephedrine are thought to have been in use in China for more than 2000 years. However, it was only in the 1920s that ephedrine was introduced

185

into Western medicine, more than 20 years after adrenaline had been identified and first used in the treatment of asthma. Both drugs can be given
subcutaneously or by inhalation and, in addition, ephedrine is active by
mouth. However, neither drug is long acting and both produce potentially
hazardous cardiovascular side-effects. Although both adrenaline and
ephedrine are still available in a wide variety of formulations, they have
been superceded by synthetic drugs with the marked advantages of metabolic stability and pharmacological selectivity. Nevertheless, subcutaneous
adrenaline is still the preferred treatment for systemic anaphylactic reactions, where its vascular as well as its bronchodilator actions are valuable.

No significant advances over ephedrine and adrenaline emerged until
isoprenaline became available in the 1940s[1]. Although inactive by mouth it
could be given by inhalation and ultimately pressurized aerosol formulations were developed. Isoprenaline is an effective bronchodilator of short
duration, with fewer cardiovascular side-effects than ephedrine and adrenaline, but still with pronounced positive chronotropic and inotropic
effects which, because of efficient buccal and pulmonary absorption, are
noticeable shortly after inhalation.

Although the concept of drugs acting at specific receptors had been
proposed long before the introduction of isoprenaline[2], no rationale for the
many and varied responses to the natural catecholamines and their synthetic analogues had yet been formulated. However, in 1948 Ahlquist[3]
demonstrated that responses to catecholamine-like drugs could be subdivided into two classes (α and β) on the basis of the differential activity of
noradrenaline (α) and isoprenaline (β), and proposed the existence of distinct α- and β-adrenotropic receptors through which these responses were
exerted.

In the 1960s two significant advances were made. Firstly Lands and his
colleagues[4-6], using the same techniques as Ahlquist, showed that the
responses mediated through the β-adrenoceptor could be subdivided into
two groups (β_1 and β_2). Cardiac β_1 responses (chronotropy and inotropy)
could be separated to a great degree from the β_2 responses, of which
relaxation of bronchial smooth muscle was the most important. This work
led to the first β_2-selective bronchodilator, isoetharine[7] and also focused
the attention of the medicinal chemist on the value of N-substitution for
enhancing β_2 selectivity, by highlighting the activity of t-butyl-
noradrenaline. Secondly, the work of many groups[8,9], emphasized the
importance of uptake mechanisms and catechol-O-methyltransferase in the
metabolic inactivation of both natural and synthetic catecholamines. This
work identified the catechol nucleus as a target for medicinal chemists aim-
ing to produce drugs with enhanced metabolic stability and consequent
oral activity and long duration of action.

These two approaches were followed virtually simultaneously. The outcome has been reviewed extensively, particularly by Brittain et al.[10] and
will only be summarized here:

(1) Replacement of the 3-hydroxyl group with hydroxymethyl (e.g. salbu-
     tamol), methane sulphonamide (e.g. soterenol) or amino-based substi-
     tuents such as urea (e.g. carbuterol), movement of the 4-hydroxyl to
     the 5-position to form a resorcinol (orciprenaline, terbutaline,

fenoterol) or replacement of the 3,4-dihydroxy grouping with 3,5-dichloro-4-amino substituents (clenbuterol) has given compounds of metabolic stability and long duration of action, particularly in the last case[11,12]. Fortuitously, modifications designed to reduce O-methylation have also reduced O-sulphation[13], thus promoting oral activity and general metabolic stability.

(2) Both the 4-hydroxy-3-hydroxymethyl and the 3,5-dichloro-4-amino analogues of isoprenaline are to a degree β_2 selective. Thus, these modifications provide some specificity as well as stability.

(3) N-Alkyl substitution depresses α activity and enhances β activity (cf. noradrenaline and adrenaline). As the size of the substituent increases, β_2 activity is maintained or enhanced selectively (cf. orciprenaline and terbutaline). N-Aralkyl substitution has the same effect (e.g. fenoterol). The N-alkyl substituent can be cyclized (e.g. rimiterol).

(4) Ethyl substitution on the α-carbon of the phenethanolamine side-chain enhances selectivity although absolute potency falls (cf. isoetharine and isoprenaline).

(5) The aromatic nucleus can be modified in a variety of ways. In some compounds (e.g. pirbuterol, procaterol), the side-chain remains intact, in others (e.g. trimetoquinol) it is incorporated into the modification.

Currently available drugs and other interesting compounds are summarized in *Table 10.1* and *Figure 10.1*.

TABLE 10.1 β-Adrenoceptors agonists in common use in asthma

Approved name (US equivalent)	Selectivity	Dose and route of administration		
		Oral (mg)	Inhaled (μg)	Duration (h)
Adrenaline (epinephrine)	No	—	250	0.5–1
Ephedrine	No	10–50	—	1–2
Isoprenaline (isoproterenol)	No	—	80–160	0.5–1
Isoetharine	Yes	10	350	1–2
Rimiterol	Yes	10	200	1–2
Orciprenaline (metaproterenol)	Poor	20	750	1–3
Terbutaline	Yes	5	250	4–6
Fenoterol	Yes	—	200	4–8
Reproterol	Yes	20	500	3–6
Salbutamol (albuterol)	Yes	2–4	200	4–6
Pirbuterol	Yes	10–15	200	4–6
Procaterol	Yes	50	—	6–8
Clenbuterol	Yes	10–20 μg	—	> 12

Combination of these two advances has led to a range of potent long-acting β_2-selective bronchodilators active locally by inhalation and in most cases orally. They provide excellent bronchodilatation with virtual lack of side-effects by inhalation and readily tolerated, pharmacologically mediated side-effects by the oral route. These side-effects are skeletal muscle tremor, which appears to be a β_2-mediated response, and tachycardia which is a combination of a reflex response to β_2-mediated peripheral vasodilatation[14] and direct positive chronotropy exerted through a minority population of β_2-receptors in the sino-auricular node of the heart.

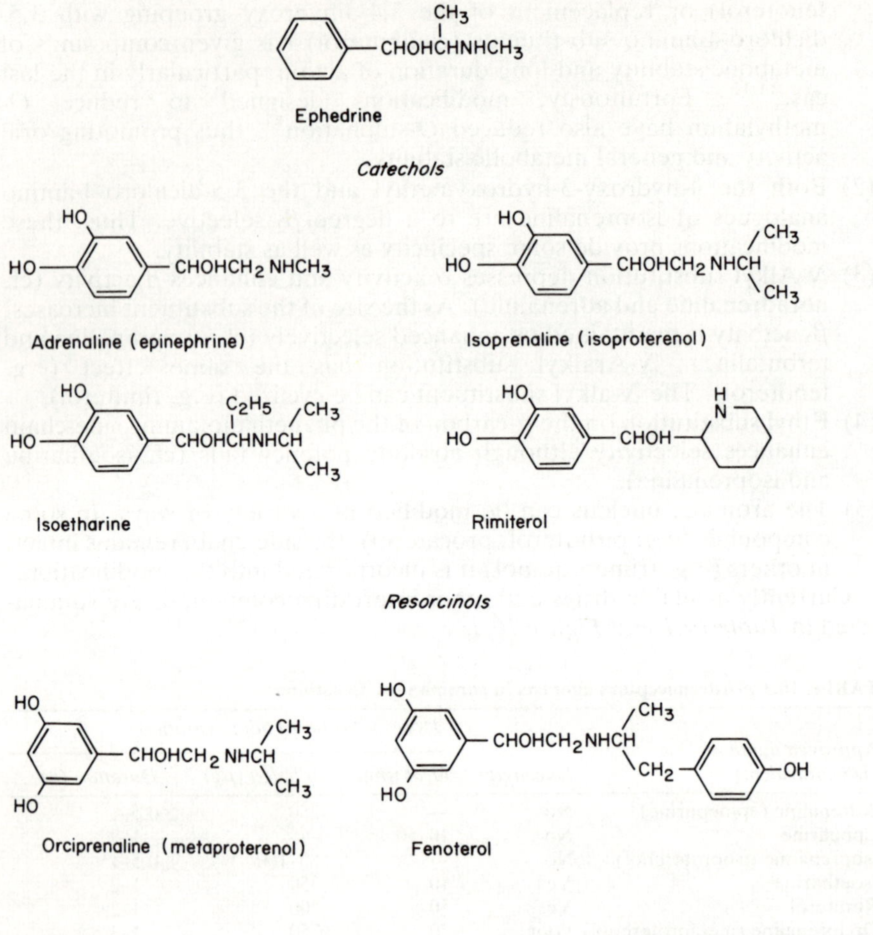

Ephedrine

Catechols

Adrenaline (epinephrine)

Isoprenaline (isoproterenol)

Isoetharine

Rimiterol

Resorcinols

Orciprenaline (metaproterenol)

Fenoterol

Terbutaline

Reproterol

Figure 10.1 β-Adrenoceptor stimulant bronchodilators in common use.

In recent years, attention has turned to the ability of β_2-adrenoceptor stimulants to inhibit the release of histamine and SRS-A, two of the putative mediators of allergic asthma, from human lung sensitized to and challenged with antigen. Inhibition of the release of histamine from lung by catecholamines is a well-established observation[15]. Recently it has been

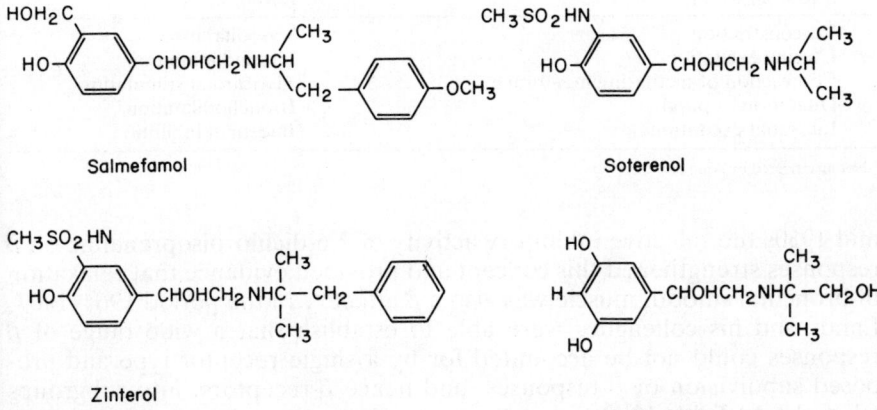

Figure 10.1 (continued)

shown that this is mediated via a β_2-receptor and that the human mast cell is virtually devoid of functional β_1-receptors[16]. At concentrations of these drugs that cause bronchodilatation, release of histamine and SRS-A is inhibited[17] and it has been proposed that giving these drugs in a prophylactic regimen will prevent asthmatic attacks as well as provide bronchodilatation.

Receptor classification: the pharmacological basis for selectivity of action

Brief reference was made above to the fundamental work of Ahlquist[3] and of Lands et al.[4-6] in demonstrating that physiological and biochemical responses to catecholamines could be subdivided and ascribed to actions at distinct receptor subtypes. It is now clear that the classification of catecholamine receptors is considerably more complex than was imagined by these workers or indeed by most of the pharmacologists and medicinal chemists that capitalized on their discoveries. However, most of the recent work on the subdivision of α-receptors does not impinge on the treatment of asthma by β_2-selective agonists and need not be discussed here. The purpose of this section is to review in more detail the pharmacological basis for the selectivity that makes β_2-adrenoceptor stimulants such useful drugs.

Two important techniques have contributed to receptor classification. Firstly, comparison of the rank order of potency of a series of agonists in a range of pharmacological preparations, a difference in rank order between two preparations indicating that the responses may be exerted through different receptors. Secondly, as suitable drugs have become available, comparison of the effects of selective and non-selective antagonists on responses to a range of agonists allowed confirmation of results obtained by comparison of potency.

As early as 1939 evidence was obtained that adrenaline might exert its varied effects by acting at two distinct receptors[18]. Ahlquist's studies reinforced this evidence and allowed him to propose the existence of α- and β-adrenotropic receptors mediating distinct responses (Table 10.2)[3]. In the

TABLE 10.2 Separation of responses to catecholamines into α and β effects (after Ahlquist[3])

α Responses	β Responses
Vasconstriction	Vasodilatation
Uterine excitation	Uterine inhibition
Contraction of nictitating membrane	Myocardial stimulation
Dilatation of pupil	Bronchodilatation*
Intestinal excitation	Intestinal inhibition

* Not investigated by Ahlquist.

mid 1950s the selective inhibitory activity of 2,6-dichloroisoprenaline on β responses strengthened this concept and provided evidence that relaxation of bronchial smooth muscle was also a β effect[19]. In the period 1964–1967, Lands and his colleagues were able to establish that a wide range of β responses could not be accounted for by a single receptor type and proposed subdivision of β responses, and hence β-receptors, into subgroups (β_1 and β_2) (Table 10.3)[4-6].

The synthesis of β_1-selective antagonists and β_2-selective agonists gave a major boost to this subdivision as a working hypothesis; however, rigorous pharmacological analysis suggested that it was an oversimplification and that perhaps further subtypes existed[20]. The work of Carlsson et al. clarified the situation by indicating that both β_1 and β_2-adrenoceptors could exist in the same tissue[21]. The pharmacological evidence for this proposal

TABLE 10.3 Subdivision of β responses according to Lands et al.[4-6]

β_1	β_2
Lipolysis	Bronchodilatation
Cardiac stimulation	Vasodilatation
Intestinal inhibition	Uterine inhibition

has been reviewed recently by Levy and his colleagues[22,23] and has been supported by ligand-binding studies in several species[24,25]. It provides a rational explanation for several apparently inconsistent results. For example, the presence of a significant minority of β_2-receptors in the cat atrium explains why salbutamol is a potent full agonist in this tissue[26] and, in this species, lacks the selectivity for bronchial muscle *in vitro* and *in vivo* that is so clearly demonstrable in the guinea-pig[27].

Recent work has demonstrated clearly that a selective response *in vivo* does not always reflect selectivity at the receptor level but may depend on tissue or organ selectivity[28,29]. This is particularly true of partial agonists of low intrinsic efficacy. These may show apparent receptor-selective activity in a tissue that contains a large receptor pool or operates the receptor–effector coupling system more efficiently. However, there is no clear evidence that apparently selective β_2-adrenoceptor stimulants owe their selectivity to this mechanism. Nevertheless, it has been noted that some agonists, such as soterenol, fenoterol and salbutamol, bind with equal affinity to both β_1 and β_2-receptors and apparently owe their selectivity to greater efficacy at the latter, while other agonists, such as procaterol, show greater affinity for β_2-receptors[30,31].

The biochemical basis of pharmacological activity: receptor–ligand interaction and activation of adenylate cyclase

At the time that Lands was demonstrating that β-receptors could be divided into β_1 and β_2 subtypes, it was becoming clear that β-receptors were linked to adenylate cyclase and exerted their pharmacological actions through an elevation of intracellular adenosine cyclic $3':5'$-monophosphate (cyclic AMP or cAMP) activation of cAMP-dependent protein kinases and phosphorylation of specific proteins[32]. While that basic mechanism of action remains valid, the past 15 years have seen major advances in our knowledge of the molecular and biochemical mechanisms involved in these events. Those that are relevant to establishing the mechanism of adenylate cyclase activation will be reviewed in this section and the consequences of elevating cyclic AMP in the following section.

Three factors govern the pharmacological response to an agonist:
(1) The affinity of the agonist for the receptor[33,34]. This controls the proportion of receptors occupied at a given concentration of agonist.
(2) The number of receptors present on the cell. Although maximal responses to full agonists can usually be achieved with only a fraction of the receptors occupied, all the receptors contribute to the mass action equation governing the number of receptor sites occupied[35]. A response will be achieved at a lower agonist concentration in tissues

carrying large number of 'spare receptors' than in a tissue carrying few receptors. Factors 1 and 2 thus determine the number of receptors occupied at a given concentration.

(3) The efficacy of the drug. This is a measure of the ability of the drug to activate the receptor[36]. Factors 2 and 3 can be combined to give the intrinsic efficacy (efficacy/receptor number)[37], which is a measure of efficacy that is independent of tissue type[28,29]

The key to present knowledge of the mechanism by which adenylate cyclase is activated was the discovery, by Rodbell and his coworkers, of the obligatory role of guanosine 5'-triphosphate (GTP) in the activation of the cyclase[38]. This led to the identification of GTP-binding protein, characterization of its GTPase activity and the realization that this protein provides the mechanism by which receptor occupancy is coupled to cyclase activation and the mechanism through which cyclase activation is controlled[39-41].

The use of ligand–receptor binding and ligand displacement studies, particularly in association with measurement of adenylate cyclase, has in the past few years provided models of the mechanism of cyclase activation. It is beyond the scope of this article to discuss the relative merits of these models and the evidence for them but there are, in summary, two models in common currency.

(a) *Collision coupling model (mobile receptor model)*[42,43]

In this model the receptor and cyclase components of the system are considered to be independently mobile in the lateral plane of the membrane. On collision between receptor and cyclase, the enzyme is only activated if the receptor is occupied by drug (DR) and the cyclase is associated with the nucleotide-binding protein (E_{GTP}). Such an interaction produces a transient complex DRE_{GTP} that is in equilibrium with an activated state DRE^*_{GTP} from which the activated enzyme E^*_{GTP} dissociates. This activated state is terminated by the hydrolysis of GTP to GDP (*Figure 10.2*). This model permits a single drug–receptor complex to activate more than one cyclase molecule.

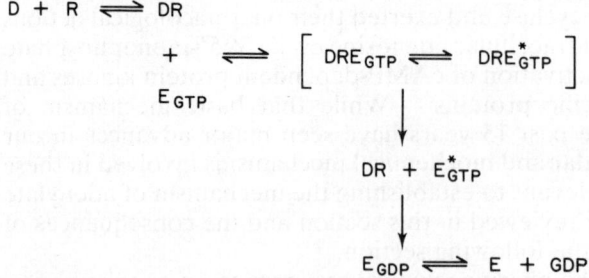

Figure 10.2 Collision coupling model of adenylate cyclase activation. D—drug or natural agonist; R—receptor; E_{GTP} cyclase enzyme complex; E^*_{GTP} cyclase complex in activated state.

(b) *Dynamic receptor affinity model*[44-46]

In contrast, this model allows a single drug–receptor complex to activate only one cyclase molecule. Coupling between receptor and cyclase is mediated through the nucleotide-binding protein and the function of the agonist–receptor complex is to supply active nucleotide-binding protein (N_{GTP}) to activate the cyclase. There is no direct interaction between receptor and cyclase. The mechanism is visualized as a series of interacting cycles (*Figure 10.3*).

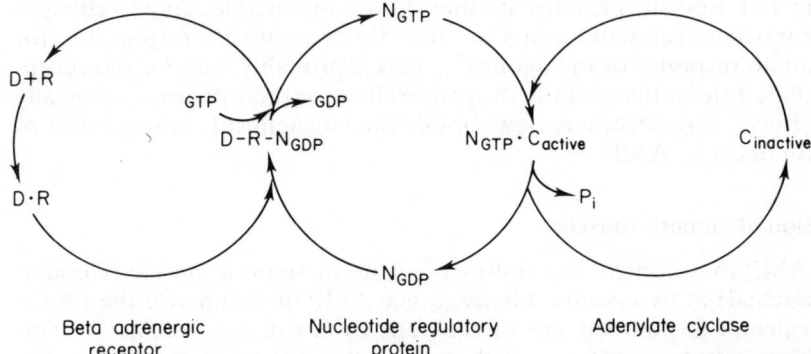

Figure 10.3 Dynamic receptor affinity model of adenylate cyclase activation (modified from Lefkowitz and Hoffman[46]). D—drug or natural agonist; R—receptor; N—nucleotide-binding protein; C—catalytic unit of adenylate cyclase. From Lefkowitz, R.J. and Hoffman, B.B., 1980, *Trends in Pharmacological Sciences*, Vol. 1, p. 317, by courtesy of the authors and publisher.

Ligand displacement experiments have shown that the interaction of agonist with the receptor induces a high affinity state of the receptor. This high affinity state interacts with nucleotide-binding protein carrying $GDP(N_{GDP})$ forming a complex ($D \cdot RN_{GDP}$) from which GDP is displaced by GTP ($D \cdot RN_{GTP}$). This binding of GTP reduces the affinity of the receptor for agonist and the complex dissociates, liberating agonist, receptor and the nucleotide-binding protein charged with $GTP(N_{GTP})$. In this form, the binding protein interacts with the catalytic unit of the cyclase activating it. Activity persists until the GTP is hydrolysed to GDP at which stage the cyclase-binding protein complex dissociates liberating N_{GDP} which can again inter-react with the agonist–receptor complex.

Agonists induce the high affinity GTP-sensitive state of the receptor to an extent that correlates with their intrinsic activity as activators of adenylate cyclase. Antagonists fail to alter affinity or induce sensitivity to N_{GTP}. Experiments involving preincubation with agonists indicate that desensitization is a combination of a reduction in the ability of the receptor to form this high-affinity N_{GTP}-sensitive state and a reduction in the numbers of binding sites[45–47].

Correlation between ligand binding and activation of adenylate cyclase has shown that β_2-adrenoceptor selective drugs can achieve their selectivity in one of two ways. In the first case, procaterol, zinterol and salmefamol (*Figure 10.1*) bind selectively at β_2-adrenoceptors and subsequently activate them. In the second case, drugs such as salbutamol, terbutaline, fenoterol and soterenol (*Figure 10.1*) bind with approximately equal affinity to both β_1 and β_2-receptors but are efficacious only at the latter[30,31,48].

The biochemical basis of pharmacological activity: consequences of elevating cyclic AMP

Agonists acting at β-adrenoceptors exert their actions by raising the intracellular concentration of cyclic AMP. Elevation of intracellular cyclic AMP leads to activation of specific cyclic AMP-dependent protein kinases by dissociation of the inhibitory regulatory subunit of the enzyme from the catalytic unit. Specific proteins are thus phosphorylated leading to changes in their biochemical activity that are directly or indirectly responsible for the ultimate response of the agonist[49]. This is probably true for the receptor-mediated side-effects of the drugs as well as for their pharmacologically useful effects. This section reviews briefly the biochemical consequences of elevation of cyclic AMP.

Relaxation of smooth muscle

Cyclic AMP may control the contractile state of smooth muscle (vascular and bronchial) at two points. Firstly, cyclic AMP may enhance the rate at which calcium is pumped out of the cells by a calcium ATPase[50]. This mechanism may be analogous to that controlling relaxation in the cardiac cell. Here it has been shown that cAMP-dependent phosphorylation of phospholamban leads to the activation of the calcium ATPase of the sarcoplasmic reticulum and enhanced sequestration of calcium ions[51,52]. Secondly, a cAMP-dependent protein kinase may indirectly inhibit the formation of the contractile actin–myosin complex[53]. In order for myosin to interact with actin, the light chain of myosin must be phosphorylated.

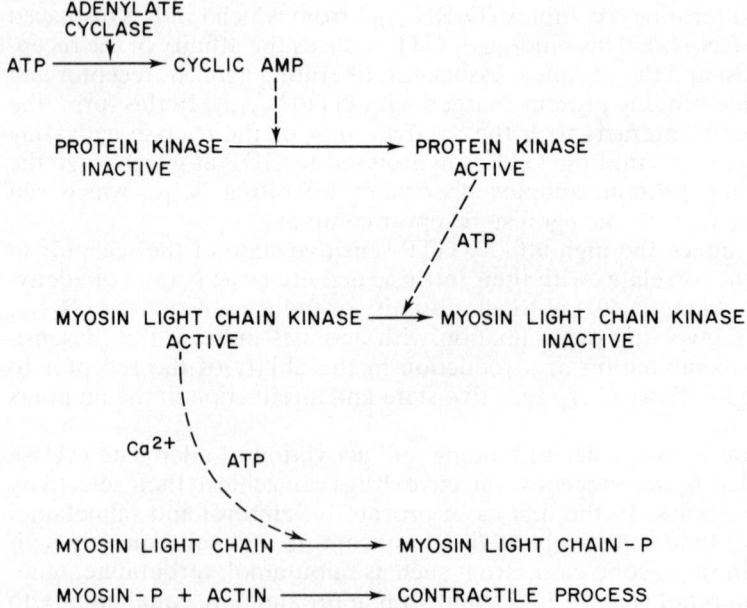

Figure 10.4 Inhibition of smooth muscle contraction by cyclic AMP.

This is controlled by a calcium–calmodulin-dependent myosin light chain kinase. The activity of myosin light chain kinase is itself controlled by a phosphorylation–dephosphorylation cycle in which the phosphorylated form of the enzyme is inactive. Phosphorylation of light chain kinase is catalysed by a cAMP-dependent protein kinase so that, as the intracellular concentration of cyclic AMP is raised, the inhibitory kinase is activated, myosin phosphorylation is prevented and contraction inhibited or reversed (*Figure 10.4*).

Inhibition of the release of spasmogens from mast cells

The role of cyclic AMP in preventing spasmogen release from mast cells has not yet been worked out, but clues as to the function of cyclic AMP can be obtained from other cells and tissues where knowledge is more extensive. Cyclic AMP may inhibit the uptake of extracellular calcium. Lapetina and his colleagues have proposed that, in platelets, the uptake of extracellular calcium in response to aggregatory stimuli may be controlled by the production of an endogenous ionophore, phosphatidic acid, from phosphatidylinositol[54]. In this system, cyclic AMP prevents the accumulation of phosphatidic acid by promoting its reconversion to phosphatidylinositol[55], thus reducing the concentration of ionophore and preventing calcium uptake. Calcium appears to have two functions in the platelet: to trigger 5-hydroxytryptamine release and to initiate the generation of arachidonic acid from which thromboxanes are synthesized. These functions are analogous to the release of histamine and the generation of arachidonic acid for the synthesis of leukotrienes by the mast cell and a similar cAMP-sensitive mechanism may operate in this cell.

Positive chronotropy

Part of the positive chronotropic response to β_2-adrenoceptor agonists is a reflex response to peripheral vasodilatation which, we have already noted, is likely to be mediated by cyclic AMP. These agonists also exert a direct positive chronotropic effect by acting at a minority of β_2-receptors in the myocardium. While one of the important responses to these drugs is accelerated relaxation of the myocardium due to enhanced sequestration of calcium by the sarcoplasmic reticulum (*see above*)[51,52], the contribution of this to increased heart rate is likely to be at the physiological level, allowing adequate refilling during diastole[56]. Effects on pacemaker activity appear to be mediated by increasing the rate of diastolic depolarization so that the depolarization threshold is reached more rapidly[57]. This may be controlled by cAMP-dependent phosphorylation of specific proteins.

Skeletal muscle tremor

Skeletal muscle tremor appears to be caused by a decrease in the recovery time following contraction[58]. As in smooth and cardiac muscle, one effect of cyclic AMP may be to enhance resequestration of calcium released to trigger the contractile process increasing the recovery rate of the fibre.

Clinical activity of drugs acting at β_2-receptors

There is no doubt that drugs of this class are effective bronchodilators both experimentally and clinically. Those commonly prescribed are included in *Table 10.1* and *Figure 10.1*. However, their use as treatments for asthma varies throughout the world. In the United Kingdom, for example, they are the drugs of choice in both acute and chronic reversible bronchospasm and are considered to be extremely safe as well as effective. In the United States, however, where they were introduced much later than in Europe, they are not yet so widely prescribed as the many theophylline-based preparations. It will be interesting and instructive to follow the relative futures of these two types of bronchodilator over the next few years.

The range of β_2 stimulants available now, in oral preparations, metered dose aerosols, dry powder inhalers and nebulizer solutions, offers the physician the opportunity to provide the patient with that type of therapy most suited to their condition and pharmacological responsiveness. In the United Kingdom, the inhaled route of administration is favoured over the oral route, for the entirely rational reasons that it provides maximally effective bronchodilatation with minimal exposure to drug and lack of side-effects. Increasingly, these drugs are given by inhalation in a prophylactic regimen. However, despite the advantages of inhaled therapy the oral route is preferred in many countries. Metabolic stability provides a long duration of action by the oral route but other factors may control duration by the inhaled route. Clenbuterol is metabolically very stable[12,59] and can provide a very long-lasting bronchodilatation by the oral route[11], but inhalation of quite large doses fails to extend the duration beyond about six hours[60,61].

Because the clinical effectiveness of this class of drug is so well established and has been reviewed extensively by others, the remainder of this section will deal with only four aspects of clinical activity: prophylactic use, desensitization, safety and scope for improvement.

Prophylaxis

Although Schild[62] showed, as long ago as 1936, that adrenaline inhibited the release of histamine from guinea-pig lung sensitized to and challenged with antigen, it was more than thirty years later before catecholamines were shown to inhibit anaphylactic release of histamine from human basophils and fragments of human lung[63,64]. Since then there have been many confirmatory reports that β-adrenoceptor agonists inhibit the release of both histamine and SRS-A from human lung. The use of a range of agonists and both selective and non-selective antagonists has shown that the human mast cell carries predominantly β_2-receptors[16]. Because of this, the potency of β_2-selective agonists, such as salbutamol, as inhibitors of spasmogen release is at least as great as their spasmolytic potency[17]. This suggests that doses of drug that cause significant bronchodilatation, if given in a prophylactic regimen, will also reduce significantly the release of these mediators and prevent not only bronchoconstriction but also pulmonary inflammation and the bronchial hyper-reactivity that appears to be associated with it[65].

Only in the past few years has evidence that β_2-adrenoceptor agonists have prophylactic activity been sought seriously. Understandably, this search has been complicated by the bronchodilator activity of these drugs and much of the available evidence for and against is circumstantial. However, on balance, the evidence from widely differing studies favours the use of these drugs prophylactically. In the first instance there are a series of studies designed to investigate the drugs in a challenge situation. Several groups have demonstrated that topically applied β_2-adrenoceptor agonists (fenoterol, salbutamol terbutaline, KWD 2131) inhibit allergic reactions in the nose[66–69]. In another study, KWD 2131 at doses which failed to give bronchodilatation provided some, albeit marginal, protection of asthmatics exposed to an inhaled challenge with antigen[70]. Martin, in a detailed study using terbutaline in a prophylactic regimen, was able to correlate protection from antigen challenge with inhibition of the release of histamine and NCFA (neutrophil chemotactic factor of anaphylaxis) into the plasma after challenge[71]. However, in contrast to these findings, Orr and his colleagues were unable to inhibit the NCFA response to antigen in patients treated acutely with inhaled salbutamol[72]. In addition, numerous studies by Pepys[73] have failed to demonstrate a protective effect of β stimulants given acutely against the late response to antigen.

Anderson and her colleagues compared the effects of inhaled and oral salbutamol in asthmatics and found that, while by either route the drug provided good bronchodilatation, much better protection against postexercise bronchospasm was provided by the inhaled drug[74]. A later study[75] showed that inhaled terbutaline would not only protect against exercise-induced asthma, but also inhibited the rise in plasma histamine that accompanies the bronchoconstriction. This has been interpreted by several commentators as evidence for an inhibitory effect of these drugs on the release of spasmogens from mast cells[76,77]. A much more extensive trial was reported in outline by VanAs[78] in which prophylactic treatment with β-stimulant bronchodilators for a period of twelve months was superior to treatment with either disodium cromoglycate or prednisone, both given regularly with bronchodilators on demand. From this and other reports[76,79], it seems that regular prophylactic treatment with β_2 stimulants provides better control of asthma than does treatment of symptoms alone. Current views of the pathobiology of allergic asthma[80,81] emphasize the central role of the mast cell and, in particular, the function of the luminal mast cells as the first sensitized cells to be exposed to antigen[82] and this underlines the value of the inhaled route of administration in the control of asthma.

Desensitization (tachyphylaxis)

Desensitization and supersensitivity are well-known pharmacological phenomena[83]. In all probability they are manifestations under extreme conditions of a subtle homeostatic mechanism that tailors the sensitivity of the receptor mechanism to the level of stimulus it normally receives[84]. At the molecular level, the phenomenon of desensitization is probably better understood for the β-adrenoceptor–adenylate cyclase–cyclic AMP system than for any other example of transmembrane signalling. For this system it has been established that receptor-specific desensitization is a two stage process. Firstly, there is a rapid readily reversible 'uncoupling' of the receptor from the cyclase, as a result of which the agonist can no longer induce the high-affinity GTP-sensitive state of the receptor with its original efficiency and loses some of its ability to activate cyclase[85,86]. Secondly, on more prolonged exposure to agonists, there is loss of receptor number[85,86] which is reversed more slowly. During this stage receptors appear to be internalized[87,88]. There is also evidence that receptor–drug affinity falls. The immediate consequence of densensitization is a reduction in the ability of the cell to respond to a given stimulus by synthesizing cyclic AMP. The key questions are firstly, whether desensitization occurs in patients taking β_2 stimulants and, secondly, if it does occur is it of clinical significance?

The natural variablity of asthma complicates any studies other than simple acute investigations. In addition it is important to carry out experiments on desensitization under conditions designed to minimize the effects of previous or current medication. Thus, it is not surprising that both experimental results and clinical opinions vary considerably. Reports that subsensitivity can develop following either short or long-term administration of these drugs are balanced by others claiming that desensitization does not occur in the asthmatic airway (*Table 10.4*).

TABLE 10.4 Tachyphylaxis to β_2-selective bronchodilators

Evidence for	Evidence against
Nelson et al.[89]	Larsson et al.[97]
Jenne et al.[90]	Sims[98]
Plummer[91]	Peel and Gibson[99]
Holgate et al. (normal subjects)[92]	Harvey et al. (asthmatic airway only)[100]
Falliers[93]	Tashkin et al. (histamine)[96]
Conolly et al.[94]	Repsher et al.[101]
Weber[95]	
Tashkin et al. (antigen)[96]	

On balance clinical evidence favours the view that if desensitization takes place at all, then, at normal doses of these drugs, it is at most of minor significance[102,103].

Toxicity and side-effects

The idea that desensitization to β-adrenergic bronchodilators might have clinical significance originally arose from attempts to analyse the increase in deaths from asthma that occurred in the United Kingdom in the mid 1960s[104]. This coincided with the introduction of high-dose metered-dose aerosols of isoprenaline and declined with the subsequent reduction in their use. The introduction of the β_2-selective bronchodilators in 1969 and the steady increase in their use over the past thirteen years has not been accompanied by an increase in deaths from asthma; indeed the death rate from asthma in the United Kingdom has stayed essentially constant since 1969[105], even though the number of subjects diagnosed as asthmatic and treated as such has increased considerably over this period.

Many commentators have attempted to analyse the cause of the increase in deaths in the 1960s. What seems beyond doubt is that the victims died of asthma. Crompton[106] has pointed out that the earlier work of Hume and

Gandevia[107] clearly identified the limitations of bronchodilators in severe asthma. He and many others underline the point that the increased use of bronchodilator is an accurate index of deteriorating asthma and that it is the duty of the physician to make the patient aware of this and to act on it. It seems most likely that lack of appreciation of this, combined with some increase in the severity of asthma and the introduction of new but still short-acting bronchodilators, combined together to produce the increase in deaths.

The β_2-adrenoceptor bronchodilators are remarkably non-toxic. A survey of attempted poisonings with salbutamol failed to identify a single death, even at doses up to 75 times the recommended oral dose[108]. Side-effects at normal oral doses are mild and receptor related. Mild tachycardia and muscle tremor are observed in some patients, but tolerance or adaptation to tremor develops rapidly in most subjects[109,110]. By the inhaled route even these side-effects are eliminated. In contrast, the theophylline-based bronchodilators have a low therapeutic index that necessitates very careful control of the concentration of drug in the plasma.

Scope for improvements

The β_2-adrenoceptor stimulant bronchodilator drugs are clearly highly effective non-toxic drugs which, by the inhaled route, are virtually free of side-effects. Consequently it is very difficult to pinpoint areas where improvement might be achieved. It might be thought that improving β_2 selectivity might offer an advantage but this is probably an illusion. Firstly, skeletal muscle tremor in man and its equivalent in experimental animals appears to be mediated through β_2-receptors[22]. Secondly, the tachycardia that these drugs induce also appears to be mediated, directly and indirectly, through β_2-receptors (*see* p. 195)[14].

The synthetic β_2-adrenoceptor agonists are all of considerably longer duration of action than isoprenaline by inhalation and are active orally. Enhanced duration of action could be of value, particularly in a prophylactic regimen. Metabolic stability enhances duration by the oral route as is shown by clenbuterol[11,12], but other factors such as absorption may govern duration by the inhaled route.

Recently, Paterson *et al.* have pointed out one area where improvement may be obtained[103]. The efficacies of β_2-adrenoceptor agonists differ considerably. At low levels of bronchoconstriction, this is unlikely to be significant as all will appear to be full agonists, but as the severity of bronchoconstriction increases compounds with low efficacy will become partial agonists before those of greater efficacy. Thus, it is argued[103] that consideration should be given to relative efficacies when new compounds are being considered for development.

α-Antagonists in the treatment of asthma

In 1968, Szentivanyi proposed that hypo-responsiveness of β-adrenoceptors and hyper-responsiveness of α-adrenoceptors were major determinants of bronchoconstriction in asthma[111]. Since then several groups have shown that human airways contain α-adrenoceptors[112,112] that may be hyper-responsive in asthmatics[114], that β blockade can produce bronchoconstriction in asthmatics[115] and that, in β-blocked normals and asthmatics, α-agonists can cause bronchoconstriction[113,116–118]. This is circumstantial evidence for an involvement of α-adrenoceptors in asthma and this proposal has been investigated both under challenge conditions and in clinical asthma using a range of α-adrenoceptor antagonists.

Thymoxamine[119,120], phentolamine and phenoxybenzamine[121] have all been shown to reduce histamine-induced bronchospasm. Phentolamine[122], thymoxamine[123] and indoramin[124] inhibit exercise-induced bronchospasm and thymoxamine[125] inhibits the bronchoconstrictor response to antigen. However, it has been pointed out that all these drugs have, in addition to their α-antagonist activity, pharmacological activity such as H_1 antagonist activity (phenoxybenzamine, thymoxamine, indoramin) or non-specific inhibitory actions on smooth muscle (phentolamine) that could contribute to their anti-bronchoconstrictor activity[126]. In contrast prazosin, which is a pharmacologically 'clean' α_1-adrenoceptor antagonist, failed to cause bronchodilatation[126]. The conclusion therefore is that α-adrenoceptors do not play a significant role in asthmatic bronchoconstriction and that α-antagonists have no useful role in controlling bronchospasm.

References

1. KONZETT, H. *Naunyn-Schmiedebergs Archiv fuer Pharmakologie und Experimentelle Pathologie*, **197**, 27 (1940)
2. LANGLEY, J.N. *Journal of Physiology*, **39**, 235 (1909)
3. AHLQUIST, R.P. *American Journal of Physiology*, **153**, 586 (1948)
4. LANDS, A.M. and BROWN, T.G. *Proceedings of the Society for Experimental Biology and Medicine*, **116**, 331 (1964)
5. LANDS, A.M., ARNOLD, A., McAULIFFE, J.P., LUDENA, F.P. and BROWN, T.G. *Nature*, **214**, 597 (1967)
6. LANDS, A.M., LUDENA, F.P. and BUZZO, H.J. *Life Sciences*, **6**, 2241 (1967)
7. COLLIER, J.G. and DORNHORST, A.C. *Nature*, **223**, 1283 (1969)
8. IVERSEN, L.L. *British Journal of Pharmacology*, **41**, 571 (1971)
9. KOPIN, I.J. *Catecholamines, Handbuch der experimentellen Pharmakologie*. Eds H. Blashko and E. Muscholl. Vol. 33, Chapter 8. Berlin: Springer (1972)
10. BRITTAIN, R.T., DEAN, C.M. and JACK, D. *Respiratory Pharmacology*. Ed. J.G. Widdicombe. Chapter 25. Oxford: Pergamon (1981)
11. ZIMMER, A. *Arzneimittel-Forschung*, **26**, 1446 (1976)
12. ANDERSON, G. and WILKINS, E. *Thorax*, **32**, 717 (1977)
13. GEORGE, C.F., BLACKWELL, E.W. and DAVIES, D.S. *Journal of Pharmacy and Pharmacology*, **26**, 265 (1974)
14. GIBSON, D.J. and COLTART, D.J. *Postgraduate Medical Journal*, **45** (Supplement), 40 (1971)
15. ASSEM, E.S.K. and SCHILD, H.O. *Nature*, **224**, 1028 (1969)
16. BUTCHERS, P.R., SKIDMORE, I.F., VARDEY, C.J. and WHEELDON, A. *British Journal of Pharmacology*, **71**, 663 (1980)
17. BUTCHERS, P.R., FULLERTON, J.R., SKIDMORE, I.F., THOMPSON, L.E., VARDEY, C.J. and WHEELDON, A. *British Journal of Pharmacology*, **67**, 23 (1979)
18. YOUMANS, W.B., AUMANN, K.W. and HANEY, H.F. *American Journal of Physiology*, **126**, 237 (1939)
19. POWELL, C.E. and SLATER, I.H. *Journal of Pharmacology and Experimental Therapeutics*, **122**, 480 (1958)
20. FURCHGOTT, R.F. *Catecholamines, Handbuch der experimentellen Pharmakologie*. Eds H. Blashko and E. Muscholl. Vol. 33. Chapter 9. Berlin: Springer (1972)

21. CARLSSON, E., ABLAD, B., BRANDSTROM, A. and CARLSSON, B. *Life Sciences*, **11**, 953 (1972)
22. LEVY, G.P. and APPERLEY, G.H. *Recent Advances in the Pharmacology of Adrenoceptors*. Eds E. Szabadi, C.M. Bradshaw and P. Bevan. p. 201. Amsterdam: Elsevier/North Holland (1978)
23. DALY, M.J. and LEVY, G.P. *Trends in Autonomic Pharmacology*. Ed. S. Kalsner. p. 347. Baltimore: Urban and Swartzenberg (1980)
24. BARNETT, D.B., RUGG, E.L. and NAHORSKI, S.R. *Nature*, **273**, 116 (1978)
25. MINNEMAN, K.P., HEGSTRAND, L.R. and MOLINOFF, P.B. *Molecular Pharmacology*, **16**, 34 (1979)
26. CORNISH, E.J. and MILLER, R.C. *Journal of Pharmacy and Pharmacology*, **27**, 23 (1975)
27. APPERLEY, G.H., DALY, M.J. and LEVY, G.P. *British Journal of Pharmacology*, **57**, 235 (1976)
28. KENAKIN, T.P. *Journal of Pharmacology and Experimental Therapeutics*, **223**, 416 (1982)
29. KENAKIN, T.P. *Trends in Pharmacological Sciences*, **3**, 153 (1982)
30. MINNEMAN, K.P., HEGSTRAND, L.R. and MOLINOFF, P.B. *Molecular Pharmacology*, **16**, 21 (1979)
31. MINNEMAN, K.P., HEDBERG, A. and MOLINOFF, P.B. *Journal of Pharmacology and Experimental Therapeutics*, **211**, 502 (1979)
32. ROBINSON, G.A., BUTCHER, R.W. and SUTHERLAND, E.W. *Annual Reviews of Biochemistry*, **37**, 149 (1968)
33. CLARK, A.J. *General Pharmacology, Handbuch der experimentellen Pharmakologie*. Vol. 4. Berlin: Springer (1937)
34. ARIENS, E.J. *Archives Internationales de Pharmacodynamie et de Thérapie*, **99**, 32 (1954)
35. LEVITSKI, A. *Receptors and Recognition*. Eds P. Cuatrecasas and M.F. Greaves. Vol. 2. p. 199. London: Chapman and Hall (1976)
36. STEPHENSON, R.P. *British Journal of Pharmacology*, **11**, 379 (1956)
37. FURCHGOTT, R.F. *Advances in Drug Research*, **3**, 21 (1966)
38. RODBELL, M., BIRNBAUMER, L., POHL, S.L. and KRANS, H.M.J. *Journal of Biological Chemistry*, **246**, 1877 (1971)
39. PFEUFFER, T. and HELMREICH, E.J.M. *Journal of Biological Chemistry*, **250**, 867 (1975)
40. CASSEL, D. and SELINGER, Z. *Biochimica et Biophysica Acta*, **452**, 538 (1976)
41. CASSEL, D. and SELINGER, Z. *Proceedings of the National Academy of Sciences of the United States of America*, **75**, 4155 (1978)
42. CUATRECASAS, P. *Annual Reviews of Biochemistry*, **43**, 169 (1974)
43. LEVITSKY, A. *Trends in Pharmacological Sciences*, **3**, 203 (1982)
44. BLOOM, B.M. and GOLDMAN, I.M. *Advances in Drug Research*, **3**, 121 (1966)
45. HOFFMAN, B.B. and LEFKOWITZ, R.J. *Annual Reviews of Pharmacology and Toxicology*, **20**, 581 (1980)
46. LEFKOWITZ, R.J. and HOFFMAN, B.B. *Trends in Pharmacological Sciences*, **1**, 314 (1980)
47. KENT, R.S., DE LEAN, A. and LEFKOWITZ, R.J. *Molecular Pharmacology*, **17**, 14 (1980)
48. RUGG, E.L., BARNETT, D.B. and NAHORSKI, S.R. *Molecular Pharmacology*, **14**, 996 (1978)
49. GLASS, D.B. and KREBS, E.G. *Annual Reviews of Pharmacology and Toxicology*, **20**, 363 (1980)
50. SILVER, P.J. and STULL, J.T. *Calcium Blockers: Mechanisms of Action and Clinical Applications*. Eds S.F. Flaim and R. Zelis. Chapter 3. Baltimore: Urban and Schwartzenberg (1982)
51. KATZ, A.M., TAZA, M. and KIRCHBERGER, M.A. *Advances in Cyclic Nucleotide Research*, **5**, 453 (1975)
52. HICKS, M.J., SHIGEKAWA, M. and KATZ, A.M. *Circulation Research*, **44**, 384 (1979)
53. STULL, J.T., BLUMENTHAL, D.K. and COOKE, R. *Biochemical Pharmacology*, **29**, 2537 (1980)
54. LAPETINA, E.G. *Trends in Pharmacological Sciences*, **3**, 115 (1982)
55. LAPETINA, E.G. and CUATRECASAS, P. *Biochimica et Biophysica Acta*, **573**, 394 (1979)
56. KATZ, A.M. *Trends in Pharmacological Sciences*, **1**, 434 (1980)
57. KATZ, A.M. *Physiology and Biophysics of the Heart*. p. 367. New York: Raven Press (1977)
58. APPERLEY, G.H. *Membership of the Institute of Biology: Thesis* (1977)
59. KOPITAR, Z. and ZIMMER, A. *Arzneimittel-Forschung*, **26**, 1435 (1976)
60. TSCHAN, M., PERROUGHOUD, A. and HERZOG, G. *European Journal of Clinical Pharmacology*, **15**, 159 (1979)

61. BARONTI, A., GRIECO, A. and VIBELLI, C. *European Journal of Respiratory Diseases*, **61**, 143 (1980)
62. SCHILD, H.O. *Quarterly Journal of Experimental Physiology*, **26**, 165 (1936)
63. LICHENSTEIN, LM. and MARGOLIS, S. *Science*, **161**, 902 (1968)
64. ORANGE, R.P., AUSTEN, W.G. and AUSTEN, K.F. *Journal of Experimental Medicine*, **134**, 1369 (1971)
65. McFADDEN, E.R., SOTER, N.A. and INGRAM, K.H. *Journal of Allergy and Clinical Immunology*, **66**, 472 (1980)
66. JORDE, W., BOHLMANN, G.-G., LINSENMANN, P. and WERDERMANN, K. *Medizinsche Klinik*, **70**, 1314 (1975)
67. BORUM, P. and MYGIND, N. *Journal of Allergy and Clinical Immunology*, **66**, 25 (1980)
68. SCHUMACHER, M.J. *Journal of Allergy and Clinical Immunology*, **66**, 33 (1980)
69. SVENSSON, G. *Acta Oto-Laryngologica*, **90**, 130 (1980)
70. HEGARDT, B., LOWHAGEN, O. and SVEDMYR, N. *Allergy*, **35**, 413 (1980)
71. MARTIN, G.L., ATKINS, P.C., DUNSKY, E.H. and SWEIMAN, B. *Journal of Allergy and Clinical Immunology*, **66**, 204 (1980)
72. ORR, T.S.C., ELLIOTT, E.V., ALTOUNYAN, R.E.C. and STERN, M.A. *Clinical Allergy*, **10** (Supplement), 491 (1980)
73. PEPYS, J. *Bronchial Asthma: Mechanisms and Therapeutics*. Eds E.B. Weiss and M.S. Segal. Chapter 17. Boston: Little, Brown (1976)
74. ANDERSON, S.D., SEALE, D.P., ROZEA, O., BANDLER, L., THEOBALD, G. and LINDSAY, D.A. *American Review of Respiratory Disease*, **114**, 493 (1976)
75. FERRIS, L., ANDERSON, S.D. and TEMPLE, D.M. *British Medical Journal*, **1**, 1697 (1978)
76. WOOLCOCK, A.J. *Drugs*, **15**, 1 (1978)
77. PATERSON, J.W., WOOLCOCK, A.J. and SHENFIELD, G.M. *American Review of Respiratory Disease*, **120**, 1149 (1979)
78. VAN AS, A. *New Directions in Asthma*. Ed. M. Stein. Chap. 25. Park Ridge, Illinois: American College of Chest Physicians (1975)
79. SHEPHERD, G.L., HETZEL, M.R. and CLARK, T.J.H. *British Journal of Diseases of the Chest*, **75**, 215 (1981)
80. ORANGE, R.P. and AUSTEN, K.F. *Progress in Immunology*, **1**, 173 (1972)
81. SKIDMORE, I.F. *Trends in Pharmacological Sciences*, **3**, 66 (1982)
82. HOGG, J.C., PARE, P.D., BOUCHER, R.C. and MICHOUD, M.-C. *Canadian Medical Association Journal*, **121**, 409 (1979)
83. BOWMAN, W.C. and RAND, M.J. *Textbook of Pharmacology*, 2nd ed. Chaps 9, 39. Oxford: Blackwell (1980)
84. PERKINS, J.P. *Trends in Pharmacological Sciences*, **2**, 326 (1981)
85. SU, Y.F., HARDEN, T.K. and PERKINS, J.P. *Journal of Biological Chemistry*, **255**, 7410 (1980)
86. WESSELS, M.R., MULLIKIN, D. and LEFKOWITZ, R.J. *Molecular Pharmacology*, **16**, 10 (1979)
87. REGGIANI, A., VERNALEONE, F. and ROBISON, G.A. *Neurosciences Abstracts*, **6**, 534 (1980)
88. CHUANG, D.M. and COSTA, E. *Proceedings of the National Academy of Sciences of the United States of America*, **76**, 3024 (1979)
89. NELSON, H.S., RAINE, E., DONER, H.C. and POSEY, W.C. *American Review of Respiratory Disease*, **116**, 871 (1977)
90. JENNE, J.W., CHICK, T.W., STRICKLAND, R.D. and WALL, F.J. *Journal of Allergy and Clinical Immunology*, **59**, 383 (1977)
91. PLUMMER, AL., *Chest*, **73** (Supplement), 949 (1978)
92. HOLGATE, S.T., BALDWIN, C.J. and TATTERSFIELD, A.E. *Lancet*, **ii**, 375 (1977)
93. FALLIERS, C.J. *Annals of Allergy*, **47**, 387 (1981)
94. CONOLLY, M.E., TASHKIN, D.P., HUI, K.K.P., LITTNER, M.R. and WOLFE, R.M. *Journal of Allergy and Clinical Immunology*, **70**, 423 (1982)
95. WEBER, R.W., SMITH, J.A. and NELSON, H.S. *Journal of Allergy and Clinical Immunology*, **70**, 417 (1982)
96. TASHKIN, D.P., CONOLLY, M.E., DEUTSCH, R.I., HUI, K.K.P., LITTNER, M.R., SCARPACE, P. et al. *American Review of Respiratory Disease*, **125**, 185 (1982)
97. LARSSON, S., SVEDMYR, N. and THIRINGER, G. *Journal of Allergy and Clinical Immunology*, **59**, 93 (1977)
98. SIMS, B.A. *British Journal of Clinical Pharmacology*, **1**, 291 (1974)
99. PEEL, E.T. and GIBSON, G.J. *American Review of Respiratory Diseases*, **121**, 973 (1980)
100. HARVEY, J.E., BALDWIN, C.J., WOOD, P.J., ALBERTI, K.G.M.M. and TATTERSFIELD, A. *Clinical Science*, **60**, 579 (1981)

101. REPSHER, L.H., MILLER, T.D. and SMITH, S. *Annals of Allergy*, **47**, 405 (1981)
102. TATTERSFIELD, A.E. *New Concepts in the Topical Treatment of Asthma and Related Disorders.* p. 33. Boston: Glaxo Inc. (1982)
103. PATERSON, J.W., LULICH, K.M. and GOLDIE, R.G. *Trends in Pharmacological Sciences*, **4**, 67 (1983)
104. CONOLLY, M.E., DAVIES, D.S., DOLLERY, C.T. and GEORGE, C.F. *British Journal of Pharmacology*, **43**, 389 (1971)
105. CLARK, T.J.H. *New Concepts in the Topical Treatment of Asthma and Related Disorders.* p. 31. Boston: Glaxo Inc. (1982)
106. CROMPTON, G.K. *New Concepts in the Topical Treatment of Asthma and Related Disorders.* p. 10. Boston: Glaxo Inc. (1982)
107. HUME, K.M. and GANDEVIA, B. *Thorax*, **12**, 276 (1957)
108. PRIOR, J.G., COCHRANE, G.M., RAPER, S.M., ALI, C. and VOLANS, G.N. *British Medical Journal*, **282**, 1932 (1981)
109. LARSSON, S. and SVEDMYR, N. *Scandinavian Journal of Respiratory Diseases, Supplementum*, **88**, 54 (1974)
110. JENNE, J.W. *New Concepts in the Topical Treatment of Asthma and Related Disorders.* p. 28. Boston: Glaxo Inc. (1982)
111. SZENTIVANYI, A. *Journal of Allergy*, **42**, 203 (1968)
112. MATHE, A.A., ASTROM, A. and PERSSON, N.-A. *Journal of Pharmacy and Pharmacology*, **23**, 905 (1971)
113. SIMONSON, B.G., SVEDMYR, N. and SKOOG, B.E. *Scandinavian Journal of Respiratory Diseases*, **53**, 227 (1972)
114. HENDERSON, W.R., SHELHAMER, J.H., REINGOLD, D.B., SMITH, L.J., EVANS, R. and KALINER, M. *New England Journal of Medicine*, **300**, 642 (1979)
115. GRIECO, M.H. and PIERSON, R.N. *Journal of Allergy and Clinical Immunology*, **48**, 143 (1971)
116. PRIME, F.J., BIANCO, S., GRIFFIN, J.P. and KAMBUROFF, P.L. *Bulletin European de Physiopathologie Respiratoire—Clinical Respiratory Physiology*, **8**, 99 (1972)
117. PATEL, K.R. and KERR, J.W. *Clinical Allergy*, **3**, 349 (1973)
118. SNASHALL, P.D., BOOTHER, F.A. and STERLING, G.M. *Clinical Science and Molecular Medicine*, **54**, 282 (1978)
119. GADDIE, U., LEGGE, J.S., PETRIE, G. and PALMER, K.N.V. *British Journal of Diseases of the Chest*, **66**, 141 (1972)
120. BIANCO, S., GRIFFIN, J.P., KAMBUROFF, P.H. and PRIME, F.J. *British Journal of Diseases of the Chest*, **66**, 27 (1972)
121. KERR, J.W., GOVINDARAJ, M. and PATEL, K.R. *British Medical Journal*, **2**, 139 (1970)
122. BEIL, M. and DE KOCK, M.A. *Respiration*, **35**, 78 (1975)
123. PATEL, K.R., KERR, J.W., McDONALD, E.B. and MacKENZIE, A.M. *Journal of Allergy and Clinical Immunology*, **57**, 285 (1976)
124. BIANCO, S., GRIFFIN, J.P., KAMBUROFF, P.H. and PRIME, F.J. *British Medical Journal*, **4**, 18 (1974)
125. PATEL, K.R. and KERR, J.W. *Clinical Allergy*, **5**, 311 (1975)
126. BARNES, B.J., IND, P.W. and DOLLERY, C.T. *Thorax*, **36**, 378 (1981)

Chapter 11

Theophylline

M. Cushley and S.T. Holgate

Introduction

Theophylline is a naturally occurring plant alkaloid deriving its name from the Greek for 'divine leaf' in tribute to the leaves of the tea plant, *Thea (Camellia) sinensis*. Structurally, it is 1,3-dimethylxanthine and is related to two other alkaloids—theobromine (3,7-dimethylxanthine) found in cocoa seeds, and caffeine (1,3,7-trimethylxanthine) found in coffee beans, tea leaves and cola nuts (*Figure 11.1*).

The potential medicinal and stimulatory properties of these compounds were first noted by the Prior of an Arabian convent when 'shepherds reported that goats that had eaten the berries of the coffee plant gambolled

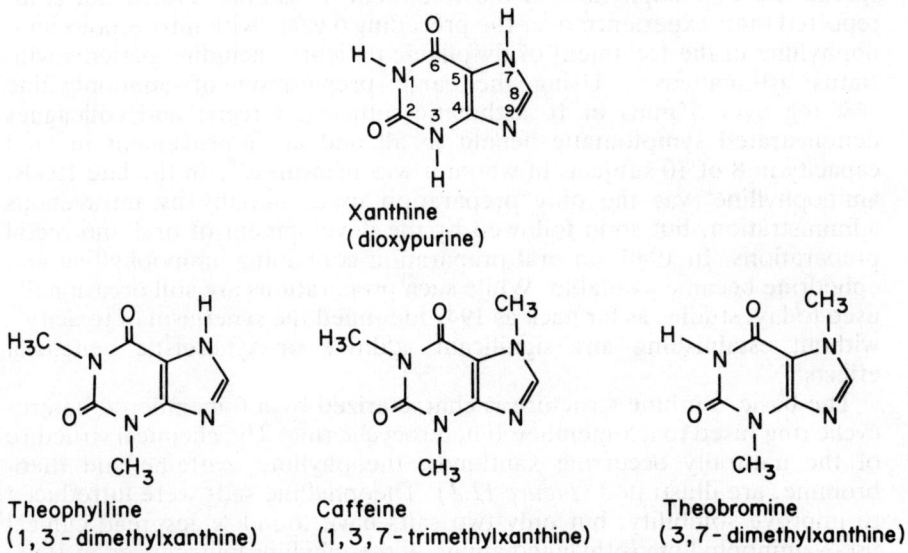

Xanthine
(dioxypurine)

Theophylline
(1,3-dimethylxanthine)

Caffeine
(1,3,7-trimethylxanthine)

Theobromine
(3,7-dimethylxanthine)

Figure 11.1 Structural formulae of the xanthine molecule and the naturally occurring methylated xanthines.

205

and frisked about all through the night instead of sleeping'. The Prior saw the advantage of this and used the berries in a beverage to help him stay awake through the long nights of prayer[1]. The first definite use of xanthines in the treatment of asthma was reported in the *Edinburgh Medical Journal* in 1859 when strong black coffee was described as one of the commonest and best reputed remedies for attacks of asthma[2]. In 1888, the active agent was extracted from tea leaves and named theophylline[3]. Seven years later theophylline was identified chemically as 1,3-dimethylxanthine[4].

Following this initial enthusiasm, general acceptance of the xanthines as useful therapeutic agents in asthma was slow. Caffeine was reported to prevent exercise-induced dyspnoea in 1890[5] and the bronchodilatory effect of caffeine was repeatedly studied in animals from 1912 to 1915[6-8]. One of the problems encountered with theophylline was its poor water solubility and, in 1908, a more soluble preparation, aminophylline (the ethylenediamine salt of theophylline) was formulated enabling the drug to be investigated in more detail. In 1921 Macht and Ting reported a study of the antispasmodic effect of drugs based on many of the folklore remedies[9]. Prompted by Salter's report[2] they investigated caffeine and found that it had only a weak relaxant effect on isolated bronchial smooth muscle, but that the related xanthine, theophylline, was much more effective. Within a few months of this report Hirsch published the relaxant effect of theophylline on bovine bronchial muscle strips *in vitro* and the beneficial effect of a theophylline/theobromine preparation in two patients with asthma[10]. Despite this clear evidence of the *in vitro* and *in vivo* relaxant effects of theophylline on airways tone, no further reports appeared until 1936. In this year a series of anecdotal studies were published on the use of theophylline in relieving attacks of asthma, especially those which were adrenaline resistant[11-14]. Twelve months later 2 reports heralded the widespread use of theophylline in the treatment of asthma. Herrmann *et al.* reported their experience over the preceding 6 years with intravenous aminophylline in the treatment of dyspnoeic patients, including patients with status asthmaticus[15]. Using the same preparation of aminophylline (480 mg over 5 min) in 16 asthmatic subjects, Greene and colleagues demonstrated symptomatic benefit in all and an improvement in vital capacity in 8 of 10 subjects in whom it was measured[16]. In the late 1930s, aminophylline was the only preparation used, initially by intravenous administration, but soon followed by the development of oral and rectal preparations. In 1940, an oral preparation containing aminophylline and ephedrine became available. While such preparations are still occasionally used today, studies as far back as 1942 identified the synergism of toxicity[17] without establishing any significant additive or synergistic beneficial effects[18].

The basic xanthine structure is characterized by a 6-membered heterocyclic ring fused to a 5-membered heterocyclic ring. The chemical structure of the naturally occurring xanthines, theophylline, caffeine and theobromine, are illustrated (*Figure 11.1*). Theophylline salts were introduced to improve solubility, but only two salts have found widespread clinical use—aminophylline (ethylenediamine + theophylline) introduced in 1908, and choline theophyllinate (choline + theophylline) in 1954. These preparations dissociate, following administration, into free theophylline and the

TABLE 11.1 Theophylline content of the theophylline salts

Salt	Theophylline content (%)*
Theophylline	100
Aminophylline (theophylline + ethylenediamine)	85
Choline theophyllinate (oxtriphylline)	64
Theophylline sodium glycinate	50
Theophylline calcium salicylate	48

* Theophylline content given by weight.

respective cation. From a therapeutic standpoint such salts should be regarded in terms of their theophylline content (*Table 11.1*).

In the 1940s a number of N-7 substituted methylxanthine derivatives were developed in an attempt to improve solubility and reduce gastrointestinal side-effects. However, preparations introduced over the next 10 years, such as diprophylline (1946), acephylline piperazine (1949), etophylline (1951) and proxyphylline (1956), although still used, are less efficacious than theophylline and often have poor absorption characteristics[19,20]. Comparative studies with theophylline are few, but Svedmyr demonstrated that proxyphylline required a 5-fold and diprophylline a 9-fold higher concentration than theophylline to produce the same relaxant response on human bronchial muscle *in vitro*[1].

Serum levels and clinical effects

Toxicity of the methylxanthines, which on occasions resulted in death, was first noted in adult patients in 1943[22], confirmed in 1948[23] and documented in children in 1950[24]. The early deaths were mainly in patients with cardiac problems, but, in children, serious toxic effects and death were noted when aminophylline was given by intravenous, rectal and oral routes[25]. It has been the unacceptable and often unpredictable side-effects of methylxanthines which has concerned clinicians. While deaths attributable to methylxanthines still occur[26], the introduction of efficient and reliable assays for measuring plasma levels of theophylline has meant that this group of drugs may now be used in a more rational and safe manner.

In 1949, Schack and Waxler developed a spectrophotometric assay for theophylline in biological fluids[27]. Since that time the technique has been modified and other methods have been introduced based on gas chromatography[28], high-performance liquid chromatography[29], and immunoassay [two commercially available methods: radioimmunoassay (RIA)[30] and enzyme immunoassay (EMIT)[31]].

Over the last 10 years a better understanding of the pharmacokinetics of methylxanthines has stimulated their wider use. The first correlation between serum or plasma drug levels and clinical effect was by Truitt who investigated the diuretic effect of theophylline[32]. In 1957, Turner-Warwick reported that a plasma level of 10 μg/ml (55 μM) was necessary for subjective relief of bronchospasm in asthma[33], whilst Jackson and colleagues showed that plasma levels of 12 μg/ml were necessary before objective improvement of pulmonary function could be detected[34]. Detailed pharmacokinetic studies were initiated in 1972[35] and based on these and similar studies (*Figure 11.2*) the first dosage recommendations were introduced[36,37]. It is now widely asserted that, in asthma, both subjective and objective improvement occur with plasma levels greater than 5 μg/ml[38]. The recommended plasma theophylline range of 5–20 μg/ml represents a compromise between efficacy and toxicity. Theophylline has a narrow therapeutic index and adverse effects occur with increased severity and frequency at concentrations greater than 20 μg/ml[39]. Resistant seizures, arrhythmias and deaths can occur without warning symptoms[40,41]. It is now

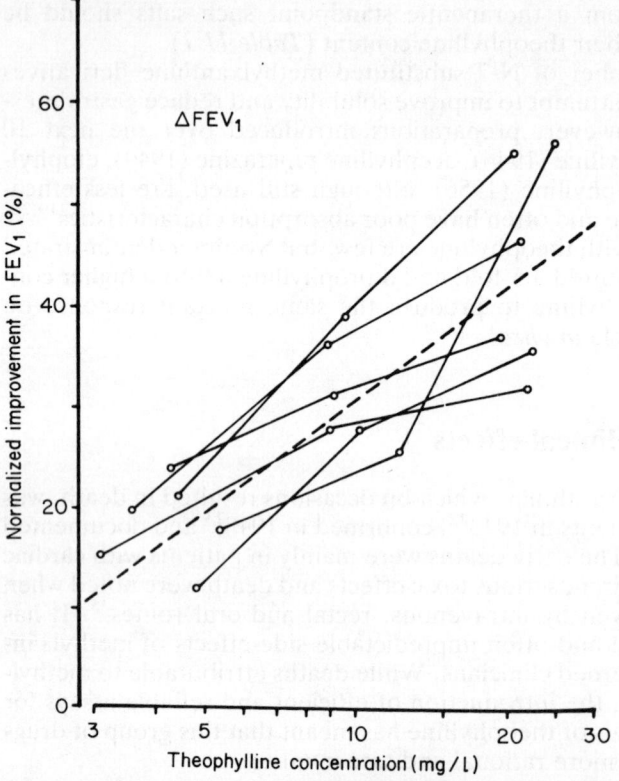

Figure 11.2 Relationship between the logarithm of the plasma theophylline concentration and change in FEV_1. From Mitenko, P.A. and Ogilvie, R.I., 1973, *New England Journal of Medicine*, Vol. 289, p. 600, by courtesy of the authors and publisher.

clear that the original recommendation of Mitenko and Ogilvie for intravenous aminophylline (5.6 mg/kg loading, 0.9 mg/kg per h maintenance infusion) is too high for many patients with severe asthma, who may have reduced drug clearance and who may be on a wide variety of other medications with which theophylline may interact.

Theophylline is principally (90%) metabolized by the liver through oxidation and demethylation to 3-methylxanthine, 1,3-dimethyluric acid and 1-methyluric acid, the remaining 10% being excreted unchanged in the urine (*Figure 11.3*).

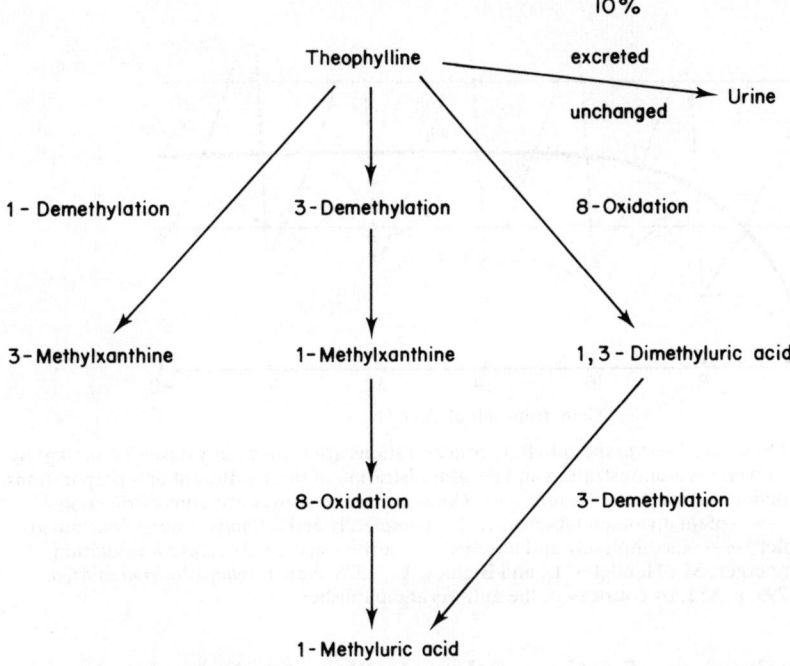

Figure 11.3 Hepatic metabolism of theophylline.

Hepatic metabolism shows marked interindividual variation and may also be affected by liver disease, cardiac failure and fever (reduced clearance), smoking (increased clearance) and other factors, such as sex, age, diet, and drug interactions[42,43]. As a consequence, the dosage recommendation has been revised and a reasonable compromise for parenteral aminophylline appears to be a loading dose of 6 mg/kg over 30 minutes followed by 0.5 mg/kg per h maintenance at maximum (reduced to 0.2 mg/kg per h if liver disease or congestive cardiac failure are present)[44]. This regime produces peak plasma theophylline levels of 10 μg/ml, but it should be noted that the 95% confidence limits are wide (4.4–22.5 μg/ml) and, to obtain a maximum benefit with reduced risk of toxicity, infusion rates for individual patients should be adjusted in response to the plasma theophylline levels[45].

Pharmacokinetic studies have also influenced oral prescribing. The early 1970s saw the development of rapid dissolution oral theophylline preparations which were completely and consistently absorbed from the gastrointestinal tract. However, to maintain serum concentrations between 10 and 20 μg/ml, 6-hourly administration was necessary (*Figure 11.4*). Less frequent dosing caused cyclical overdose and underdose with an increase in side-effects. Reliable sustained release formulations reduced the fluctuations in serum concentrations, thereby permitting longer dosing intervals with twice daily regimes and possibly once daily preparations[46,47].

Theophylline is reliably absorbed from rectal preparations, but intramuscular routes are not advised on account of pain and unreliable absorption[48].

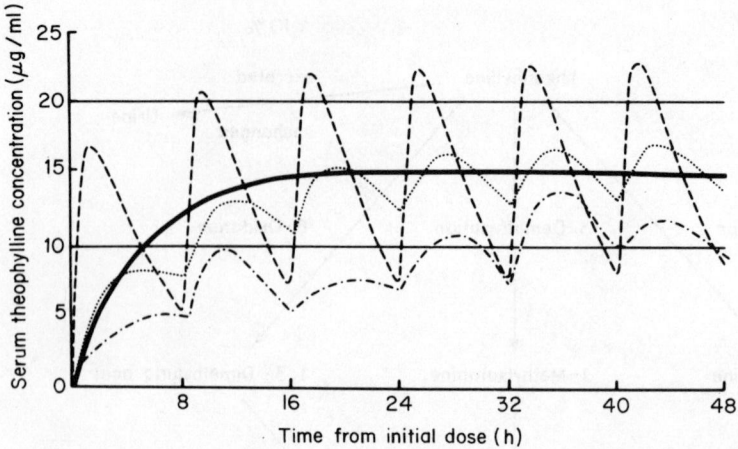

Figure 11.4 Simulated serum theophylline concentrations after same daily dose (9.6 mg/kg) by constant intravenous administration and by administration of three different oral preparations in equally divided doses every 8 hours. —— Constant rate as with continuous intravenous infusion; – – – – plain uncoated tablet; .. .. completely and reliably absorbed sustained-release tablet; –·–·– incompletely and unreliably absorbed sustained-release formulation. From Weinberger, M., Hendeles, L. and Bighley, L., 1978, *New England Journal of Medicine*, Vol. 299, p. 852, by courtesy of the authors and publisher.

The mechanism of action of theophylline at cellular level

Phosphodiesterase inhibition

Adenosine cyclic 3':5'-monophosphate (cyclic AMP) was initially discovered as the intracellular mediator of the glycogenolytic effect of adrenaline and glucagon in the liver[49]. It has since been recognized as a second messenger mediating a variety of hormonal effects, including the bronchodilator action of the β-adrenoceptor agonists[50]. Adrenaline and more selective β_2-adrenergic agonists relax airways smooth muscle by increasing cellular levels of cyclic AMP. This is achieved by activation of receptor-linked adenylate cyclase which catalyses the conversion of adenosine triphosphate (ATP) to cyclic AMP (cAMP) (*Figure 11.5*). Cyclic AMP mediates its effect by activating cAMP-dependent protein kinases which selectively phosphorylate proteins to inhibit calcium-dependent excitation–contraction coupling in smooth muscle. How this is achieved is not completely understood. One suggestion involves cAMP-dependent protein kinase phosphorylation of myosin light chain kinase.

An enzyme activity capable of biologically inactivating cyclic AMP was detected in various mammalian tissues in 1958[51]. Investigations showed that this activity was due to a magnesium-dependent phosphodiesterase which catalyses the hydrolysis of the cyclic nucleotide at the 3'-position, yielding adenosine 5'-monophosphate (AMP). Partially purified preparations of this enzyme were found to be competitively inhibited by the methylxanthines. In 1962, the inhibition of a more soluble phosphodiesterase extracted from beef heart was studied[52]. Theophylline was found to produce competitive inhibition of cyclic AMP phosphodiesterase and was 6.7 and 5.8 times more potent than theobromine and caffeine,

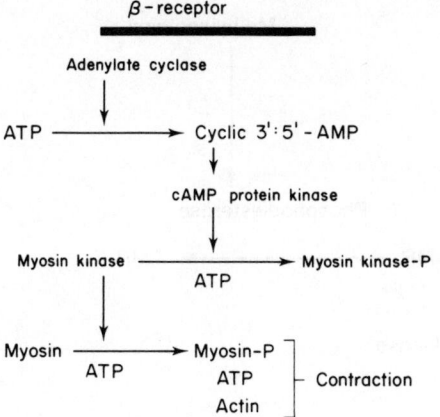

Figure 11.5 Proposed action of β agonists on smooth muscle.

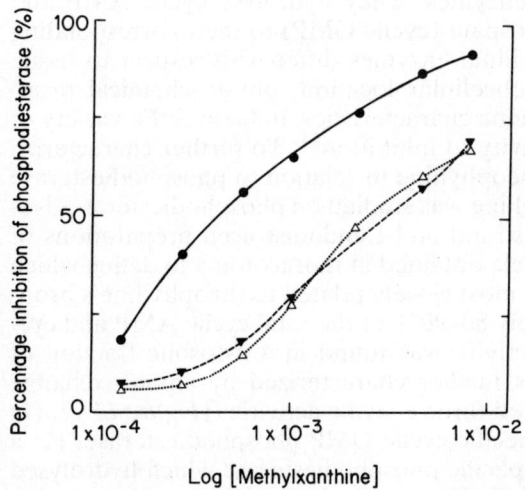

Figure 11.6 Relative potencies of the methylxanthines. (●—●) Theophylline; (△...△) caffeine; (▼– – –▼) theobromine. From Butcher, R.W. and Sutherland, E.W., 1962, *Journal of Biological Chemistry*, Vol. 237, p. 1244, by courtesy of the authors and publisher.

respectively (*Figure 11.6*). It subsequently became accepted that the therapeutic effects of the methylxanthines, theophylline and aminophylline, in heart failure and bronchial asthma were related to inhibition of phosphodiesterase and to a rise in intracellular cyclic AMP levels producing more forceful myocardial contraction and bronchodilatation[53]. Since both β-adrenoceptor agonists and theophylline increase cellular levels of cyclic AMP by different methods, a unified and attractive concept for the bidirectional role of cyclic AMP as a second messenger in maintaining smooth muscle tone was born.

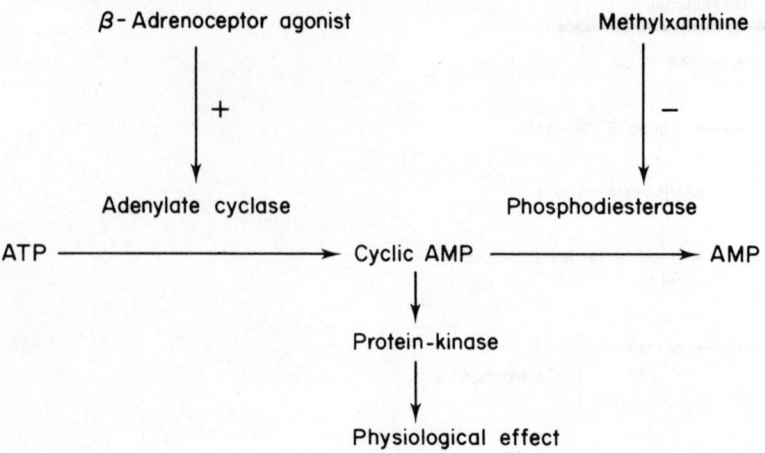

Following the initial partial purification of phosphodiesterase, further work has established that the cyclic nucleotide phosphodiesterases constitute a heterogenous class of enzymes. They hydrolyse cyclic AMP and guanosine cyclic 3':5'-monophospate (cyclic GMP) to their corresponding 5'-monophosphates. The individual enzymes differ with respect to tissue and/or cellular distribution, subcellular location, physicochemical properties, substrate specificity, kinetic characteristics, influence of a variety of modulators *in vitro* and sensitivity to inhibition[54]. To further characterize the bronchodilator action of theophylline in relation to phosphodiesterase inhibition the effect of theophylline was studied on phosphodiesterases isolated from lung tissue[55]. Bergstrand and Lundquist used preparations of human lung and bronchial muscle obtained at thoracotomy to define which phosphodiesterase activity was most closely related to theophylline's bronchodilator effect. Approximately 80–90% of the total cyclic AMP and cyclic GMP phosphodiesterase activity was found in a cytosolic fraction of human lung. This activity was further characterized by anion exchange chromatography which separated three enzyme activities (*Figure 11.7*). (1) a high-affinity (K_m 0.4 μM) specific cyclic GMP phosphodiesterase; (2) a low-affinity (K_m 25 μM) non-specific phosphodiesterase which hydrolysed both cyclic GMP and cyclic AMP; (3) a high-affinity (K_m 0.4 μM) specific cyclic AMP phosphodiesterase (K_m = the substrate concentration giving half the maximum velocity of the enzyme reaction). Theophylline was non-specific in inhibiting all three enzyme fractions to a similar extent[56].

If theophylline produces its effects principally by inhibiting the hydrolysis of cyclic AMP by phosphodiesterase one might expect to demonstrate that: (1) theophylline is a phosphodiesterase inhibitor, (2) there is a correlation between the smooth muscle relaxation and phosphodiesterase inhibition, (3) therapeutic concentrations of theophylline would be associated with phosphodiesterase inhibition, (4) smooth muscle relaxation might be associated with elevation of cyclic AMP levels, (5) other phosphodiesterase inhibitors should produce smooth muscle relaxation, and (6) synergy between drugs increasing the formation of cyclic AMP (β-adrenoceptor agonists) and those inhibiting the breakdown of cyclic AMP (methylxanthines).

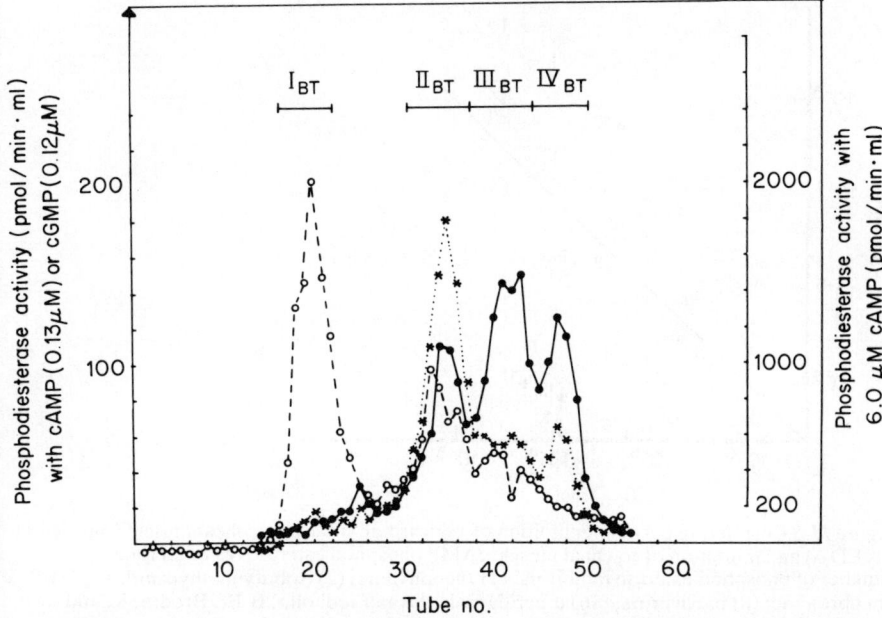

Figure 11.7 Separation and characterization of phosphodiesterase activity from human lung tissue by chromatography. Fraction I = high-affinity cGMP-specific phosphodiesterase; fraction II = low-affinity non-specific phosphodiesterase for cAMP and cGMP; fraction III = high-affinity cAMP-specific phosphodiesterase; fraction IV = probably a subunit of fraction III. (●—●—●) 0.13 μM cAMP; (○---○---○) 0.12 μM cGMP; (*---*---*) 6.0 μM cAMP. From Bergstrand H. and Lundquist, B., 1978, *Molecular and Cellular Biochemistry*, Vol. 21, p. 9, by courtesy of the authors and publisher.

Several studies have shown a significant correlation between *in vitro* phosphodiesterase activity and the capacity to produce relaxation of a variety of animal tracheal preparations. However, in most of these studies the concentration of theophylline required to produce significant inhibition of phosphodiesterase was 10–20-fold higher than required to produce airways smooth muscle relaxation $(2 \times 10^{-5}M)$[57–59]. Extrapolation of these concentrations to equivalent values *in vivo* should take account of the availability of free theophylline, since approximately 60% of the drug is bound to plasma proteins[60]. Assuming there is no additional theophylline binding to intracellular proteins, the free concentration available for phosphodiesterase inhibition would be in the range of $(2–4) \times 10^{-5}$ M. Over this concentration range *in vitro*, theophylline inhibits phosphodiesterase from human lung by 10–12.5%, and, even at 10^{-4} M (a concentration well into theophylline's toxic range), only 14–20% inhibition occurs[61].

Studies relating airways smooth muscle relaxation to cyclic AMP levels have produced conflicting results. Lohmann found that, *in vitro*, at theophylline concentrations producing complete relaxation of bovine trachea (10^{-3} M), no increase in cellular levels of cyclic AMP could be detected[62]. In man, neither oral theophylline[63] nor continuously infused theophylline[64] produced significant increases in plasma cyclic AMP levels,

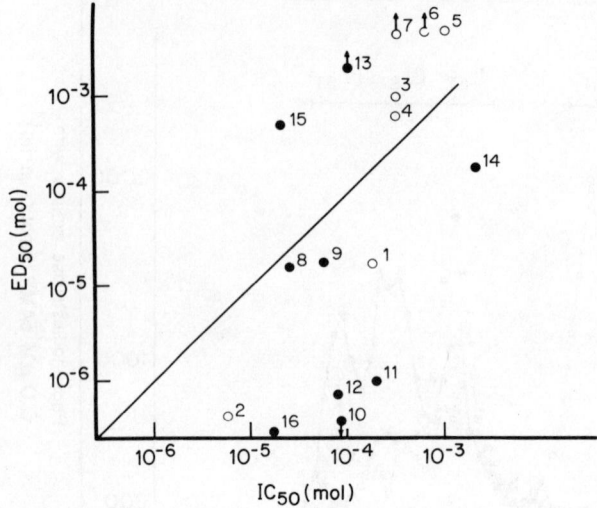

Figure 11.8 Correlation between inhibition of pilocarpine-induced tracheal muscle contraction (as ED_{50}) and inhibition of tracheal muscle cAMP phosphodiesterase (as IC_{50}) for a number of phosphodiesterase inhibitors: (1) theophylline; (2) isobutylmethylxanthine; (7) theobromine; (8) papaverine; (16) dipyridamole. From Fredholm, B.B., Brodin, K. and Strandberg, K., 1979, *Acta Pharmacologica et Toxicologica*, Vol. 45, p. 336, by courtesy of the authors and publisher.

whereas with a single intravenous bolus of aminophylline 5.6 mg/kg, a 50% increase in plasma cyclic AMP levels occurred[65,66].

Theophylline is only one of many drugs which inhibit phosphodiesterase. Fredholm has compared the effects of 16 compounds on relaxation of guinea-pig tracheal tone and inhibition of cyclic AMP phosphodiesterase[59] (*Figure 11.8*). A weak positive correlation was found ($r = 0.46$). Two drugs, papaverine and dipyridamole, were potent cyclic AMP phosphodiesterase inhibitors, but had no detectable relaxant effect on tracheal tone. This lack of effect could not be due to a preferential effect on cyclic GMP phosphodiesterase (*Table 11.2*), although selective effects of each agent on different cyclic AMP phosphodiesterase isoenzymes could not be excluded (*Table 11.2*).

If β-adrenoceptor agonists and theophylline act by increasing intracellular cyclic AMP levels as commonly proposed, one might expect a synergistic interaction when the two drugs are used in combination. This has been demonstrated on relaxation of guinea-pig isolated trachea[67], cyclic AMP levels in human lung fragments[68], rabbit cardiac inotropic responses[69] and inhibition of histamine release from human leucocytes[70]. However, *in*

TABLE 11.2. Inhibition of cyclic AMP and cyclic GMP hydrolysis by various phosphodiesterase inhibitors

Inhibitor	cAMP	cGMP	cAMP/cGMP
Isobutylmethylxanthine	5×10^{-6}	8×10^{-6}	0.6
Papaverine*	3×10^{-5}	1×10^{-4}	0.3
Theophylline	1.2×10^{-4}	2×10^{-4}	0.6
Dipyridamole*	3×10^{-5}	6×10^{-4}	0.05

* Potent phosphodiesterase inhibitor, but negligible bronchodilating activity. Values given are the molar concentrations that produce 50% inhibition of hydrolysis.

vivo, only the study by Campbell, using inhaled isoprenaline and intravenous aminophylline in asthma, showed a greater than additive effect and this was only at a single time point using the rate of maximal airflow at half vital capacity as an index of airways calibre[65]. The administration of drugs by different routes to investigate pharmacological interaction is undesirable since intravenous aminophylline may in itself produce bronchodilatation and increase the access of an inhaled β-adrenoceptor agonist to its proposed site of action. All other studies in asthma and chronic bronchitis have, at most, shown additive effects when both drugs are given orally, intravenously or by a combination of inhaled and intravenous routes[70–75].

Theophylline is a phosphodiesterase inhibitor, albeit relatively weak, and one cannot exclude that at least part of its pharmacological effect on airways smooth muscle is by this action. Because of the postulated cascade nature of cAMP-mediated activities, it is possible that small changes in levels of cyclic AMP may be amplified to produce substantially larger effects in the cell. Cellular compartments may exist which contain species of phosphodiesterases which may be more sensitive to theophylline and have not yet been studied. Other explanations might include accumulation of theophylline in cellular compartments producing levels not reflected by plasma levels, or that a metabolite of theophylline may be producing part of its effect. 3-Methylxanthine, one of the major theophylline metabolites, is as effective at relaxing guinea-pig tracheal muscle and stimulating cardiac muscle as theophylline. Its effect as an inhibitor of cyclic AMP phosphodiesterase varies with substrate concentration, being as effective as theophylline at low substrate concentrations (1.4 μM), but less active at high substrate concentrations (400 μM)[76].

Adenosine antagonism

The evidence for inhibition of phosphodiesterase as the sole mechanism of action for methylxanthines in asthma is not strong and it is reasonable to look for alternative pharmacological activities for this group of drugs.

An action of theophylline which has aroused recent interest is antagonism of endogenously produced adenosine. Adenosine is a naturally occurring purine nucleoside comprising the purine ring, adenine, linked at its 9-position to the 1′-carbon atom of the sugar ribose (*Figure 11.9*). Adenosine is formed from adenosine monophosphate (AMP) by the action of the membrane-bound ectoenzyme 5′-nucleotidase. Its relevance in asthma is not completely defined, but *in vitro* adenosine is released from lung tissue following antigen challenge[77] and under conditions of ischaemia and hypoxia[78]. In asthmatic subjects, adenosine is also released into the circulation in significant amounts following antigen-induced bronchoconstriction[79] suggesting that it may serve as an additional mediator in this disease. At a molecular level, adenosine decreases or increases cellular cyclic AMP levels by stimulating specific cell surface receptors which either inhibit (Ri or A_1) or stimulate (Ra or A_2) adenylate cyclase, respectively[80]. Adenosine potentiates IgE-dependent mediator release from rat[81] and human[82] mast cells challenged with antigen, inhibits sympathetic and cholinergic neurotransmission pre- and postsynaptically[83–86] and stimulates afferent nerve endings[87].

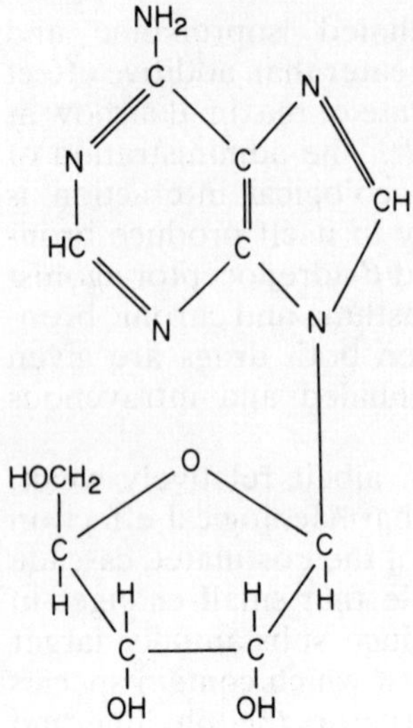

Figure 11.9 Structure of adenosine.

In man, adenosine has a bronchoconstrictor effect when given by inhalation to subjects with asthma[88]. This effect is likely to be specific since it also occurs with the parent nucleotide AMP, but not with inosine, the principal breakdown product of adenosine, or the related nucleoside guanosine[89]. Theophylline competitively inhibits the effects of adenosine at external receptor sites (A_1 and A_2) in all tissues studied[90,91]. This action occurs at concentrations which are similar to those found therapeutically in man and lower than those required to produce phosphodiesterase inhibition. In asthma, low concentrations of inhaled theophylline which produce little bronchodilatation significantly inhibited adenosine-induced bronchoconstriction with an effect which was four-fold greater than achieved on nonspecific bronchoconstriction induced by inhaled histamine[92].

Antagonism of adenosine has been proposed as the mechanism by which theophylline causes central nervous system stimulation[93], cardiac excitability[94] and diuresis[95]. It has recently been claimed that the xanthine, enprofylline (3-propylxanthine), is a more potent bronchodilator than theophylline in man and has no adenosine antagonistic properties[96]. However, in at least one tissue, the hippocampus, enprofylline has proved to be a potent A_2 adenosine antagonist[97].

Other mechanisms

There is increasing evidence that theophylline has an effect on sympathetic activity, either by a direct effect on the adrenal medulla causing catecholamine release, or indirectly through a postural effect and reflex increased sympathetic activity. High concentrations of theophylline *in vivo* produced significant release of catecholamines from the adrenal gland[98,99] and, in dogs, Westfall and Fleming found that pretreatment with either reserpine or propranolol depressed the chronotropic response to aminophylline[100]. In man, Atuk demonstrated an increase in urinary catecholamines with intravenous aminophylline and oral theophylline[101] and Mackay showed that in normal subjects pretreatment with propranolol significantly inhibited the bronchodilator and cyclic AMP response following intravenous aminophylline[66]. The recent availability of sensitive techniques for plasma catecholamine assay has confirmed that clinically relevant concentrations of theophylline, administered orally or intravenously, are associated with elevated catecholamine levels[102,103]. The increases are small and the bronchodilator effects of intravenous aminophylline and oral theophylline are only partially inhibited by pretreatment with propranolol[66,104].

There is less data available on the redistribution of intracellular calcium and prostaglandin antagonism. Kolbeck has described the effect of therapeutic concentrations of theophylline on the translocation of calcium in guinea-pig and dog trachea[105]. A redistribution of calcium occurred at theophylline concentrations which did not affect cyclic AMP levels. In rat mesenteric artery preparations, methylxanthines interact with indomethacin to inhibit prostaglandin generation[106].

Thus, at a cellular level, theophylline is a phosphodiesterase inhibitor and an adenosine antagonist. It may relax airways smooth muscle in asthma by both these mechanisms and also through the secondary release of catecholamines. It is therefore likely that the bronchodilator effect of theophylline is a function of more than one mechanism.

Other beneficial effects which may be relevant in respiratory disease include increased diaphragm contractility, especially under conditions of fatigue[107], improved tracheobronchial mucociliary clearance[108], an effect on reducing pulmonary oedema[109], inhibition of mediator release from mast cells[110,111], improvement in biventricular function in subjects with chronic obstructive pulmonary disease[112], and a stimulatory effect on respiratory control[113]. How all these actions can be related to the overall clinical efficacy of drugs such as theophylline remains to be answered.

Future developments

The way ahead must be to define more clearly the relevant actions of the methylxanthines in asthma, be it phosphodiesterase inhibition, adenosine antagonism, an effect on calcium redistribution or some action not yet apparent. Phosphodiesterase inhibition, adenosine antagonism and smooth muscle relaxation are not interdependent. Powerful phosphodiesterase inhibitors such as dipyridamole[114] and papaverine[115] have no bronchodilator effect, and dipyridamole actually potentiates the effects of adenosine at its external receptor[116] by inhibiting adenosine uptake by cells. Similarly, 8-phenyltheophylline is a potent adenosine antagonist with virtually no phosphodiesterase inhibitory activity, whereas 7-benzylisobutylmethylxanthine has less activity as an adenosine antagonist and appears to be a relatively selective agent for inhibiting calcium-dependent phosphodiesterases and membrane-located phosphodiesterases[117] (*Table 11.3*).

TABLE 11.3. Comparison of potency of selected alkylxanthines as adenosine antagonists and phosphodiesterase inhibitors

| Xanthine | IC_{50} (μM) of phosphodiesterase | | | | | | |
	A calcium dependent	B calcium independent	C membrane	D adenosine elicited cAMP accumulation	A/D	B/D	C/D
3-Isobutyl-1-methylxanthine	7.5	40	65	60	0.1	0.7	1.0
Theophylline	950	500	1000	60	16	8	17
8-Phenyltheophylline	>100*	>100*	—	6	>17	>17	—
7-Benzyl-isobutyl-1-methylxanthine	1.5	100	12	100	0.02	1	0.1

* Solubility prevented determination of actual IC_{50}.

IC_{50} = concentration required to produce 50% inhibition of enzyme activity.

Study of structure–activity relationships should allow manipulation of the xanthine rings to select analogues with more specific effects[118]. That small changes in the chemical structure bring about significant changes in activity is exemplified by the naturally occurring xanthines theophylline, caffeine and theobromine. Persson has summarized current knowledge regarding alkyl substitution at the various positions in the xanthine molecule[119–121] (*Figure 11.10*).

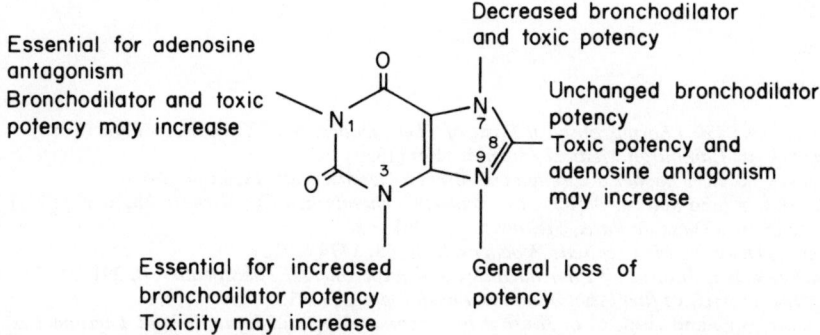

Essential for adenosine
antagonism
Bronchodilator and toxic
potency may increase

Decreased bronchodilator
and toxic potency

Unchanged bronchodilator
potency
Toxic potency and
adenosine antagonism
may increase

Essential for increased
bronchodilator potency
Toxicity may increase

General loss of
potency

Figure 11.10 Features of alkyl substitution at various positions in the xanthine molecule. From Persson, C.G.A., 1982, *Trends in Pharmacological Sciences*, Vol. 3, p. 312, by courtesy of the authors and publisher.

The commercially available chemical derivatives of theophylline with substitution at the 7-position on the xanthine ring, although being neutral and less irritant, are also less potent and absorption is unreliable[20]. Removal of methyl groups from theophylline produces the monomethyl-xanthines—3-methylxanthine and 1-methylxanthine, both of which produce the same maximal relaxation of guinea-pig tracheal muscle as theophylline, although at higher concentrations[76]. Alkyl substitution at position 3 with groups larger than $-CH_3$, such as benzyl, isoamyl or iso-butyl, bring about a 4–16-fold increase in cyclic AMP and cyclic GMP phosphodiesterase inhibitor potency, whilst substitution at position 7 or 8 greatly reduces potency against cyclic GMP phosphodiesterases[122,123].

The recognition of adenosine receptor subtypes has opened up new avenues of research. A wide variety of xanthine derivatives appear to have a similar effect on the A_1 and the A_2 receptor, but it is likely that xanthines will be developed which will distinguish between these receptors. 3-Propylxanthine is a new bronchodilator approximately five times as potent as theophylline, but lacking its central nervous system stimulant and diuretic effects[120]. It was thought to have no significant adenosine antagonistic properties, but it now seems that it is as potent as theophylline as an antagonist of the A_2 receptor in at least one cell system tested[97]. The tissue distribution of the adenosine receptor subtypes will reveal the significance of activities selective for A_1 or A_2 receptors and future development will undoubtedly include theophylline derivatives with little adenosine antagonistic activity and derivatives specific for A_1 and/or A_2 adenosine receptors, with little phosphodiesterase inhibitory activity[124].

Less promising areas of research involve different formulations of available preparations and different techniques of administration. The advent of the sustained release preparations with reliable and almost complete bioavailability suggests that there will be no future for any new salts of theophylline. The methylxanthine preparations are exceptional in the treatment of asthma in that they are not administered by inhalation. At best they appear to be weak bronchodilators via this route and are unpalatable[125-128]. Only the development of more soluble, less irritant preparations will further research in this area.

References

1. RALL, T.W. *The Pharmacological Basis of Therapeutics*. New York: Macmillan (1980)
2. SALTER, H. *Edinburgh Medical Journal*, 1109 (1859)
3. KOSSEL, A. *Berichte der deutschen chemischen Gesellschaft*, **21**, 2164 (1888)
4. FISCHER, E. and ACH, L. *Berichte der deutschen chemischen Gesellschaft*, **28**, 3135 (1895)
5. PARISOT, H., *Thèse de Paris, Steinheit*, 1 (1890)
6. PAL, J. *Deutsche Medizinische Wochenschrift*, **38**, 1774 (1912)
7. JACKSON, D.E. *Journal of Pharmacology and Experimental Therapeutics*, **4**, 291 (1913)
8. MEYER, F. *Archive fuer Anatomie und Physiologie*, **1**, (1915)
9. MACHT, D.I., and TING, G.-C. *Journal of Pharmacology and Experimental Therapeutics*, **18**, 373 (1921)
10. HIRSCH, S. *Klinische Wochenschrift*, **1**, 615 (1922)
11. TUFT, L. and BRODSKY, A.B. *Journal of Allergy*, **7**, 238 (1936)
12. EFRON, B.G. *Journal of Allergy*, **7**, 249 (1936)
13. HAJOS, K. *Weiner Klinische Wochenschrift*, **49**, 737 (1936)
14. FEINBERG, S.M. *Journal of Allergy*, **8**, 280 (1937)
15. HERRMANN, G., AYNESWORTH, M.B. and MARTIN, J. *Journal of Laboratory and Clinical Medicine*, **23**, 135 (1937)
16. GREENE, J.A., PAUL, W.D. and FELLER, A.E. *Journal of the American Medical Association*, **109**, 1712 (1937)
17. RICHARDS, R.K. *Journal of Pharmacology and Experimental Therapeutics*, **72**, 33 (1942)
18. WEINBERGER, M. and BRONSKY, E. *Clinical Pharmacology and Therapeutics*, **17**, 585 (1975)
19. FLEETHAM, J.A., OWEN, J.A., MAY, B., MUNT, P.W. and NAKATSU, K. *Thorax*, **34**, 540 (1979)
20. ZUIDEMA, J. and MERKUS, F.W.H.M. *Current Medical Research and Opinion*, Suppl. **6**, 14 (1979)
21. SVEDMYR, N. *Scandinavian Journal of Respiratory Diseases Suppl.* **101**, 125 (1977)
22. MERRILL, G.A. *Journal of the American Medical Association*, **123**, 1115 (1943)
23. BRESNICK, E., WOODARD, W.K. and SAGEMAN, C.B. *Journal of the American Medical Association*, **136**, 397 (1948)
24. GARDNER, R.A., HANSEN, A.E., EWING, P.L. and EMERSON, G.A. *Texas Medical Journal*, **46**, 516 (1950)
25. ROUNDS, W.J. *Paediatrics*, **14**, 528 (1954)
26. CAMARATA, S.J., WEIL, M.H., HANASHIRO, P.K. and SHUBIN, H. *Circulation*, **44**, 688 (1971)
27. SCHACK, J.A. and WAXLER, S.H. *Journal of Pharmacology and Experimental Therapeutics*, **97**, 283 (1949)
28. SHAH, V.P. and RIEGELMAN, S. *Journal of Pharmaceutical Sciences*, **63**, 1283 (1974)
29. THOMPSON, R.D., NAGASAWA, H.T. and JENNE, J.W. *Journal of Laboratory and Clinical Medicine*, **84**, 584 (1974)
30. COOK, C.E., TWINE, M.E., MYERS, M., AMERSON, E., KEPLER, J.A. and TAYLOR, G.F. *Research Communications in Chemical Pathology and Pharmacology*, **13**, 497 (1976)
31. GUSHAW, J.B., HU, M.W., SINGH, P., MILLER, J.G. and SCHNEIDER, R.S. *Clinical Chemistry*. **21**, 1144 (1977)
32. TRUITT, E.B., McKUSICK, V.A. and KRANTZ, J.C. *Journal of Pharmacology*, **100**, 309 (1950)
33. TURNER-WARWICK, M. *British Medical Journal*, 67 (1957)
34. JACKSON, R.H., McHENRY, J.I., MORELAND, F.B., RAYMER, W.J. and ETTER, R.L. *Diseases of the Chest*, **45**, 78 (1964)

35. JENNE, J.W., WYZE, E., ROOD, F.S. and MacDONALD, F.M. *Clinical Pharmacology and Therapeutics*, **13**, 349 (1972)
36. MITENKO, P.A. and OGILVIE, R.I. *New England Journal of Medicine*, **289**, 600 (1973)
37. NICHOLSON, D.P. and CHICK, T.W. *American Review of Respiratory Disease*, **108**, 241 (1973)
38. PIAFSKY, K.M. and OGILVIE, R.I. *New England Journal of Medicine*, **23**, 1218 (1975)
39. HENDELES, L., BIGHLEY, L., RICHARDSON, R.H., HEPLER, C.D. and CARMICHAEL, J. *Drug Intelligence and Clinical Pharmacy*, **11**, 12 (1977)
40. ZWILLICH, C.H., SUTTON, F.D., NEFF, T.A., COHNS, W.M., MATTHAY, R.A. and WEINBERGER, M. *Annals of Internal Medicine*, **82**, 784 (1975)
41. JACOBS, M.H., SENIOR, R.M. and KESSLER, G. *Journal of the American Medical Association*, **235**, 1983 (1975)
42. OGILVIE, R.I. *Clinical Pharmacokinetics*, **3**, 267 (1978)
43. McELNAY, J.C., SMITH, G.D. and HELLING, D.K. *Drug Intelligence and Clinical Pharmacy*, **16**, 533 (1982)
44. *FDA Drug Bulletin*, **10**, 4 (1980)
45. EDITORIAL, *Lancet*, **i**, 746 (1980)
46. DASTA, J., MIRTALLO, J.M. and ALTMAN, M. *American Journal of Hospital Pharmacy*, **36**, 613 (1979)
47. NOLTE, D. and NEUMANN, M. *British Journal of Clinical Practice*, Suppl. 23 (1983)
48. SEGAL, M.S., LEVINSON, L., BRESNICK, E. and BEAKY, J.P. *Journal of Clinical Investigation*, **28**, 1190 (1949)
49. SUTHERLAND, E.W. and RALL, T.W. *Journal of Biological Chemistry*, **232**, 1077 (1958)
50. SUTHERLAND, E.W., ROBISON, G.A. and BUTCHER, R.W. *Circulation*, **37**, 279 (1968)
51. BUTCHER, R.W. and SUTHERLAND, E.W. *Pharmacologist*, **1**, 63 (1959)
52. BUTCHER, R.W. and SUTHERLAND, E.W. *Journal of Biological Chemistry*, **237**, 1244 (1962)
53. EDITORIAL, *Lancet*, **ii**, 1119 (1970)
54. STRADA, S.J. and THOMPSON, W.J. *Advances in Cyclic Nucleotide Research*, **9**, 265 (1978)
55. BERGSTRAND, H. and LUNDQUIST, B. *Molecular and Cellular Biochemistry*, **21**, 9 (1978)
56. BERGSTRAND, H. *European Journal of Respiratory Disease*, Suppl. 109, 37 (1980)
57. NEWMAN, D.J., COLELLA, D.F., SPAINHOUR, C.B., BRANN, E.G., ZABKO-POTAPOVICH, B. and WARDELL, J.R. *Biochemical Pharmacology*, **27**, 729 (1978)
58. POLSON, J.B., KRZANOWSKI, J.J., FITZPATRICK, D.F. and SZENTIVANYI, A. *Biochemical Pharmacology*, **27**, 254 (1978)
59. FREDHOLM, B.B., BRODIN, K. and STRANDBERG, K. *Acta Pharmacologica et Toxicologica*, **45**, 336 (1979)
60. MANGIONE, A., IMHOFF, T.E., LEE, R.V., SHUM, L.Y. and JUSKO, W.J. *Chest*, **73**, 616 (1978)
61. POLSON, J.B., KRZANOWSKI, J.J., GOLDMAN, A.L. and SZENTIVANYI, A. *Clinical and Experimental Pharmacology and Physiology*, **5**, 535 (1978)
62. LOHMANN, S.M., MIECH, R.P. and BUTCHER, F.R. *Biochimica et Biophysica Acta*, **499**, 238 (1977)
63. PARROTT, F.H., GRABENKORT, W.R., PASCHAL, T.C., BRANSOME, E.D., SPEIR, W.A., VALLNER, J.J. et al. *American Review of Respiratory Disease*, **113**, 156 (1976)
64. TREMBATH, P.W. and SHAW, J. *British Journal of Clinical Pharmacology*, **6**, 499 (1978)
65. CAMPBELL, I.A., MIDDLETON, W.G., McHARDY, G.J.R., SHOTTER, M.V., McKENZIE, R. and KAY, A.B. *Thorax*, **32**, 424 (1977)
66. MACKAY, A.D., BALDWIN, C.J. and TATTERSFIELD, A.E. *American Review of Respiratory Disease*, **127**, 609 (1983)
67. BOKSAY, I. and BOLLMAN, V. *Archives Internationales de Pharmacodynamie et de Thérapie*, **194**, 174 (1971)
68. KALINER, M.A., ORANGE, R.P., KOOPMAN, W.J., AUSTEN, K.F. and LAVAIA, P.J. *Biochimica et Biophysica Acta*, **252**, 160 (1971)
69. RALL, T.W. and WEST, T.C. *Journal of Pharmacology and Experimental Therapeutics*, **139**, 269 (1963)
70. LICHTENSTEIN, L.M. and MARGOLIS, S. *Science*, **161**, 902 (1968)
71. BARCLAY, J., WHITING, B., MEREDITH, P.A. and ADDIS, G.J. *British Journal of Clinical Pharmacology*, **11**, 203 (1981)
72. BILLING, B., DAHLQVIST, R., GARLE, M., HORNBLAD, Y. and RIPE, E. *European Journal of Respiratory Disease*, **63**, 399 (1982)
73. HANDSLIP, P.D.J., DART, A.M. and DAVIES, B.H. *Thorax*, **36**, 741 (1981)

74. WOLFE, J.D., TASHKIN, D.P., CALVARESE, B. and SIMONS, M. *New England Journal of Medicine*, **298**, 363 (1978)
75. MARLIN, G.E., HARTNETT, B.J.S., BEREND, N. and HACKET, N.B. *British Journal of Clinical Pharmacology*, **5**, 45 (1978)
76. WILLIAMS, J.F., LOWITT, S., POLSON, J.B. and SZENTIVANYI, A. *Biochemical Pharmacology*, **27**, 1545 (1978)
77. FREDHOLM, B.B. *Acta Physiologica Scandinavica*, **111**, 507 (1981)
78. MENTZER, R.M., RUBIO, R. and BERNE, R.M. *American Journal of Physiology*, **229**, 1625 (1975)
79. MANN, J.S., RENWICK, A.G. and HOLGATE, S.T. *Clinical Science*, **65**, 22P (1983)
80. WOLFF, J., LONDOS, C. and COOPER, D.M.F. *Advances in Cyclic Nucleotide Research*, **14**, 199 (1981)
81. HOLGATE, S.T., LEWIS, R.A. and AUSTEN, K.F. *Proceedings of the National Academy of Sciences of the United States of America*, **77**, 6800 (1980)
82. CHURCH, M.K., HUGHES, P.J. and HOLGATE, S.T. *Federation Proceedings*, **42**, 1342 (1983)
83. VERHAEGE, R.H., VANHOUTTE, P.M. and SHEPHERD, J.T. *Circulation Research*, **40**, 208 (1977)
84. WAKADE, A.R. and WAKADE, T.D. *Journal of Physiology*, **282**, 35 (1978)
85. SILINSKY, E.M. *British Journal of Pharmacology*, **71**, 191 (1980)
86. BURNSTOCK, G. *British Medical Bulletin*, **35**, 255 (1979)
87. BLEEHEN, T. and KEELE, C.A. *Pain*, **3**, 367 (1977)
88. CUSHLEY, M.J., TATTERSFIELD, A.E. and HOLGATE, S.T. *British Journal of Clinical Pharmacology*, **15**, 161 (1983)
89. CUSHLEY, M.J., TATTERSFIELD, A.E. and HOLGATE, S.T. *Agents and Actions*, **13**, 109 (1983)
90. ALLY, A.I. and NAKATSU, K. *Journal of Pharmacology and Experimental Therapeutics*, **199**, 208 (1976)
91. FREDHOLM, B.B. *European Journal of Respiratory Disease*, **61**, Suppl. 109, 29 (1980)
92. CUSHLEY, M.J., TATTERSFIELD, A.E. and HOLGATE, S.T. *American Review of Respiratory Disease*, **125**, 62 (1983)
93. DALY, J.W., BRUNS, R.F. and SNYDER, S.H. *Life Sciences*, **28**, 2083 (1980)
94. SZENTMIKLOSI, A.J., NEMETH, M., SZEGI, J., PAPP, J. GY., and SZEKERES, L. *Naunyn-Schmiedeberg's Archives of Pharmacology*, **311**, 147 (1980)
95. OSSWALD, H. *Naunyn-Schmiedeberg's Archives of Pharmacology*, **288**, 79 (1975)
96. PERSSON, C.G.A., ERJEFALT, I. and KARLSSON, J.A. *Acta Pharmacologica et Toxicologica*, **49**, 317 (1981)
97. FREDHOLM, B.B. and PERSSON, C.G.A. *European Journal of Pharmacology*, **81**, 673 (1982)
98. POISNER, A.M. *Biochemical Pharmacology*, **22**, 469 (1973)
99. PEACH, M.J. *Proceedings of the National Academy of Sciences of the United States of America*, **69**, 834 (1972)
100. WESTFALL, D.P. and FLEMING, W.W. *Journal of Pharmacology and Experimental Therapeutics*, **159**, 98 (1968)
101. ATUK, N.O., BLAYDES, M.C., WESTERVELT, F.B. and WOOD, J.E. *Circulation*, **35**, 745 (1967)
102. HIGBEE, M.D., KUMAR, M. and GALANT, S.P. *Journal of Allergy and Clinical Immunology*, **70**, 377 (1982)
103. WARREN, J.B., TURNER, C., DALTON, N., THOMPSON, A., COCHRANE, G.M. and CLARK, T.J.H. *British Journal of Clinical Pharmacology*, **16**, 405 (1983)
104. STUBBS, A., CUSHLEY, M.J. and TATTERSFIELD, A.E. *Clinical Science*, **66**, 57P (1984)
105. KOLBECK, R.C., SPEIR, W.A., CARRIER, G.O. and BRANSOME, E.D. *Lung*, **156**, 173 (1979)
106. HORROBIN, D.F., MANKIN, M.S., FRANKS, D.J. and HAMET, P. *Prostaglandins*, **13**, 33 (1977)
107. AUBIER, M. DE TROYER, A., SAMPSON, M. MACKLEM, P.T. and ROUSSOS, C. *New England Journal of Medicine*, **305**, 249 (1981)
108. MATTHYS, H. and KOHLER, D. *European Journal of Respiratory Disease*, **61**, Suppl. 109, 98 (1980)
109. PERSSON, C.G.A., EKMAN, M. and ERJEFALT, I. *Acta Pharmacologica et Toxicologica*, **44**, 216 (1979)
110. KALINER, M. and AUSTEN, K.F. *Cyclic AMP, Cell Growth and the Immune Responses*. New York: Springer-Verlag (1974)
111. MIDDLETON, E. *Journal of Pharmaceutical Sciences*, **69**, 243 (1980)
112. MATTHAY, R.A., BERGER, H.J., DAVIES, R., LOKE, J., GOTTSCHALK, A. and ZARET, B.L. *American Heart Journal*, **104**, 1022 (1982)
113. SANDERS, J.S., BERMAN, T.M., BARTLETT, M.M. and KRONENBERG, R.S. *Chest*, **78**, 279 (1980)

114. RUFFIN, R.E. and NEWHOUSE, M.T. *European Journal of Respiratory Disease*, **62**, 123 (1981)
115. ENDRES, P. *Praxis und Klinik der Pneumologie*, **30**, 751 (1976)
116. COLEMAN, R.A. *British Journal of Pharmacology*, **57**, 51 (1976)
117. SMELLIE, F.W., DAVIS, C.W., DALY, J.W. and WELLS, J.N. *Life Sciences*, **24**, 2475 (1979)
118. KARLSSON, J.-A. and PERSSON, C.G.A. *British Journal of Pharmacology*, **74**, 783P (1981)
119. PERSSON, C.G.A., KARLSSON, J.A. and ERJEFALT, I. *Life Sciences*, **30**, 2181 (1982)
120. PERSSON, C.G.A. *Agents and Actions*, Suppl. 13, 115 (1983)
121. PERSSON, C.G.A. *Trends in Pharmacological Sciences*, **3**, 312 (1982)
122. GARST, J.E., KRAMER, G.L., WU, Y.J. and WELLS, J.N. *Journal of Medicinal Chemistry*, **19**, 499 (1976)
123. KRAMER, G.L., GARST, J.E., MITCHEL, S.S. and WELLS, J.N. *Biochemistry*, **16**, 3316 (1977)
124. DALY, J.W. *Journal of Medicinal Chemistry*, **25**, 197 (1982)
125. STEWART, B.N. and BLOCK, A.J. *Chest*, **69**, 718 (1976)
126. KANDT, D., IVAINSKY, H. and SEHRT, I. *Respiration*, **42**, 278 (1981)
127. GREGER, G. *Zeitschrift fuer Erkrankungen der Atmungsorgane*, **157**, 270 (1981)
128. CUSHLEY, M.J. and HOLGATE, S.T. *Thorax*, **38**, 223 (1983)

Chapter 12

Prostaglandins and related compounds

Jehan Bagli

Introduction

Prostaglandins (PGs) belong to a group of autocoids that have been shown to exercise major influences on pulmonary function.

The presence in lung tissue of enzyme systems for the formation and deactivation of this class of compounds was demonstrated early in their history[1]. The synthesis and release of PGs and related substances have been demonstrated to occur both *in vitro* and *in vivo*[2] as a result of a variety of mechanical, chemical and immunochemical stimuli. The PGs of the E series have, in general, a relaxant effect on bronchial smooth muscle and also lower pulmonary vascular resistance[3]. In contrast, both in intact animals as well as in a variety of isolated lung tissue preparations, $PGF_{2\alpha}$ consistently produces constrictor and/or contractile responses[3]. The contractile and relaxant responses produced by PGs are independent of α- or β-adrenergic receptor activation.

Levels of PGE and PGF in lung parenchyma and in the isolated airways are balanced by the rates of their biosynthesis and their enzymatic degradation[4,5]. This balance in pulmonary tissue may play a role in maintaining the patency of the airways. A disturbance of this equilibrium by allergic or bronchospastic stimuli could, in part, be responsible for the manifestation of asthmatic syndromes.

The effect of natural prostaglandins on isolated human bronchial muscle has been reported[6]. More recently, the bronchodilator properties of PGE in intact animals have been demonstrated by Rosenthale and coworkers[7].

The observation that the inhalation of aerosolized PGE by asthmatic individuals resulted in an increase in the vital capacity and forced expiratory volume[8] highlighted the therapeutic potential of PGs in the treatment of asthmatic conditions.

It soon became apparent, however, that the natural prostaglandins of the E series had several disadvantages: (*a*) a limited shelf-life as a result of their decomposition under atmospheric conditions, (*b*) a short pharmacological half-life due to rapid metabolic deactivation and (*c*) an apparent ability to induce cough and irritation of the upper respiratory tract. These limitations on the use of the endogenous PGs have opened the door for the development of a plethora of syntheses leading to PG analogues with a more acceptable profile of activity.

Chemistry

Chemically, the PGs constitute a class of twenty carbon fatty acids, the parent member of which has come to be recognized as prostanoic acid (1).

The natural PGs of the E series, abbreviated PGE (1a), have a carbonyl function at C-9 and an α-hydroxyl group at C-11. In contrast, those of the PGF (1b) series possess an α-hydroxyl function both at C-9 and C-11. The compounds of the PG_1 series have a *trans*-double bond at C-13, whereas those of the PG_2 series have an additional *cis*-double bond at C-5. All natural prostaglandins have an α-hydroxyl at C-15. For a detailed discussion of

Scheme 1

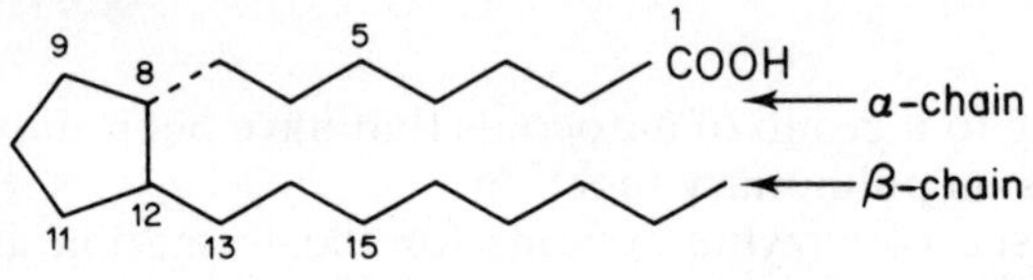

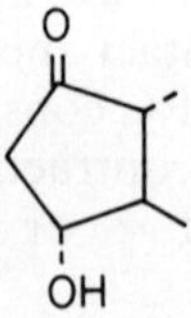

PGE (1a) 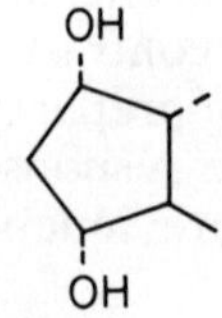   PGF (1b) 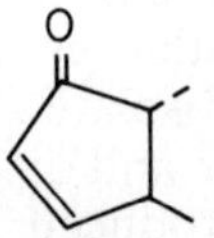   PGA (1c)

the nomenclature, readers are urged to refer to the original article by Nelson[9]. There are two alkyl chains present in these molecules: the one attached to C-8 has α orientation and the other attached to C-12 has β orientation. For convenience, the former will be referred to as the α-chain and the latter as the β-chain (*Scheme 1*).

The syntheses of prostaglandins have been adequately reviewed[10-13] in recent years. For the purposes of this chapter, only the highlights of the reactions employed in the syntheses of PG congeners having significant bronchodilator activities will be discussed.

The most useful strategy for PG synthesis may be divided into two principal pathways as follows: (*a*) construction of a cyclopentane ring with an α-chain followed by the elaboration of the β-chain and (*b*) generation of a synthon with both α- and β-chain residues incorporated into it with stereochemical control. In the case of approach (*a*), the β-chain was elaborated in the earlier synthesis[14] by using a single carbon conjugate addition followed by additional reactions to introduce the remaining fragment.

With the recent advances in the field of organometallic chemistry, conjugate addition of the entire β-chain with proper control of the hydroxyl function at C-15 has been extensively utilized. Approach (*b*) was the result of an imaginative synthetic strategy developed at Harvard[15]. All the stereochemical centres on the cyclopentane ring are correctly predisposed, and suitable ring cleavage at the right time unravels the latent functionalities. In this approach, the control of the stereochemistry at C-15 was achieved by the use of suitable protecting groups and specially designed[16] reducing agents.

11-Deoxy-11-substitued prostaglandins

It was evident from the earlier studies[17] that the absence of a hydroxyl function at C-11 in the prostaglandin molecule yields compounds with a significant degree of biological activity. In addition, this structural change also imparts a greater stability to the molecule. The slightly reduced potency of the derived products is a disadvantage in some cases. One of the key intermediates in the synthesis of 11-deoxy-prostaglandins is 5-oxo-1-cyclopentene-1-heptanoic acid ester (2). The synthesis (*Scheme 2*) of this compound was first reported[18] by the Ayerst group. Subsequently, several other syntheses of (2) have been published[10]. Irradiation of enone (2) with

Scheme 2

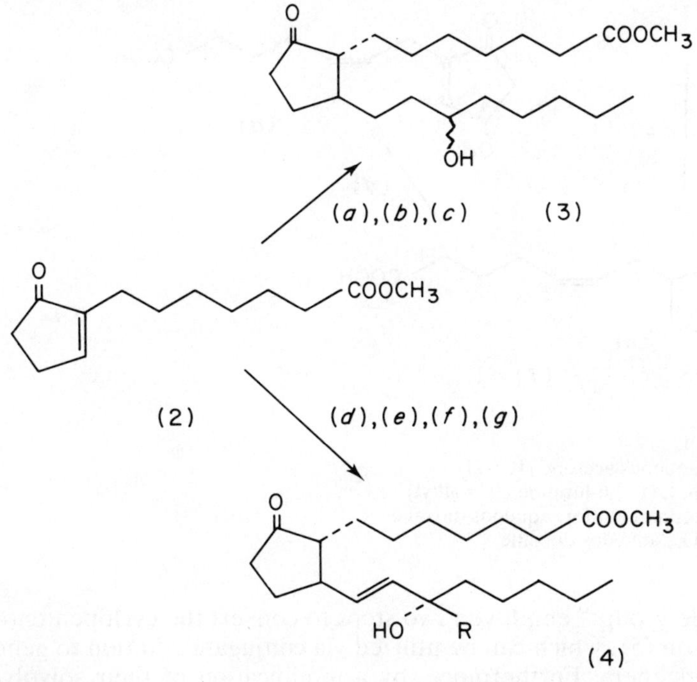

(*a*),(*b*),(*c*)   (3)

(2)

(*d*),(*e*),(*f*),(*g*)

(4)

(*a*) *hv*
(*b*) Zn/AcOH
(*c*) NaBH$_4$

(*d*) CH$_3$NO$_2$
(*e*) H$^+$ (Nef reaction)
(*f*) Wittig reaction
(*g*) NaBH$_4$ or CH$_3$MgBr

1-chloro-3-oxo-oct-1-ene led to a bicyclo[3.2.0]heptane derivative. This was cleaved with zinc-acetic acid to yield 9,15-diketoprostanoic acid ester, which was transformed to a mixture of C-15 alcohols (3) by suitable manipulation. In contrast, treatment of cyclopentenone (2) with nitromethane[19], followed by exposure to the conditions of the Nef reaction, yielded the corresponding aldehyde. A similar approach was also reported by Syntex[19b] and May and Baker[19c] scientists. A Wittig reaction, followed by suitable manipulation at the C-15 oxygen, led to 11-deoxy-PGE$_1$ derivatives (4).

Scheme 3

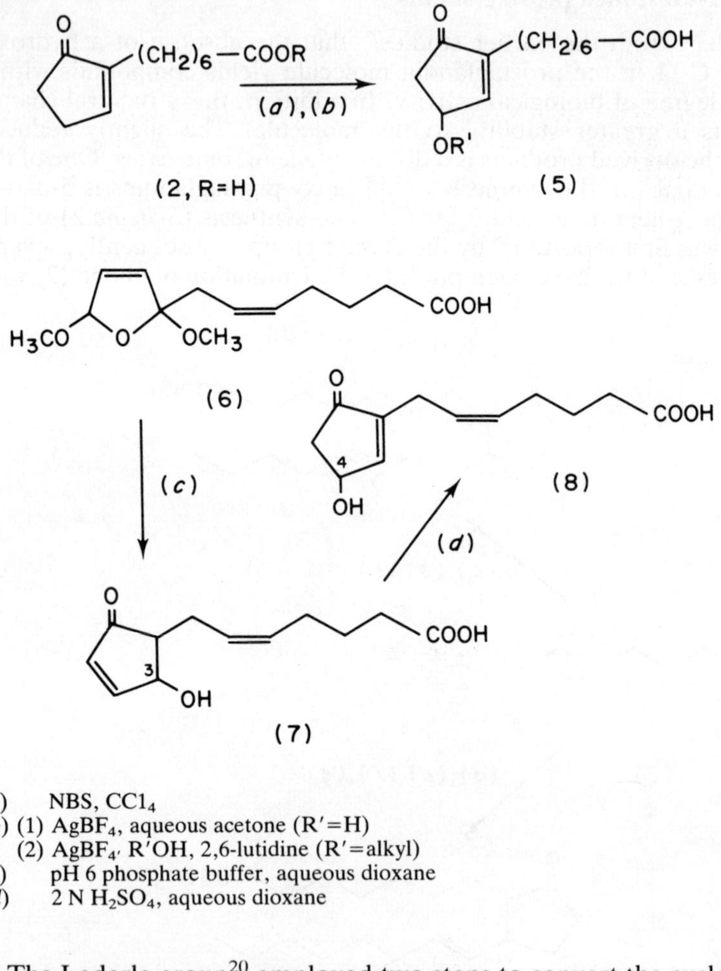

O
‖
(CH$_2$)$_6$—COOR
——(a),(b)——→

(2, R=H)

O
‖
(CH$_2$)$_6$—COOH

OR'

(5)

H$_3$CO   O   OCH$_3$ COOH

(6)

| (c)

O
‖
         COOH

3
OH

(7)

O
‖
         COOH

4
OH

(8)

(d)

(a)   NBS, CCl$_4$
(b)   (1) AgBF$_4$, aqueous acetone (R'=H)
       (2) AgBF$_4$, R'OH, 2,6-lutidine (R'=alkyl)
(c)   pH 6 phosphate buffer, aqueous dioxane
(d)   2 N H$_2$SO$_4$, aqueous dioxane

The Lederle group[20] employed two steps to convert the cyclopentenone (2) to a synthon (5), which can be utilized via conjugate addition to generate PGE$_1$ congeners. Furthermore, by a modification of their solvolytic procedure, they were able to introduce a variety of alkoxy functions which ultimately yielded 11-deoxy-11-α-alkoxy-prostaglandin congeners (*Scheme 3*).

As the allylic bromination procedure was not applicable for the corresponding PG_2 precursor, a novel route to 4-hydroxycyclopentenone (8) was devised. A crucial step in this process involved the quantitative rearrangement of 3-hydroxycyclopentenone to the more stable 4-hydroxy isomer. Thus, a suitable furan derivative (6) was rearranged in phosphate buffer to the 3-hydroxy derivative (7), which was transformed with acid catalysis to the desired synthon (8) in excellent yield. The interconversion of 3- and 4-hydroxy isomers with suitable manipulation allows the synthesis of precursors for a variety of 11-substituted PGE_2 derivatives. Thus, treatment of

Scheme 4

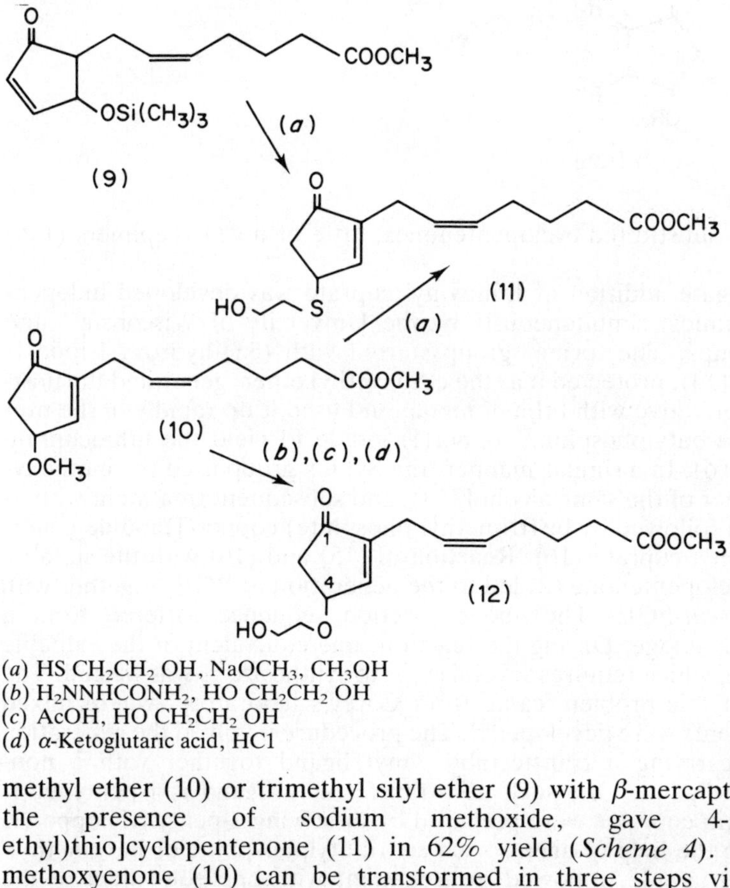

(a) HS CH_2CH_2 OH, NaOCH$_3$, CH$_3$OH
(b) H$_2$NNHCONH$_2$, HO CH_2CH_2 OH
(c) AcOH, HO CH_2CH_2 OH
(d) α-Ketoglutaric acid, HCl

methyl ether (10) or trimethyl silyl ether (9) with β-mercaptoethanol, in the presence of sodium methoxide, gave 4-[(2-hydroxy-ethyl)thio]cyclopentenone (11) in 62% yield (*Scheme 4*). In contrast, methoxyenone (10) can be transformed in three steps via the semicarbazone to 4-(2-hydroxyethoxy)cyclopentenone (12) in an overall yield of 37%. When suitably protected, these alcohols generate substrates for conjugate addition reactions.

Conjugate addition of a 'vinyl ate' complex to the β-position of the conjugated cyclopentenone precursor described above represents an efficient way to generate, in a stereospecific manner, α- and β-chains of prostaglandins. A key feature of this addition reaction is that it proceeds from the less hindered side. This produces a cyclopentanone (13a) (*Scheme 5*) with the two chains disposed in a *trans* relationship to each other. Furthermore, in

Scheme 5

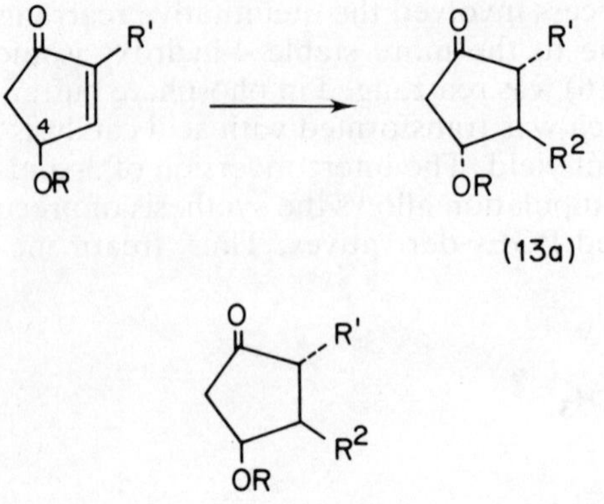

(13a)

(13b)

the case of 4-substituted cyclopentenones, little or no 11-β-epimers (13b) are formed.

The conjugate addition of lithiovinyl cuprate was developed independently and almost simultaneously by the University of Wisconsin[21] and Syntex[22] groups. The former group started with (3S)-hydroxy-1-iodo-1-*trans*-octene (14), protected it as the ethoxyethyl ether, generated the unstable lithio derivative with lithium metal, and used it up rapidly in the presence of tri-*n*-butylphosphine copper(I) iodide to yield the lithiocuprate (15) (*Scheme 6*). In a similar manner, the Syntex group used the methoxy-isopropyl ether of the same alcohol (14), and subsequent treatment with *n*-butyl lithium followed by bis(trimethyl phosphite) copper(I) iodide generated the divinyl cuprate (16). Reaction of (15) and (16) with the suitably protected cyclopentenone (2) led to the generation of PGE$_1$ together with some 15-*epi-ent*-PGE. The above reaction sequence suffered from a serious disadvantage. During the reaction, one equivalent of the valuable vinyl alcohol, which requires several steps to synthesize[22], was wasted. The resolution of this problem came from Corey's laboratory, where mixed cuprate reagents were developed[23]. The procedure involved the generation of cuprate carrying a transferrable vinyl ligand together with a non-transferrable ligand. One such non-transferrable ligand is 1-pentyne. 1-Pentynyl lithio cuprates were prepared by dissolving 1-pentynyl copper(I) in ether with the help of agents such as tributylphosphine or hexamethylphosphorus triamide, followed by treatment with one equivalent of the vinyl lithium reagent generated from the protected iodo-alcohol (14). The above sequence led to the preparation of 1-pentynyl lithio cuprate (18). In a similar manner, the reaction of a suitable vinyl lithium with copper(I) thiophenoxide[24] yielded the corresponding vinyl cuprate (17), where thiophenoxide served as the non-transferrable ligand.

Nucleophilic vinylation via readily available vinyl stannanes was first demonstrated by Corey and his colleagues[25]. This procedure has been utilized by other workers to prepare precursors for the introduction of the β-chain. Starting with 3-triethylsilyloxy-1-octyne (19) and reacting[26] it with

Scheme 6

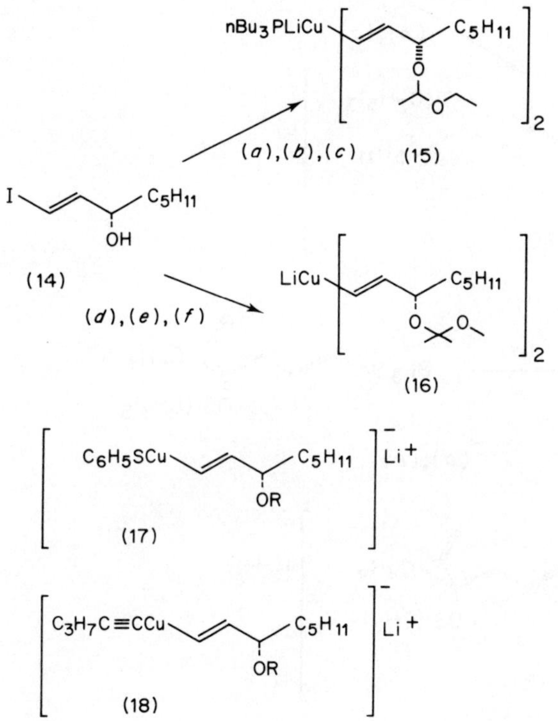

nBu$_3$PLiCu — [CH=CH—CH(C$_5$H$_{11}$)] $_2$ (with OC(=O)O ethyl ester)

(a),(b),(c)   (15)

I—CH=CH—CH(OH)—C$_5$H$_{11}$

(14)

(d),(e),(f)

LiCu — [CH=CH—CH(C$_5$H$_{11}$)] $_2$ (with acetonide O–C(CH$_3$)$_2$–O)

(16)

[C$_6$H$_5$SCu—CH=CH—CH(OR)—C$_5$H$_{11}$] $^-$ Li$^+$

(17)

[C$_3$H$_7$C≡CCu—CH=CH—CH(OR)—C$_5$H$_{11}$] $^-$ Li$^+$

(18)

(a) CH$_2$=CH-O-CH$_2$CH$_3$, HCl
(b) Li, ether
(c) nBu$_3$PCuI, ether

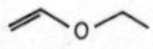

(d) (CH$_3$)$_2$C(OCH$_3$)O
(e) nBuLi, hexane
(f) ((CH$_3$O)$_3$P)$_2$CuI

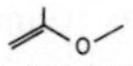

tributylstannane in the presence of azo-bisisobutyronitrile gave the hydrostannation product in excellent yield. This adduct was lithiated with butyl lithium and then treated with pentynyl copper to yield the mixed lithiocuprate (20) (*Scheme 7*). Starting with the octyne (21), a similar sequence of reactions was utilized to synthesize the β-chain precursor (22) for 15-deoxy-16-alkyl-16-hydroxy derivatives[26b]. It must be noted that, in the case of the ethynyl alcohol of type (21), the hydrostannation reaction yields a small amount of *cis*-vinyl stannane together with *trans*-olefin as a major product. The reaction in the case of alcohol (19), however, proceeds essentially stereospecifically to yield the *trans*-octene. Similar reactions were also employed by the Searle group[26c] to prepare C-17 unsaturated PG analogues.

Scheme 7

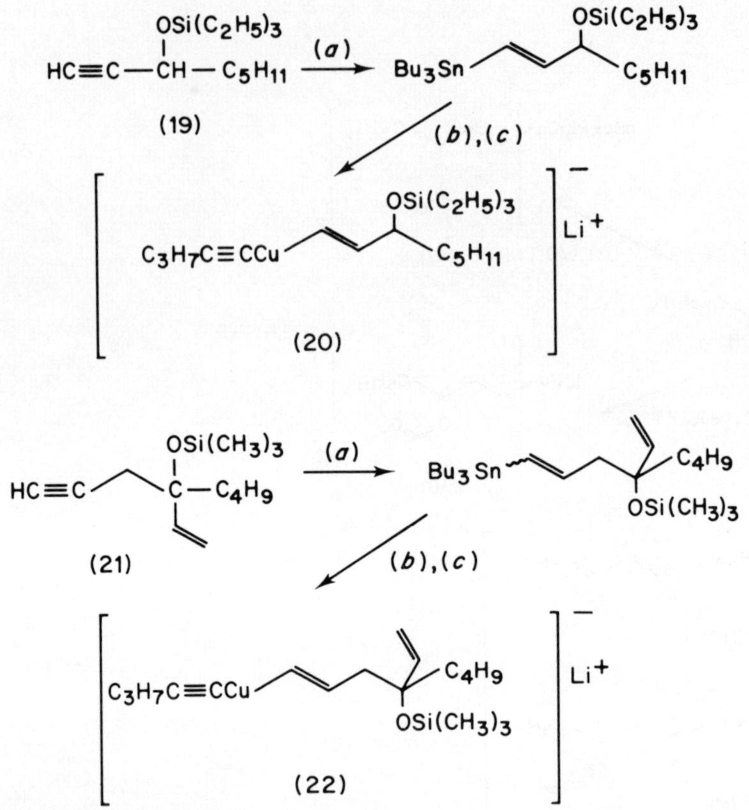

(a) Bu$_3$SnH, azo-bisisobutyronitrile
(b) BuLi
(c) C$_3$H$_7$C≡CCu, hexamethylphosphorus triamide

The use of alanates for the conjugate addition was successfully explored by the Lederle group[27]. The terminal alkyne of the type (23), which is readily available from the condensation of ethynyl Grignard with the corresponding carbonyl compound, was used in the development of two processes (*Scheme 8*) for the synthesis of alanates. Initially, *cis*-hydroalumination of (23) with diisobutyl aluminium hydride provided the *trans*-vinylalane (24). It is of critical importance to have a bulky protecting group on the hydroxyl function in order to minimize the formation of *cis*-vinylalane. Subsequent treatment with methyl lithium furnished the desired trialkyl vinyl alanate (25). The yields in the above process were low due to extensive side reactions (C-O bond cleavage). In an alternative process, the terminal acetylene (23) was transformed to the 1-iodo-*trans*-1-alkene (26) using a previously described procedure[22]. This intermediate was then exposed to alkyl lithium, and the resulting vinyl lithio reagent was treated with trimethyl aluminium to provide lithio alkenyl alanate (27) for the conjugate addition. These alanates undergo regiospecific 1,4-addition reactions with an appropriate cyclopentenone, without generating any 1,2-addition products at the carbonyl carbon of a methyl ester or cyclopentenone.

Scheme 8

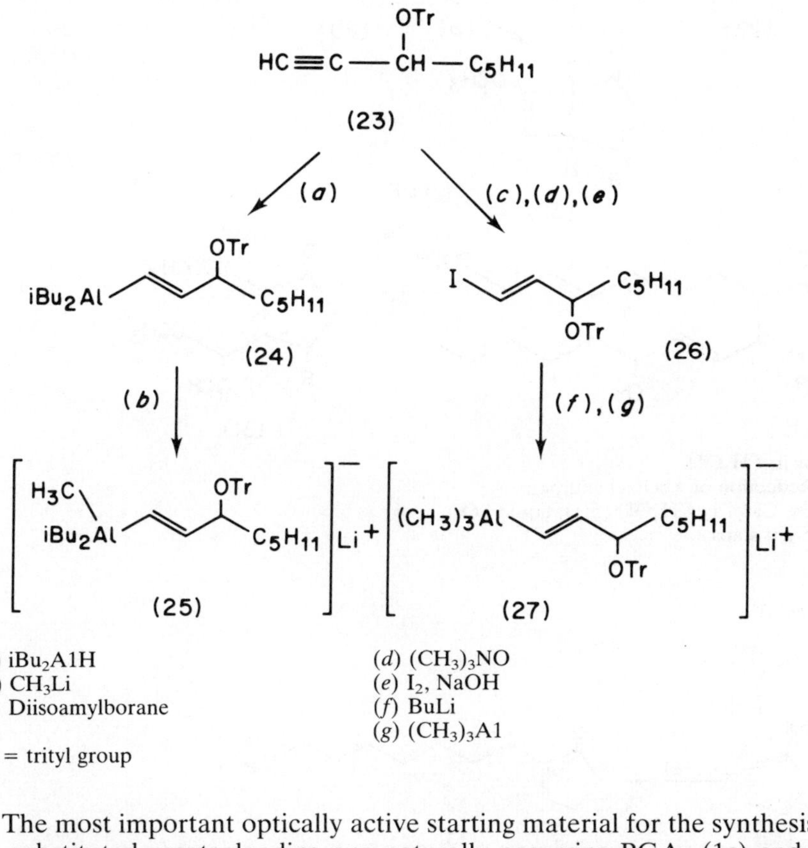

(a) iBu_2AlH
(b) CH_3Li
(c) Diisoamylborane

(d) $(CH_3)_3NO$
(e) I_2, NaOH
(f) BuLi
(g) $(CH_3)_3Al$

Tr = trityl group

The most important optically active starting material for the synthesis of 11-substituted prostaglandins was naturally occurring PGA_2 (1c) and 15-*epi*-PGA_2. The 15-*epi*-PGA_2 was isolated from *Plexaura homomalla* (esper) gathered from Florida waters[28]. In contrast, the species collected from Caribbean waters[29] was found to possess as high as 2% of the dry weight of PGA_2. Two groups, Lederle[30] and Wyeth[31], were involved in extensive exploration of Michael-type additions of a wide variety of nucleophiles. This furnished a large number of 11-deoxy-11-substituted PG derivatives. These included 11-alkyl, 11-alkenyl, 11-aryl, 11-thioalkyl and several kinds of functionalized alkyl derivatives.

A recent detailed report describes the use of α-tropolone methyl ether as a starting material which also leads to the synthesis of 11-deoxy and 11-substituted PG derivatives[32]. The first step involves the irradiation of α-tropolone methyl ether (28) (*Scheme 9*) which furnishes the rearranged 7-methoxy-bicyclo[3.2.0]hepta-3,6-dien-2-one (29). The double bond at C-3 can be selectively hydrogenated to yield the mono-olefin (30, R = H).

Scheme 9

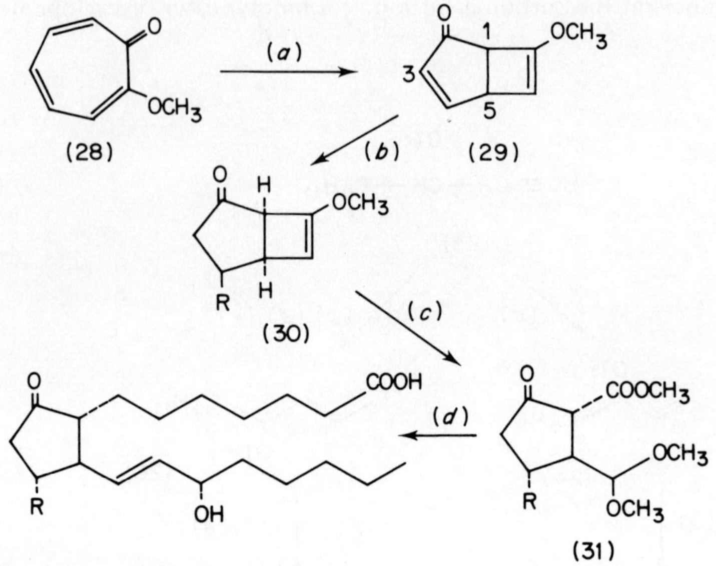

(a) $h\nu$ in CH_3OH
(b) Reduction or Michael addition
(c) O_3, CH_2Cl_2:CH_3OH (5:1), liquid SO_2
(d) Eight steps

Scheme 10

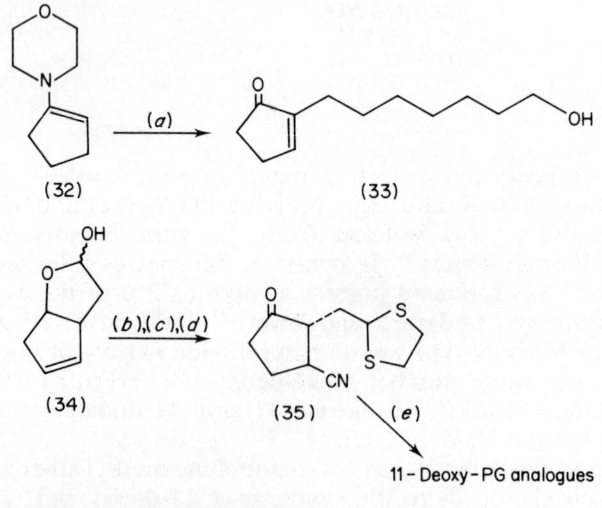

11 – Deoxy – PG analogues

(a) $OHC-(CH_2)_5CH_2OH$
(b) 1,2-Ethanedithiol, BF_3-etherate
(c) Dicyclohexylcarbodiimide, dimethylsulphoxide
(d) Acetone cyanohydrin
(e) Nine steps

Ozonolysis, followed by treatment with sulphur dioxide yielded the β-keto ester (31) in about 50% overall yield from α-tropolone methyl ether. The C-2 position in (31) is suitably activated for an alkylation with an appropriate nucleophile to generate the α-chain directly. Interestingly, the carbomethoxy function is decarboxylated with sodium cyanide–hexamethylphosphoric triamide, with the retention of the acetal function. Alternatively, (29) can be alkylated in a Michael fashion using a variety of alkyl or aryl cuprates to furnish C-11 substituted PG derivatives. 20-Ethyi-11-deoxy-PGE$_1$ [M&D 26693 (113)] was synthesized[19c] in a manner very similar to that described earlier by the Ayerst group, the key difference being the mode of generation of the cyclopentenone (33), which was obtained by a condensation of cyclopentanone morpholino enamine (32) with 7-hydroxyheptanal (*Scheme 10*). Another 11-deoxy-prostaglandin analogue that was tested clinically came from the Hoechst group[33]. The compound HR-102 (106) was synthesized in a manner involving a shift at the C-5 double bond of PGE$_2$ to the C-4 position. Their synthetic strategy is briefly outlined in *Scheme 10* [(34)→(35)].

Modified natural prostaglandins

A large number of modifications of the C-1 carboxylic acid functions have been reported. One such effort provided the derivative CP-27,987 (105), which was submitted for clinical evaluation. The Pfizer group[34] utilized the optically active hemiacetal (36) and, following the well-known Corey proc-

Scheme 11

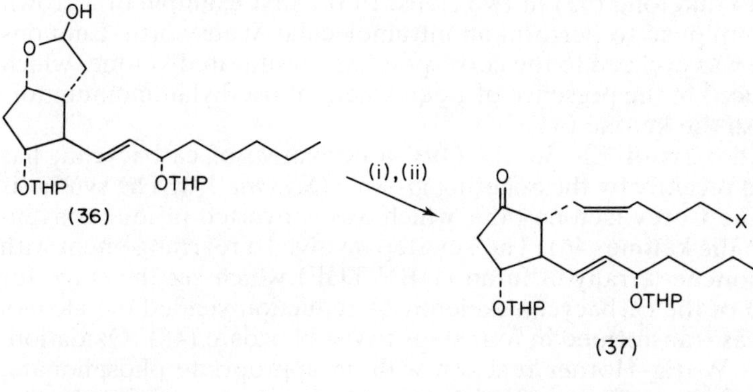

(i) (Ph)$_3$P$^+$(CH$_2$)$_3$ X Br
(ii) Oxidation
THP = tetrahydropyran

(a) X = CH$_2$CN$_4$H
(b) X = CH$_2$CONHSO$_2$CH$_3$
(c) X = CH$_2$CONHSO$_2$C$_6$H$_5$
(d) X = CH$_2$CONHCOCH$_3$
(e) X = CH$_2$CONHCOC$_6$H$_5$
(f) X = CH$_2$CONH$_2$

edure, generated a series of $PGF_{2\alpha}$ analogues by condensing (36) with the requisite ylide derived from the appropriate phosphonium salt. It was noted that ylides with a strongly acidic δ function (for example see (a), (b), (c) in Scheme 11) participated readily in a Wittig reaction. In contrast, those with weaker acidic functions (for example see (d) and (e) in Scheme 11) underwent a significant degree of intramolecular acylation. As expected, no Wittig product was isolable from ylide (f), which underwent intramolecular condensation exclusively. Each $PGF_{2\alpha}$ derivative was transformed to the corresponding PGE_2 (37) in the conventional manner. 16,16-Dimethyl derivatives were similarly synthesized. Using similar synthetic sequences, C-20 isopropylidene PGE_2 CS-412 (112) and PGE_1 derivatives[35] were also produced.

Prostacyclin congeners

The discovery of prostacyclin[36] generated a new surge of interest in prostanoid chemistry. The desirable biological profile and the molecular lability[37] of prostacyclin stimulated the search for analogues with biological activity coupled with enhanced stability. Recently, prostacyclin has been extensively tested for its potential as a bronchodilator (see pp. 255–257). Some highlights of the synthesis of prostacyclin analogues are discussed below.

Soon after the structure of prostacyclin (38) was confirmed by synthesis[38], the first synthesis of a carba analogue appeared[39]. cis-Bicyclo[3.3.0]octane-3,7-dione (39), the starting compound, was transformed into the aldehyde (40) in seven steps. This synthon has built into it the C-13 and C-6 carbonyl functions needed to complete the synthesis via Wittig-type reactions. After suitable deprotection of the hydroxyl group, this synthesis furnished the carbocyclic analogue (41) (Scheme 12). More recently, a unique modification[40] of the Wadsworth–Emmons reaction was used to generate an intermediate (44) which can furnish compound (41). Optically active lactone (42), which by then was readily accessible, was transformed to diketone (43) in two steps. In the first example of a crown ether being employed to perform an intramolecular Wadsworth–Emmons reaction, (43) was cyclized to the corresponding unsaturated ketone, which was then reduced in the presence of 1 equivalent of triethylammonium formate to furnish the ketone (44).

A novel synthesis of ZK 36 374 (49), a derivative of carbacyclin, has been reported recently by the Schering group[41] (Scheme 13). The synthesis started with the Corey lactone (45), which was converted in four conventional steps to the ketone (46). The key step involved a rearrangement with diazabicyclononene-tetrahydrofuran (DBN-THF) which set the stage for the formation of the carbacyclin skeleton. A reduction yielded the alcohol (47), which was transformed in four steps to the benzoate (48). Oxidation, followed by a Wittig–Horner reaction with an appropriate phosphonate, generated the β-chain. The synthesis was finished using conventional steps, the final one being a Wittig reaction which generated ZK 36 374 (49) and its isomer. The configuration of the C-5 double bond was tentatively assigned based on the biological profile of the isomer.

A group of congeners which had various heteroatoms interposed in place of the enol ether function was reported by the Hoechst group[42] (Scheme

Scheme 12

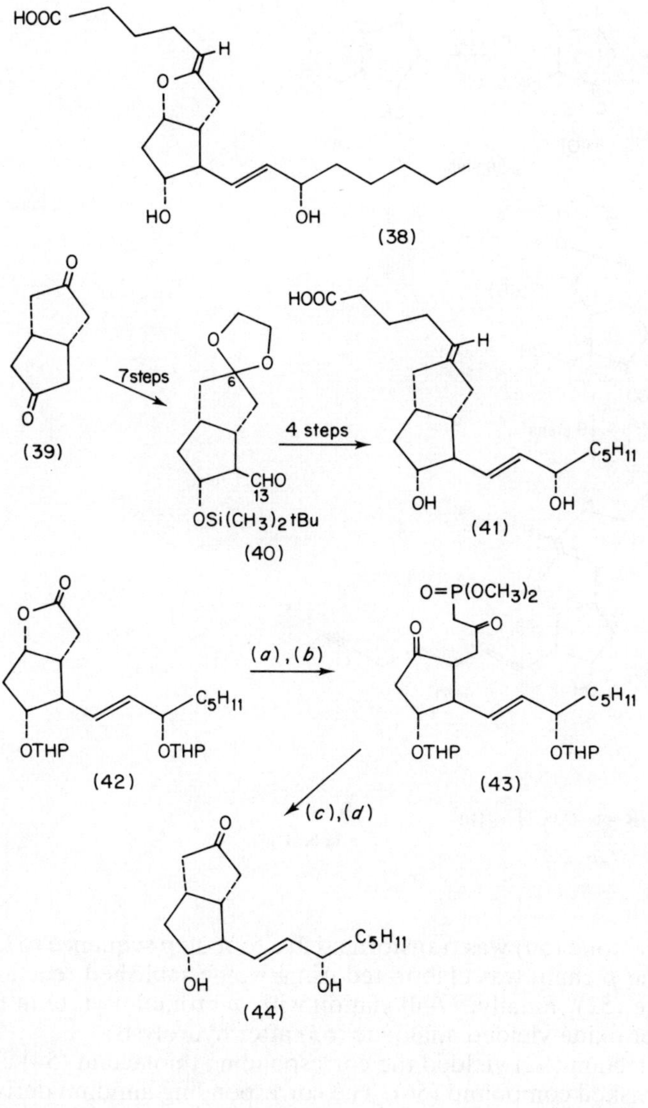
HOOC
H
O
HO
OH
(38)
O
O
(39)
7steps
O
O
6
CHO
13
OSi(CH3)2tBu
(40)
4 steps
HOOC
H
C5H11
OH
OH
(41)
O
O
C5H11
OTHP
OTHP
(42)
(a), (b)
O=P(OCH3)2
O
O
C5H11
OTHP
OTHP
(43)
(c),(d)
O
C5H11
OH
OH
(44)

(*a*) $LiCH_2\text{-}\overset{\displaystyle O}{\overset{\|}{P}}\text{-}(OCH_3)_2$, tetrahydrofuran
(*b*) CrO_3-Py, CH_2C1_2
(*c*) K_2CO_3, 18-Crown-6, toluene
(*d*) $Et_3NH^+HCO_2^-$, 5% Pd/C, toluene
THP = tetrahydropyran

Scheme 13

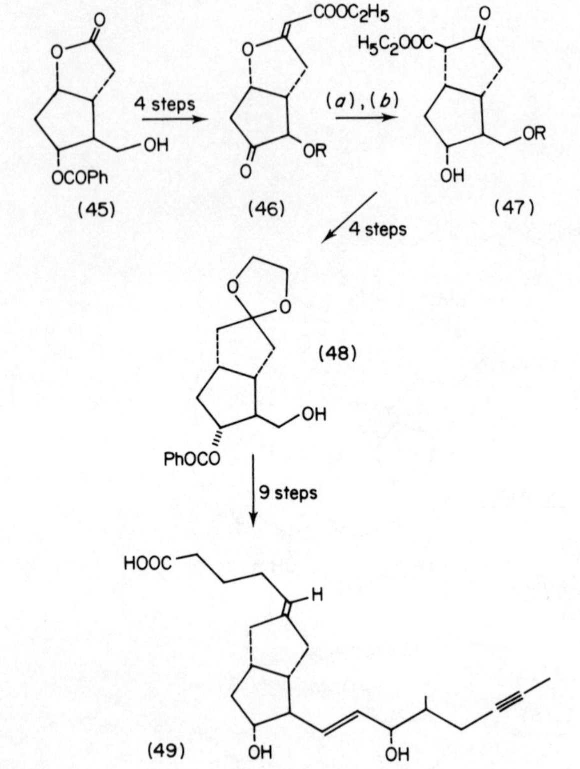

$$R = -Si(CH_3)_2tBu$$

(*a*) DBN-THF   (*b*) NaBH$_4$

14). The Corey lactone (50) was transformed in a four-step sequence to lactam (51), and the β-chain was elaborated using well-established reactions to yield diacetate (52). Finally, O-alkylation with ω-bromobutyrate in the presence of silver oxide yielded analogue (53) after hydrolysis.

Thiolation of lactam (52) yielded the corresponding thiolactam (54) and S-alkylation furnished compound (56). The corresponding amidino derivative (57) was obtained via the imino-S-methyl derivative (55), which was furnished by the alkylation of the thiolactam with methyl iodide–dimethoxyethane.

In an effort to improve the stability of prostacyclin, the five-membered furan ring was expanded to a pyran ring. This was achieved by the Schering

Scheme 14

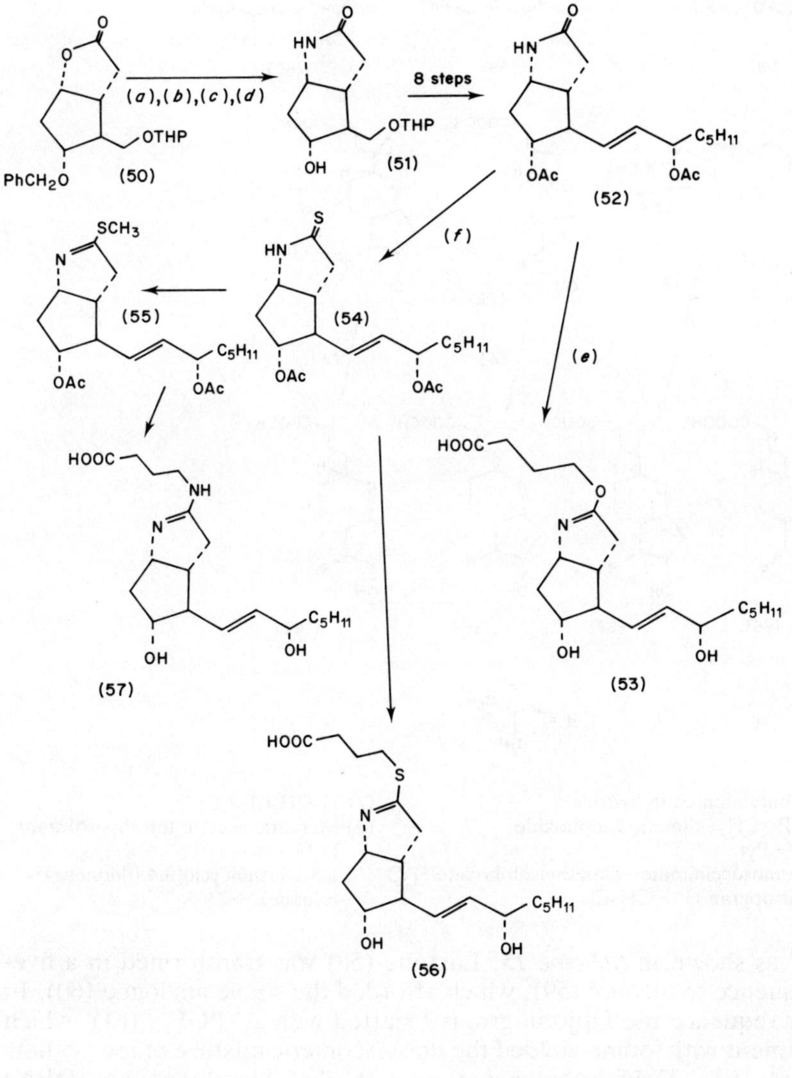

(a) Aminolysis−NH₃
(b) Jones' oxidation
(c) PhSH, chlorotrimethylsilane−Pyr−CH₂Cl₂

(d) Raney Ni-*t*BuOH
(e) ω-Bromobutyrate, AgO−xylene
(f) P₄S₁₀−Pyr/Pyridine

Scheme 15

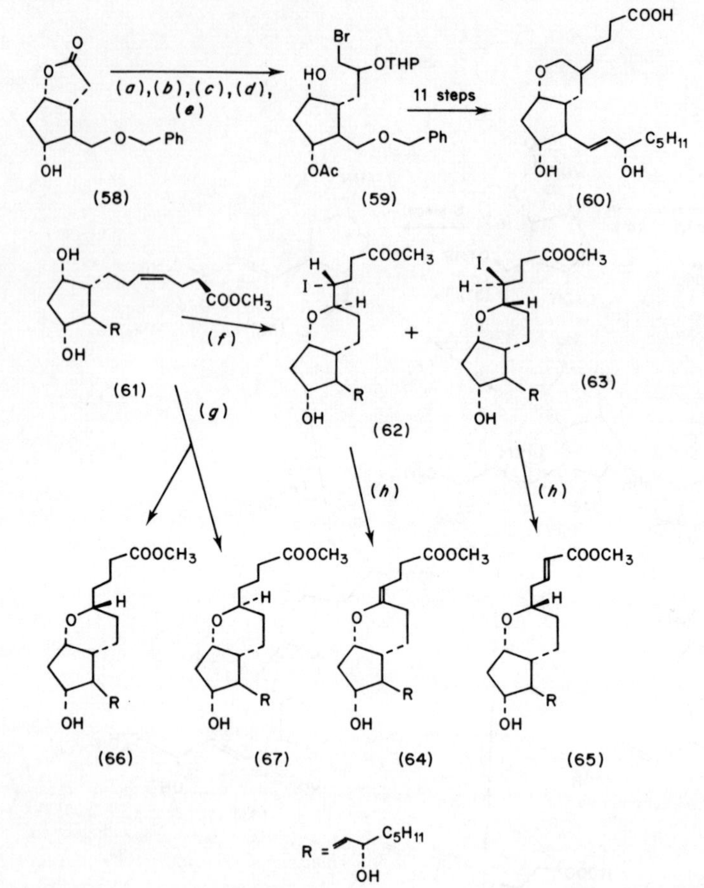

(a) Diisobutylaluminum hydride
(b) $(Ph)_3P=CH_2$-dimethylsulphoxide
(c) Ac_2O-Pyr
(d) N-Bromosuccinimide-dimethylsulphoxide/H_2O
(e) Dihydropyran/H^+-CH_2Cl_2

(f) I_2-CH_2Cl_2
(g) Mercuric acetate-tetrahydrofuran/H_2O
(h) 1,5-Diazabicyclo[3.4.0]nonene-5-toluene

group[43] as shown in *Scheme 15*. Lactone (58) was transformed in a five-step sequence to alcohol (59), which afforded the stable analogue (60). In another sequence the Upjohn group[44] started with Δ^4-$PGF_{1\alpha}$ (61), which on treatment with iodine yielded the diastereomeric mixture of iodo-ethers (62) and (63). Dehydrohalogenation with diazabicyclononene (DBN) yielded (4Z)-9-deoxy-5,9α-epoxy-Δ^4-PGF_1 methyl ester (64) from (62) and the unsaturated ester (65) from (63). Corresponding saturated analogues (66) and (67) were obtained by sequential treatment of (61) with mercuric acetate and sodium borohydride.

In another approach directed towards stabilizing the prostacyclin structure, Japanese workers[45] incorporated electron-withdrawing functions in the vicinity of the enol ether function. Their efforts led to the synthesis of analogues (68)–(71) (*Scheme 16*). An elegant synthesis of 10,10-difluoro-13-dehydroprostacyclin (72) was recently reported[46]. The metabolic deactivation of prostacyclin occurs through dehydrogenation at C-15 and reduction[47] of the double bond at C-13. In order to prevent this enzymatic process from taking place, Novak and coworkers[48] replaced the double bond with heteroatoms such as sulphur and oxygen. This led to the synthesis of compounds (75) and (76) (*Scheme 16*).

Epoxyalcohol (73) was converted to 13-oxa-13,14-dihydro-PGF$_{2\alpha}$ (74, X = O) using an excess of the sodium salt of (2S)-hydroxy-1-heptanol. Compound (74) was transformed via iodo etherification and subsequent dehydrohalogenation with DBN to yield 13-oxaprostacyclin (75). The synthesis of the 13-thia derivative (76) proceeded in an analogous manner.

Most of the prostacyclin analogues described above were available in limited quantities. In most cases, bioassays were used only to measure the ability of these analogues to inhibit platelet aggregation or to lower blood pressure. To date, no data are available regarding the action of these compounds on the pulmonary system *in vitro* or *in vivo*.

Scheme 16

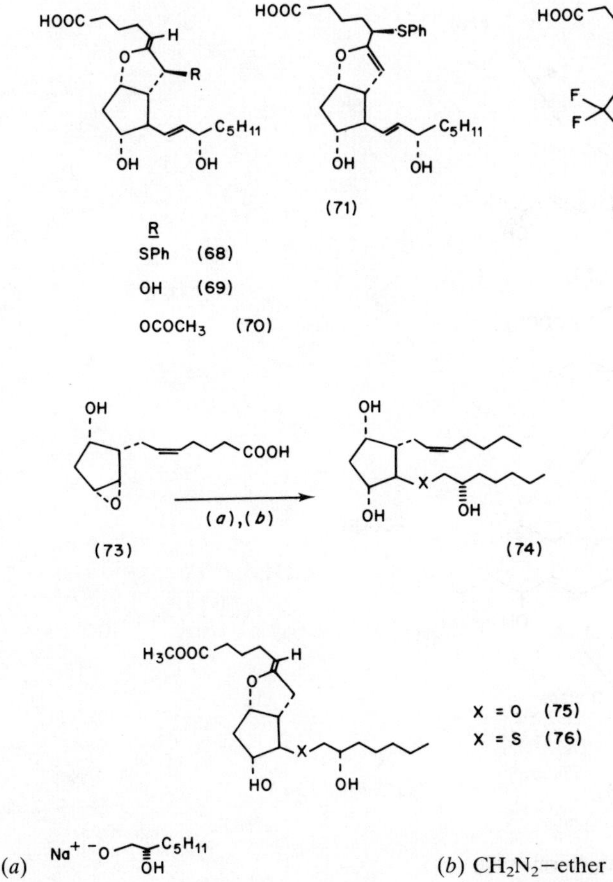

Novel synthesis of PGE₁

One of the most difficult challenges for the organic chemist is to devise methods that simulate natural biogenetic pathways. Recently, workers at Hokkaido University[49] developed a method of synthesis of PGE$_1$ which mimics the biogenetic pentannulation and provides four of the five asymmetric centres in a stereocontrolled manner. In an experiment to test this strategy, the triene (77) was cyclized to the cyclopentanol (78) as shown in *Scheme 17*. The two isomers at C-15 (PG numbering) could be separated and the bromomercury group was replaced by a hydroxy function using oxygen–sodium borohydride to give (79). The stereochemistry at the asymmetric centres at C-8, C-9, and C-12 was proven by degradative experiments and it was shown that, with the exception of C-11, the stereochemistry was as desired.

Scheme 17

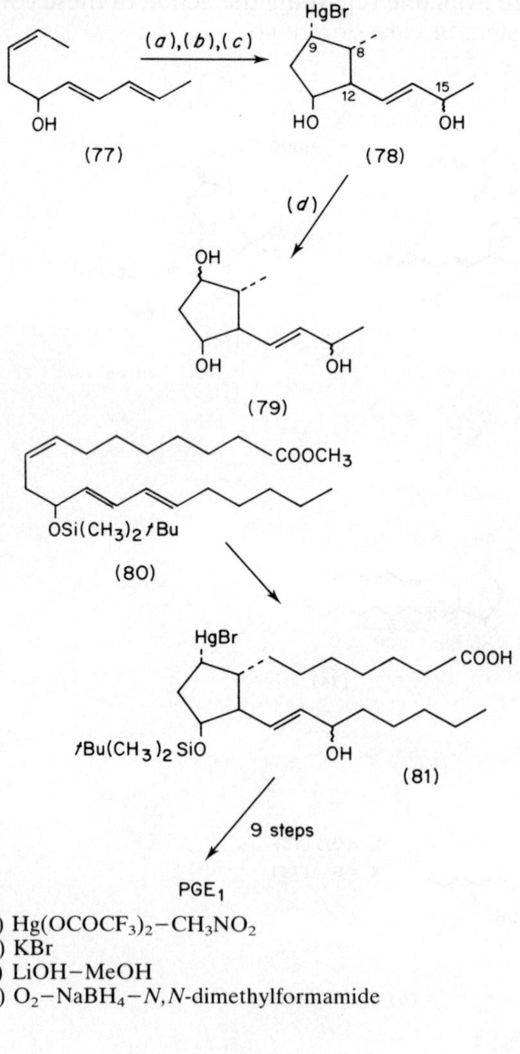

(a) Hg(OCOCF₃)₂–CH₃NO₂
(b) KBr
(c) LiOH–MeOH
(d) O₂–NaBH₄–N,N-dimethylformamide

The trienoic acid methyl ester (80) was similarly transformed to the corresponding bromomercury derivative (81) in 48% yield. Nine steps were required to transform (81) to PGE_1, which was found to be identical to the natural product in all respects.

Biology

The potent contractile or relaxant effects exerted by prostaglandins on bronchial smooth muscles vary depending on their structures. Due to the rapid metabolic deactivation of natural prostaglandins on passage through the pulmonary circulation, a variety of modified congeners has been synthesized and tested for their bronchodilator activity in animals and humans.

Screening methods

The technique most commonly used to screen PG analogues for bronchodilator activity was introduced by Konzett and Rossler[50]. In this procedure, anaesthetized guinea-pigs are artificially ventilated and bronchoconstriction is induced by the intravenous (i.v.) injection of either acetylcholine, histamine, or 5-hydroxytryptamine. The test drug is injected intravenously or given by aerosol and is assessed for its ability to inhibit or reverse the induced bronchoconstriction. This assay, with modifications, is used by most workers in the field.

Bronchodilator activity is also assessed in two canine models. In one method[51], anaesthetized, pilocarpine-bronchoconstricted dogs are monitored for drug-related effects on airways resistance and on cardiovascular parameters. The drug is generally administered as an aerosol. This model is viable for a number of hours, thus allowing the duration of action of the compound to be evaluated. In the second model[52], male collie dogs are rendered bronchitic by inhaling a mixture of air and sulphur dioxide. The procedure can be carried out in conscious animals, and the test drug is administered as an aerosol.

In yet another model[53], anaesthetized cats are artificially ventilated and bronchoconstriction is induced with an i.v. infusion of 5-hydroxytryptamine. The ability of the test compound to reverse the induced bronchoconstriction and decrease the airways resistance is taken as an indication of bronchodilator activity.

A major drawback of the pharmacological methods described above is that none of them can adequately measure the possible irritation and cough-inducing properties of the test compounds. The identification of a PG analogue for clinical study is therefore critically impeded by this deficiency. Several attempts have been made to overcome this limitation. The May and Baker group[19c] have used metered doses of the drug administered as an aerosol to study the susceptibility of young beagles to PGE_2-induced coughing. An average of 4 out of 25 animals responded in a reproducible manner. M&B 26693 (113) was chosen for clinical studies[54] on the basis of these experiments but was found to be irritant in humans. Similar efforts using cats[55] and monkeys[56] have also been reported. However, the reproducibility of the results obtained from such experiments and their applicability to clinical situations have yet to be determined.

PGE$_1$ has been found[57] to have bronchodilator activity in healthy as well as in asthmatic subjects. In contrast, PGE$_2$ has been shown to be a bronchoconstrictor in some patients and a bronchodilator in others. Strandberg[58] has shown that PGE$_1$ consistently caused relaxation of isolated human bronchi, whereas in some experiments PGE$_2$ induced relaxation which was followed by contraction. These results have been subsequently confirmed[59] in other *in vitro* studies using human tracheal, bronchial, and bronchiolar strips. Thus, contradictory evidence was obtained: PGE$_2$ was found to act as a bronchodilator in animal models but did not consistently relax human bronchial muscles *in vitro*. These observations suggest that clinical efficacy may be more accurately predicted with the results obtained from the *in vitro* studies using human bronchial tissue.

The route of administration of the prostaglandins to animals affects their relative potencies, for example the effects of structurally modified prostaglandins on the bronchial system were recently reported by workers from Wyeth Laboratories[60]. They found that when they administered PGE$_1$ and PGE$_2$ as aerosols, the compounds were equipotent in reversing acetylcholine-induced bronchoconstriction in anaesthetized guinea-pigs.

In contrast, Lederle workers[61] found a significant difference between the bronchodilator activities of the two compounds (*Table 12.1*). An important difference between the two methodologies was that the Wyeth group administered the PGs as aerosols, whereas the Lederle group injected them intravenously. It is well documented that the natural prostaglandins are several times more potent when administered by the aerosol route than when given i.v. This is believed to be due to the enzymatic deactivation which occurs in the pulmonary circulation.

Structure–activity relationships

Substitution at C-11

It has been shown that the removal of the 11α-hydroxyl group generally lowers the bronchodilator potency of PGs in animals (*Table 12.1*). Wyeth workers found that 11-deoxy-PGE$_1$ and PGE$_1$ were equipotent with respect to bronchodilator activity. In contrast, results obtained by Greenberg[62] indicated that DL-11-deoxy-PGE$_1$ administered as an aerosol was 0.59 times as potent as PGE$_2$ in preventing histamine-induced bronchoconstriction in guinea-pigs. However, the Wyeth workers did not state whether their test compounds were racemic or optically pure. 11-Deoxy-PGE$_2$ and the fully saturated 11-deoxy-PGE$_0$ were found to be much less potent in similar studies (*Table 12.1*).

Substitution of the 11α-hydroxyl group by other functionalities has given, in some instances, compounds that have displayed moderate bronchodilator activity in animals. Some of the results obtained by Lederle workers[61] are shown in *Table 12.2*. It is clear from the data (*Table 12.2*) that the α-stereochemistry is crucial for the retention of biological activity. The replacement of the terminal hydroxyl group of the hydroxyethylthio group of (86) by a sulphydryl as in (90), or the exchange of a sulphur for an oxygen atom as in (89), led to significant reduction in or total loss of biological activity. The L-11-deoxy-11α-(2-hydroxyethylthio)-PGE$_2$ (DHET-PGE$_2$) methyl ester (86) was selected as a candidate for further study. This

TABLE 12.1. Bronchodilator activity of some 11-deoxy-PG derivatives relative to PGE₁*

Compound	Acetylcholine†	5-Hydroxytryptamine†	Histamine‡
L-PGE$_1$ (C-5 saturated)	1	1	1
L-PGE$_2$	1	0.18	0.52
11-Deoxy-PGE$_1$	1	0.44	0.13
11-Deoxy-PGE$_2$	0.001	0.084	0.065
11-Deoxy-PGE$_0$ (no double bond)	0.001	0.15	1.35

* Measured in the anaesthetized guinea-pig by the method of Konzett–Rossler.
† PGs administered as an aerosol[60].
‡ PGs administered i.v.[61].

TABLE 12.2. Bronchodilator activity of some 11-substituted PGE analogues*

R	Relative potency against	
	5-Hydroxytryptamine	Histamine
(82) α-OH (PGE$_2$)	1	1
(83) α-H	0.19	0.16
(84) α-CH$_3$	0.004	0.017
(85) α/β-CN	0.27	0.16
(86) L-α-S-CH$_2$CH$_2$OH (methyl ester)	0.16	0.18
(87) L-β-S-CH$_2$-CH$_2$-OH (methyl ester)	0.016	0.018
(88) DL-α-S-CH$_2$CH$_2$OH (methyl ester)	0.053	0.054
(89) DL-α-O-CH$_2$-CH$_2$-OH (methyl ester)	0.008	0.005
(90) α/β-S-CH$_2$-CH$_2$SH (methyl ester)	Inactive	
(91) α/β-S-CH$_2$-CH$_2$OH (no C-5 double bond)	0.18	0.18

* Measured by the Konsett–Rossler procedure using guinea-pigs, and the test compounds were administered i.v.

DHET - PGE$_2$ (86)

compound inhibited the bronchoconstriction induced by 5-hydroxytryptamine, histamine and acetylcholine in anaesthetized guinea-pigs; furthermore, it displayed bronchodilator activity against pilocarpine-induced bronchoconstriction in anaesthetized dogs and against chronic bronchoconstriction induced in conscious dogs by inhalation of a mixture of air and sulphur dioxide[63]. When aerosol doses 1000 times greater than that needed for effective bronchodilatation were tested, (86) did not cause any cardiovascular, respiratory, or gastrointestinal side-effects. The results of *in vitro* studies using isolated canine bronchial strips demonstrated that (86) could relax carbachol-induced contractions of the tissue (*Table 12.3*).

TABLE 12.3. Effect of DHET-PGE$_2$ and other bronchodilators on isolated dog bronchi*

Compound†	Decrease in tension (%)‡
DHET-PGE$_2$ (86)	38.8 ± 13.7 (10)
L-PGE$_1$	91.3 ± 7.3 (10)
L-PGE$_2$	93.4 ± 8.4 (10)
Salbutamol	60.0 ± 7.5 (10)
Isoprenaline	93.5 ± 5.5 (10)

* Bronchial strips were contracted with carabachol 10^{-6}M.
† Compounds were tested at 10^{-4}M concentration.
† Means ± s.e.m. (number of bronchi tested).

After the administration of compound (86) to 21 patients with reversible obstructive bronchospastic disease, bronchodilatation was observed in only 5 patients, all of whom had received the high dose. On the other hand, both the low and high doses caused bronchoconstriction in 12 patients. It was later shown that DHET-PGE$_2$ (86) caused further contraction of the isolated carbachol-contracted human bronchus (*Table 12.4*). The latter finding reinforces the claim[59] that the results of *in vitro* studies using human bronchial tissue may more reliably indicate the selection of a candidate for *in vivo* human studies.

TABLE 12.4. Effect of DHET-PGE$_2$ and other bronchodilators on isolated human bronchi*

Compound†	Increase or decrease in tension (%)‡
DHET-PGE$_2$ (86)	+ 20 (5)
PGE$_2$	+ 31 (15)
Salbutamol	− 38 (5)
Isoprenaline	− 125 (10)

* Bronchial strips or rings were contracted with carbachol 10^{-6}M.
† Compounds were tested at 10^{-4}M concentration.
‡ Number in brackets indicates the number of preparations tested.

The Wyeth[31,60] and the Lederle[61] workers demonstrated that the analogues in which the 11α-hydroxy function had been replaced by a group with small steric requirement, e.g. methyl or thiol, retained a small degree of bronchodilator activity. 11α-Methyl or 11α-mercapto derivatives were shown to be one-tenth as potent as PGE$_2$.

In another series of C-11 substituted analogues, Syntex workers synthesized[64] a variety of 11-deoxy-11α, 12α-methano-PGs. The results of the studies on bronchodilatation in animals led to the conclusion that (*a*) the compounds of the 9-keto series were more potent than the corresponding 9-hydroxy derivatives, (*b*) the analogues with α-orientation of the difluoromethylene group were consistently superior in their activity to those with β-stereochemistry and (*c*) the introduction of a C-15 methyl group made little difference in the biological profiles of these analogues.

Some of the results obtained from the animal studies are listed in *Table 12.5*. It is of interest to note that the saturation of the C-13 double bond, as in (93), has little influence on the biological activity. On the other hand, if the C-5 double bond is saturated and the 13,14-unsaturation is retained (E_1 series), the activity drops to one-tenth of that of compound (92). Moreover, when compounds (92) and (94) were administered as aerosols to guinea-pigs, they were found to be much less potent (one-seventeenth and one-fourth, respectively) than when given i.v. In asthmatic patients, however, neither (92) nor (94) showed any bronchodilator activity.

TABLE 12.5. Bronchodilator activity of some 11-deoxy-11α, 12α-methano-PG analogues*

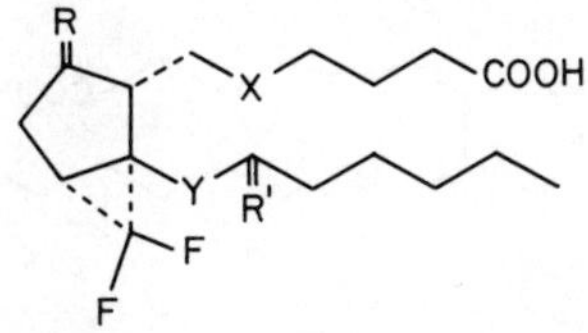

Compound	X	Y	R	R'	Relative potency
PGE$_2$					1
(92)	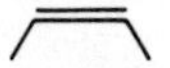	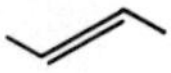	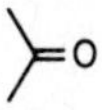 =O	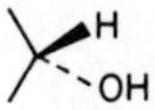 H, OH	5
(93)	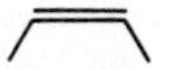	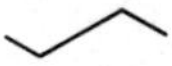	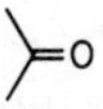 =O	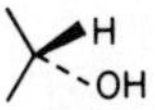 H, OH	~6
(94)	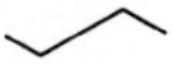	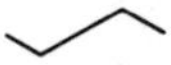	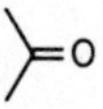 =O	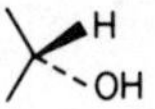 H, OH	4
(95)		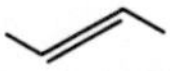	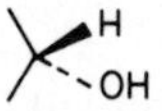 H, OH	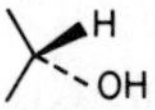 H, OH	0.05
(96)†	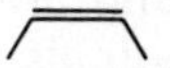	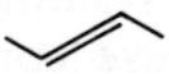	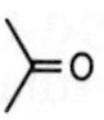 =O	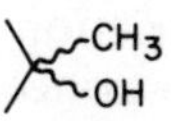 CH$_3$, OH	1–2
(97)	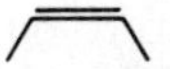	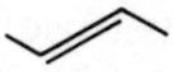	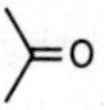 =O	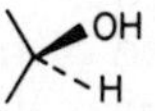 OH, H	1

* Konzett–Rossler assay in the anaesthetized guinea-pig—effect of intravenously administered drug on histamine-induced bronchoconstriction.
† Tested as methyl ester.

Substitution at C-9

In some analogues of the 11-deoxy series, modification of the C-9 ketone function to oxime, hydrazones or ketal results in the retention of a significant degree of bronchodilator activity.

Scheme 18

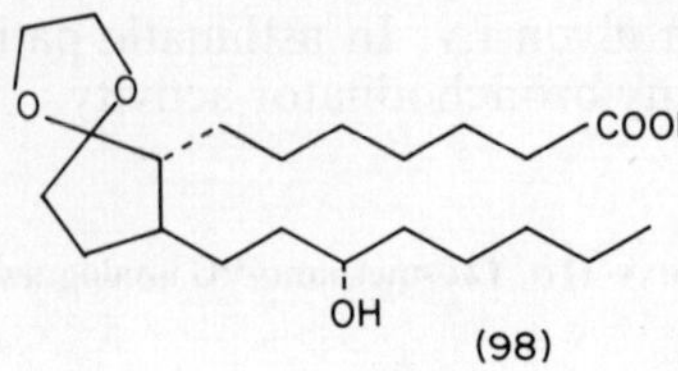

(98)

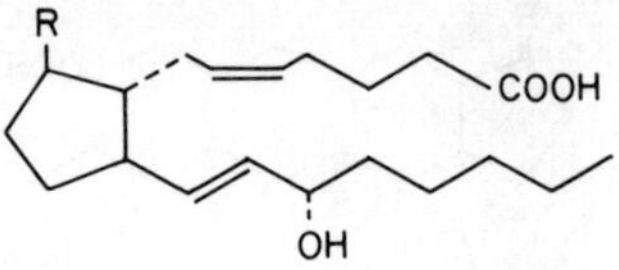

R

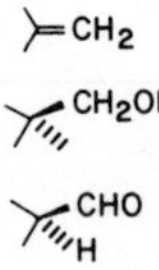

(99)

(100)

(101)

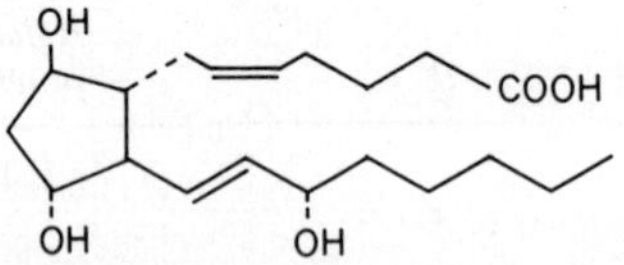

(102)

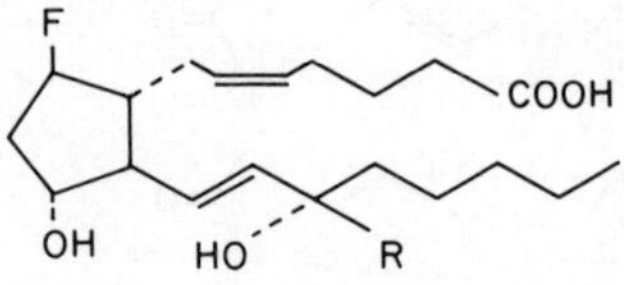

R

H (103)

CH_3 (104)

In the Konzett–Rossler assay in the guinea-pig[61], the ketal analogue (98) was 0.8 and 0.36 times as potent as the corresponding ketone in reversing the bronchoconstriction induced by histamine and 5-hydroxytryptamine, respectively. It is conceivable that these compounds may serve as pro-drugs, generating the parent ketone in the body. In contrast, none of the three carba analogues (99,100,101) displayed any activity[61].

A C-9 substituted compound that was observed to have potent bronchodilator properties was the C-9 epimer (102) of $PGF_{2\alpha}$. The animal studies on this compound have been reported earlier[65]. $PGF_{2\beta}$ (102) was capable of reversing the bronchoconstriction induced by either acetylcholine or $PGF_{2\alpha}$ in guinea-pigs and cats. The compound exerted no perceptible effect when administered as an aerosol (up to 200 mg) to healthy volunteers[66]. However, when given to asthmatics with higher bronchial reactivity, $PGF_{2\beta}$ produced immediate bronchoconstriction. Other effects, including cough, were also noted.

Syntex workers[64] reported that a variety of C-9 halogenated PG analogues had potent bronchodilator activity. The most interesting derivatives were the 9β-fluoro analogues (103) and (104). Both these compounds were four times as potent as PGE_2 when given i.v. to guinea-pigs with histamine-induced bronchoconstriction. The potencies of these compounds were much reduced when they were administered as aerosols. Replacement of the fluorine atom by chlorine caused the activity to drop to one-eighth of its previous level. This suggests that there is a limit to the steric bulk allowed at the site of action. Compound (103) was selected for clinical studies based on the results obtained in animals, but it was found to cause irritation of the upper respiratory tract when given as an aerosol to normal volunteers. This result precluded further studies.

Changes in the α-chain

During the metabolism of PGs, the α-chain is degraded mainly via the β-oxidation of the carboxylic acid group. Efforts to prevent this metabolic deactivation have involved changing the nature of this terminal acid group. The carboxylic acid group has been replaced by sulphonic acid, phosphonate, amines, carbinol, and amides. Many of the terminal carbinols have been demonstrated[67] to retain significant bronchodilator activity; however, no clinical data is available for these compounds at the present time. Similarly, there is no evidence which indicates whether these alcohols are active *per se* or must be metabolized to the acid to produce their effect.

In an effort to generate pro-drug equivalents of the carboxylic acid function, the Pfizer group synthesized[34] various imides. Compound CP-27,987 (105), a member of this series, was found to be a potent bronchodilator in animals and was subsequently tested in human volunteers. When 12 asthmatics received (105), as an aerosol at doses ranging from 6 to 140 μg, the drug had an onset of action of less than 5 minutes and caused a mean increase of about 15% in the forced expiratory volume for 90 minutes post-treatment[68]. At higher doses (105 μg), significant decreases in the systolic blood pressure were observed. Throat irritation and dry mouth were reported with the placebo as well as with the drug. It was concluded that CP-27,987 may prove useful in treating certain asthmatic patients.

It is of interest to note that a metabolic study[69] using tritiated carboximide showed that (105) was readily biotransformed to PGE_2. When given intratracheally to rats, no unchanged drug could be detected in the serum. In contrast, serum levels of PGE_2 were significantly increased. Also, the major metabolite detected was 15-keto-13,14-dihydro-PGE_2. It was also demonstrated in an *in vitro* study with plasma that CP-27,987 was readily hydrolysed to PGE_2[69]. The enzymatic hydrolysis of PG esters is well documented; however, hydrolysis of PGs with amide functions has not yet been reported. A point worthy of note is that, whereas PGE_2 has proved unsuitable as an anti-asthmatic agent in human subjects, (105), a pro-drug that generates PGE_2, appears to be more promising. Further studies will be needed before the therapeutic value of this compound is established.

A variety of alkyl[70] and/or alkoxy substituents has been incorporated in the α-chain of PGs. Most of these compounds showed little or no bronchodilator activity. The Hoechst group[70], however, has synthesized C-5 and C-6 methyl derivatives which display a marked level of bronchodilator activity. At present, there is no evidence which suggests that the activity of these analogues is associated with the reduced rate of β-oxidation of the α-chain.

Another modification reported[70] by the Hoechst chemists is embodied in the structure of HR 102 (106) which is a mixture of stereoisomers at C-15. Although the C-15-*nat* isomer was much more potent as a bronchodilator than the C-15-*epi* isomer, the mixture (1:1) was found to be more potent against histamine-induced bronchospasm in guinea-pigs than either of the two isomers separately. This activity was superior to that of PGE$_2$. In human trials, however, the compound was found to be ineffective and induced cough in some of the asthmatics.

Scheme 19

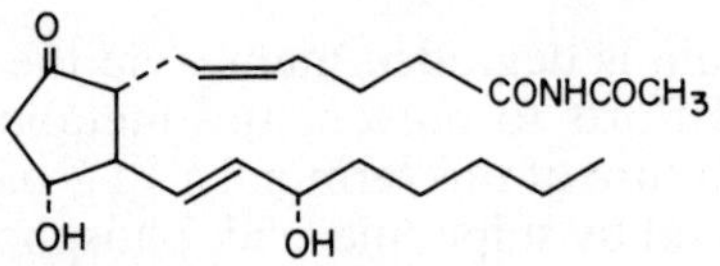

CP–27,987 (105)

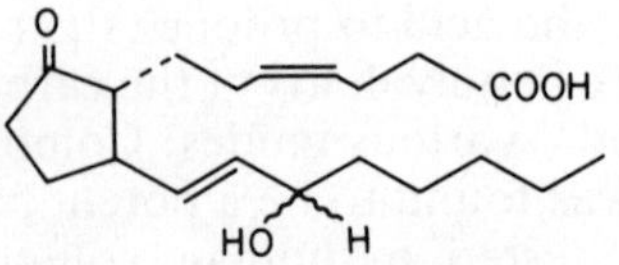

HR–102 (106)

From the results obtained with PGE$_1$ and PGE$_2$, it is clear that saturation of the C-5 double bond improves the bronchodilator potency. The Konzett–Rossler assay was used to determine the biological potencies of compounds in the 11-deoxy series. It was demonstrated[71] that Doxaprost (107) was a potent bronchodilator, whereas the corresponding C-5 unsaturated derivative (108) was a bronchoconstrictor.

Changes in the β-chain

The β-chain of the prostaglandin molecule is known to be enzymatically metabolized in three different ways: (a) ω-oxidation at C-20, (b) dehydrogenation at C-15 and (c) reduction of the C-13 double bond.

In an effort to block ω-oxidation at C-20, various terminal cycloalkyl derivatives were synthesized[61]. The 16-cyclopentyl-17,20-tetranor analogues appeared to have significant bronchodilator activity. In the Konzett–Rossler assay, the DL-11-deoxy derivative (110) was 3.78 times as

Scheme 20

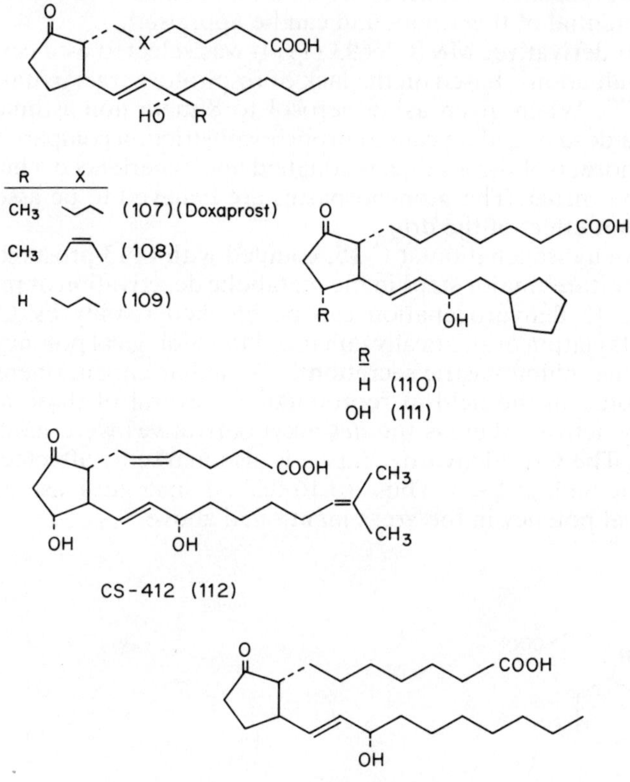

R	X	
CH₃	∿	(107)(Doxaprost)
CH₃	⌇	(108)
H	∿	(109)

R
H   (110)
OH   (111)

CS-412 (112)

M & B   26693 (113)

potent as PGE_2 in inhibiting histamine-induced bronchoconstriction. On the other hand, the PGE_1 analogue (111) given i.v. was 1.95 times more potent than PGE_2 in preventing 5-hydroxytryptamine-induced broncho-constriction in guinea-pigs. These compounds were also active against pilo-carpine-induced bronchoconstriction in dogs. However, the compounds had a short duration of action which precluded further studies.

In another series of compounds, a double bond was introduced at C-20 to block the ω-oxidation. This led to the identification of CS-412 (112) as a potential bronchodilator in humans. The compound was 5.4 times more potent than PGE_2 in preventing histamine-induced bronchoconstriction in guinea-pigs[72]. In anaesthetized cats it inhibited the bronchoconstriction induced by 5-hydroxytryptamine. When cats received an i.v. dose of CS-412, it was 1.9 times as potent as PGE_2, but when the compound was given as an aerosol, it was 0.85 times as potent as PGE_2[73].

C-20-Isopropylidene PGE_2 (112) was tested in 18 patients with bronchial asthma. A significant increase in specific airways conductance (SGaw) was observed 5, 15 and 30 minutes after the inhalation of a dose of 50 μg. A dose-dependent rise in SGaw was noted with increasing doses (maximum of 200 μg) of (112). There was no evidence of irritation of the upper respiratory tract or any vascular side-effects during these studies. These encouraging findings must be confirmed by additional clinical data before the therapeutic potential of this compound can be appraised.

A C-20 bishomo derivative, M&B 26693 (113), was selected as a candidate for clinical evaluation[54] based on the lack of respiratory tract irritation in animal studies[19c]. When given as an aerosol to 8 male non-asthmatic subjects, (113) at a dose of 250 μg caused bronchoconstriction compared to placebo. Furthermore, 6 of the 8 subjects coughed and experienced a burning sensation in the throat. The bronchospasms are believed to be associated with the irritant effect of the drug.

The enzymatic dehydrogenation at C-15, coupled with C-13 prostaglandin reductase, constitutes major steps in the metabolic deactivation of prostaglandins. The C-15 dehydrogenation can be blocked readily by C-15 alkylation. Such alkylation dramatically enhanced the biological potency of PG analogues which inhibit gastric secretion[74]. A similar enhancement in potency is also noted in the field of reproduction. Several of these analogues were orally active, whereas the des-alkyl derivatives were ineffective by this route. The C-15 dehydrogenation is also markedly affected by the increased steric bulk at C-16. Thus, 16,16-dialkyl analogues also have enhanced biological potency in the areas mentioned above.

Scheme 21

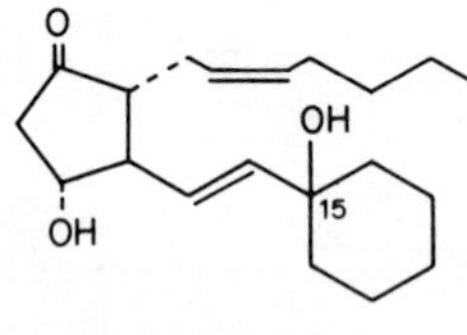

(114)

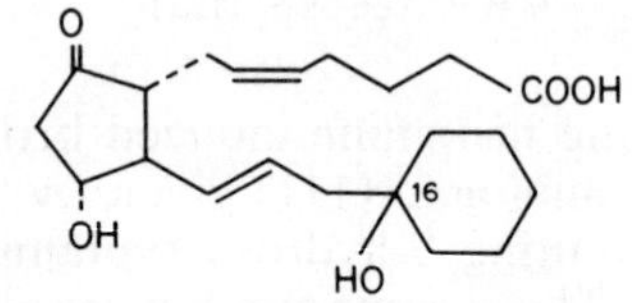

(115)

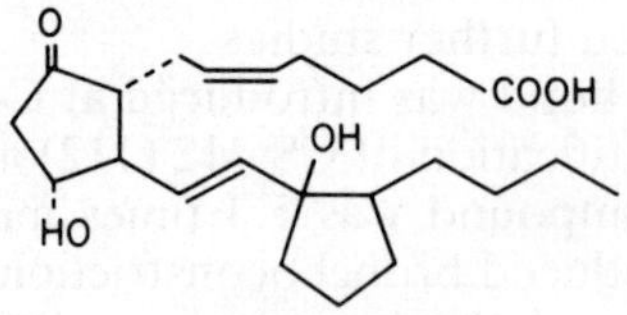

(116)

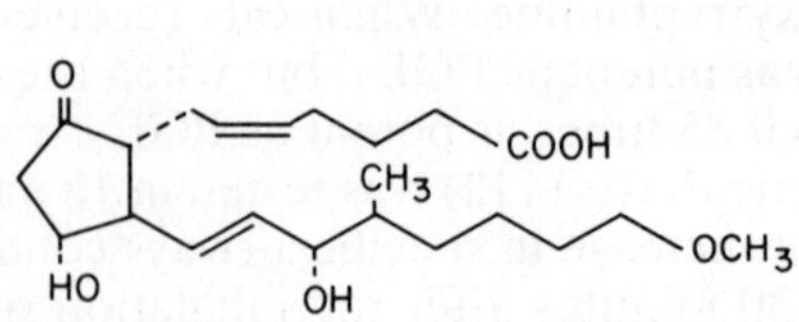

YPG-209 (117)

However, the efforts to improve bronchodilator potency using this type of modification were less fruitful. Methylation of PGE_2 at C-15 resulted in a derivative with weaker bronchodilator potency[61]. Cycloalkyl derivatives such as (114) and (115) were uninteresting in the Konzett–Rossler assay in the guinea-pig and in dogs with pilocarpine-induced bronchoconstriction. Cycloalkyl derivative (116) was highly effective in both assays but induced transient pulmonary hypertension in dogs. The 16-methyl-20-methoxy derivative (117) has been shown to have potent bronchodilator properties in guinea-pigs[92]. This is the only bronchodilator reported to have oral activity. Further studies on this derivative are warranted. In clinical studies[75], 15-methyl-PGE_2 200 μg administered as an aerosol to 6 normal subjects was found to be non-irritant but produced no perceptible bronchodilator effect. In 6 asthmatic patients, the compound had no effect on the airways tone or forced expiratory volume.

However, the 15-methyl analogues of the 11-deoxy series did show greater activity than the des-methyl derivatives[53]. The 11-deoxy-15-methyl-PGE_1 (107) administered as an aerosol was found to be 73.5 times more potent than the corresponding des-methyl analgoue (109) in inhibiting histamine-induced bronchoconstriction in guinea-pigs. When administered i.v., compound (107) was only 32.5 times as potent as (109), and both drugs demonstrated transient hypotensive effects.

Doxaprost (107) was administered[71] to 3 asthmatics and 3 patients with chronic bronchitis. Two of the 6 patients responded favourably to aerosol doses of 10 and 20 μg, 2 others worsened, and the other 2 remained unchanged. Mild throat irritation occurred in 3 patients. No serious adverse symptoms or haemodynamic changes were noted.

In contrast to 15-alkylated analogues, 16,16-dialkylated compounds exerted marked bronchodilator effects. The results[76] obtained with 16,16-trimethylene derivatives were of particular interest (*Table 12.6*). These

TABLE 12.6. Bronchodilator potency of 16,16-trimethylene-PG analogues*

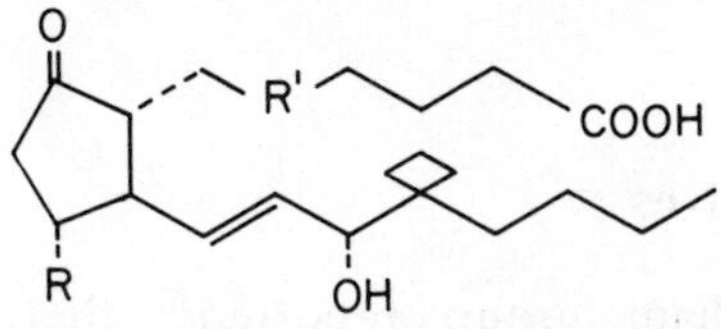

Compound	R	R'*	Relative potency against:	
			5-Hydroxytryptamine	Histamine
PGE_2			1.0	1.0
(118)	H	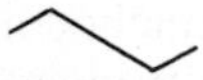	0.26	2.2
(119)	H	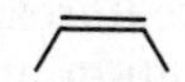	0.68	2.4
(120)	OH	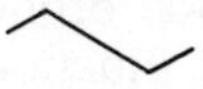	1.62	0.76
(121)	OH	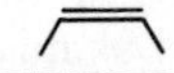	0.56	0.38

* Measured by the Konsett–Rossler procedure using guinea-pigs, the test compounds being administered i.v.

compounds were also potent bronchodilators when tested in dogs with pilocarpine-induced bronchoconstriction. However, some of the compounds of this series induced pulmonary hyptertension at similar doses to those required for bronchodilatation.

Due to the lack of efficacy of 15-alkylated derivatives in clinical studies, it is pertinent to consider the results obtained with these compounds in the *in vitro* assay[59] using bronchial tissue. It is clear from the results (*Table 12.7*) that C-15 and C-16 alkylated compounds exert significant broncho-constrictor effects on human bronchial tissues. Based on the above results,

TABLE 12.7. Effect of C-15 and C-16 substituted PG analogues on human respiratory muscle *in vitro*

		Relative potency*		
Compound	Effect	Tracheal	Bronchial	Bronchiolar
PGE_1	Relaxation	1	1	1
PGE_2	Relaxation	0.6	0.95	0.8
	Contraction	0.55	0.6	0.45
$PGF_{2\alpha}$	Contraction	1	1	1
(15S)-15-Methyl-PGE_1	Contraction	0.07	0.07	0.06
(15S)-15-Methyl-PGE_2	Contraction	0.39	0.45	0.57
16,16-Dimethyl-PGE_1	Contraction	1.98	3.11	5.7
16,16-Dimethyl-PGE_2	Contraction	6.33	11.04	30.3
11-Deoxy-16,16-dimethyl-PGE_1	Contraction	41.85	64.5	53.45

* Mean of three preparations; comparison reference for relaxation is $PGE_1 = 1$, and for contraction is $PGF_{2\alpha} = 1$.

the 16,16-dialkylated analogues are not likely to be of any therapeutic utility. It thus follows that 16,16-disubstituted derivatives used for the inhibition of gastric secretion or as an abortifacient must be used with caution in the case of asthmatics.

Miscellaneous Derivatives

Recently, the Beecham group reported[77] that some 8,10,12-triaza-prostaglandins of types (122) and (123) have bronchodilator activity. These compounds are simple to synthesize and have good stability.

These analogues were tested for their bronchodilator activity using the Konzett–Rossler method. The drugs were administered i.v. and tested against 5-hydroxytryptamine-induced bronchoconstriction in guinea-pigs.

There was a correlation between the bronchodilator activities of these compounds and the following structural features: (*a*) an α side-chain consisting of seven carbon atoms; (*b*) saturation at the C-5, C-6 bond (the unsaturation at this bond did not preclude bronchodilator activity), (*c*) a methyl group at N-10 and (*d*) an alkyl function at C-15 (this generally improved the bronchodilator profile). From the available literature, it appears that these compounds were tested as mixtures of stereoisomers at C-15 and were, in general, less potent than PGE_1 or PGE_2.

Scheme 22

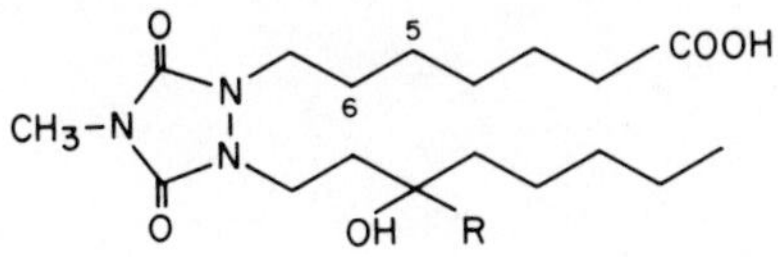

COOH

CH₃–N

R = H or CH₃   (122)

COOH

CH₃ –N

HO   CH₃

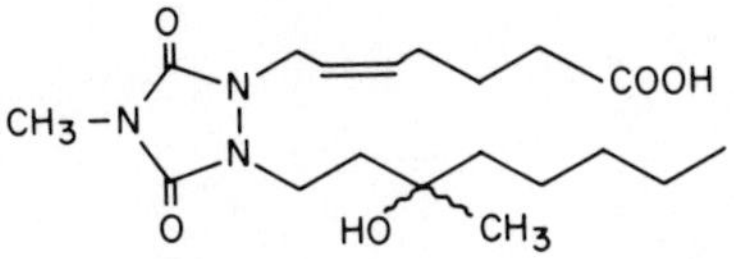

(123)

Prostacyclins

Prostacyclin (PGI_2) (124) represents a recent member of the prostaglandin family to be discovered by Vane and coworkers[78]. It was found to be a potent inhibitor of platelet aggregation as well as a potent vasodilator[79]. Since the compound is endogenously produced[80] in lung tissue, its effect on respiratory physiology is of particular interest. The first report of the respiratory effect of PGIs in animals came from Wassermann and coworkers[81]. PGI_2 inhibited the carbachol-induced contractions of the isolated guinea-pig trachea. A similar but much weaker effect was exerted by 6-keto-$PGF_{1\alpha}$ (125), a metabolite of PGI_2.

Since thromboxane A_2 has been shown to be a potent bronchoconstrictor[82], and is often considered to be the biological antithesis of PGI_2, it was of interest to study the bronchodilator effect of PGI_2. It was observed that PGI_2 at doses of 0.002–0.2% in aerosol form, or 0.3–30 μg/kg via parenteral injection, reversed the bronchoconstriction induced by $PGF_{2\alpha}$ in anaesthetized dogs in a dose-dependent manner. The effect was more pronounced in central airways than in peripheral ones. Pretreatment with PGI_2 also afforded significant protection to guinea-pigs challenged with histamine and to animals sensitized by an aerosol of ovalbumin.

In the Konzett–Rossler assay in the guinea-pig, the Lederle group[61] noted weak bronchodilator activity associated with PGI_2. This low activity may be partly due to the rapid degradation of the injected drug to 6-keto-$PGF_{1\alpha}$ (125) (*Scheme 23*). The iodo analogue (126) was found to retain a significant degree of bronchodilator activity in the guinea-pig model.

Recently, it was reported[83] that an i.v. infusion of PGI_2 2–50 μg/kg per min in healthy human volunteers produced profound changes in the circulatory system. In another study[84], a PGI_2 aerosol inhaled by healthy volunteers (0.3–30 μg) and asthmatic patients (200–400 μg) caused dispersion of circulating platelet aggregates and vasodilatation comparable to that seen when the drug was administered i.v. The appearance of systemic effects after aerosol administration may be explained by the fact that PGI_2 is not rapidly metabolized by the pulmonary circulation[85]. However, the compound had no effect on pulmonary function when it was administered

Scheme 23

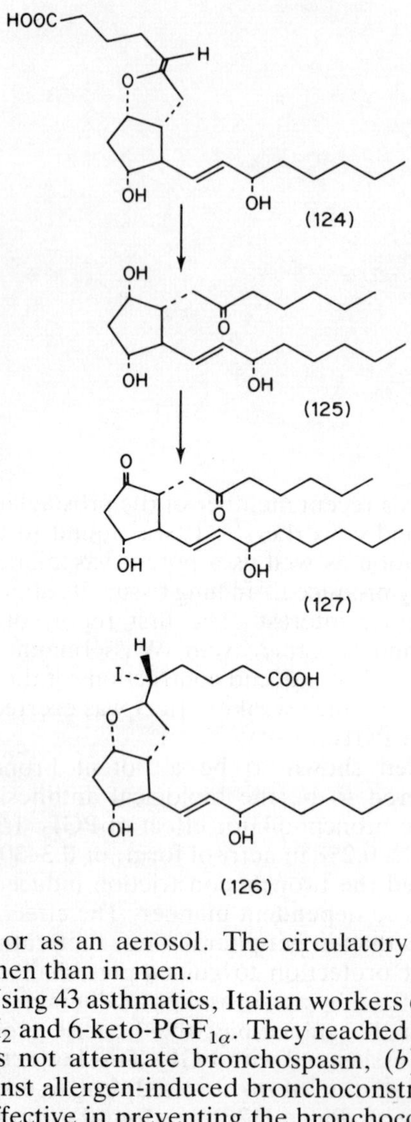

i.v. or as an aerosol. The circulatory effects were more pronounced in women than in men.

Using 43 asthmatics, Italian workers carried out a comparative study[86] of PGI_2 and 6-keto-$PGF_{1\alpha}$. They reached the following conclusions: (*a*) PGI_2 does not attenuate bronchospasm, (*b*) PGI_2 does not afford protection against allergen-induced bronchoconstriction and (*c*) at lower doses, PGI_2 is effective in preventing the bronchoconstriction evoked by ultrasonically generated water mist or exercise[87]. In contrast, 6-keto-$PGF_{1\alpha}$ was found to be devoid of any beneficial effects. PGI_2 thus afforded significant protection against non-specific bronchoconstrictor stimuli and had little effect on bronchial muscle tone. These results suggest little, if any, potential for PGI_2 as an anti-asthmatic.

An analogue, 20-methyl-Δ^6-prostacyclin, was also tested[88] in humans. This compound was also found to provide protection in patients in whom bronchoconstriction was induced by ultrasonically generated water mist or by exercise. This analogue also produced cardiovascular effects similar to those of PGI_2.

Prostacyclin is metabolically degraded to 6-keto-PGF$_{1\alpha}$ (125). 9-Hydroxyprostaglandin dehydrogenase[89] may transform this metabolite to 6-keto-PGE$_1$. This transformation, however, has not been conclusively proven. An account of the bronchodilator activity of 6-keto-PGE$_1$ (127) has recently appeared[90], and it was shown that compound (127) inhibited the 5-hydroxytryptamine-induced bronchoconstriction in the cat. 6-Keto-PGE$_1$ produced a response similar to that caused by PGI$_2$. When given i.v. both compounds lowered the central airways resistance and reduced contractions of the peripheral region of the lung. In this respect 6-keto-PGE$_1$ appeared to be 3–10 times more potent than prostacyclin. Furthermore, at the doses employed, 6-keto-PGE$_1$ had a minimal effect on the vasomotor activity in the lung, whereas PGI$_2$ significantly reduced the pressure in the pulmonary artery.

When PGI$_2$ and its metabolites were tested *in vitro* for their effects on isolated human bronchial muscle, the results[59] were rather surprising. Both PGI$_2$ and 6-keto-PGE$_1$ produced relaxation, whereas 6-keto-PGF$_{1\alpha}$ was inactive. Although PGI$_2$ did not produce any bronchodilator effects in human subjects, the compound was found to be about 3.56 and 4.33 times more potent than PGE$_1$ in relaxing isolated human tracheal and bronchial tissues, respectively. Prostacyclin appears to be the first compound where the *in vitro* results obtained with human lung muscles are contradictory to those observed in human subjects.

Conclusions

In conclusion, the results obtained from pharmacological and clinical studies of the effects of PGs on respiratory physiology and pathophysiology indicate that these compounds may become viable alternatives to β-sympathomimetic agents in reversing acute bronchoconstriction.

To date, the anti-asthmatic potential of the PGs has not been achieved. This may be explained, in part, by the suggested existence of two opposed[91] receptors for prostaglandins, i.e. one which responds to PGE$_1$ (leading to tissue relaxation) and the other to PGF$_{2\alpha}$ (leading to tissue contraction). Variation in receptor numbers and differences in sensitivity may lead to undesirable responses. Thus PGE$_2$ behaves as a bronchodilator in some subjects and produces bronchoconstriction in others. The same principle may hold true for some of the analogues tested. Since there appears to be a high correlation between the clinical results produced by PGs and their effects on isolated human bronchial muscle, this *in vitro* screening procedure may be of significant use in the selection of potential candidates for clinical study. Compounds such as (105) and (112), which were essentially devoid of undesirable effects in the initial clinical studies, require additional clinical data to confirm the results obtained.

Acknowledgments

I wish to thank Mr G. Medawar for his assistance in the retrieval of the literature and Miss C. Aks for editorial assistance. I also wish to gratefully acknowledge the careful constructive criticism of the biology section by Dr D. Grimes.

References

1. ANGGARD, E., GREEN, K. and SAMUELSSON, B. *Journal of Biological Chemistry*, **240**, 1932 (1965)
2. PIPER, P. and VANE, J. *Annals of the New York Academy of Sciences*, **180**, 365 (1971)
3. KADOWITZ, P.J., JOINER, A.L. and HYMAN, A.L. *Annual Review of Pharmacology*, **15**, 285 (1975)
4. MATHÉ, A.A., YEN, S.S. and SOHN, R.J. *Biochemical Pharmacology*, **26**, 181 (1977)
5. YEN, S.S., MATHÉ, A.A. and DUGAN, J.J. *Prostaglandins*, **11**, 227 (1976)
6a. SWEATMAN, W.J.F. and COLLIER, H.O.J. *Nature*, **217**, 69 (1968)
6b. SHREAD, P.J. *Journal of Pharmacy and Pharmacology*, **20**, 232 (1968)
7. ROSENTHALE, M.E., DERVINIS, A., BEGANY, A.J., LAPIDUS, M. and GLUCKMAN, M.I. *Experientia (Basel)*, **26**, 119 (1970)
8a. CUTHBERT, M.F. *British Medical Journal*, **4**, 723 (1969)
8b. CUTHBERT, M.F. *Proceedings of the Royal Society of Medicine*, **64**, 15 (1971)
8c. HERXHEIMER, H. and ROETSCHER, I. *European Journal of Clinical Pharmacology*, **3**, 123 (1971)
9. NELSON, N.A. *Journal of Medicinal Chemistry*, **17**, 911 (1974)
10. BINDRA, J.S. and BINDRA, R. *Prostaglandin Synthesis*. New York: Academic Press Inc. (1977)
11. MITRA, A. *The Synthesis of Prostaglandins*. New York: John Wiley and Sons (1977)
12. CRABBÉ, P. *Prostaglandin Research*. New York: Academic Press (1977)
13. *Chemistry, Biochemistry and Pharmacological Activity of Prostanoids*. Eds S.M. Roberts and F. Scheinmann. Oxford: Pergamon Press (1979)
14. BINDRA, J.S. and BINDRA, R. *Prostaglandin Synthesis*. p. 386. New York: Academic Press Inc. (1977)
15. COREY, E.J., RAVINDRANATHAN, T. and TERASHIMA, S. *Journal of the American Chemical Society*, **93**, 4326 (1971)
16. COREY, E.J., BECKER, K.B. and VERMA, R.K. *Journal of the American Chemical Society*, **94**, 8616 (1972)
17. BAGLI, J. and BOGRI, T. *Tetrahedron Letters*, 1639 (1969)
18. BAGLI, J. and BOGRI, T. *Journal of Organic Chemistry*, **37**, 2132 (1972)
19a. BAGLI, J. and BOGRI, T. *Tetrahedron Letters*, 3815 (1972)
19b. ALVAREZ, F.S. and WREN, D. *Tetrahedron Letters*, 569 (1973)
19c. CATON, M.P.L. and CROWSHAW, K. *Biochemical Aspects of Prostaglandin and Thromboxanes*. p. 75. Santa Monica, California: Intra-Science Research Foundation Symposium (1976)
20. FLOYD, M.B., SCHAUB, R.E., SIUTA, A.J., SKOTNICKI, J.S. GRUDZINSKAS, C.V. and WEISS, M.J. *Journal of Medicinal Chemistry*, **23**, 903 (1980)
21a. SIH, C.J., SALOMON, R.G., PRICE, P., SOOD, R. and PERUZZOTTI, G. *Journal of the American Chemical Society*, **97**, 857 (1975)
21b. SIH, C.J., HEATHER, J.B., SOOD, R., PRICE, P., PERUZZOTTI, G., HSU LEE, L.F. *et al. Journal of the American Chemical Society*, **97**, 865 (1975)
22. KLUGE, A.F., UNTCH, K.G. and FRIED, J.H. *Journal of the American Chemical Society*, **94**, 7827 (1972)
23. COREY, E.J. and BEAMES, D.J. *Journal of the American Chemical Society*, **94**, 7210 (1972)
24. HALLETT, W.A., WISSNER, A., GRUDZINSKAS, C.V. and WEISS, M.J. *Chemistry Letters*, 51 (1977)
25. COREY, E.J. and WOLLENBERG, R.H. *Journal of Organic Chemistry*, **40**, 2265 (1975)
26a. CHEN, S.-M.L., SCHAUB, R.E. and GRUDZINSKAS, C.V., *Journal of Organic Chemistry*, **43**, 3450 (1978)
26b. BIRNBAUM, J.E., CERVONI, P., CHOM, P.S., CHEN, S.-M.L., FLOYD, M.B., GRUDZINSKAS, C.V. *et al. Journal of Medicinal Chemistry*, **25**, 492 (1982)
26c. COLLINS, P.W., JUNG, C.J., GASIECKI, A. and PAPPO, R. *Tetrahedron Letters*, 3187 (1978)
27. BERNARDY, K.F., FLOYD, M.B., POLETTO, J.F. and WEISS, M.J. *Journal of Organic Chemistry*, **44**, 1438 (1979)
28. WEINHEIMER, A.J. and SPRAGGINS, R.L. *Tetrahedron Letters*, 5185 (1969)
29. SCHNEIDER, W.P., HAMILTON, R.D. and RHULAND, L.E. *Journal of the American Chemical Society*, **94**, 2122 (1972)
30. GRUDZINSKAS, C.V. and WEISS, M.J. *Tetrahedron Letters*, 141 (1973)
31. STRIKE, D.P. and KAO, W. Personal communication

32. GREENE, A.E., TEIXEIRA, M.A., BARREIRO, E., CRUZ, A. and CRABBÉ, P. *Journal of Organic Chemistry*, **47**, 2553 (1982)
33. BARTMANN, W., BECK, G. and LERCH, U. *Tetrahedron Letters*, 2441 (1974)
34. SCHAAF, T.K. and HESS, H.J. *Journal of Medicinal Chemistry*, **22**, 1340 (1979)
35. United States Patent 4064351, Dec. 20 (1977)
36. JOHNSON, R.A., MORTON, D.R., KINNER, J.H., GORMAN, R.R., McGUIRE, J.C., SUN, F.F. *et al. Prostaglandins*, **12**, 915 (1976)
37. CHIANG, Y., KRESGE, A.J. and CHO, M. *Journal of the Chemical Society. Chemical Communications*, 129 (1979)
38. COREY, E.J., KECK, G.E. and SZÉKLEY, I. *Journal of the American Chemical Society*, **99**, 2006 (1977)
39. NICOLAU, K.C., SIPIO, W.J., MAGOLDA, R.L., SEITZ, S. and BARNETTE, W.E. *Journal of the Chemical Society. Chemical Communications*, 1067 (1978)
40. ARISTOFF, P.A. *Journal of Organic Chemistry*, **46**, 1954 (1981)
41. SKUBALLA, W. and VORBRUGGEN, H. *Angewandte Chemie International Edition in English*, **20**, 1046 (1981)
42. BARTMANN, W., BECK, G., KNOLL, J. and RUPP, R.H. *Angewandte Chemie International Edition in English*, **19**, 819 (1980)
43. SKUBALLA, W. *Tetrahedron Letters*, 3261 (1980)
44. JOHNSON, R.A. and NIDY, E.G. *Journal of Organic Chemistry*, **45**, 3802 (1980)
45. BANNAI, K., TORU, T., OBA, T., TANAKA, T., OKAMURA, N., WATANABE, K. *et al. Tetrahedron Letters*, 1417 (1981)
46. FRIED, J., MITRA, D.K., NAGARAJAN, M. and MEHROTRA, M.M. *Journal of Medicinal Chemistry*, **23**, 235 (1980)
47. SUN, F.F. and TAYLOR, B.M. *Prostaglandins*, **21**, 307 (1981)
48. NOVAK, L., ASZODI, J. and SZANTAY, C. *Tetrahedron Letters*, **23**, 2135 (1982)
49. SATO, C., IKEDA, S., SHIRAHAMA, H. and MATSUMOTO, T. *Tetrahedron Letters*, **23**, 2099 (1982)
50. KONZETT, H. and ROSSLER, R. *Archiv fuer Pharmakologie und Experimentelle Pathologie*, **195**, 71 (1940)
51. LULLING, J., EL SAYED, F. and LIEVENS, P. *Medicina et Pharmacologia Experimentalis*, **16**, 481 (1967)
52. LULLING, J., PRIGNOT, J. and LIEVENS, P. *Archiv fuer Pharmakologie und Experimentelle Pathologie*, **261**, 1 (1968)
53. GREENBERG, R., SMORONG, K. and BAGLI, J.F. *Prostaglandins*, **11**, 961 (1976)
54. CATON, M.P.L. and WALKER, J.L. In *Medicinal Chemistry, Proceedings of the 6th International Symposium on Medicinal Chemistry*. Ed. M.A. Simpkins. p. 385. Oxford: Cotswold Press Ltd (1978)
55. GARDINER, P.J., COPAS, J.L., ELLIOTT, R.D. and COLLIER, H.O.J. *Prostaglandins*, **15**, 303 (1978)
56. WEISSBERG, R.H., BRADSHAW, J.B. and GARAY, G.L. *Journal of Pharmacology and Experimental Therapeutics*, **205**, 246 (1976)
57. MATHÉ, A.A., HEDQVIST, P., STRANDBERG, K. and LESLIE, C.A. *New England Journal of Medicine*, Vol. 296, p. 910, April 21 (1977)
58. STRANDBERG, K. and HEDQVIST, P. *Acta Physiologica Scandinavica*, **100**, 172 (1977)
59. KARIM, S.M.M., ADAIKAN, P.G. and KOTTEGODA, S.R. *Advances in Prostaglandin and Thromboxane Research*, **7**, 969 (1980)
60. ROSENTHALE, M.E., DERVINIS, A. and STRIKE, D. *Advances in Prostaglandin and Thromboxane Research*, **1**, 477 (1976)
61. GRUDZINSKAS, C.V., SKOTNICKI, J.S., CHEM, S.-M.L., FLOYD, M.B., HALLETT, W.A., SCHAUB, R.E. *et al.* In *Drugs Affecting the Respiratory System*. Ed. D.L. Temple. p. 301. Washington: The American Chemical Society (1980)
62. GREENBERG, R. and SMORONG, K. *Canadian Journal of Physiology and Pharmacology*, **53**, 799 (1975)
63. BIRNBAUM, J.E., BIRKHEAD, N.C., ORONSKY, A.L., DESSY, F., RIHOUX, J.P. and VAN HUMBUCK, L. *Prostaglandins*, **21**, 457 (1981)
64. MUCHOWSKI, J.M. In *Chemistry, Biochemistry and Pharmacological Activity of Prostanoids*. Eds S.M. Roberts and F. Schienmann. p. 39. Oxford: Pergamon Press (1979)
65. ROSENTHALE, M.E., DERVINIS, A., KASSARICH, J., SINGER, S. and GLUCKMAN, M.I. *Advances in Biosciences*, Vol. 9. p. 229. International Conference on Prostaglandins, Vienna. Oxford: Pergamon Press (1973)

66. HAMOSH, P. and DA SILVA, A.M. *Prostaglandins*, **10**, 599 (1975)
67. ARNDT, H.C., GARDINER, P.J., HONG, E., KLUENDER, H.C., MYERS, C. and WOESSNER, W.D. *Prostaglandins*, **16**, 67 (1978)
68. SPECTOR, L.S. and BALL, R.E. *Annals of Surgery*, **38**, 302 (1976)
69. FALKNER, F.C. *Prostaglandins*, **18**, 779 (1979)
70. BARTMANN, W., BECK, G., LERCH, U., TEUFEL, H., BABEJ, M., BICKEL, M. *et al.* In *Chemistry, Biochemistry and Pharmacology of Prostanoids.* Eds S.M. Roberts and F. Schienmann. p. 194. Oxford: Pergamon Press (1979)
71. AYERST LABORATORIES. Unpublished results
72. YAMAGUCHI, T., SAKAI, K., YUSA, T. and YAMAZAKI, M. *Prostaglandins*, **20**, 521 (1980)
73. MURAO, M., UCHIYAMA, K., SHIDA, A., SAKAI, K., YUSA, T. and YAMAGUCHI, T. *Advances in Prostaglandin and Thromboxane Research*, **7**, 985 (1980)
74. ROBERTS, A. and MAGERLEIN, B.J. *Advances in Biosciences*. Vol. **9**, p. 247. International Conference on Prostaglandins, Vienna. Oxford: Pergamon Press (1963)
75. SMITH, A.P. *International Research Communications System (IRCS)*, **2**, 1457 (1974)
76. SKOTNICKI, J.S., SCHAUB, R.E. and WEISS, M.J. *Journal of Medicinal Chemistry*, **20**, 1042 (1977)
77. ADAMS, D.R., BARNES, A.F. and CASSIDY, F. *Advances in Prostaglandin and Thromboxane Research*, **7**, 989 (1980)
78. MONCADA, S., HIGGS, E.A. and VANE, J.R. *Lancet*, **i**, 18 (1977)
79. SCHRÖR, K.S., MONCADA, S., UBATUBA, F.B. and VANE, J.R. *Naunyn-Schmiedesberg's Archives of Pharmacology*, **297**, R 31 (1977)
80. GRYGLEWSKI, R.J., KORBUT, R. and OCETKIEWIEZ, A. *Nature*, **273**, 765 (1978)
81. WASSERMAN, M.A., DUCHARME, D.W., WENDLING, M.G., GRIFFIN, R.L. and DEGRAAF, G.L. *European Journal of Pharmacology*, **66**, 53 (1980)
82. SVENSSON, J., STRANDBERG, K., TUREMO, T. and HAMBERG, M. *Prostaglandins*, **14**, 425 (1977)
83. SZCZEKLIK, A., GRYGLEWSKI, R.J., NIZANKOWSKI, R., MUSIAL, J., PIETON, R. and MRUK, J. *Pharmacological Research Communications*, **10**, 545 (1978)
84. SZCZEKLIK, A., GRYGLEWSKI, R.J., NIZANKOWSKI, E., NIZANKOWSKI, R. and MUSIAL, J. *Prostaglandins*, **16**, 651 (1978)
85. DUSTING, G.J., MONCADA, S. and VANE, J.R. *British Journal of Pharmacology*, **62**, 414P (1978)
86. PARSARGIKLIAN, M. and BIANCO, S. *Advances in Prostaglandin and Thromboxane Research*, **7**, 943 (1980)
87. BIANCO, S., ROBUSCHI, R., CESERANI, R. and GANDOLFI, C. *European Journal of Respiratory Diseases*, Suppl. **106**, 81 (1980)
88. BIANCO, S., ROBUSCHI, R., CESERANI, R., GANDOLFI, C. and KAMBUROFF, P.L. *Pharmacological Research Communications*, **10**, 657 (1978)
89. WONG, P. Y.-K., LEE, W.H., REISS, R.F. and McGIFF, J.C. *Federation Proceedings*, **39**, 392 (1980)
90. SPANNHAKE, E.W., LEVIN, J.L., HYMAN, A.L. and KADOWITZ, P.J. *Prostaglandins*, **21**, 267 (1981)
91. GARDINER, P.J. and COLLIER, H.O.J. *Prostaglandins*, **19**, 819 (1980)
92. TOMIOKA, K., TERAI, M. and MAENO, H. *Archives Internationales de Pharmacodynamie et de Thérapie*, **226**, 224 (1977)

Section 3   Inhibitors of mediator release

Chapter 13

Disodium cromoglycate and compounds with similar activities

D.R. Buckle

Introduction

In common with many other therapeutically useful compounds, disodium cromoglycate (DSCG), the disodium salt of 1,3-bis(2-carboxychromon-5-yloxy)-2-hydroxypropane (1), was first shown to have beneficial effects in man and, subsequent to this, attempts were made to elucidate the mode of action responsible for this benefit.[1] Despite a considerable amount of effort by a large number of research groups, the activities shown by DSCG that are relevant to its clinical effect are still far from certain. The failure to determine the relevant mode of action, not only of DSCG but of many other drugs, highlights the difficulties facing the medicinal chemist today. It is now necessary to demonstrate that a compound shows potential benefit in the human disease using animals or other test systems before proceeding to evaluate the compound in man. Even with this potential indicated, progression into man is only possible after lengthy and expensive toxicity studies in animals.

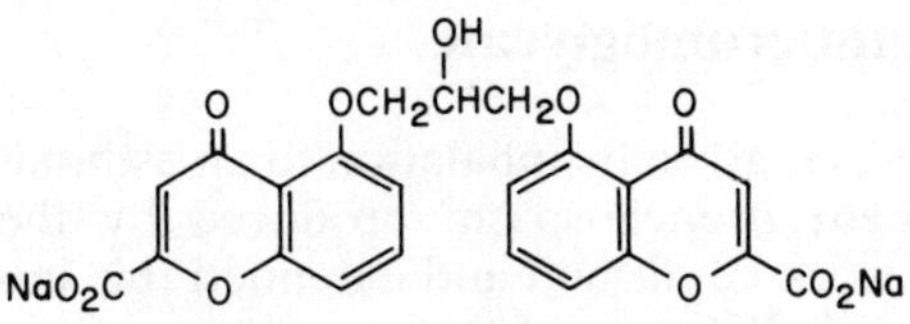

(1) Disodium cromoglycate, Intal *

Disodium cromoglycate was first introduced as a medicine in the United Kingdom in 1967 as a result of a programme designed to modify the naturally occurring chromone khellin (2)[2,3]. Khellin, an isolate from the seeds of the Eastern Mediterranean plant *Ammi visnaga*[1], was known for its coronary vasodilatory and smooth muscle relaxant properties, and had found

---

* Intal is a trademark of Fisons p.l.c.

some use both in the treatment of angina and as a bronchodilator[4,5]. Unfortunately the clinical value of khellin is limited by its propensity to cause nausea and vomiting and by its low aqueous solubility. Earlier attempts by Schönberg and Sina[6] to improve the efficacy of the drug as a bronchodilator, mainly by modification of the alkyloxy groups, had proved unsuccessful.

Using a different approach, based on 2-carboxychromones, Altounyan's group soon identified compounds without the bronchodilatory activity of khellin, but with an unexpected prophylactic protection against provoked bronchospasm in an asthmatic volunteer[1,7]. The lack of suitable animal models hindered progress in the early stages, especially since the synthetic compounds were inactive in all the conventional test systems. Evaluation was, therefore, dependent on the unusual expedient of testing compounds as inhibitors of antigen-induced bronchospasm in man. With the discovery of high potency in a series of 5-alkyloxychromones, especially the 5-(2-hydroxypropoxy) derivative (3), came the eventual cross-linked products, the bis-chromones of the DSCG type[2,3].

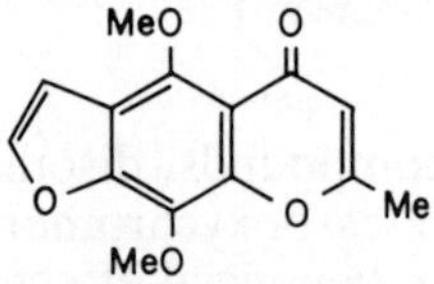

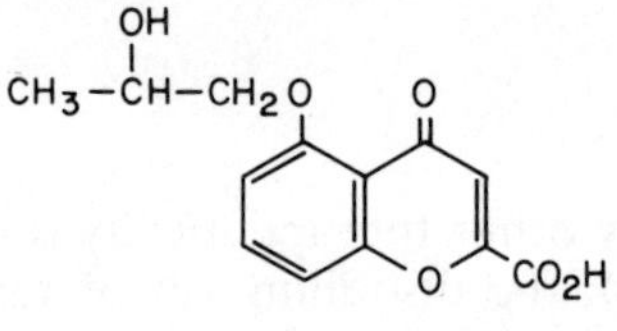

Disodium cromoglycate does have disadvantages, however, and the research effort expended by a large number of pharmaceutical companies to find improved drugs with a similar mode of action has been enormous. A number of promising candidates have been clinically evaluated, but to date there has been no commercial successor to DSCG. This lack of success is a reflection of our poor understanding of asthma, and more especially of the mode of action of DSCG relevant to its therapeutic activity. Current research in a number of areas should lead to a greater insight into the apparent uniqueness of DSCG, and perhaps, to better drugs.

Mechanism of action of disodium cromoglycate

It was shown by Altounyan, that DSCG, given by inhalation to an asthmatic, could protect against subsequent bronchospasm produced by the inhalation of antigen[3]. Subsequent work confirmed and extended this initial observation and showed also that DSCG was of therapeutic benefit in asthma[8]. In extensive animal studies DSCG was shown to have few pharmacological activities[1]. It was not an antagonist of possible mediators of asthma, nor did it show bronchodilatory activity. DSCG was, however, shown to be capable of stabilizing mast cells[2] at some stage subsequent to antigen–antibody interaction on the cell surface[1,9,10]

There is, however, some dispute as to whether or not mast cell stabilization is relevant to the therapeutic effects of DSCG. The arguments against this relevance seem to be largely:

(1) Many compounds with similar, and often more potent, mast-cell-stabilizing activity to that shown by DSCG have been prepared by the pharmaceutical industry but, if one excludes those compounds with predominant H_1 antihistamine activity, none of these has reached the market.

(2) DSCG is of benefit in the treatment of intrinsic or cryptogenic asthma in which there is no evidence for the involvement of antigen or sensitized mast cells[11].

(3) DSCG can protect asthmatics against bronchospasm induced by exercise[12] and sulphur dioxide[13] in which the evidence for mast cell involvement is questionable[13,14].

(4) It is not very effective in stabilizing human mast cells *in vitro* in that it provides only partial protection against the antigen-induced release of mast cell products from passively sensitized human lung, and only then at a relatively high dose and with a bell-shaped dose–response curve[1,13,15].

These arguments can, of course, be countered. Those compounds with similar activities to DSCG might have failed in man for a number of reasons, such as inappropriate pharmacokinetics, toxicity, or because of inappropriate evaluation in the clinic. Mast cells might be involved in cryptogenic asthma, and DSCG might be more active *in vivo* than *in vitro*. The latter is certainly true in the rat in which DSCG completely inhibits the antigen-induced release of histamine in the peritoneal cavity[16], but is less potent and usually provides only partial inhibition from isolated rat peritoneal mast cells[17].

The evidence for the involvement of the mast cell in asthma, even atopic asthma, is still circumstantial and attempts are being made to obtain direct evidence by measuring mast cell products, such as histamine, in the blood of asthmatics during bronchospasm[18]. The measurement of histamine levels in blood plasma is technically difficult and complicated by leakage from basophils, although it has recently been suggested that plasma histamine levels, reliably measured using a double isotope radioenzymatic assay, are a potentially useful index of the rate of mast cell and basophil degranulation[18,19]. However, it is not presently possible to distinguish between the contributions of these two cell types to the total histamine levels[18,19].

Currently attempts are being made to estimate the blood levels of other mast cell products, such as the leukotrienes and PGD_2[20]. It has been shown that levels of neutrophil chemotactic factor of anaphylaxis (NCFA) can increase in the blood of asthmatics during exercise or antigen-induced bronchospasm, and that both the bronchospasm and increase in NCFA levels can be prevented by prior inhalation of DSCG[21–23]. There is always the argument that NCFA may not be released from mast cells, but, nevertheless, these types of study might ultimately provide direct evidence for the involvement of the mast cell in asthma and support mast cell stabilization as the relevant mode of action of DSCG.

In this review, the possible mechanisms by which DSCG stabilizes mast cells will be discussed, followed by a brief outline of alternative mechanisms that might be involved in the therapeutic benefit provided by DSCG.

Mast cell stabilization

The precise mechanism by which DSCG exerts its action on mast cells is still not fully understood, but it seems likely that its action occurs at the cell membrane[23]. Support for this idea has recently been provided from experiments with DSCG covalently bound to fluorescent beads, where image-intensified fluorescence microscopy clearly showed the localization of the drug–bead conjugates on the cell surface under conditions which produced inhibition of histamine release[24].

Several possibilities for the action of DSCG and similar drugs exist:

(1) The inhibition of cellular metabolism[16,23,25]
(2) The inhibition of calcium transport, either by a direct effect or by prevention of the calcium gating mechanism[26–29]
(3) The inhibition of membrane-bound phosphodiesterases[23,30]
(4) The regulation of protein phosphorylation[31,32]
(5) Stabilization of the mast cell membrane[33,34]
(6) Promotion of disaggregation of microtubules[35]

From early studies, it was evident that the antigen-induced release of histamine from mast cells was dependent on a metabolically viable cell, a number of metabolic poisons having been shown to prevent histamine release[25]. Even today it is possible that many compounds claimed as being able to stabilize mast cells may, in reality, owe this action to their toxic effects on cell metabolism. It is unlikely, however, that any drug sufficiently toxic to affect cell metabolism would be of therapeutic value in asthma.

The dependence of antigen-induced mast cell degranulation on the presence of exogenous calcium has been claimed by a number of workers and, until recently, the influx of calcium ions into the cell was considered to be a necessary prerequisite to mediator release[36–38]. The idea that DSCG prevented this influx by some action on the calcium gating mechanism, either by a direct or an indirect effect, has received considerable support[26–29].

Early experiments had shown that DSCG and its congenors did not inhibit the calcium ionophore-induced release of histamine from rat mast cells (a process which circumvents the calcium gating mechanism[27]) while inhibiting the antigen-induced release[26]. More recent work by Pearce and his coworkers, however, has demonstrated that these apparent differences may simply reflect variations in experimental technique[39–41]. In particular, high concentrations of ionophore release a considerably larger percentage of the available histamine than that normally observed on antigen induction. Using concentrations of ionophore which produced a submaximal release of histamine, at levels more akin to the antigen response, a dose-dependent inhibition of ionophore-induced release of histamine was observed with DSCG[39,42]. A similar finding has also been reported by other workers[43].

Experiments with radiolabelled calcium have demonstrated that DSCG will prevent the intracellular accumulation of labelled cation in stimulated mast cells, an observation which has been attributed to a decreased influx of calcium[23]. This may not be a direct effect of DSCG, however, and it has been argued that accumulation studies alone are insufficient to allow this conclusion since other effects, such as increased efflux, would produce a similar result[39]. Furthermore, it has been shown that extracellular calcium is not required for exocytosis of the mast cell[39,40,44].

These results have been rationalized by Pearce who has provided evidence for the existence of a number of calcium pools within the mast cell which together control exocytosis[45]. There seems to be little doubt that the release of histamine from the mast cell is triggered by an increase of calcium ions in the cytosol[44,46] and it would appear that the source of this calcium, whether it be from intra- or extracellular sources, depends to a large extent on the nature of the calcium environment and on the stimulus itself[44]. These findings have led to the suggestion that DSCG does not stabilize mast cells by the inhibition of the calcium gating mechanism, but that it might activate membrane pumps to extrude the cation from the cytosol or promote a sequestration of the ion into internal stores[39,40,44]. Whether this effect occurs directly, or as a result of an increase in intracellular cyclic AMP or some other factor, is not known. Despite these arguments, however, the requirement for extracellular calcium ions is essential for optimal histamine release from mast cells[41].

DSCG is a known inhibitor of cyclic-nucleotide phosphodiesterase[47,48], which could promote increased levels of cyclic AMP, and it has been suggested that DSCG may exert its action in this way[20,30,33]. Its ability to inhibit the release of mediators at low concentrations, relative to its inhibition of cyclic-nucleotide phosphodiesterase, however, would tend to suggest that its action on phosphodiesterase is not a relevant mode of action. Despite this, it has been argued that the topical mode of administration of DSCG could result in sufficiently high localized concentrations of the drug for phosphodiesterase inhibition to be a significant factor[23].

The suggestion that DSCG and similar acting drugs might be involved in the regulation of protein phosphorylation in the plasma or perigranular membrane of the mast cell and so prevent the fusional changes necessary for exocytosis, has been put forward by several workers[31,32]. Exocytosis of rat mast cells with Compound 48/80 or the calcium ionophore A23187 is known to result in the phosphorylation of cellular proteins. In particular, three proteins of molecular weight less than or equal to 68 000 are rapidly phosphorylated and it has been suggested that these might be involved in the release process, whilst a fourth protein of molecular weight 78 000, which is phosphorylated more slowly, might be involved in the termination of secretion[49a]. DSCG, even in the absence of challenge, is able to induce phosphorylation of this higher-molecular-weight protein giving rise to the notion that DSCG might stabilize the mast cell by the activation of a natural control mechanism[32]. In continuance of this idea, it was shown that anti-IgE produces a similar pattern of protein phosphorylation to that observed for Compound 48/80 and that phosphorylation of the protein of molecular weight 78 000 by DSCG and some related compounds reflected their potencies as inhibitors of anti-IgE-induced histamine release[49b]. Furthermore, the same workers demonstrated also that dibutyryl-guanosine cyclic 3':5'-monophosphate (dibutyryl-cGMP) induces phosphorylation of this protein, but that compounds which inhibit histamine release by raising levels of adenosine cyclic monophosphate do not. It was concluded that DSCG might activate an endogenous control mechanism for stabilizing mast cells by a mechanism mediated by cyclic GMP[49b].

Detailed studies by Hirata and Axelrod[50] have identified enzymatic cascades, resulting from the activation of phospholipid methyltransferases after IgE cross-linking on the mast cell surface, which lead to a subsequent perturbation of the membrane and exocytosis. It is conceivable that DSCG may act on any one of these stages.

Disodium cromogylcate will stabilize mast cells activated by agents other than cross-linked IgE antibody, and it has been shown to protect the mast cell against degranulation induced by surface active agents, such as melittin[34]. In these studies, DSCG was shown to inhibit histamine release from isolated rat peritoneal mast cells when applied simultaneously with the inducer, and did so at concentrations similar to those shown to prevent IgE-mediated secretion[34]. This led to the suggestion that DSCG might act by a general stabilization of the mast cell membrane, although no mechanism for this action has been proposed.

A number of other hypotheses, such as the idea that DSCG may act by promoting disaggregation of the mast cell microtubules[35], have been suggested, but little experimental work has been presented to support them and the current situation remains something of an enigma.

Relevance of mast cell stabilization to the therapeutic activity of DSCG and other mechanisms that might be involved

As discussed earlier, the significance of the ability of DSCG to stabilize mast cells to its therapeutic utility in asthma is questionable, especially when one considers those manifestations of the disease in which the role of the mast cell is unimportant or doubtful. There is no doubt, however, that mast cell products, such as histamine, are potent inflammatory and bronchoconstrictor agents and as such are likely to play an important part in the disease state.

The suggestion that DSCG may exert actions in addition to mast cell stabilization is not new, despite the knowledge that the drug is a relatively pharmacologically inert compound[1]. In order to rationalize its effectiveness in exercise-induced asthma, the concept of irritant receptor blockade has been proposed[51]. In anaesthetized dogs, DSCG suppressed the response of sensory 'C' fibre endings to capsaicon[52], but had no effect on the resting discharge of irritant receptors or their ability to respond to histamine[53]. The blockade of irritant receptors has also been proposed as the mechanism of the protective action of DSCG against bronchospasm induced by bronchial irritants such as sulphur dioxide[54]. A possibility that DSCG has α-adrenoceptor blocking activity[55,56] has been questioned[57]. Altounyan has proposed that there are two different receptors for DSCG in the lung and that it therefore has two modes of action: mast cell stabilization, and the blocking of irritant receptors[13]. This argument has been used to explain the action of DSCG in both antigen-induced and exercise-induced asthma.

Possibly one of the more important properties of DSCG is its ability to induce a long-term reduction of bronchial hypersensitivity in man[57-59]. In clinical studies in both adults[58] and children[59], a significant reduction in bronchial hyper-reactivity to histamine was observed on extended DSCG treatment. It has been suggested that the probable action of DSCG in reducing this hyper-reactivity is by the indirect action of its inhibitory effects on the immediate response[13].

It is of interest that DSCG has been claimed to inhibit both the early and late reactions when given prior to antigen challenge, but has no effect on the latter when administered after the immediate reaction. In these studies, DSCG was distinguished from the β-adrenoceptor stimulants and the corticosteroids which inhibit only the early and late reactions, respectively[60–62].

Pharmacokinetics and clinical results of DSCG

Despite the lack of understanding surrounding the mechanism of action of DSCG, there is little doubt that it is of value in the treatment of asthma[8]. It is somewhat disappointing, however, that not all asthmatics are responsive to the drug, and that those who benefit often do not get complete relief[11]. DSCG treatment will frequently reduce the need for alternative anti-asthmatic preparations, such as bronchodilators and the corticosteroids, and as such is a useful adjunct to other therapies[11].

In general, young people, especially those with overt atopic or exercise-induced asthma, are claimed to be the ones most likely to respond to DSCG treatment[11]. Those asthmatics with clearly defined IgE-mediated reactions fall within the sphere of likely responders, whereas those with IgG-mediated reactions and no demonstrable IgE levels are least likely to be improved[63].

The clinical evaluation of drugs of the DSCG type is difficult for a number of reasons, not the least of which is the variable nature of asthma[64]. Moreover, the observation that benefit from treatment with DSCG may not be noticed until the drug has been taken for some time, and then may extend for several weeks after drug withdrawal, are notable problems in the organization of clinical trials[8,65,66].

DSCG itself has a number of significant disadvantages, one being its lack of oral absorption[1,67]. Indeed, plasma levels of DSCG have been measured in a number of species following oral administration of the drug and all were found to be extremely low[68]. In man, ^{14}C-labelling studies have demonstrated that less than 1% of the administered oral dose is absorbed[67]. Furthermore, plasma levels following intravenous administration show a very short half-life because of rapid excretion, although the drug appears to be metabolically inert[67].

Although DSCG has moderate water solubility[1], its low potency necessitates the administration of relatively large amounts of drug. As a consequence of this the drug is introduced as a dry micronized powder directly into the lungs using a specially designed inhaler[69]. This, in itself, introduces a number of problems in that young people particularly find the inhaler difficult to use effectively, frequently receiving insufficient drug either due to improper use or through impaired bronchial function[70,71]. However, new formulations which may circumvent this are being introduced[72,73]. Moreover, DSCG has shown remarkably few side-effects in man and those which do occur tend to be associated with the inhalation of a dry solid[30].

Possibly one of the more intriguing properties of DSCG is its propensity to give bell-shaped dose–response curves in many *in vitro* test systems used for the assessment of similar drugs and, indeed, in some animal models of anaphylaxis[15]. This has been explained in terms of a rapid onset of tolerance or tachyphylaxis which can be demonstrated *in vivo* in the rat passive cutaneous anaphylaxis test. In this test, rats predosed with a bolus injection of DSCG suffer a reduction in potency of subsequent doses[16]. It has been suggested that the effect of the bolus predose is to trigger and subsequently block the effective receptor site[16]. Fortunately, there is no evidence in clinical practice for bell-shaped dose–response curves[13], the absence of this having been attributed to a rapid clearance of the drug from the bronchial mucosa into the blood stream, such that overdosage or saturation of the submucosal receptors cannot be achieved[13].

The clinical activity of DSCG in numerous trials has been collated in an excellent review by Brogden, Speight and Avery[11] and has recently been reappraised by Altounyan[13].

Biological test systems for drugs of the DSCG type

Since DSCG was discovered as a result of its prophylactic effect in man, and was subsequently shown to have a mode of action different from other anti-asthmatic drugs, the attempt to develop biological screens to identify similar drugs occurred later. As yet, there is no commercial successor to DSCG despite the efforts of many groups over a number of years, and this has led to the conclusion that the currently available models of DSCG activity may not be of clinically predictive value[15,30] The problem is compounded by the inactivity of DSCG in many classical biological systems and the doubt surrounding the mechanism by which it exerts its benefit in asthma. These inherent problems have forced researchers attempting to evaluate drugs of this kind to use screens of limited proven usefulness. The need for a meaningful test system is of primary importance. In the absence of this ideal test system, there can be no guarantee that a candidate drug will be of eventual clinical benefit for the prophylaxis and/or treatment of asthma.

Several model systems have been developed for the characterization and purported identification of DSCG-like compounds[15], some of which are described below.

Rat passive cutaneous anaphylaxis

The model most frequently used to demonstrate the effects of DSCG is the rat passive cutaneous anaphylaxis (PCA) test[74] which arose out of pioneering work by Ovary and Bier[75]. Even today this test frequently ranks as a primary screening procedure for the evaluation of similar compounds and as such deserves reasonable mention.

The test, as normally carried out, involves the intradermal injection of dilutions of rat serum containing specific IgE antibody into the shaved backs of recipient rats whereby the antibody attaches to the mast cells at the injection site. After an appropriate sensitization time, usually 24–72 hours, antigen is injected intravenously together with a vital blue dye to label plasma proteins. The antigen combines with the mast-cell-bound IgE antibody triggering the release of vasoactive materials. This results in the extravasation of dye-labelled plasma proteins and the formation of blue wheals at the antibody injection sites. Compounds are evaluated for their ability to inhibit the wheals when given to the rats prior to antigen. The rat PCA test is, therefore, dependent upon IgE antibody being triggered by antigen to activate mast cells and, in this sense, may have a similar aetiology to allergic asthma.

DSCG produces a marked inhibition of rat PCA when given just prior to antigen challenge, but this activity rapidly diminishes when the time between drug administration and challenge is increased[76,77]. Moreover, predosing at 30 minutes before challenge with a dose of DSCG sufficient to be inhibitory when given just prior to challenge, whilst producing no inhibition itself, can reduce the inhibitory action of subsequent doses given just before challenge[76]. The tolerance to a dose of DSCG fades with increasing time after injection and has been rationalized as a triggering and blocking of the receptor site for DSCG, full return of activity only occurring after desorption of the drug from the receptor[76,78].

A major disadvantage of the rat PCA test is its lack of specificity, in that a number of compounds with activities different from that of DSCG can inhibit the PCA response. Particular examples are the β-adrenoceptor stimulants, which act as functional antagonists[79], and competitive antagonists such as the H_1 antihistamines, especially if they also show anti-5-hydroxytryptamine activity[79].

Cross-reacting tachyphylaxis has been shown for DSCG and a number of drugs (e.g. see [77,80]) and this has been used to identify compounds acting by a common pathway with DSCG[15,16]. By the use of this procedure, specificity in the rat PCA test can be achieved.

Rat passive peritoneal anaphylaxis

This test (rat PPA test) is similar to the rat PCA test, except that antiserum containing IgE antibody is injected into the peritoneal cavities of rats instead of intradermally. After sensitization, a vital blue dye is again injected intravenously, simultaneously with an intraperitoneal injection of antigen. The rats are killed at an appropriate time after challenge and the peritoneal fluids are collected for assay. This allows direct measurements to be made *in vivo* of the mediators of an allergic reaction such as histamine and slow-reacting substance of anaphylaxis (SRS-A). In addition, the pathology of the reaction can be measured directly as an increase in concentration in the peritoneal fluids of extravasated dye-labelled plasma proteins. The effects of injecting drugs prior to antigen on the release of histamine and SRS-A has been studied by many groups and has been reviewed[81].

The system can be used to identify compounds with a similar mode of action to DSCG. The intraperitoneal injection of DSCG just before antigen inhibits extravasation only at doses at which it inhibits histamine release, suggesting that mast-cell stabilization may be relevant to its ability to inhibit the pathology of the reaction. This contrasts with the activities of the H_1 antihistamines and β-adrenoceptor stimulants which inhibit extravasation at doses that have no effect on histamine release[82], showing that in this system at least, their anti-allergy effects are due to competitive or functional antagonism of the released mediators.

Stabilization of isolated rat mast cells

DSCG will inhibit histamine release by antigen from rat peritoneal mast cells *in vitro* and it is more potent and more effective when passively sensitized, rather than actively sensitized, cells are used[83]. However, it only produces a partial inhibition of histamine release, even from passively sensitized cells, and it is less potent and less effective as an inhibitor of histamine release *in vitro* than it is in the rat PPA system[17]. The system lacks specificity, but again this can be attained with the use of cross-reacting tachyphylaxis[76]. Histamine release by antigen from rat peritoneal mast cells is an energy-dependent process and depends on the viability of the cells. Compounds that interfere with the metabolism of the cells will be likely, therefore, to inhibit histamine release even though the metabolic step that is poisoned may not be directly involved in the release process. This rather obvious fact tends to be forgotten and should be considered when compounds are claimed to stabilize mast cells. In many cases, compounds are likely to inhibit histamine release merely through their toxicity to the treated cell.

Antigen-induced bronchospasm in the rat

DSCG will inhibit bronchospasm in the actively or passively sensitized rat, but is only partially active in the former and produces a bell-shaped dose–response curve[84]. The passively sensitized rat system, however, has been used to evaluate a series of DSCG-like compounds from which the rank order of potency was shown to be similar to that shown in rat PCA[85]. Since the measurement of bronchospasm is more difficult than the measurement of PCA, and there are no apparent compensating advantages, this test is of limited usefulness.

Anaphylaxis in species other than the rat

It has proved to be difficult to achieve reproducible inhibition of anaphylactic reactions with DSCG in animal species other than the rat[30]. Some inhibition of antigen-induced bronchospasm in actively sensitized monkeys[86], passively sensitized marmosets[1] and actively sensitized dogs[87] has been observed, but the variability of the effects reported is too great for the method to have any value as a primary screening procedure[15,87]

Stabilization of human basophils and mast cells

DSCG has no effect on the release of histamine from human basophils[88], but at high doses it will inhibit the antigen-induced release of histamine and SRS-A from passively sensitized human lung fragments. The inhibition is only partial, however, with the drug sometimes producing a bell-shaped dose–response curve, and the effects are variable[33,89,90]. Compounds such as the β-adrenoceptor stimulants, with different modes of activity, are more effective and more potent[91]. The system therefore lacks specificity and is too variable to be useful as a screen for DSCG-like activity.

Cardiovascular effects in the dog

One of the few other pharmacological effects of DSCG is the production of a transient bradycardia and fall in blood pressure when injected intravenously into the dog, a response to which tachyphylaxis rapidly develops[1]. Intravenously administered DSCG is also able to block the reflex bronchoconstriction produced in the anaesthetized dog by the inhalation of histamine, and there is evidence that these effects are all produced by stimulation of a DSCG responsive receptor in the left ventricle of the heart[53]. The hypotension and bradycardia produced in the dog by the stimulation of this receptor by drugs, i.e. the production of the Bezold–Jarisch reflex, and cross-reacting tachyphylaxis with DSCG has been used to identify compounds with similar activities[7,15]. Some compounds that produce cross-reacting tachyphylaxis with DSCG in the rat PCA test also produce the Bezold–Jarisch reflex in the dog[30] and it is not clear whether this reflex and tachyphylaxis with DSCG identifies distinct classes of compounds or rank orders of potency different from those found by the rat PCA test.

Summary

The only reported laboratory tests used to screen compounds for activities similar to DSCG that are reliably reproducible, and that can evaluate sufficient compounds for the determination of structure–activity correlations, remain those that make use of the rat. The obvious criticism of these tests is that they are possibly, and even probably, not relevant to the therapeutic activity of DSCG. Nevertheless, they have been used, particularly the rat PCA test, to evaluate many different structural classes of compound and these will be reviewed in the next section.

Compounds with activities similar to DSCG in biological test systems

The clinical success of DSCG has stimulated considerable interest in compounds having a similar mechanism of action, and the bulk of this interest has centred on the development of compounds which, unlike DSCG, are effective when given orally.

In this section only the scientific literature will be reviewed, the patent literature having been adequately covered in a recent article[92], and the activities of the compounds discussed are those in the rat PCA test unless stated otherwise.

Chromone-2-carboxylic acids

DSCG (1) the clinical pioneer of all compounds of this type, is one of a series of similar bis-chromones which have been described[93], and all are strong acids with a pK_a range of 1.3–2.0. Cross-linking across all but the C-8 positions of the chromone nucleus was found to be compatible with activity in the rat PCA test, and the nature of the bridging moiety had little effect, provided that the total number of bridging atoms did not exceed eight. A single methylene bridge caused a considerable drop in potency, presumably because in this instance coplanarity of the two chromone rings, which is believed to be a prerequisite for activity, is not possible[93].

The benzodipyranones (4–6), which can be regarded as two chromones in which the benzenoid ring is common to both, also show PCA activity, and in this series the linear derivatives (4) and (5) were more potent than their angular counterpart (6)[94]. Some of these compounds were markedly more potent than DSCG, but it is unlikely that any were better orally absorbed.

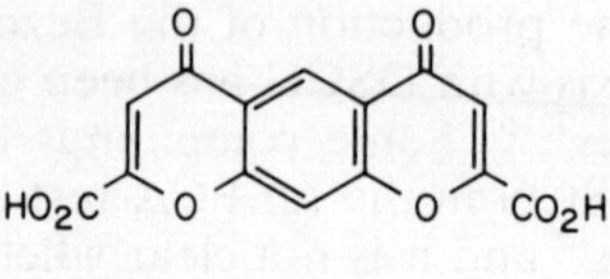

(4)

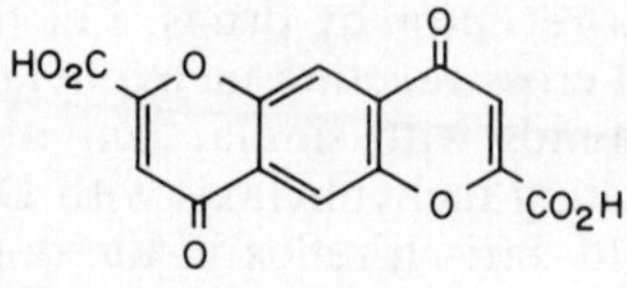

(5)

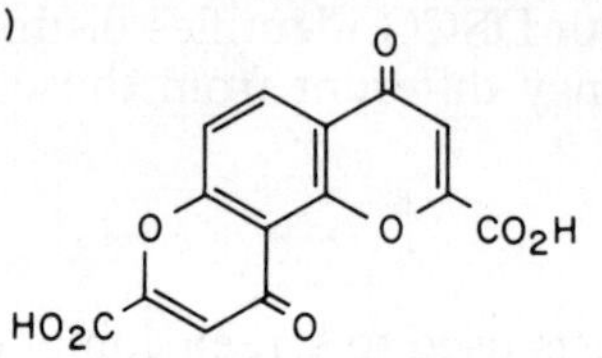

(6)

Only in mono-chromones has oral activity been reported and, in general, this property is a function of greatly increased lipophilicity[7]. One of the first compounds described was the 6,8-di-t-butyl analogue, FPL 52791 (7) with a potency some six times that of DSCG in the rat PCA test and with additional moderate analgesic and anti-inflammatory properties[95]. Soon afterwards two other lipophilic chromones, FPL 52757 (8) and FPL 57787 (9), were reported which, although orally active, were noticeably less

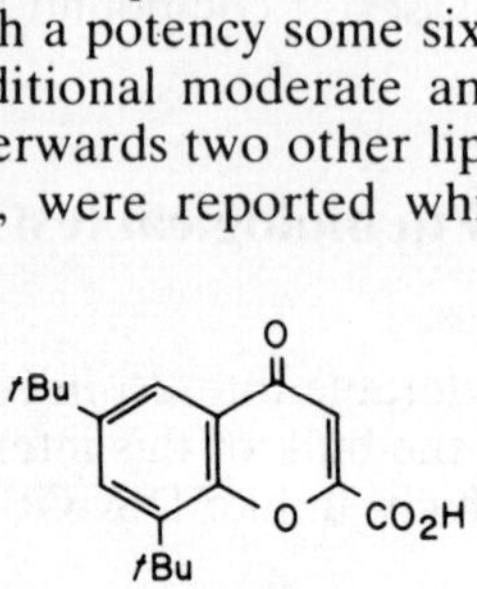

(7)

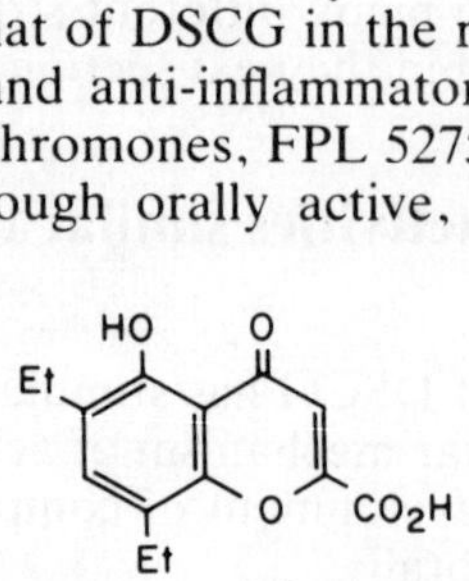

(8)

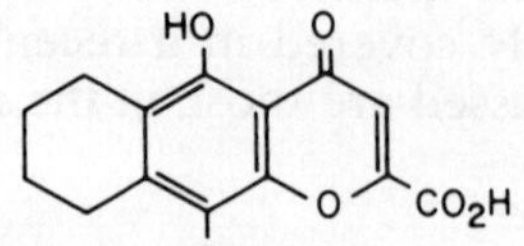

(9)

potent than DSCG[80]. These two compounds were shown to exhibit cross-reacting tachyphylaxis with DSCG, suggesting a similar mode of action, and (8) was active when given by inhalation or orally in bronchial provocation tests in man[80]. The hepatotoxicity shown by (8) has resulted in no further clinical work[96].

Of much greater interest is the tricyclic chromone (9), proxicromil, which has shown efficacy in both antigen-induced[97] and exercise-induced[98] asthmatics and was due for marketing in early 1982 when unfortunate side-effects in long-term toxicology studies in animals necessitated its withdrawal.

The mono-chromone FPL 52694 (10) has been evaluated for inhibitory effects on gastric acid secretion and shown to have weak but significant effects[99]. It appears unlikely, however, that this will be a useful property of this type of compound due to the lack of responsiveness to DSCG of isolated intestinal mucosal mast cells of the rat[100].

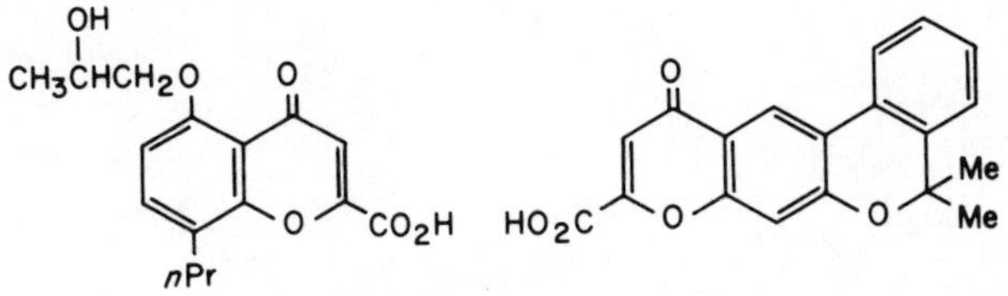

(10)   (11)

The highly lipophilic tetracyclic chromone (11), PR-D-92-Ea, one of a series of similar compounds[101], has been shown to antagonize several of the mediators of anaphylaxis in addition to its ability to inhibit mediator release[102]. The compound has also been shown to inhibit antigen-induced bronchoconstriction in ascaris-sensitive Rhesus monkeys after oral administration[103] and to be reasonably well absorbed orally in man[104]. No clinical data on PR-D-92-Ea has yet been published.

As an extension to chromone-2-carboxylic acids, Ellis and coworkers have replaced the carboxylic acid moiety by the equally acidic 5-tetrazolyl group to give compounds such as (12)[105]. Some of these compounds show enhanced PCA activity over that of DSCG and it was an encouraging result to find that chromone-carboxylic acids were not uniquely active.

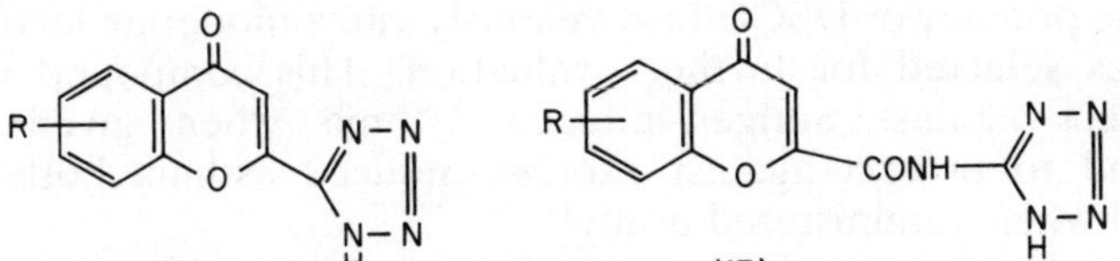

(12)   (13)

This work has been extended to include N-tetrazolylcarboxamides of type (13) which have also been shown to be potent inhibitors of rat PCA[106]. The parent compound, (13, R=H), apparently showed activity similar to DSCG in the clinic[106].

Xanthone-2-carboxylic acids

Soon after the introduction of DSCG, it was realized that structures other than chromone derivatives shared similar biological properties. In particular, among this new generation of compounds were the xanthone-2-carboxylic acids, such as (14), which were born out of the realization that the O–C=C–C=O moiety was common to both nuclei[107]. In the early studies, the requirement for the carboxyl group to be at C–2 was identified in addition to the enhancement of rat PCA activity observed with substituents at the C–5 and C–7 positions[107]. Some of these xanthones, especially 7-alkyloxy derivatives, were orally effective in animal tests and two, AH 7725 (14) and xanoxic acid (15), have inhibited provoked bronchospasm in asthmatics[30].

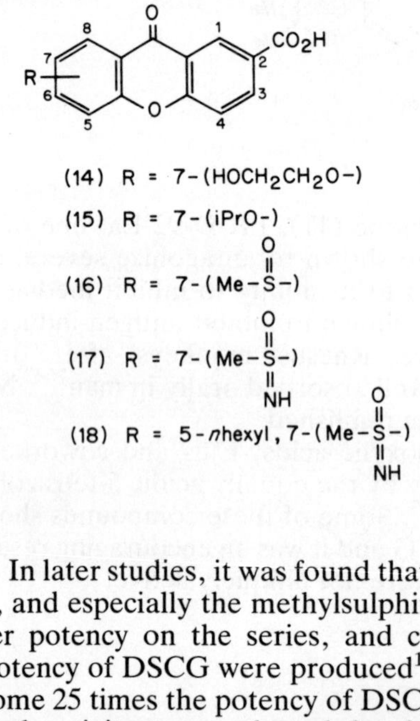

(14) R = 7-(HOCH$_2$CH$_2$O–)

(15) R = 7-(iPrO-)

(16) R = 7-(Me–$\overset{\text{O}}{\overset{\|}{\text{S}}}$–)

(17) R = 7-(Me–$\overset{\text{O}}{\overset{\|}{\underset{\|}{\underset{\text{NH}}{\text{S}}}}}$–)

(18) R = 5-$n$hexyl, 7-(Me–$\overset{\text{O}}{\overset{\|}{\underset{\|}{\underset{\text{NH}}{\text{S}}}}}$–)

In later studies, it was found that electron-withdrawing substituents at C-7, and especially the methylsulphinyl group, could impart somewhat greater potency on the series, and compounds having up to 260 times the potency of DSCG were produced[108]. From this series tixanox (16), having some 25 times the potency of DSCG intravenously and a moderate level of oral activity, was selected for further evaluation. This compound was shown to protect against antigen-induced asthma when given by inhalation[109], and to protect against exercise-induced asthma both by inhalation[110] and when administered orally[111].

Encouraged by these results, a large number of xanthone-2-carboxylic acids and their esters and amides have been prepared[112–114], but only one compound, the sulphoximide (18), with some 260 times the potency of DSCG, has emerged as a clinical candidate[114]. It is of interest that the 2-(S-methylsuphonimidoyl)-xanthone (19), prepared as a biological isostere of xanthone-2-carboxylic acid, was devoid of rat PCA activity, whereas the combined derivative (17) had some 30–40 times the potency of DSCG[114].

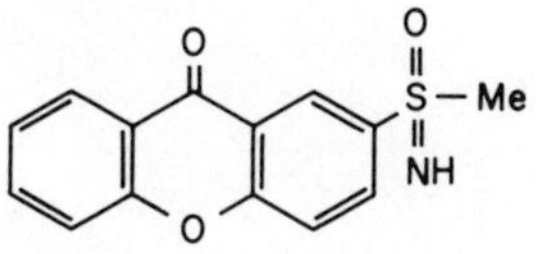

(19)

More recently, an aza analogue of the xanthone carboxylic acids has been reported, in which the carboxylic acid moiety is replaced by the acidic tetrazole group[115]. This compound, Y-12,141 (20), embodies a number of structural features characteristic of DSCG-like compounds (see below) and, although only 5 times the potency of DSCG, is orally active and of low toxicity[115]. No clinical data are currently available on this compound.

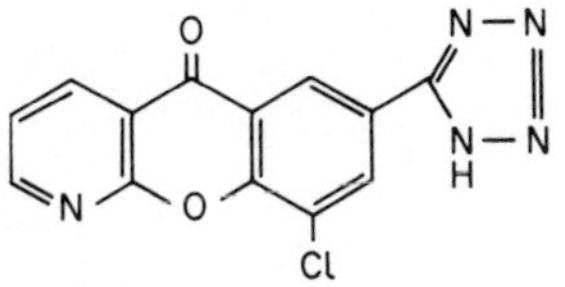

(20) 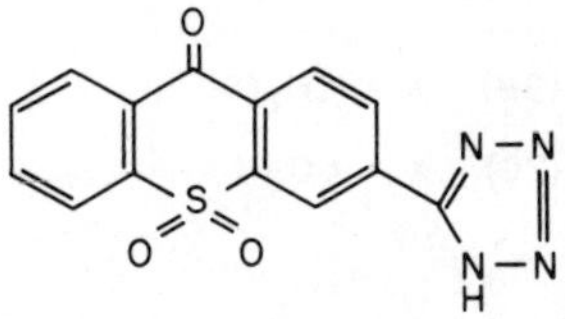   (21)

A related compound, doxantrazole (21), in which the xanthone bridging oxygen atom is replaced by the sulphonyl group, was one of the earlier compounds of the DSCG type reported to be orally effective[116]. This compound, with an oral dose producing 50% maximal response (ED$_{50}$) of 10 mg/kg in the rat PCA test[30,116], was of added interest because of its extended duration of activity, a 30 mg/kg p.o. dose resulting in activity lasting up to 7 hours[116]. Initial clinical studies with doxantrazole against antigen-induced bronchospasm offered encouragement[117], but later studies at both 200 mg and 400 mg doses failed to elicit significant protection[118]. Furthermore, a 14-day repeat dose study (400 mg three times daily) failed to demonstrate a beneficial effect[118]. The absence of useful activity against exercise-induced bronchospasm[119] has resulted in a curtailment of further development.

Flavones and other pyranone derivatives

Based on the knowledge that extracts containing the flavonoid baicalein (22) and its disodium phosphate (23) have anti-anaphylactic properties[120], attempts have been made by Nohara and his colleagues to improve the potency of these natural materials[121,122]. Preliminary studies by this group identified enhanced potency in chromones bearing carbonyl substituents at the C-3 position, although simple aldehydes and carboxylic acids, such as (24) and (25), respectively, did not inhibit rat PCA[121,122]. In contrast to these results, however, the 3-hydroxymethyl chromone (28) (W-8011) was active in rat PCA but was inactive in vitro, suggesting that the carboxylic acid (29) is the active species[123].

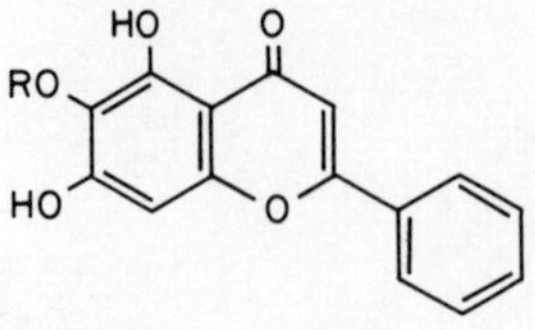

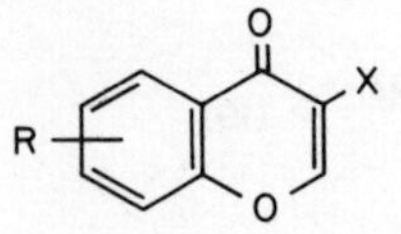

(22)   R = H
(23)   R = PO(ONa)$_2$

(24)   X = CHO
(25)   X = CO$_2$H
(26)   X = CH=CHCO$_2$H
(27)   X = CH$_2$CH$_2$CO$_2$H

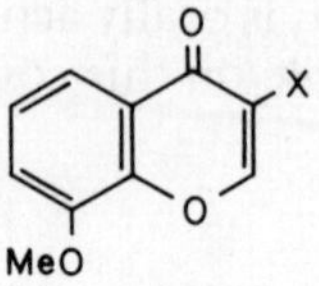

(28)   X = CH$_2$OH
(29)   X = CO$_2$H

The loss of activity in the carboxylic acids (25), considered to be a reflection of intramolecular hydrogen bonding of the 4-keto group with the acid, and consequent reduction of acidity, was avoided in the vinologous acrylic acids (26) in which this hydrogen bonding is not possible[124]. Structure–activity studies on this acrylic acid series[121] revealed a loss of activity in the propanoate derivatives (27) and a strong steric preference for the *E* geometric isomer. Although members of this series show oral activity, there are no reports of any further evaluation.

Additional studies in which the carboxyl group of (25) was replaced by a 5-tetrazolyl moiety, however, tend to be more promising[124]. From this series, the 6-ethyl homologue, AA-344 (30), was selected for more detailed evaluation[125,126] and clinical benefit in human asthma has been reported[122].

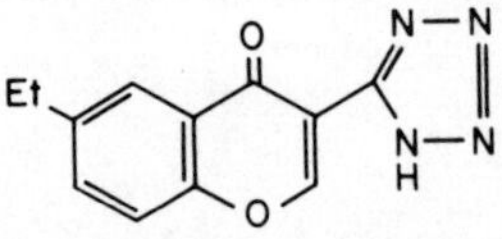

(30)

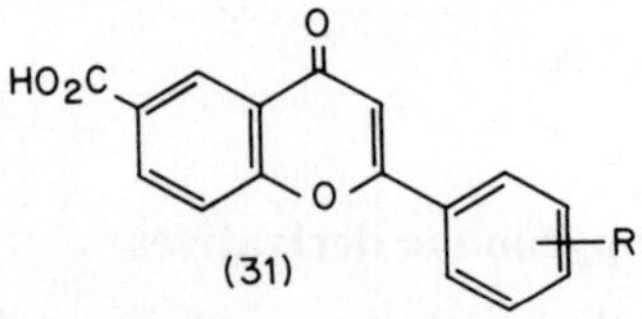

(31)

In addition to the developments outlined above, a number of workers have concentrated on carboxylated flavones[127–130], most of which fall within the general scope of formula (31) and have a strong analogy with xanthone-2-carboxylic acids[127,128]. A number of modifications, including replacement of the pendant phenyl ring of (31) by aromatic heterocycles[129], and vinologous extention of the appended ring[130] have been studied. In general, none of these modifications offer a great advantage over DSCG although oral activity has been observed[129,130]. Some derivatives of (31) have been shown to inhibit histamine-induced gastric secretion[127], but whether or not this action is of therapeutic value is not known.

Annellated 4-pyranones

4-Pyranone-2-carboxylic acids annellated with heterocyclic rings have received attention by several groups[131–134], but the resulting compounds, (32) and (33), are generally of equal or diminished potency to DSCG. Possibily the most interesting class of compounds are the pyranoindoles (32, X = NR') in which the carboxyl group is replaced by the 5-tetrazolyl group. These compounds display a reasonable level of oral PCA activity and are potential candidates for further evaluation[132].

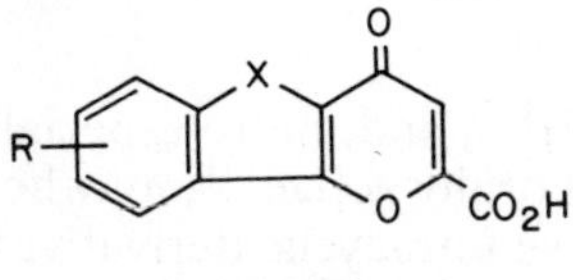

(32)   X = O, S, NR'

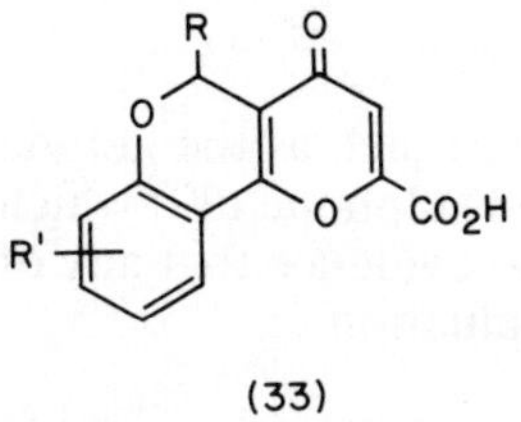

(33)

Quinoline carboxylic acids and related compounds

Apart from the modifications of DSCG which have retained the 4-pyranone moiety (*see* previous sections), a considerable amount of interest has been shown in the related pyridone analogues, and especially in derivatives of 1,4-dihydro-4-oxoquinoline-2- and 3-carboxylic acids of the general type (34)[135–138].

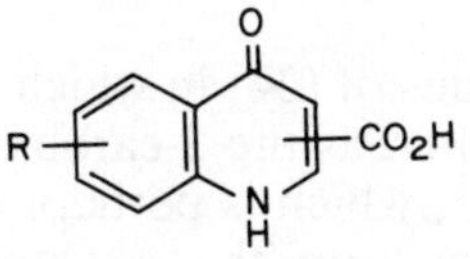

(34)

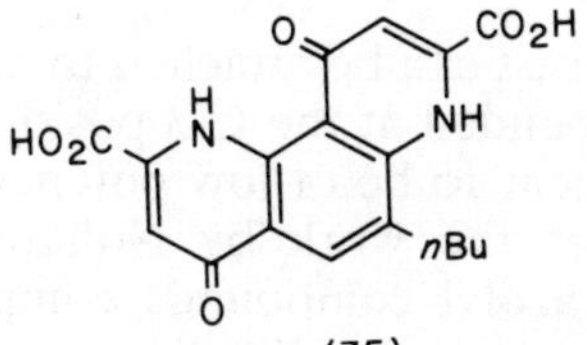

(35)

Much of this interest was initiated in the early 1970s when the simultaneous work of two groups first identified compounds with PCA activity in a series of 1,4-dihydro-4-oxoquinoline-2-carboxylic acids[135,136]. Subsequently this work led to studies on bis-quinolines more akin to the structure of DSCG itself and finally to tri- and tetracyclic compounds[135,139] from which bufrolin (35) (ICI 74,917) was selected for further evaluation[135]. Bufrolin, which is the most potent compound of its type so far reported, has some 300 times the potency of DSCG when administered i.v. in the rat

PCA test and, like DSCG, has no anti-mediator properties[135]. Unfortunately, the compound has no oral activity and its poor performance in clinical trials resulted in its withdrawal from further development[30].

Later work on other 2-carboxylic acid derivatives has failed to identify compounds with a markedly improved profile to that of bufrolin, although weak oral activity has been reported for the related linear derivative (36) (U-38,650)[140].

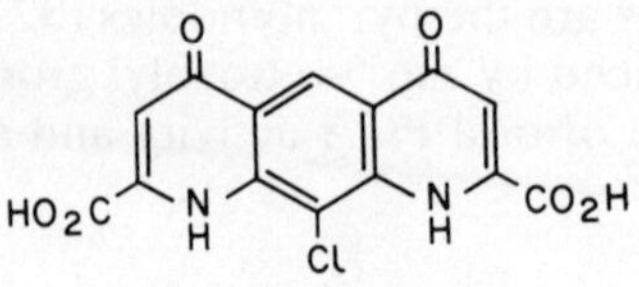

(36)

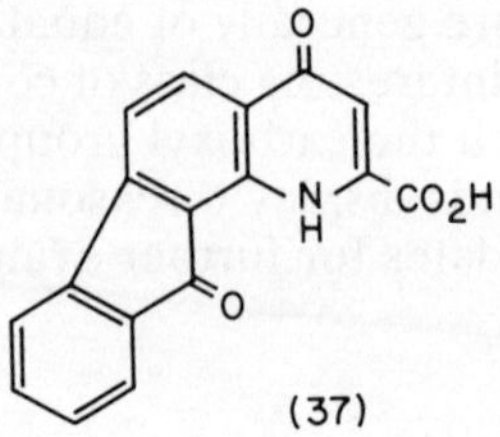

(37)

Annellated derivatives such as the ketone (37)[137], and, more especially, the sulphoxide (38) and sulphone (39) which are orally active[141], may be of interest, but there is no evidence that any of these tetracyclic derivatives is undergoing further evaluation.

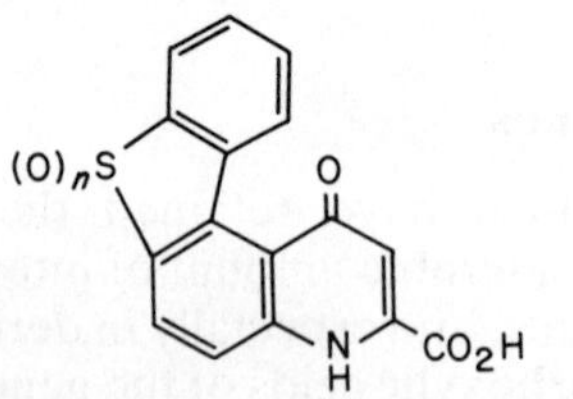

(38) n = 1
(39) n = 2

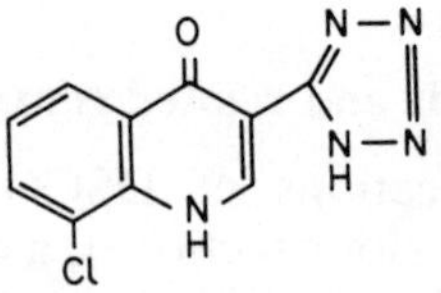

(40)

Possibly more interest can be attached to analogues of (34) in which the acidic function is appended at the C-3 position. Whereas the 3-carboxylic acids themselves appear to be of low potency[136,138], which is perhaps not surprising in view of the work by Nohara's group on the analogous chromones[124], 5-tetrazolyl compounds comprise a potent group. Specifically, the 8-chloro derivative (40), having some 33 times the potency of DSCG when given i.v. and with additional oral activity, was selected for further study but later abandoned because of low solubility and its tendency to cause crystalluria[138].

Oxamates, quinazolines and related derivatives

Once DSCG-like activity was demonstrated in the quinoline carboxylic acids, a further incremental step led to the related quinazolines. In one study, the detailed evaluation of the 5-methoxy derivative (41) led to the identification of an acyclic contaminant, the oxamate (42) (Wy-16,922), of unexpectedly greater potency in the rat PCA test[142]. Although (42) was of low potency relative to DSCG, its oral activity led to its further progression. The pharmacology of compound (42) has been discussed in detail[143] but its clinical performance was disappointing[144].

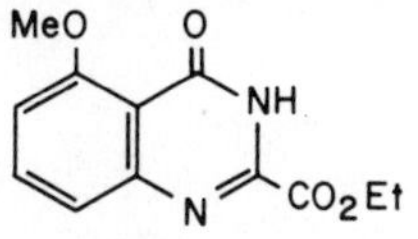

(41)

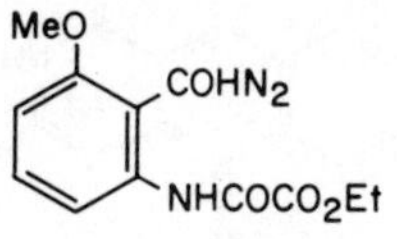

(42)

Further modification of the aromatic substituents, however, has resulted in analogues with a marked improvement in potency and one compound, the methylamino derivative (43) (Wy-41,195) with an oral ED_{50} of 0.07 mg/kg in the rat PCA has been extensively studied as a potential clinical candidate[145].

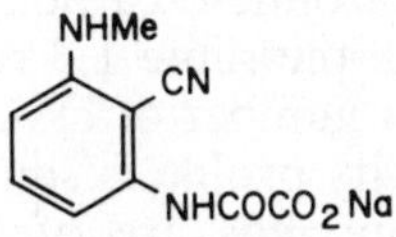

(43)

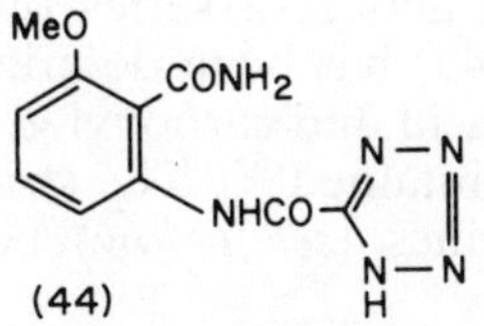

(44)

Tetrazole analogues of (43) have also been prepared[146], but these appear to offer no advantage. The preferred compound from a series was the analogue (44)[146].

A considerable improvement in potency has been achieved by coalescing the oxamate moiety with quinoline-2-carboxylic acids, as in (45), which have up to 25 times the potency of DSCG[147], but it is unlikely that oral absorption is retained.

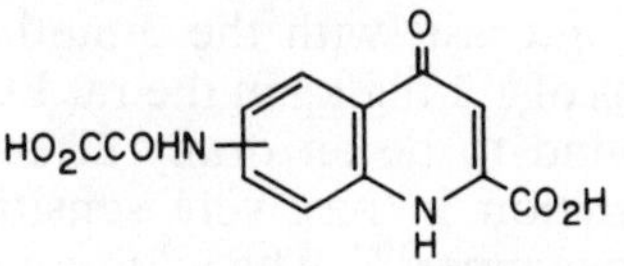

(45)

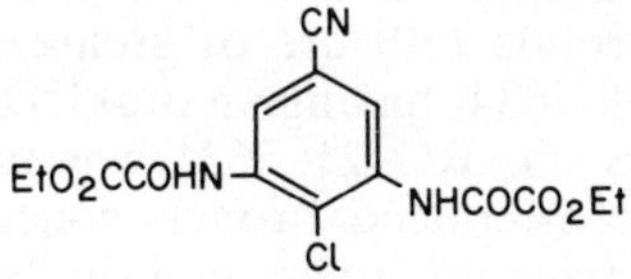

(46)

A more profitable approach using bis-oxamate functionality has led to some of the most potent inhibitors of rat PCA known. One of these compounds, lodoxamide ethyl (46), has some 2500 times the potency of DSCG given intravenously and shows activity when given orally[148]. This compound, and the di-tromethamine salt of its diacid (lodoxamide), have shown benefit in the clinic against bronchial provocation and exercise-induced bronchospasm[149,150].

More recently a series of N-troponyloxamic acid esters, of which the parent compound (47) was preferred, have been shown to inhibit rat paw anaphylaxis[151]. This compound was of comparable potency to that of DSCG but in contrast was orally effective.

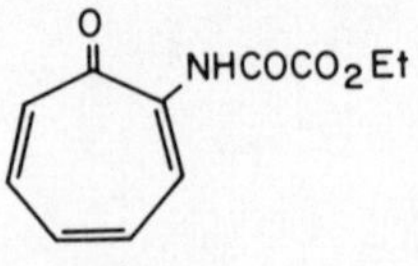

(47) 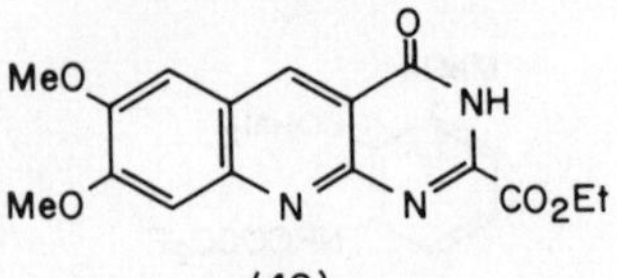   (48)

In addition to the oxamate developments, a number of workers have reported on the further elaboration of 3,4-dihydro-4-oxoquinazoline-2-carboxylic acid. By successive modification of the parent system, the potency of this weakly active compound was increased several-fold and led to the development of pirolate (48), a pyrimidoquinoline which has some 84 times the potency of DSCG in the rat PCA screen and is orally effective with an ED_{50} of 1.0 mg/kg[152-154].

Using a somewhat different approach, but one which may be likened to the flavones discussed above, a series of 2-arylquinazoline-6-carboxylic acids of general type (49) has been described in which the same 1,3 relationship of carboxylic acid and carbonyl group, as in a number of DSCG-like compounds, is maintained[155]. The structure–activity profile is similar to that of the azapurines (see below) but the compounds are of low potency.

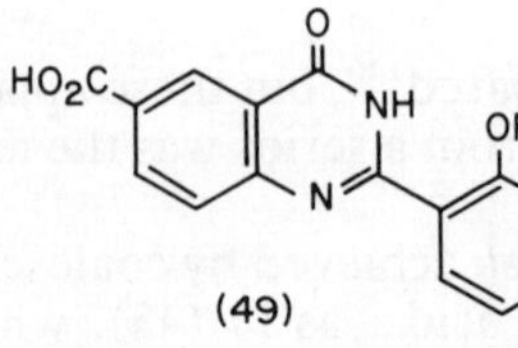

(49) 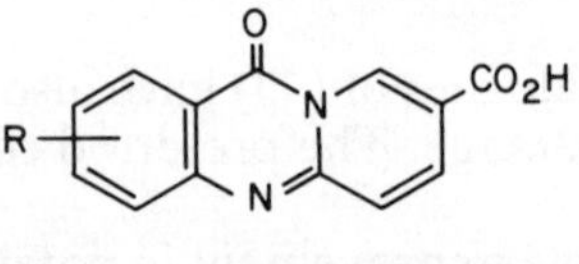   (50)

Annellation of the pyrimidine ring in the quinazolines has produced a number of compounds of interest[156-158] and the structure–activity profile for these tricyclic derivatives has been reasonably well defined. In general, compounds of formula (50) are of greatest interest, with the 3-methoxy compound, RO 21–7634, having an oral ED_{50} of 1.1 mg/kg in the rat PCA. In contrast to DSCG, RO 21–7634 was found to be an orally effective inhibitor of antigen-induced bronchoconstriction in passively sensitized rats[159], although it appears to act in a similar manner[160]. The addition of a further nitrogen atom to compounds of type (50) has also been studied, but the resulting compounds, (51), despite having a similar intravenous potency to that of the deaza analogues, are orally inactive[161].

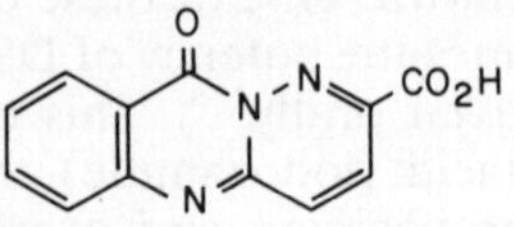

(51) 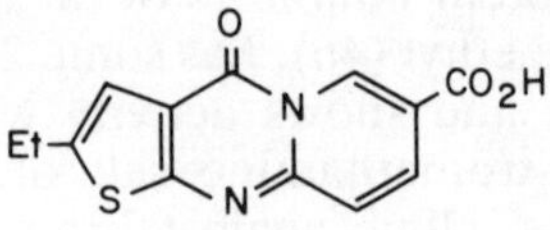   (52)

Compounds with moderate oral activity have been prepared by substitution of a thienyl ring for the benzenoid ring of (50). Thus, (52) and tetrazole-derived compounds have been identified as the most potent in this series[162].

In a similar vein, the bicyclic pyrimidine (53) has shown moderate oral PCA activity[163], but again it is unlikely that compounds of this type offer any advantage over some of the more potent compounds described above.

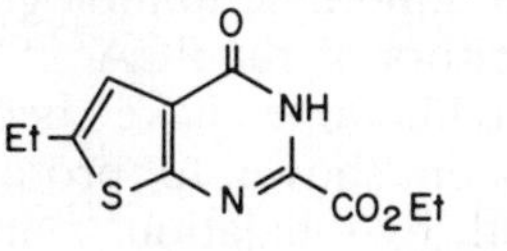

(53) 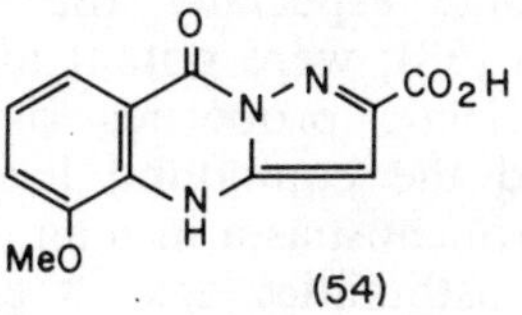   (54)

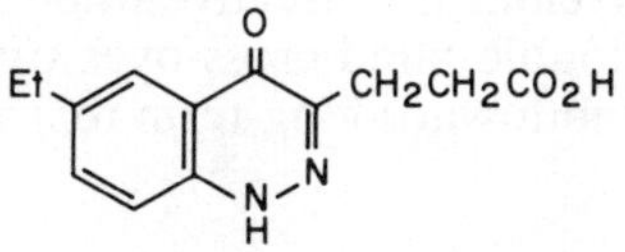

(55)

A number of potent compounds have been identified in an extensive series of pyrazoloquinolinone-2-carboxylic acids and the related (N-tetrazolyl)-carboxamides and tetrazoles, and one compound, the 5-methoxy derivative (54) with 250 times the intravenous potency of DSCG in the rat PCA screen, has been described[164]. Members of this series also show oral activity, but there is no indication that any compound is undergoing further evaluation.

Oral activity has also been observed in a series of cinnoline-3-propionic acids, although the potency of the group as a whole is low[165]. Within this series, the preferred compounds are the 6-ethyl homologue (55) and its ethyl ester, which are some two-fold less potent than DSCG. The possibility that these compounds owe their activity to β-oxidation to the corresponding cinnoline-3-carboxylic acids, whose structure is closer to that of known DSCG-like compounds, cannot be discounted, but no evidence is available to support this suggestion[165].

Slightly better potency has been reported for the hydrazono-pyrido-pyrimidinone, Chinoin-1045 or UCB.L140 (56), which is one of a series of similar compounds developed from the analgesic rimazolium (57)[166]. Few of the analogues of (56) have noteworthy activity, however, but it is of interest that the activity of (56) itself is exclusive to the ($6S$)-isomer. On the basis of its oral efficacy, Chinoin-1045 has undergone extensive pharmacological evaluation[167] and has been selected for clinical study[166].

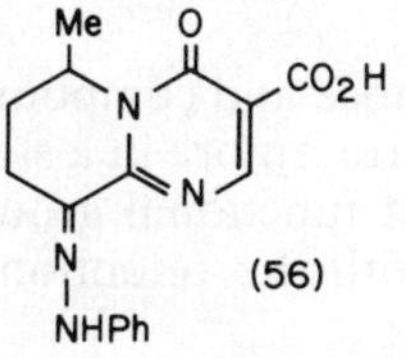

(56) 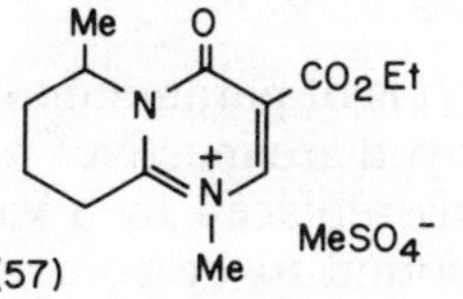   (57)

Nitro- and cyano-1,3-dicarbonyl compounds

From the previous sections, it will have been noticed that compounds with DSCG-like activity have generally been acidic compounds, or latentiated derivatives thereof, and that this acidity has usually been imparted by the carboxyl or tetrazolyl moieties. However, activity of the type shown by DSCG is not exclusive to compounds containing one or other of these two functional groups and, in 1973, it was shown that another acidic class, the 2-nitroindan-1,3-diones, and especially the 5,6-dimethyl homologue (nivimedone, BRL 10833) (58), were potent inhibitors of rat PCA[77,168]. The detailed anti-anaphylactic properties of nivimedone have been described[77,82,83,169–171] and the compound has been shown to protect against antigen-induced bronchospasm in man, both by inhalation[172] and orally[173], and to protect asthmatics against exercise-induced broncho-constriction[174]. Nivimedone was also clinically effective when administered orally to asthmatics in a six-week double-blind cross-over trial[66], but was subsequently withdrawn because of untoward long-term toxicity in rats[66].

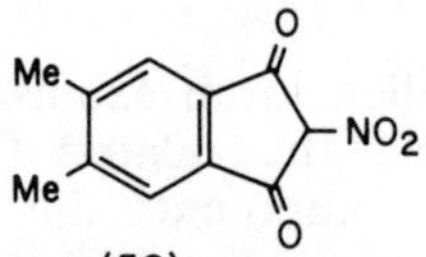

(58) 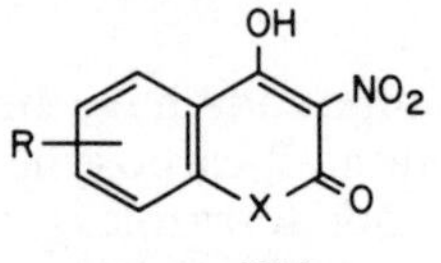   (59) 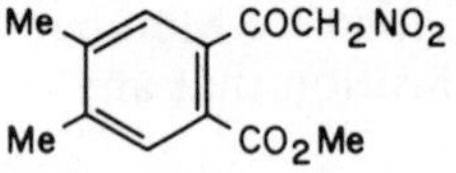   (60)

A number of compounds similar to nivimedone have also been described. Many of these fall within the general formula (59) in which X is an oxygen[175] or nitrogen[176] atom, or a carbonyl group[177], and were generally potent, orally effective compounds with a similar structure–activity profile to that of the nitroindan-1,3-diones in the rat PCA test. Analogous compounds of formula (59), in which X is a carbon atom bearing one or two alkyl groups, were inactive[177]. From these studies it was evident that, in this system at least, the requirement of a planar system was an essential prerequisite for biological activity[176,178].

In related work, activity was also observed in a monocyclic system based on 2-(nitroacetyl)benzoic acid, but a detailed study on the most potent compound (60) clearly showed that this compound was readily metabolized to the corresponding nitroindan-1,3-dione (58) and that this was the most likely reason for its activity[179].

The acidity of (58) and (59) is of paramount importance and compounds in which this acidity is destroyed are inactive[168,179]. Furthermore in a study in which the nitro group was replaced by a variety of functional groups, only the cyano group was found to be compatible with the retention of reasonable potency[180].

Purines, pyrimidines and related compounds

Compositions containing theophylline (61) have a long history of use as bronchodilators in the treatment of asthma, but bronchodilatation is just one of the many activities of this drug. Although relatively weak, theophylline and other methylxanthines such as caffeine (62), are also known to inhibit rat PCA[181]. During attempts to improve this activity of these compounds, it was soon realized that 8-aza analogues were some ten times more potent in this respect, and that within a series of general type (63) those derivatives having bulky substituents, e.g. benzyl, at the 3-position were optimal[181].

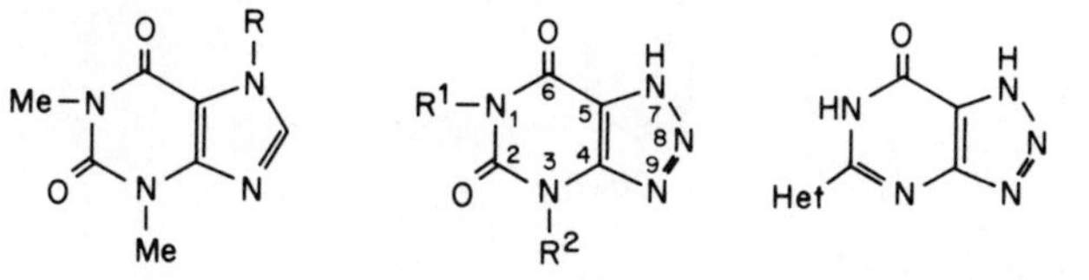

(61)   R = H   (63)   (64)

(62)   R = Me

A further improvement in PCA activity was demonstrated in the related 8-azahypoxanthines (64), in which a bulky heteroaromatic group replaced the carbonyl group at the 2-position[182]. In this series, it was suggested that coplanarity of the purine nucleus and the pendant aromatic ring were conducive to enhanced potency. Even so, within the small range of derivatives studied only a two-fold improvement over DSCG was observed[182]. A significant advance in this interesting approach came with the study of analogues of (64) in which the pendant ring was benzenoid[183]. In this series, a linear free-energy correlation was successfully used to identify the 2-*n*-propyloxy derivative, M&B 22948 (65), as the most potent compound within the series, having some 40 times the intravenous potency of DSCG. Again the high potency of this compound correlated well with coplanarity of the two ring systems, which was favoured by strong hydrogen bonding between the purine N-H and the ethereal oxygen atom[183]. The coplanarity within this compound was subsequently confirmed by X-ray crystallographic studies[184].

In addition to its PCA activity, which is also evident orally, M&B 22948 has been shown to be more potent than DSCG at inhibiting the anaphylactic release of both histamine and SRS-A from human lung tissue[185]. Furthermore, the compound has been reported to antagonize some of the purported mediators of the allergic response, histamine, SRS-A and $PGF_{2\alpha}$, on isolated bronchial muscle[185]. M&B 22948 has progressed into man and preliminary results suggest that it is effective at preventing antigen-induced bronchospasm when given at a 5-mg dose by metered aerosol[186].

A number of related derivatives have been studied by other workers and two, the azahypoxanthine (66) and the aza-adenine (67) have shown low PCA activity by the intraperitoneal route, but are devoid of oral activity[187,188].

Pyrimidine analogues of (65) have also been extensively studied. In a series of acids and esters of general formula (68), potent oral activity in the rat PCA test was observed with structure–activity correlations paralleling those found for the analogous purines[189]. More recently this series was the subject of quantitative structure–activity relationship (QSAR) studies which reinforced the original conclusions[190].

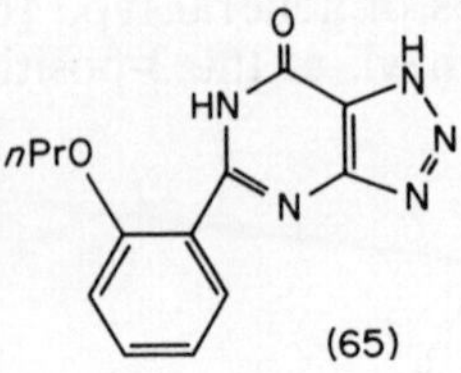

(65)

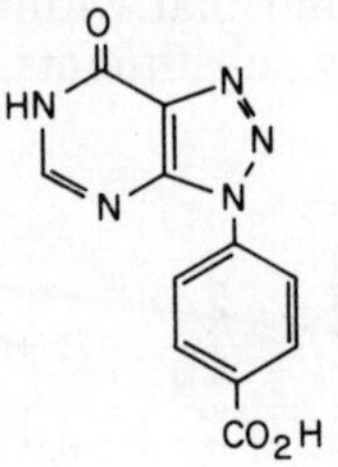

(66)

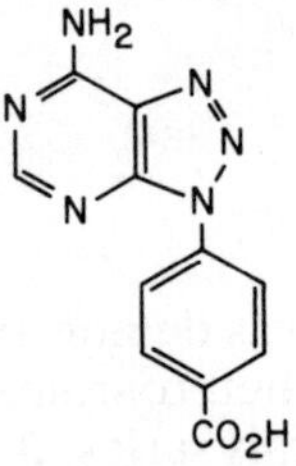

(67)

Of somewhat greater interest, however, are the related 5-tetrazolyl ana-logues of (68) which again follow the expected structure–activity profile[191]. These derivatives were shown to have some 5–10 times the oral potency of the corresponding carboxylic acids in the rat PCA test, with BL-5255 (69), having an intravenous potency approximately 50 times that of DSCG[191,192]. BL-5255 has been the subject of more extensive study[192] and is reported to be undergoing clinical assessment[191].

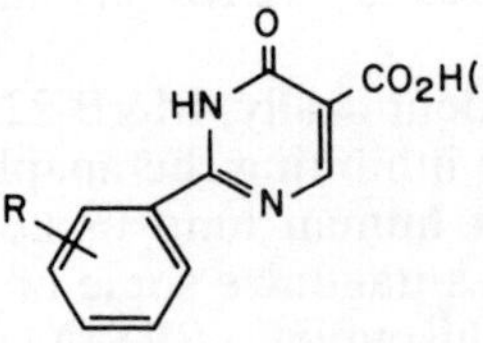

(68)

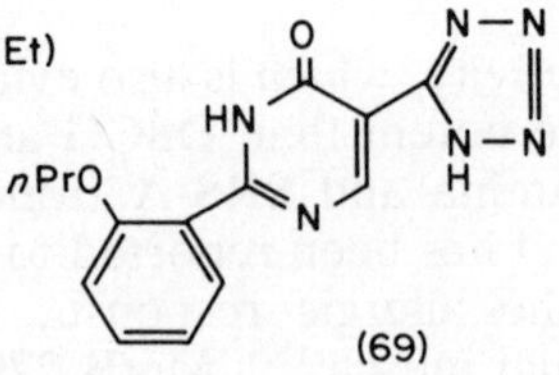

(69)

More distantly related compounds, such as the triazoloquinolines (70), which like M&B 22948 utilize the acidity of the triazole nucleus, have been reported to show activity of the DSCG type[193], and more extensive studies on the isosteric benzopyranotriazoles (71) have identified compounds with intravenous potencies of some 10 times that of DSCG in the rat PCA test[194].

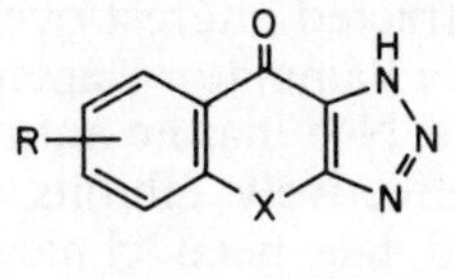

(70)   X = NH

(71)   X = O

(72)   X = CO

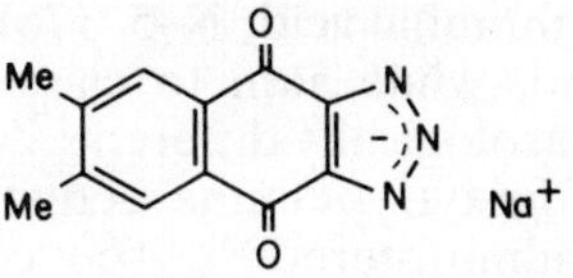

(73)

Of markedly greater importance, however, are the allied naphtho-triazoles (72) which, in general, are more potent than the other two series[195], and one compound, BRL 22321A (73), is currently undergoing clinical assessment. This compound has some 50 times the intravenous potency of DSCG in the rat PCA reaction and is a potent inhibitor when orally administered[195]. More detailed studies have shown cross-reacting tachyphylaxis with DSCG in the rat PCA test[17]. The additional smooth muscle relaxant activity reported for BRL 22321A and its ability to stabilize mast cells of species other than the rat were additional factors leading to its selection for further evaluation[17].

Miscellaneous compounds

Apart from the well-defined groups of DSCG-like compounds set out on pp. 271–285, a large number of structural types have been described which are not readily rationalized in terms of a unifying set of structural features. Since it is an impossible task to list all of these variants in a meaningful way, only those compounds which are of structural or clinical interest have been selected for inclusion in this section.

Perhaps one of the most interesting approaches is that which led to the development of the pyranenamines. A large number of these derivatives have been studied using QSAR techniques and a compound (74) with some 1000 times the potency of DSCG was identified[196–198]. As a result of more detailed analysis, a less potent compound, SK&F 78729-A (75), was chosen for further evaluation[196].

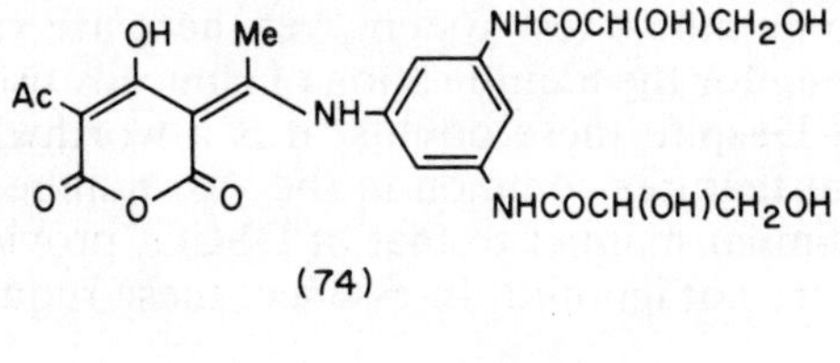

(74)

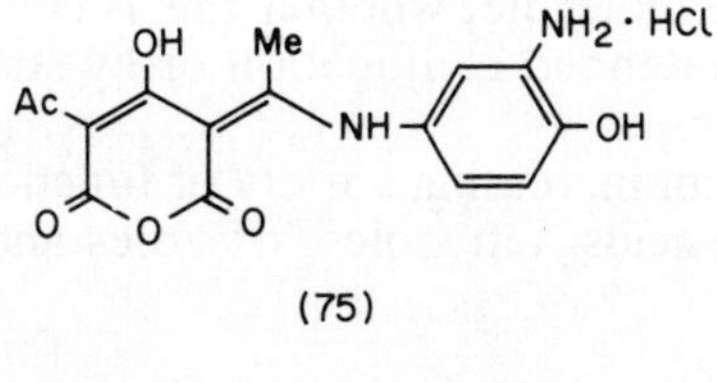

(75)

The cinnamoyl anthranilic acid, N–5' (76), has attracted interest over a number of years and, while akin to classical anti-inflammatory agents, appears to be pharmacologically different[199,200]. Thus, N–5' has no antihistamine or anti-5-hydroxytryptamine activity but effectively inhibits rat PCA when orally administered[200]. The compound has been clinically evaluated in a large group of asthmatic children over a four-week period and showed significant benefit when administered orally in three daily doses totalling 6 or 10 mg/kg per day[201].

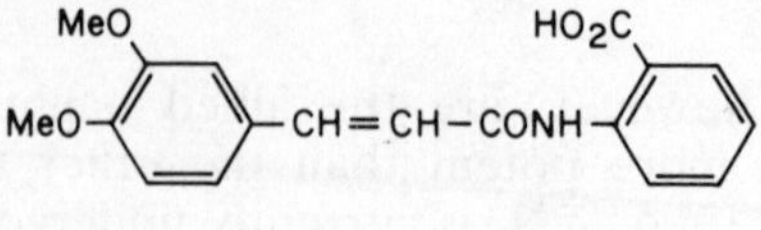

MeO

MeO—⟨ ⟩—CH = CH—CONH—⟨ ⟩—HO_2C

(76)

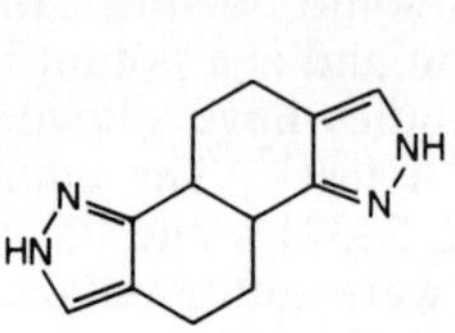

(77)

The bis-pyrazole LC–6 (77) is yet another structurally unique compound which inhibits rat PCA when administered orally, but its intrinsic potency is weak[202,203]. The compound shows an extended duration of activity compared to most DSCG-like compounds and, although it is suggested that its action is similar to that of DSCG, its failure to show cross-tachyphylaxis might suggest an alternative mode of action[204].

Structural rationalization of DSCG-like compounds

Throughout the previous sections an underlying trend toward a structural pattern, albeit sometimes far from obvious, is generally evident. A number of workers have attempted to unify the structural parameters essential for DSCG-like activity[92,142,205,206] and, within the series based on the 2-nitro-1,3-dicarbonyl moiety, we ourselves have tried to define the precise constraints for biological activity[177]. In all these correlations the rat PCA reaction has featured strongly as the definitive test system, yet there are valid doubts as to the value of this screen for the identification of clinically useful compounds of the DSCG type. Despite these doubts, it is a worthwhile exercise to summarize the salient features common to the vast number of compounds claimed to act in a similar manner to that of DSCG, provided that the associated reservations are not ignored. In essence, these requirements are:

(a) **Planarity** of a substantial part of the molecule, whether this is conferred by aromaticity or π overlap in extended conjugation or by strong intramolecular hydrogen bonding.

(b) **Acidity,** usually imparted by one of an increasing variety of functional groups among which are carboxylic acids, tetrazoles, triazoles and 2-nitro-1,3-dicarbonyl moieties.

(c) **Carbonyl groups** and/or **heteroatoms**. Most DSCG-like compounds have at least one carbonyl group which is usually conjugated to an aromatic ring and through which the acidic moiety is frequently attached. In addition, heterocyclic systems are often the carrier ring of the carbonyl function with the most notable exceptions being those compounds containing two symmetrical homoannular carbonyl groups (e.g. nitroindandiones[168] and naphthotriazoles[195]).

These requirements are epitomized in structure (78) in which the ring A may be an aromatic ring, or a saturated or partially saturated derivative thereof, or a pendant aromatic nucleus hydrogen bonded to the parent ring system such that coplanarity is attained. In the parent ring system, X may be a heteroatom, a carbonyl group, or a carbonyl group equivalent (e.g. SO_2), and Y may be a bond, a carbon atom or a nitrogen atom. The acidic function, depending on its character, may be pendant or fused to the parent ring or may be conjugated to it via vinylation or an aromatic ring.

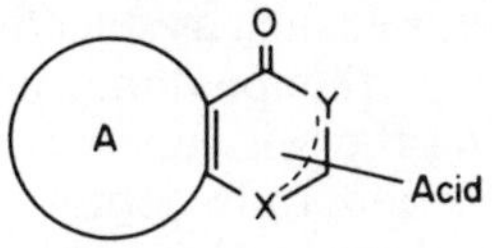

(78)

Apart from the miscellaneous compounds discussed here, the most notable exceptions to this generalized (and possibly ambitious) unified structure are the oxamates discussed on p. 279, although even within this class the cyclic analogues, the quinazolines, fall within the framework of structure (78).

Conclusion and possible future developments

The underlying concern about all compounds with purported DSCG-like activity is the lack of suitable biological screening models capable of predicting clinical efficacy and, until a drug selected from the currently available screens demonstrates real clinical benefit, this concern is likely to remain. To date, proxicromil is the only compound of its type that has come close to being marketed and it is unfortunate that this compound failed in a late stage of toxicity studies.

An understanding of the mechanism by which DSCG shows its activity might allow the development of more relevant tests. There have been numerous attempts to correlate the activity of DSCG and similar compounds with physical parameters, such as acidity[93], and with the inhibition of a variety of enzyme systems, such as cyclic nucleotides[207], oxidative enzymes[208], and alkaline phosphatase[209], but the significance of these correlations is not clear. Most laboratory screens to detect DSCG-like compounds in animals involve the administration of a single dose of the compound under test. When given in a single dose to asthmatics, DSCG can protect against provoked bronchospasm, but this might not be relevant to its therapeutic benefit, which sometimes only becomes apparent after repeat dosing for some time, often weeks[11]. Tests involving chronic dosing to animals might give results with greater relevance to the clinical situation than those from single dose studies, although such tests would reduce the number of compounds that could be evaluated.

But what can be done in the absence of proven predictive tests, and do we need to look more closely at the current methods of clinical evaluation? Clearly these are difficult questions to answer, but it might prove of value to reappraise present-day clinical assessment since the situation today is considerably more complex than in 1967 when DSCG was first shown to be of benefit. At that time in the United Kingdom, asthmatic patients were probably undertreated with drugs. There was a reluctance to prescribe oral corticosteroids or theophylline because of their side-effects, and there was a well-publicized apparent association between the use of inhaled isoprenaline and an increase in deaths from asthma[210,211]. Inhaled corticosteroids and inhaled selective β-adrenoceptor stimulants were not available at this time and there was a need for a new effective drug treatment. It is likely that, because of this restricted drug usage, the clinical benefit threshold was low. Today, however, most patients selected for clinical trials are already controlled by some form of maintenance therapy, such as selective β_2-adrenoceptor stimulants, inhaled corticosteroids or theophylline, and the benefit threshold by comparison is greater than in otherwise uncontrolled patients. Moreover, this maintenance therapy is generally continued throughout the clinical evaluation of new candidate drugs and it is likely that the drug would have to be markedly effective to produce a measurable improvement. Possibly in this present-day environment, new DSCG-like drugs might only show real clinical efficacy if given to patients previously removed from all other drug treatment when the benefit threshold would again be basal. It is doubtful, however, that normal ethics would allow such a practice to be carried out, if indeed the patients were prepared to comply.

Much of the effort devoted to finding a successor to DSCG has been directed towards orally effective drugs, and again this may not be the best approach. It is possible that compounds lacking oral absorption, but of high potency, may be preferred since these materials could be administered directly to the lung by aerosol with little concern for the majority of the material which ultimately enters the stomach. Orally absorbed materials, on the other hand, might yield undesirable side-effects due to increased systemic absorption.

Since DSCG is not of benefit to all patients, there is a need for drugs with activities additional to those shown by DSCG. Some of these drugs obviously form a part of other chapters within this book, but there are others which bridge the conceptual boundaries of asthma therapy and deserve mention here. One such approach has been adopted in our own laboratories over the past few years in which we have attempted to combine mast-cell-stabilizing properties with specific mediator antagonism. Since DSCG does not equally inhibit the release of all mediators of anaphylaxis and, in particular, is poor at inhibiting the release of SRS-A from non-mast cell sources[16,170,212,213] nitrocoumarins, such as (79) have been studied which effectively combine the inhibition of histamine release with specific SRS-A antagonism[214]. Similar combined effects have been reported for PR-D-92-Ea (11), and M&B 22948 (65) which are somewhat less potent and specific as SRS-A antagonists[101,102,185].

An alternative and complimentary approach is offered by isamoxole (80), which is one of a series of similar oxazoles[215]. Isamoxole, while not inhibiting the rat PCA reaction, was reported to inhibit the release of both histamine and SRS-A from chopped guinea-pig and human lung, suggesting that this might be a more effective overall inhibitor of mediator release[215].

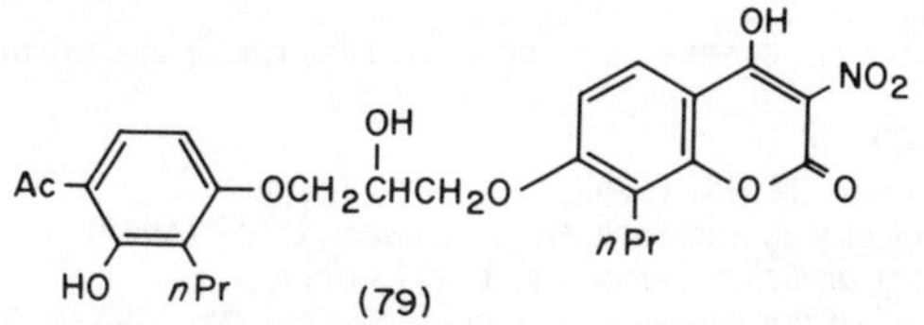

(79)

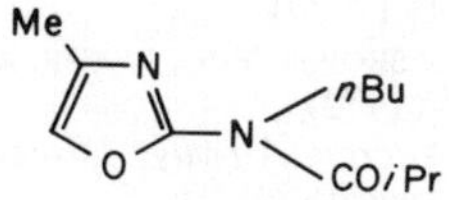

(80)

The addition of smooth muscle relaxant activity to DSCG-like compounds is an interesting and potentially useful concept which has been recently studied. The identification of bronchodilatory activity of some four times that of theophylline in the imidazolylpurinone (81), in addition to modest oral PCA activity[216], led to the development of a considerably more potent compound, the pyrimidobenzothiazolone (82) with some 60 times the intravenous potency of DSCG[217]. The good oral PCA activity of (82), coupled with its ability to inhibit the methacholine-induced bronchospasm in anaesthetized rats, makes this a compound of interest[217].

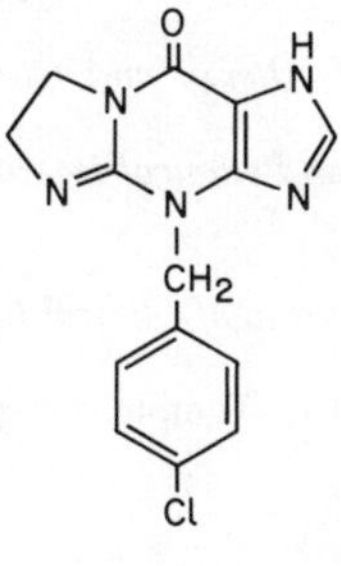

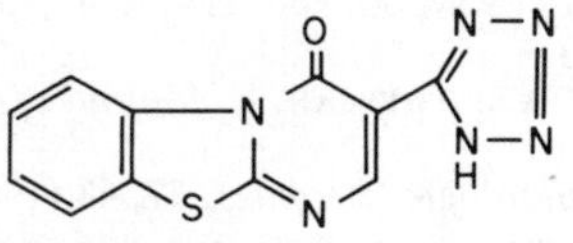

(82)

(81)

The recently described BRL 22321A (73), one of a series of naphthotriazoles[195], has also been shown to possess smooth muscle relaxant properties in addition to its ability to inhibit mediator release[17] and is currently undergoing further evaluation.

It is possible that these multiple activity compounds will hold the key to new generation anti-asthma drugs, but a more detailed understanding of the nature of the disease will probably produce the greatest advances in our ability to treat this complex debilitating disease.

Acknowledgements

I am indebted to Dr H. Smith for his helpful advice and constant encouragement throughout the preparation of this review and to my other colleagues at Beecham for their useful discussions and suggestions.

References

1. COX, J.S.G., BEACH, J.E., BLAIR, A.M.J.N., CLARKE, A.J., KING, J., LEE, T.B. *et al. Advances in Drug Research*, **5**, 115 (1970)
2. COX, J.S.G. *Nature*, **216**, 1328 (1967)
3. ALTOUNYAN, R.E.C. *Acta Allergologica*, **22**, 487 (1967)
4. ANREP, G.V., BARSOUM, G.S., KENAWY, M.R. and MISRAHY, G. *Lancet*, **i**, 557 (1947)
5. BAGOURI, M.M. *Journal of Pharmacy and Pharmacology*, **1**, 177 (1949)
6. SCHÖNBERG, A. and SINA, A. *Journal of the American Chemical Society*, **72**, 3396 (1950)
7. CAIRNS, H. In *Drugs Affecting the Respiratory System*, Ed. D.L. Temple. Chap. 5. Washington DC: American Chemical Society (1980)
8. BERNSTEIN, I.L., SIEGEL, S.C., BRANDON, M.L., BROWN, E.B., EVANS, R.E., FEINBERG, A.R. *et al. Journal of Clinical Immunology*, **50**, 235 (1972)
9. COX, J.S.G. In *Disodium Cromoglycate in Allergic Airways Disease*. Eds J. Pepys and A.W. Frankland. pp. 13–15. London: Butterworth (1970)
10. FOREMAN, J.C., MONGAR, J.L. GOMPERTS, B.D. and GARLAND, L.G. *Biochemical Pharmacology*, **24**, 538 (1975)
11. BROGDEN, R.N., SPEIGHT, T.M. and AVERY, G.S. *Drugs*, **7**, 164 (1974)
12. DAVIES, S.E. *British Medical Journal*, **3**, 593 (1968)
13. ALTOUNYAN, R.E.C. In *The Mast Cell, Its Role in Health and Disease*. Eds J. Pepys and A.M. Edwards. p. 199. London: Pitman Medical (1979) and references therein
14. ALTOUNYAN, R.E.C. *Schweizerische Medizinische Wochenschrift*, **110**, 179 (1980)
15. CAIRNS, H. In *The Mast Cell, its Role in Health and Disease*. Eds J. Pepys and A.M. Edwards. p. 172. London: Pitman Medical (1979)
16. SMITH, H. In *Fundamentals in Respiratory Diseases*. Eds R. Pauwels, M. van der Straeten and M. Radermecker. Vol 2, p. 123. Ghent: Belgian Society of Allergology and Clinical Immunology (1978)
17. SPICER, B.A., CLARKE, G.D., HARLING, E.J., HASSALL, P.A., ROSS, J.W., SMITH, H. *et al. Agents and Actions*, **13**, 301 (1983)
18. IND, P.W., BARNES, P.J., BROWN, M.J., CAUSON, R. and DOLLERY, C.T. *Clinical Allergy*, **13**, 61 (1983) and references cited therein
19. BROWN, M.J., IND, P.W., CAUSON, R. and LEE, T.H. *Journal of Allergy and Clinical Immunology*, **69**, 20 (1982)
20. ATKINS, P.C., NORMAN, M.E. and ZWEIMAN, B. *Journal of Allergy and Clinical Immunology*, **62**, 149 (1978)
21. NAGY, L. *Allergie und Immunologie (Leipzig)*, **27**, 48 (1981)
22. LEE, T.H., NAGY, L., NAGAKURA, T., WALPORT, M.J. and KAY, A.B. *Journal of Clinical Investigation*, **69**, 889 (1982)
23. FOREMAN, J.C. In *Drugs Affecting the Respiratory System*. Ed. D.L. Temple. Chap. 2. Washington DC: American Chemical Society (1980)
24. MAZUREK, N., BERGER, G. and PECHT, I. *Nature*, **286**, 722 (1980)
25. MONGAR, J.L. and SCHILD, H.O. *Physiological Reviews*, **44**, 226 (1962)
26. GARLAND, L.G. and MONGAR, J.L. *International Archives of Allergy and Applied Immunology*, **50**, 27 (1976)
27. FOREMAN, J.C. and GARLAND, L.G. *British Medical Journal*, 820 (1976)
28. FOREMAN, J.C., HALLETT, M.B. and MONGAR, J.L. *British Journal of Pharmacology*, **59**, 437P (1977)
29. ECKSTEIN, F. and FOREMAN, J.C. *FEBS Letters*, **91**, 182 (1978)
30. CHURCH, M.K. *Drugs of Today*, **14**, 281 (1978) and references therein
31. SULLIVAN, T.J. and PARKER, C.W. *American Journal of Pathology*, **85**, 437 (1976)
32. THEOHARIDES, T.C., SIEGHART, W., GREENGARD, P. and DOUGLAS, W.W. *Science*, **207**, 80 (1980)
33. WILHELMS, O.H. and ROESCH, E. *Naunyn-Schmiedeberg's Archives of Pharmacology*, **297** (Suppl. 2), R44 (1977)

34. PEARCE, F.L. and CLEMENTS, J. *Biochemical Pharmacology*, **31**, 2247 (1982)
35. GILLESPIE, E. and LICHTENSTEIN, L.M. *Journal of Clinical Investigation*, **52**, 2941 (1972)
36. MONGAR, J.L. and SCHILD, H.O. *Journal of Physiology*, **140**, 272 (1958)
37. LICHTENSTEIN, L.M. and OSLER, A.G. *Journal of Experimental Medicine*, **120**, 507 (1964)
38. FOREMAN, J.C. and MONGAR, J.L. *Journal of Physiology*, **224**, 753 (1972)
39. PEARCE, F.L. and TRUNEH, A. *Agents and Actions*, **11**, 44 (1981)
40. ENNIS, M., TRUNEH, A., WHITE, J.R. and PEARCE, F.L. *Nature*, **289**, 186 (1981)
41. PEARCE, F.L. *Progress in Medicinal Chemistry*, **19**, 59 (1982)
42. ENNIS, M., ATKINSON, G. and PEARCE, F.L. *Agents and Actions*, **10**, 222 (1980)
43. JOHNSON, H.G. and BACH, M.K. *Journal of Immunology*, **114**, 514 (1975)
44. WHITE, J.R. and PEARCE, F.L. *Immunology*, **46**, 361 (1982)
45. PEARCE, F.L., ENNIS, M., TRUNEH, A. and WHITE, J.R. *Agents and Actions*, **11**, 51 (1981)
46. FOREMAN, J.C., GARLAND, L.G. and MONGAR, J.L. In *Calcium in Biological Systems*. Ed. C.J. Duncan. p. 193. Cambridge: Cambridge University Press (1976)
47. ROY, A.C. and WARREN, B.T. *Biochemical Pharmacology*, **23**, 917 (1974)
48. LAVIN, N., RACHELEVSKY, G.S. and KAPLAN, S.A. *Journal of Allergy and Clinical Immunology*, **57**, 80 (1976)
49a. SIEGHART, W., THEOHARIDES, T.C., ALPER, S.L., DOUGLAS, W.W. and GREENGARD, P. *Nature*, **275**, 329 (1978)
49b. WELLS, E. and MANN, J. *Biochemical Pharmacology*, **32**, 837 (1983)
50. HIRATA, F. and AXELROD, H. *Science*, **209**, 1082 (1980) and references therein
51. JACKSON, D.M. and RICHARDS, I.M. *British Journal of Pharmacology*, **61**, 257 (1977)
52. DIXON, M., JACKSON, D.M. and RICHARDS, I.M. *British Journal of Pharmacology*, **70**, 11 (1980)
53. DIXON, M., JACKSON, D.M. and RICHARDS, I.M. *British Journal of Pharmacology*, **67**, 569 (1979)
54. HARRIES, M.G. *Annals of Allergy*, **46**, 156 (1981)
55. MARCELLE, R. *Respiration*, **27** (Suppl.) 369 (1970)
56. DE KOCK, M.A. *Bronchitis III. Proceedings of the Third International Symposium on Bronchitis*. Eds N.G.M. Ovie and R. Van der Lende. p. 354. Assen, Netherlands: Royal Van Goreum Ltd (1970)
57. ALTOUNYAN, R.E.C. *Acta Allergologica*, **30** (Suppl. 12), 65 (1975)
58. ALTOUNYAN, R.E.C. In *Disodium Cromoglycate in Allergic Airways Disease*. Eds J. Pepys and A.W. Frankland. p. 47. London: Butterworth (1970)
59. DIXON, W. In *Disodium Cromoglycate in Allergic Airways Disease*. Eds J. Pepys and A.W. Frankland. p. 105. London: Butterworth (1970)
60. ORIE, N.G.M., VAN LOOKEREN CAMPAGNE, J.G., KNOL, K., BOOIJ-NOORD, H. and DE VRIES, K. In *Intal in Bronchial Asthma*. Eds J. Pepys and Y. Yamamura. Loughborough: Fisons (1973)
61. PEPYS, J., HARGREAVE, F.E., CHAN, M. and MCHARDY, D.S. *Lancet*, **ii**, 134 (1968)
62. BOOIJ-NOORD, H., ORIE, N.G.M. and DE VRIES, K. *Journal of Allergy and Clinical Immunology*, **48**, 344 (1971)
63. BRYANT, D.H., BURNS, M.W. and LAZARUS, L. *British Medical Journal*, 589 (1973)
64. GRANT, I.W.B., CHANNEL, S. and DREVER, J.C. *Lancet*, **ii**, 673 (1967)
65. KENNEDY, M.C.S. *British Journal of Diseases of the Chest*, **63**, 96 (1969)
66. LUMB, E.M., MCHARDY, G.J.R. and KAY, A.B. *British Journal of Clinical Pharmacology*, **8**, 65 (1979)
67. WALKER, S.R., EVANS, M.E., RICHARDS, A.J. and PATERSON, J.W. *Journal of Pharmacy and Pharmacology*, **24**, 525 (1972)
68. ASHTON, M.J., CLARK, B., JONES, K.M., MOSS, G.F., NEALE, M.G. and RITCHIE, J.T. *Toxicology and Applied Pharmacology*, **26**, 319 (1973)
69. WHEATLEY, D. *Clinical Trials Journal*, **11**, 21 (1974)
70. MORRISON-SMITH, J. and PIZZARRO, Y.A. *Clinical Allergy*, **2**, 143 (1972)
71. MORRISON-SMITH, J. *British Medical Journal*, 303 (1973)
72. LAL, S., MALHOTRA, S.M. and GRIBBEN, M.D. *Clinical Allergy*, **12**, 197 (1982)
73. AMLIE, P., LEEGAARD, J., LIER, P. and WEFRING, K. *Modern Problems in Paediatrics*, **21**, 113 (1982)
74. GOOSE, J. and BLAIR, A.M.J.N. *Immunology*, **16**, 749 (1969)
75. OVARY, A. and BIER, O.G. *Proceedings of the Society for Experimental Biology and Medicine*, **81**, 584 (1952)
76. THOMSON, D.S. and EVANS, D.P. *Clinical and Experimental Immunology*, **13**, 537 (1973)

77. SPICER, B.A., ROSS, J.W. and SMITH, H. *Clinical and Experimental Immunology*, **21**, 419 (1975)
78. CHAKRIN, L.W., KRELL, R.D., MENGEL, J., YOUNG, D., ZAKER, C. and WARDELL, J.R. *Agents and Actions*, **4**, 297 (1974)
79. ANKIER, S. *International Archives of Allergy and Applied Immunology*, **41**, 163 (1971)
80. AUGSTEIN, J., CAIRNS, H., HUNTER, D., LEE, T.B., SUSCHITZKY, J., ALTOUNYAN, R.E.C. *et al.* *Agents and Actions*, **7**, 443 (1977)
81. ORANGE, R.P. and AUSTEN, K.F. *International Archives of Allergy and Applied Immunology*, **41**, 79 (1971)
82. SMITH, H., SPICER, B.A. and ROSS, J.W. *International Archives of Allergy and Applied Immunology*, **54**, 414 (1977)
83. SHARPE, T.J., ROSS, J.W. and SPICER, B.A. *Agents and Actions*, **8**, 199 (1978)
84. STOTLAND, C.M. and SHARE, N.N. *Canadian Journal of Physiology and Pharmacology*, **52**, 1119 (1974)
85. FARMER, J.B., RICHARDS, I.M., SHEARD, P. and WOODS, A.M. *Naunyn-Schmiedeberg's Archives of Pharmacology*, **269** (Suppl.), R35 (1973)
86. PATTERSON, R., TALBOT, C.H. and BRANDFONBRENER, M. *International Archives of Allergy and Applied Immunology*, **41**, 592 (1971)
87. KRELL, R.D., CHUKRIN, C.W. and WASDELL, J.R. In *Immunopharmacology*. Eds M.E. Rosenthal and H.C. Mansmann. p. 125. New York: Spectrum Publications (1975)
88. LICHTENSTEIN, L.M. and ADKINSON, N.F. *Journal of Immunology*, **103**, 866 (1969)
89. SHEARD, P. and BLAIR, A.M.J.N. *International Archives of Allergy and Applied Immunology*, **38**, 217 (1970)
90. ORANGE, R.P. and AUSTEN, K.F. *Progress in Immunology. Proceedings of the 1st International Congress on Immunology*. Ed. B. Amos. p. 173. London: Academic Press (1971)
91. AUSTEN, K.F., LEWIS, R.A., STECHSCHULTE, D.J., WASSERMAN, S.I., LEID, R.W. and GOETZL, E.J. *Progress in Immunology. Proceedings of the 2nd International Congress on Immunology*. Ed. B. Amos. p. 61. London: Academic Press (1974)
92. LUNT, E. In *Progress in Pharmaceutical Research. Critical Reports on Applied Chemistry*. Ed. K.R.H. Wooldridge. Vol. 4. p. 41. Oxford: Blackwell Scientific Publications (1982)
93. CAIRNS, H., FITZMAURICE, C., HUNTER, D., JOHNSON, P.B., KING, J., LEE, T.B. *et al.* *Journal of Medicinal Chemistry*, **15**, 583 (1972)
94. BANTICK, J.R., CAIRNS, H., CHAMBERS, A., HAZARD, R., KING, J., LEE, T.B. *et al.* *Journal of Medicinal Chemistry*, **19**, 817 (1976)
95. AUGSTEIN, J., CAIRNS, H., CHAMBERS, A., BURNS, J.W. and RADZIWONIK, H. *Journal of Pharmacy and Pharmacology*, **28**, 919 (1976)
96. EASON, C.T., PARKE, D.V., CLARK, B. and SMITH, D.A. *Xenobiotica*, **12**, 155 (1982)
97. GIRARD, J.P. and SULLIVAN, T.J. *Clinical Allergy*, **10**, 271 (1980)
98. THOMSON, N.C., GREEN, A.G.H. and KERR, J.W. *Clinical Allergy*, **10**, 43 (1980)
99. ALBAN DAVIES, H., RHODES, J. and THOMAS, M. *British Journal of Clinical Pharmacology*, **1**, 53 (1981)
100. PEARCE, F.L., BUFUS, A.D., GAULDIE, J. and BIENENSTOCK, J. *Journal of Immunology*, **128**, 2481 (1982)
101. DEVLIN, J.P., FRETER, K. and STEWART, P.B. *Journal of Medicinal Chemistry*, **20**, 205 (1977)
102. POSSANGA, G.J., BAUEN, A. and STEWART, P.B. *Pharmacologist*, **16**, 198 (1974)
103. EL AZAB, J. and STEWART, P.B. *International Archives of Allergy and Applied Immunology*, **55**, 350 (1977)
104. JOHNSON, A.J. and BEETS, J.L. *British Journal of Clinical Pharmacology*, **7**, 511 (1979)
105. ELLIS, G.P. and SHAW, D. *Journal of Medicinal Chemistry*, **15**, 865 (1972)
106. ELLIS, G.P., BECKET, G.J.P., SHAW, D., WILSON, H.K., VARDEY, C.J. and SKIDMORE, I.F. *Journal of Medicinal Chemistry*, **21**, 1120 (1978)
107. PFISTER, J.R., FERRARESI, R.W., HARRISON, I.T., ROOKS, W.H., ROSZKOWSKI, A.P., VAN HORN, A. *et al.* *Journal of Medicinal Chemistry*, **15**, 1032 (1972)
108. PFISTER, J.R., FERRARESI, R.W., HARRISON, I.T., ROOKS, W.H. and FRIED, J.H. *Journal of Medicinal Chemistry*, **21**, 669 (1978)
109. WÜTHRICH, B. and PARROTT, D. *Respiration*, **33**, 231 (1976)
110. STENIUS, B., SALORINNE, Y. and PARROTT, D. *Scandinavian Journal of Respiratory Diseases*, **59**, 75 (1978)
111. SPRENKLE, A.C., VAN ARSDEL, P.O. and BIERMAN, C.W. *Journal of Allergy and Clinical Immunology*, **55**, 118 (1975)

112. JONES, W.D., ALBRECHT, W.D., MUNRO, N.L. and STEWART, K.T. *Journal of Medicinal Chemistry*, **20**, 594 (1977)
113. BRISTOL, J.A., ALEKEL, R., FUKUNAGA, J.Y. and STEINMAN, M. *Journal of Medicinal Chemistry*, **21**, 1327 (1978)
114. BARNS, A.C., HAIRSINE, P.W., MATHARU, S.S., RAMM, P.J. and TAYLOR, J.B. *Journal of Medicinal Chemistry*, **22**, 418 (1979)
115. GOTO, K., TERASAWA, M. and MARUYAMA, Y. *International Archives of Allergy and Applied Immunology*, **59**, 13 (1979)
116. BATCHELOR, J.F., FOLLENFANT, M.J., GARLAND, L.G., GORVIN, J.H., GREEN, A.F., HODSON, H.F. *et al. Lancet*, **i**, 1169 (1975)
117. HAYDU, S.P., BRADLEY, J.L. and HUGHES, D.T.D. *British Medical Journal*, **3**, 283 (1975)
118. PAUWELS, R., LAMONT, H. and VAN DER STRAETEN, M. *Acta Allergologica*, **31**, 471 (1976)
119. POPPIUS, H. and STENIUS, B. *European Journal of Clinical Pharmacology*, **11**, 107 (1977)
120. NOHARA, A., UMETANI, T. and SANNO, Y. *Tetrahedron*, **30**, 3553 (1974)
121. NOHARA, A., KURIKI, H., SAIJO, T., UKAWA, K., MURATO, T., KAUNO, M. *et al. Journal of Medicinal Chemistry*, **18**, 34 (1975)
122. NOHARA, A. In *Drugs Affecting the Respiratory System*. Ed. D.L. Temple. Chap. 7. Washington DC: American Chemical Society (1980)
123. DI CARLO, F.J., HERZIG, D.J., KUSNER, E.J., SCHUMANN, P.R., MELGAR, M.D., GEORGE, S. *et al. Drug Metabolism and Disposition*, **4**, 368 (1976)
124. NOHARA, A., KURIKI, H., SAIJO, T., SUGIHARA, H., KANNO, M. and SANNO, Y. *Journal of Medicinal Chemistry*, **20**, 141 (1977)
125. NOHARA, A., KURIKI, H., ISHIHIRO, T., SAIJO, T., UKAWA, K., MAKI, Y. *et al. Journal of Medicinal Chemistry*, **22**, 290 (1979)
126. KANAI, Y., NAKAI, Y., NAKAJIMA, N. and TANAYAMA, S. *Xenobiotica*, **9**, 33 (1979)
127. PFISTER, J.R., WYMANN, W.E., SCHULER, M.E. and ROSZKOWSKI, A.P. *Journal of Medicinal Chemistry*, **23**, 335 (1980)
128. WURM, G. and GERES, U. *Arzneimittel-Forschung*, **29**, 15 (1979)
129. DORIA, G., ROMEO, C., GIRALDI, P., LAURIA, F., SBERZE, P., TIBOLLA, N. *et al. European Journal of Medicinal Chemistry*, **13**, 33 (1978)
130. DORIA, G., ROMEO, C., FORGIONE, A., SBERZE, P., TIBOLLA, N., CORNO, M.L. *et al. European Journal of Medicinal Chemistry*, **14**, 347 (1979)
131. WRIGHT, J.B. and JOHNSON, H.G. *Journal of Medicinal Chemistry*, **16**, 861 (1973)
132. UNANGST, P.C., BROWN, R.E. and HERZIG, D.J. *Journal of Medicinal Chemistry*, **23**, 1251 (1980)
133. GOERLITZER, K., DEHNE, A. and ENGLER, E. *Archiv der Pharmazie*, **315**, 249 (1982)
134. PHILLIPP, A., JIRKOVSKY, I. and MARTEL, R.R. *Journal of Medicinal Chemistry*, **23**, 1372 (1980)
135. EVANS, D.P., GILMAN, D.J., THOMSON, D.S. and WARING, W.S. *Nature*, **250**, 592 (1974)
136. HALL, C.M., JOHNSON, H.G. and WRIGHT, J.B. *Journal of Medicinal Chemistry*, **17**, 685 (1974)
137. ERICKSON, E.H., LAPPI, L.R., RICE, T.K., SWINGLE, K.F. and VAN WINKLE, M. *Journal of Medicinal Chemistry*, **21**, 984 (1978)
138. ERICKSON, E.H., HAINLINE, C.F., LENON, L.S., MATSON, C.J., RICE, T.K., SWINGLE, K.F. *et al. Journal of Medicinal Chemistry*, **22**, 816 (1979)
139. HALL, C.M., WRIGHT, J.B., JOHNSON, H.G. and TAYLOR, A.J. *Journal of Medicinal Chemistry*, **20**, 1337 (1977)
140. JOHNSON, H.G. and VAN HOUT, C.A. *International Archives of Allergy and Applied Immunology*, **50**, 446 (1976)
141. WADE, J.J., ERICKSON, E.H., HEGEL, R.F., LAPPI, L.R. and RICE, T.K. *Journal of Medicinal Chemistry*, **21**, 941 (1978)
142. SELLSTEDT, J.H., GUINOSSO, C.J., BEGANY, A.J., BELL, S.C. and ROSENTHALE, M. *Journal of Medicinal Chemistry*, **18**, 926 (1975)
143. ROSENTHALE, M.E., BEGANY, A.J., DERVINIS, A., SELLSTEDT, J., GUINOSSO, C. and GLUCKMAN, M.I. *Journal of Pharmacology and Experimental Therapeutics*, **197**, 725 (1976)
144. CHURCH, M.K. and GRADIDGE, C.F. *British Journal of Pharmacology*, **70**, 307 (1980)
145. KLAUBERT, D.H., SELLSTEDT, J.H., GUINOSSO, C.J., CAPETOLA, R.J. and BELL, S.C. *Journal of Medicinal Chemistry*, **24**, 742 (1981)
146. KLAUBERT, D.H., SELLSTEDT, J.H., GUINOSSO, C.J., BELL, S.C. and CAPETOLA, R.J. *Journal of Medicinal Chemistry*, **24**, 748 (1981)
147. WRIGHT, J.B. and JOHNSON, H.G. *Journal of Medicinal Chemistry*, **20**, 166 (1977)

148. WRIGHT, J.B., HALL, C.M. and JOHNSON, H.G. *Journal of Medicinal Chemistry*, **21**, 930 (1978)
149. JOHNSON, H.G. *Trends in Pharmacological Sciences*, **I**, 343 (1980)
150. HALL, C.M. and JOHNSON, H.G. In *Drugs Affecting the Respiratory System*. Ed. D.L. Temple. Chap. 4. Washington DC; American Chemical Society (1980)
151. BAGLI, J.F., BOGRI, T., PALAMETA, B., MARTEL, R., ROBINSON, W., PUGSLEY, T. *et al. Journal of Medicinal Chemistry*, **22**, 1186 (1979)
152. ALTHUIS, T.H., MOORE, P.F. and HESS, H.-J. *Journal of Medicinal Chemistry*, **22**, 44 (1979)
153. ALTHUIS, T.H., KADIN, S.B., CZUBA, L.J., MOORE, P.F. and HESS, H.-J. *Journal of Medicinal Chemistry*, **23**, 262 (1980)
154. ALTHUIS, T.H., KADIN, S.B., CZUBA, L.J., MOORE, P.F. and HESS, H.-J. In *Drugs Affecting the Respiratory System*. Ed. D.L. Temple. Chap. 3. Washington DC: American Chemical Society (1980)
155. DORIA, G., ROMEO, C., SBERZE, P., TIBOLLA, M., CORNO, M.-L. and CADELLI, G. *European Journal of Medicinal Chemistry*, **14**, 247 (1979)
156. SCHWENDER, C.F., SUNDAY, B.R. and HERZIG, D.J. *Journal of Medicinal Chemistry*, **22**, 114 (1979)
157. SCHWENDER, C.F., SUNDAY, B.R., HERZIG, D.J., KUSNER, E.K., SCHUMANN, P.R. and GAWLAK, D.L. *Journal of Medicinal Chemistry*, **22**, 748 (1979)
158. TILLEY, J.W., LE MAHIEU, R.E., CARSON, M., KIERSTEAD, R.W., BARUTH, H.W. and YAREMKO, B. *Journal of Medicinal Chemistry*, **23**, 92 (1980)
159. SALVADOR, R.A., CZYZEWSKI, L.B., BARUTH, H.W., HOOPER, A., MEDFORD, A., MILLER, D. *et al. Agents and Actions*, **11**, 339 (1981)
160. WELTON, A.F., HOPE, W.C., CROWLEY, H.J. and SALVADOR, R.A. *Agents and Actions*, **11**, 345 (1981)
161. SCHWENDER, C.F., SUNDAY, B.R., KERBLESKI, J.J. and HERZIG, D.J. *Journal of Medicinal Chemistry*, **23**, 964 (1980)
162. TINNEY, F.J., CETENKO, W.A., KERBLESKI, J.J., CONNOR, D.T., SORENSON, R.J. and HERZIG, D.J. *Journal of Medicinal Chemistry*, **24**, 878 (1981)
163. TEMPLE, D.L., YEVICH, J.P., COVINGTON, R.R., HANNING, C.A., SEIDELHAMEL, R.J., MACKEY, H.K. *et al. Journal of Medicinal Chemistry*, **22**, 505 (1979)
164. SIRCAR, J.C., CAPIRIS, T., KESTEN, S.J. and HERZIG, D.J. *Journal of Medicinal Chemistry*, **24**, 735 (1981)
165. HOLLAND, D., JONES, G., MARSHALL, P.W. and TRINGHAM, G.D. *Journal of Medicinal Chemistry*, **19**, 1225 (1976)
166. HERMECZ, I., BREINING, T., MESZAROS, Z., HORVATH, A., VASVARI-DEBRECZY, L., DESSY, F. *et al. Journal of Medicinal Chemistry*, **25**, 1140 (1982)
167. DE VOS, C., DESSY, F., HERMECZ, I., MESZAROS, Z. and BREINING, T. *International Archives of Allergy and Applied Immunology*, **67**, 362 (1982)
168. BUCKLE, D.R., MORGAN, N.J., ROSS, J.W., SMITH, H. and SPICER, B.A. *Journal of Medicinal Chemistry*, **16**, 1334 (1973)
169. SPICER, B.A., ROSS, J.W., SHARPE, T.J. and SMITH, H. *International Archives of Allergy and Applied Immunology*, **56**, 493 (1978)
170. ROSS, J.W., SMITH, H. and SPICER, B.A. *International Archives of Allergy and Applied Immunology*, **51**, 226 (1976)
171. SHARPE, T.J. and SMITH, H. *International Archives of Allergy and Applied Immunology*, **60**, 216 (1979)
172. PAUWELS, R., LAMONT, H. and VAN DER STRAETEN, M. *Clinical Allergy*, **6**, 463 (1976)
173. PAUWELS, R., LAMONT, H. and VAN DER STRAETEN, M. *Clinical Allergy*, **6**, 471 (1976)
174. LENNEY, W., MILNER, A.D. and TYLER, R.M. *British Journal of Diseases of the Chest*, **72**, 225 (1978)
175. BUCKLE, D.R., CANTELLO, B.C.C., SMITH, H. and SPICER, B.A. *Journal of Medicinal Chemistry*, **18**, 391 (1975)
176. BUCKLE, D.R., CANTELLO, B.C.C., SMITH, H. and SPICER, B.A. *Journal of Medicinal Chemistry*, **18**, 726 (1975)
177. BUCKLE, D.R., CANTELLO, B.C.C., SMITH, H., SMITH, R.J. and SPICER, B.A. *Journal of Medicinal Chemistry*, **20**, 1059 (1977)
178. BUCKLE, D.R., MORGAN, N.J. and SMITH, H. *Journal of Medicinal Chemistry*, **18**, 203 (1975)
179. BUCKLE, D.R., CANTELLO, B.C.C., MORGAN, N.J., SMITH, H. and SPICER, B.A. *Journal of Medicinal Chemistry*, **18**, 733 (1975)

180. BUCKLE, D.R., CANTELLO, B.C.C., SMITH, H. and SPICER, B.A. *Journal of Medicinal Chemistry*, **20**, 265 (1977)
181. COULSON, C.J., FORD, R.E., LUNT, E., MARSHALL, S., PAIN, D.L., ROGERS, I.H. *et al. European Journal of Medicinal Chemistry*, **9**, 313 (1974)
182. HOLLAND, A., JACKSON, D., CHAPLEN, P., LUNT, E., MARSHALL, S., PAIN, D.L. *et al. European Journal of Medicinal Chemistry*, **10**, 447 (1975)
183. BROUGHTON, B.J., CHAPLEN, P., KNOWLES, P., LUNT, E., PAIN, D.L. and WOOLDRIDGE, K.R.H. *Journal of Medicinal Chemistry*, **18**, 1117 (1975)
184. WILSON, S.R., WILSON, R.B., SHOEMAKER, A.L., WOOLDRIDGE, K.R.H. and HODGSON, D.J. *Journal of the American Chemical Society*, **104**, 259 (1982)
185. BROUGHTON, B.J., CHAPLEN, P., KNOWLES, P., LUNT, E., PAIN, D.L., WOOLDRIDGE, K.R.H. *et al. Nature*, **251**, 650 (1974)
186. EVANS, J., FORD, R.E., LESWELL, P.F., MARSHALL, S.M. and WALKER, J.L. *British Journal of Pharmacology*, **70**, 177P (1980)
187. DA SETTIMO, A., LIVI, O., FERRARINI, P.L. and BIAGI, G. *Il Farmaco Edizione Scientifica*, **35**, 308 (1980)
188. DA SETTIMO, A., LIVI, O., FERRARINI, P.L. and PRIMOFIORE, G. *Il Farmaco Edizione Scientifica*, **35**, 298 (1980)
189. JUBY, P.F., HUDYMA, T.W., BROWN, M., ESSERY, J.M. and PARTYKA, R.A. *Journal of Medicinal Chemistry*, **22**, 263 (1979)
190. BOREA, P.A. *Arzneimittel-Forschung*, **32**(I), 325 (1982)
191. JUBY, P.F., HUDYMA, T.W., BROWN, M., ESSERY, J.M. and PARTYKA, R.A. *Journal of Medicinal Chemistry*, **25**, 1145 (1982)
192. SIMINOFF, P., REED, F.C., SCHURIG, J.E. and JUBY, P.F. *Monographs in Allergy*, **14**, 318 (1979)
193. BUCKLE, D.R. *Journal of Chemical Research (S)*, 308 (1980)
194. BUCKLE, D.R., OUTRED, D.J., ROCKELL, C.J.M., SMITH, H. and SPICER, B.A. *Journal of Medicinal Chemistry*, **26**, 256 (1983)
195. BUCKLE, D.R., SMITH, H., SPICER, B.A. and TEDDER, J.M. *Journal of Medicinal Chemistry*, **26**, 741 (1983)
196. SNADER, K.M., CHAKRIN, L.W., CRAMER, R.D., GERLERNT, Y.M., MIAO, C.K., SHAH, D.H. *et al. Journal of Medicinal Chemistry*, **22**, 706 (1979)
197. CRAMER, R.D., SNADER, K.M., WILLIS, C.R., CHAKRIN, L.W., THOMAS, J. and SUTTON, B.M. *Journal of Medicinal Chemistry*, **22**, 714 (1979)
198. SNADER, K.M., CHAKRIN, L.W., CRAMER, R.D., GERLENT, Y.M., MIAO, C.K., SHAH, D.H. *et al.* In *Drugs Affecting the Respiratory System.* Ed. D.L. Temple. Chap. 8. Washington DC: American Chemical Society (1980)
199. KODA, A., NAGAI, H., WATANABE, S., YANAGIHARA, Y. and SAKAMOTO, K. *Journal of Allergy and Clinical Immunology*, **57**, 396 (1976)
200. AZUMA, H., BANNO, K. and YOSHIMURA, T. *British Journal of Pharmacology*, **58**, 483 (1976)
201. SHIODA, H. *Allergy*, **34**, 213 (1979)
202. VITOLO, M.J., MARQUEZ, V.E. and HURTADO, I. *Journal of Medicinal Chemistry*, **21**, 692 (1978)
203. DI PARSIA, M.T., SUAREZ, C., VITOLO, M.J., MARQUEZ, V.E., BEYER, B., URBINA, C. *et al. Journal of Medicinal Chemistry*, **24**, 117 (1981)
204. HURTADO, I., MARQUEZ, V.E. and VITOLO, M.J. *International Archives of Allergy and Applied Immunology*, **57**, 507 (1978)
205. CHENEY, B.V., WRIGHT, J.B., HALL, C.M., JOHNSON, H.G. and CRISTOFFERSEN, R.E. *Journal of Medicinal Chemistry*, **21**, 936 (1978)
206. WASLEY, J.W.F. In *Medicinal Chemistry Advances.* Eds F.G. De las Heras and S. Vega. p. 329. Oxford: Pergamon Press (1981)
207. COULSON, C.J., FORD, R.E., MARSHALL, S., WALKER, J.L., WOOLDRIDGE, K.R.H., BOWDEN, K. *et al. Nature*, **265**, 545 (1977)
208. WHITE, G.J. *Agents and Actions*, **11**, 503 (1981)
209. SCHWENDER, C.F., SUNDAY, B.R. and DECKER, V.L. *Journal of Medicinal Chemistry*, **25**, 742 (1982)
210. SPEIZER, F.E., DOLL, R. and HENF, P. *British Medical Journal*, **1**, 335 (1968)
211. INMAN, W.H.W. and ADELSTEIN, A.M. *Lancet*, **ii**, 279 (1969)
212. ORANGE, R.P. and AUSTEN, K.F. *Proceedings of the Society for Experimental Biology and Medicine*, **129**, 836 (1968)

213. ORANGE, R.P. and AUSTEN, K.F. *International Archives of Allergy and Applied Immunology*, **41**, 79 (1971)
214. BUCKLE, D.R., OUTRED, D.J., ROSS, J.W., SMITH, H., SMITH, R.J. and SPICER, B.A. *Journal of Medicinal Chemistry*, **22**, 158 (1979)
215. ROSS, W.J., HARRISON, R.J., JOLLEY, M.R.J., NEVILLE; M.C., TODD, A., VERGE, J.P. *et al. Journal of Medicinal Chemistry*, **22**, 412 (1979)
216. TEMPLE, D.L., YEVICH, J.P., CATT, J.D., OWENS, D., HANNING, C., COVINGTON, R.R. *et al. Journal of Medicinal Chemistry*, **23**, 1188 (1980)
217. YEVICH, J.P., TEMPLE, D.L., COVINGTON, R.R., OWENS, D.A., SEIDELHAMEL, R.J. and DUNGAN, K.W. *Journal of Medicinal Chemistry*, **25**, 864 (1982)

Chapter 14

Corticosteroids

S.M. Harding

Introduction

The isolation, characterization and synthesis of the corticosteroids was a slow process, due to technical difficulties and the need to handle large amounts of starting material. After almost 20 years of research, Kendall's Compound E, or cortisone, became available in sufficient quantities for clinical trial and, on 21st September 1948, the first injection was given. The patient, a woman with severe rheumatoid arthritis, was dramatically improved after two days' treatment with 100 mg intramuscularly. The value of cortisone was confirmed by extending the trial to another 13 patients, 2 of whom were also given adrenocorticotropic hormone (ACTH)[1]

Following this success, Bordley et al. tried ACTH in 5 patients with asthma[2]. Unequivocal benefit was noted in from 4 to 48 hours and treatment was continued for up to 3 weeks with further improvements. At almost the same time, Carryer et al. were performing a pilot trial of cortisone acetate 100 mg by daily injection to 3 patients with asthma and hay fever resulting from sensitivity to ragweed pollen[3]. Each experienced relief from their symptoms within 3 days and this relief was greater than had been achieved previously by other measures.

As cortisone gradually became available, it was used in a variety of diseases where its purported miraculous properties were tried, frequently under uncontrolled conditions and often in high dosage. The latter led to an appalling number of problems. The incidence of side-effects quoted by 1953 ranged from 20% to 100%[4], the commonest being: alteration in psyche, facial rounding, fluid retention, hypertrichosis, decreased glucose tolerance, increased blood pressure and acne.

Due to these systemic side-effects, cortisone was tried locally in the lung. Reeder and MacKey[5] reported the beneficial effects of nebulized cortisone in a patient with bacterial pneumonia. In the following year, 1951, Gelfand used inhaled cortisone in 5 patients with long-standing asthma[6]. They were treated for 2 weeks with daily doses of 50 mg in saline, delivered by a DeVilbiss nebulizer, and 4 of the 5 responded favourably. Thus the scene was set, not only for glucocorticoids to be used in asthma, but for these drugs to be used by inhalation.

297

Systemic steroids

In the years that followed, a number of analogues of cortisone were made in attempts to separate beneficial from unwanted systemic effects. The first of these was hydrocortisone (cortisol), the structure of which is shown in *Table 14.1*. Typical systemic analogues are given in the table which includes the essential features necessary for anti-inflammatory activity.

TABLE 14.1. The structure of cortisol (hydrocortisone) and some typical systemic analogues

(essential features indicated by dotted lines)

Steroid	Δ^1	C-6	C-9	C-16	Relative activity	
					GC/AI	MC
Cortisol	—	—	—	—	1	1
Prednisolone	+	—	—	—	5	0.5
Methylprednisolone	+	αMe	—	—	6	0.1
Triamcinolone	+	—	α-F	α-OH	6	0
Dexamethasone	+	—	α-F	α-Me	35	0
Betamethasone	+	—	α-F	β-Me	35	0

Cortisone and prednisone are 11-dehydro derivatives of cortisol and prednisolone, but possess the same respective biological potencies.
GC/AI = glucocorticoid/anti-inflammatory.
MC   = mineralocorticoid.

The first advance was the discovery of prednisone and prednisolone (1954), which were more potent anti-inflammatory agents. The consequent reduction in dose and in sodium-retaining and potassium-losing properties, hitherto associated with cortisone and cortisol, reduced the fluid retention and hypertension caused by these early compounds. In addition, by the time prednisone and prednisolone had become commercially available, there was a more rational approach to the use of corticosteroids and relative overdosage was less common. Indeed, prednisolone is still the standard oral corticosteroid.

Methylprednisolone and triamcinolone (1957) represented only small advances in clinical terms, but dexamethasone and betamethasone (1959) were yet more potent anti-inflammatory agents with no overt mineralocorticoid properties. Despite the synthesis of further analogues, no other steroids have since found popular use as systemic agents. This has been due to the failure to separate anti-inflammatory effects from glucocorticoid effects in man or in animal screens[7,8], although separation of some of the beneficial effects from hypothalamic–pituitary–adrenal axis suppression is possible. This can be achieved by dosing at a time in the circadian rhythm when the axis is less sensitive to feedback. Once a day or alternate day dosing early in the morning can considerably reduce the occurrence of endogenous cortisol suppression[9,10]. The shorter the plasma half-life of the steroid, the greater the sparing effect should be. Prednisolone, with a half-life of 2–3 h[11] may be better than dexamethasone or betamethasone in this respect (half-lives >5 h[12]). However, this posology does not always give an even 24-hour control of symptoms, nor does it spare some of the other unwanted effects not so dependent upon circadian change.

The failure of these systemic analogues to separate wanted from unwanted effects is reflected in the number of papers in which the sequelae of corticosteroids have been reported: a review by David, Grieco and Cushman in 1970[13] made reference to 848 papers in the English language alone. To avoid these systemic effects, the local use of these drugs by inhalation has been vigorously pursued.

Inhalational steroids and topical activity

Hydrocortisone became available in the UK in 1954. Shortly afterwards, Foulds et al. tried the drug as an inhaled powder in a study involving 15 patients with asthma[14]. The daily dose was 7.5 mg or 15 mg and the response assessed by the ability of the patient to reduce his isoprenaline requirements, which 11 managed to do. These results were confirmed by Brockbank and Pengelly[15] in a double-blind placebo-controlled study. Of 24 patients, 17 were improved or much improved over a 10-week period by a daily dose of only 3 mg hydrocortisone acetate. A further 7 patients were studied on a daily inhalation of prednisolone 1 mg, but only one improved.

The doses of hydrocortisone used in these studies were considerably lower than those which had previously been given orally (50–300 mg daily) and there seemed no doubt that the drug was acting locally. Helm and Heyworth[16] estimated that approximately 75% of an 'inhaled' dose was absorbed, mostly from the stomach after swallowing, and argued that this was firm evidence for local activity in the lung since the equivalent oral dose would have been totally inadequate. Indeed, Brockbank and Pengelly had drawn the analogy between the topical activity of hydrocortisone in the lung and in skin diseases, where the former had been found to be superior to prednisolone[17].

Despite the poor performance of prednisolone in low doses, Franklin et al.[18], using a Freon-propelled metered dose aerosol of prednisolone, found that 18 mg daily by inhalation was equivalent to 40 mg by mouth—again, evidence for local activity in the lung. In the 1960s, dexamethasone phosphate and dexamethasone isonicotinate were used by inhalation. Clinical trial showed that some oral steroid sparing effect could be achieved[19-23] but, as in the study by Franklin *et al.*, frequently at doses absorbed in sufficient quantity to give rise to systemic side-effects[24-27].

In parallel with these investigations in asthma, developments pertinent to the subject of local or topical activity were taking place in the chemical field. These involved the synthesis of more lipid-soluble compounds which could penetrate the epidermis and which were more potent when applied topically to the skin[8,28.] McKenzie noted that their potency appeared to correlate with the ability to produce vasoconstriction when a treated area of skin was occluded[29,30] and this was developed as a test to screen a number of esters of betamethasone for potential topical activity[31]. The test was proven to be of value when clinical trial of a number of these compounds ranked the steroids in the same order of potency as their vasoconstrictor scores[31,32]. From this programme came betamethasone valerate and beclomethasone dipropionate. Both were found to be highly effective when used in the management of dermatoses and both were effective in doses generally causing no systemic side-effects[33]. A selected list of topically active steroids and their vasoconstrictor scores is given in *Table 14.2*. The 'systemic' steroids including hydrocortisone produce little or no vasoconstriction in this test.

Although the property of topical activity was ill understood at this time, an investigation of the value of betamethasone valerate used topically in the lung and at a variety of other sites was made[34]. Unfortunately the inhaled preparation, an aqueous spray, was first used in 7 patients with some degree of fixed airways obstruction where it was found to be of little value. When first formulated as a metered dose aerosol, it was apparently effective in suppressing cough but did not improve lung function; on the positive side, it did not cause cortisol suppression. The first encouraging reports were received from Horne in 1969 who reported results from a formal study at a later date[35]. In this study, it was possible to withdraw oral prednisolone completely in 22 of 24 patients who were taking an average daily dose of prednisolone 11 mg. Repeated assessment of the hypothalamic–pituitary–adrenal axis function showed slow but progressive recovery to normality in almost all patients[36].

At the same time, beclomethasone dipropionate was formulated as a metered dose aerosol, but again met with little enthusiasm early in its development. Grant *et al.* began a trial comparison of beclomethasone dipropionate 400 μg/day and oral prednisolone 20 mg in 1968[37]. When the first eight cases were analysed it was found that only one had shown a useful degree of improvement on the aerosol, though most had responded well to oral prednisolone. Increasing the daily dose of aerosol to 2 mg was again disappointing and 5 of 8 patients showed evidence of adrenocortical suppression. However, other investigators were more optimistic. A letter to the *British Medical Journal* in 1971 by Smith, Booth and Davey[38] reported encouraging results in 5 patients using a daily dose of beclomethasone dipropionate 400 μg: normal cortisol levels and tetracosactrin tests were maintained. Brown, Storey and George[39], in an uncontrolled study in 60 patients, found that 28 of 37 patients on oral steroids and 19 of 23 not requiring oral steroids, were well controlled by inhaling beclomethasone dipropionate between 400 and 600 μg daily. They found no evidence of

TABLE 14.2. The structures of some steroid esters and acetonides

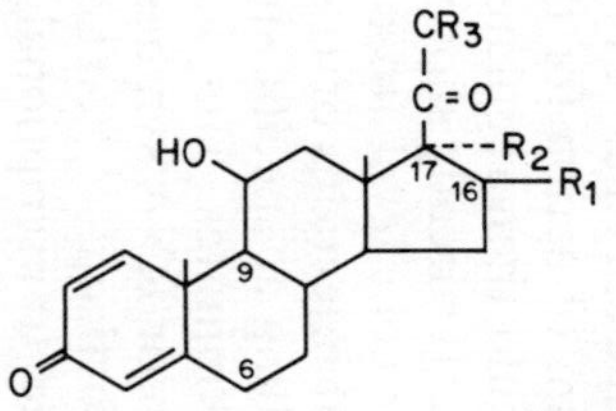

	Esters					Acetonides					
Steroid	C-6	C-9	R_1	R_2	R_3	C-6	C-9	R_1	R_2	R_3	Vasoconstrictor score*
Esters											
Fluocortin butyl ester	α-F	—	α-Me	H	$O_2C_4H_9$						+
Betamethasone valerate	—	α-F	β-Me	$OCOC_4H_9$	H_2OH						360
Beclomethasone dipropionate	—	α-Cl	β-Me	$OCOC_2H_5$	$H_2OCOC_2H_5$						500
Clobetasol propionate	—	α-F	β-Me	$OCOC_2H_5$	H_2Cl						1870
Acetonides											
Flunisolide						α-F	—	Me	Me	—	+
Triamcinolone acetonide						—	α-F	Me	Me	—	75
Fluocinolone acetonide						α-F	α-F	Me	Me	—	100
Budesonide						—	—	H (isomeric)	C_3H_7	—	+

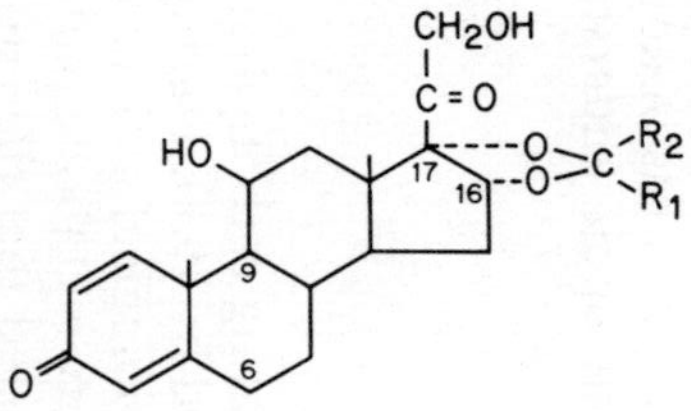

* From Phillips[28] and Wilson[33].

+ Not available; approximate values for fluocortin butyl ester and flunisolide >100, and for budesonide >500.

adrenal suppression and, indeed, mild adrenal withdrawal symptoms were a problem in some patients.

These observations were rapidly extended to include patients from many other centres in a variety of trials, controlled and uncontrolled, in the young and in the elderly, in the easily reversible asthmatic and the more chronically disabled. Symposia on betamethasone valerate[40] and beclomethasone diproprionate[41] aerosols firmly established these topical agents as valuable 'steroid-sparing' adjuncts to the therapy for asthma.

The quality of the response to these new steroids was superior to that seen with hydrocortisone, prednisolone and dexamethasone aerosols: the separation of beneficial local effects from unwanted systemic effects was far greater. Was this because these were truly topically active in some unexplained manner, as was suggested by their vasoconstrictor scores, or was it one of those fortuitous discoveries? The answer is undoubtedly the latter, for reasons that will become apparent upon understanding the mechanism of action of these drugs.

Mechanisms of action

General

The basic roles of the adrenal cortex in regulating carbohydrate metabolism and electrolyte balance had been identified by 1930. During the 1930s and 1940s, there was intense interest in the biological actions of the hormones of this gland and it was found that many metabolic pathways were influenced by them. In 1952, Dorfman suggested that the corticosteroids could regulate the activity of a number of specific enzymes[42]. From the latter grew the concept that a general mechanism of action for the steroids could be due to enzyme induction, which would then regulate, if not all effects, then at least the various metabolic effects already shown.

The first evidence for an action of a steroid at gene level arose by the recognition, by Clever and Karlson in 1960[43], that injections of 1×10^{-9} M of the insect hormone ecdysone resulted in swelling at specific sites in giant chromosomes, the change occurring within 30 minutes. This was followed by the demonstration that blockade of protein or RNA synthesis resulted in an inhibition of enzyme induction by glucocorticoids[44,45]. These findings were made shortly after the discovery of the transcriptional control of DNA to RNA and led, in the late 1960s, to an expansion of research into steroid hormone action based on transcriptional regulation.

Reviews of the next decade's discoveries culminating in the unifying theory of a common mechanism of action, applicable to all steroid classes, have been given by Rousseau[46], Baxter[47] and Munck and Leung[48]. A monograph published in 1979 also contains much useful information[49]. It has been shown that almost all cell types in the body respond, in one way or another, to glucocorticoids and that the mechanism involves steroid binding to cytosol receptors, nuclear binding and protein synthesis as shown in the simplified scheme given in *Figure 14.1*.

In brief, the steroid diffuses passively and rapidly across the cell membrane where it binds with high affinity to a class-specific soluble cytoplasmic protein receptor. The steroid–receptor complex then undergoes conformational and energy changes such that it can enter the nucleus, where

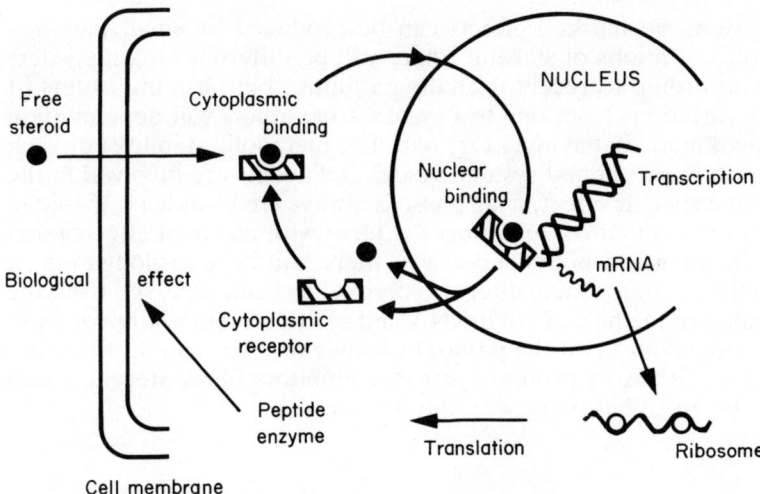

Figure 14.1 Generalized scheme of the mechanism of action of steroid hormones.

binding to nuclear acceptor sites occurs. Nuclear acceptor sites are probably not saturated in the intact cell and there is probably not sequence specificity for the stage of nuclear binding, which nevertheless also appears to be class specific. It seems highly probable, although not proven, that the glucocorticoid cytosol receptor is the same from tissue to tissue within a given species, but not necessarily between species: betamethasone valerate, for example, is inactive in the rat[50]. Whether there are differences in nuclear acceptors in different tissues of the same species is unanswered at present, but each tissue responds in a different way according to its physiological role and behaviour. Following nuclear binding, transcription of DNA sequences to messenger RNAs occurs, the mRNAs pass to ribosomal sites in the cytoplasm, and translation of the codons to peptides or proteins takes place. It is these peptides or proteins which are responsible for the expression of glucocorticoid activity.

This process confers characteristic properties which can be used in experimental situations to define whether or not a steroid response is mediated via this specific mechanism (*Table 14.3*). For example, this is an

TABLE 14.3. Features of specific and non-specific glucocorticoid effects

Specific	*Non-specific*
Occur at concn = K_d (10^{-8}–10^{-10} M)	Occur at 10^{-5} M and above
Glucocorticoid specific	Not class specific
Ranking order of potency	No rank order
Dose–response relationship	Poor dose–response effects
Inhibition by:	No inhibition by:
(i) Competitive antagonists	(i) Competitive antagonists
(ii) RNA synthesis inhibitors	(ii) RNA synthesis inhibitors
(iii) Protein synthesis inhibitors	(iii) Protein synthesis inhibitors
Time lag in onset and prolongation after steroid removed	Effects related solely to presence of steroid
Require intact and living cells	Can be demonstrated in membranes, liposomes

amplifier system, so marked effects can be produced by small (submicromolar) concentrations of steroid. There will be different ranking orders of potency according to receptor-binding affinities but absolute orders of potency, or variations from one test system to another, will depend upon the pharmacokinetic behaviour (e.g. half-life, metabolic stability) of each steroid in each experimental system. As several events are involved in the expression of a specific effect, a lag phase is always seen—at least 15 min in biochemical terms *in vitro*[51] and longer *in vivo*, with maximal effects possibly not seen for many hours. Likewise, there will be a prolongation of effect, usually for many hours after the steroid has been removed from the system, related to the half-life of mRNA and of the protein synthesized but ultimately dependent upon the pathophysiology *in vivo*. Due to the sequence of events, RNA or protein synthesis inhibitors block steroid action but have to be given before or with the steroid.

Specific

Receptor analysis has established that many actions of the corticosteroids are mediated via the glucocorticoid receptor mechanism. What we have to ask is can these actions explain the physiological and pharmacological effects attributed to steroids when used in the treatment of asthma and what, specifically, are these key beneficial effects? The effects of steroids on the various cells and components of the inflammatory response are described below and it will become clear that, whilst glucocorticoids manifestly reduce several components of the inflammatory response, it cannot be stated with surety that this is due solely to inhibition of mediator release as implied by the heading for this section of the book.

BLOOD VESSELS

The mechanisms by which steroids inhibit oedema formation and cell exudation have been reviewed recently[52-54]. The conclusions reached were that (*a*) vasoconstriction can be produced by glucocorticoids, (*b*) steroids inhibit oedema formation in several models, (*c*) this inhibition involves RNA and protein synthesis and has the time course of a specific receptor-mediated glucocorticoid action, (*d*) inhibition of oedema formation is separate from inhibition of cell migration and can be overcome by arachidonic acid or its metabolites and (*e*) suppression of neutrophil-dominated inflammation is probably due, not to inhibition of neutrophil function, but to inhibition of neutrophil–endothelial cell interaction.

No studies on vascular endothelial cells or smooth muscle have yet been carried out to identify what biochemical events are affected by glucocorticoids, nor indeed have steroid receptors been identified from these cell types. Thus, although there is little doubt that glucocorticoids can modify the vascular events occurring during inflammation, little precise data are available.

NEUTROPHILS

A neutrophil leucocytosis occurs as a result of glucocorticoid administration to man. In addition, glucocorticoids inhibit the migration of neutrophils into an inflamed site. An attractive unifying concept is that steroids inhibit the adherence of neutrophils to vascular endothelial surfaces, which occurs to some extent normally and is exaggerated at sites of injury, thereby releasing cells into the circulation and preventing emigration. Again, the specific mechanism by which this might occur has not yet been defined. In a review by Mishler[55], the conclusion was reached that it was difficult to be sure of any effect that steroids might have on neutrophils themselves, since experimental conditions made interactive mechanisms difficult to interpret and the concentrations used in many studies were suprapharmacological, i.e. 10^{-5} M or above. Braidman et al. reported that polymorphs from human rheumatoid synovial fluid do not possess steroid receptors[56], in contrast to circulating cells.

Hence, although circulating neutrophils have the ability to respond to steroids, it is possible that neutrophil function at sites of injury is unaffected. The value of steroids in acute inflammation is, therefore, probably secondary to the reduction in local neutrophil cell number and the sensitivity of neighbouring cells to products released by these cells.

MACROPHAGES

Glucocorticoids produce a profound monocytopenia and reduce migration of these cells to sites of inflammation. In high concentrations in guinea-pig lung, they inhibit bronchoalveolar aggregation[57]. However, the mechanisms for these effects have not yet been defined. Glucocorticoid receptors have been identified in a subcultured murine cell line and the inhibition of secretion of elastase, collagenase and plasminogen activator has been shown to be due to specific glucocorticoid action[58]. Similarly, inhibition of prostaglandin production from rat, mouse and guinea-pig macrophages has been shown to be due to glucocorticoid action at concentrations ranging from 3×10^{-9} M to 3×10^{-5} M[59-61].

It is apparent that the macrophage is a key cell in the chronic inflammatory process. The products of its secretion either have a direct local action or recruit other cell types to exert their effects. Glucocorticoids inhibit the migration, activity and secretion of the macrophage in a way that would be beneficial in reducing inflammation.

LYMPHOCYTES

It has been known for many years that glucocorticoids cause a lymphocytopenia (principally due to redistribution of T cells) and involution of lymphoid tissues. Many of the supposed inhibitory effects of steroids on lymphocyte behaviour in man may be secondary to these changes in circulation kinetics[62]. Although circulating human lymphocytes have been shown to possess glucocorticoid receptors[63], there are relatively few studies which demonstrate effects ex vivo or in vitro using pharmacological concentrations of steroid. Thus, antibody synthesis is only decreased when very high doses are administered in a few specific disease states[64]. By contrast, in vitro studies have shown that pharmacological concentrations of steroid enhance antibody production[65]. Studies ex vivo have shown that glucocorticoids suppress autologous, but not allogenic, mixed lymphocyte reactions[66]. Similarly, antigen-induced, but not mitogen-induced, proliferation is also suppressed by pharmacological concentrations of steroid[67].

Reversal of the decreased β-adrenergic receptor density which is found in asthmatics[68] has not been demonstrated[69].

Whilst gluococorticoids undoubtedly influence lymphocyte behaviour in man, this influence is considerably less than in rodents, animals frequently used in experimental situations. In man, it is likely that suppression of immunologically based inflammation is due more to suppression of the inflammatory consequences rather than the immune response itself.

EOSINOPHILS

Eosinopenia follows steroid administration and is so striking that, from as early as 1948, it was used as a test to measure the response to ACTH, corticosteroids or stress[70]. The eosinopenia is presumed to be due to redistribution rather than to cytolysis. Inhibition of the chemotactic response to eosinophil chemotactic factor of anaphylaxis and the complement fragment, C5a, only occurs at suprapharmacological concentrations of steroid[71].

An increased eosinophil count in the sputum and lungs of asthmatic patients is a striking feature of the pathology of this disease. In addition, blood or sputum eosinophilia in a chronic bronchitic is a feature indicating a likely favourable response to steroids[72]. Thus, alterations in transport kinetics of this cell type by steroids will obviously modify the disease process. However, why this should be so is not understood.

MAST CELLS

Corticosteroids have no apparent effects on the mast cell at pharmacological concentrations[52]. Inhibition of histamine release[73] and stabilization of mast cell or lysosomal membranes fulfil the criteria for non-specific steroid effects described in *Table 14.3*. Inhalational challenge in patients on steroids will still result in a fall in peak expiratory flow rate and skin testing will result in a wheal-and-flare response[74]. Serum IgE levels are affected little or not at all[75]. Very little is known about the kinetics of circulating basophils and the effect of steroids upon this cell type.

Why steroids do not affect the immediate response in allergic patients, yet protect these same patients in their day-to-day life, is not known. Steroids do, however, protect against the late response, in keeping with their role as anti-inflammatory agents.

ARACHIDONATE RELEASE

Mention has already been made of the effects of steroids on decreasing the production of prostaglandins from macrophages. That this is due to specific glucocorticoid action is now beyond doubt. However, the effect varies from one cell type to another and the site of inhibition is controversial[54]. The hypothesis proposed by the group from the Wellcome Foundation[76-78] is that inhibition of arachidonic acid release from cell membranes is a key feature of steroid action, thus preventing generation of vasoactive, chemotactic and bronchoconstrictive metabolites via the cyclo-oxygenase and lipoxygenase pathways. The identification of a protein molecule ('macrocortin') as the putative inhibitor is the closest any group has come to identifying the protein synthesized as a result of steroid induction[79]. However, inhibition of arachidonic acid release is not the sole mechanism for steroid action[54,80], since cellular and vascular responses of acute inflammation are discrete; furthermore, in chronic inflammation (overtly influenced by corticosteroids), the role of prostaglandins has not been clearly established. With the identification and synthesis of the leukotrienes and the considerable biochemical and pharmacological interest generated in this area of research, there is hope for further clarification in the not too distant future.

ADENYLATE CYCLASE

β-Adrenergic drugs and prostaglandin (PG) E_1, act via membrane receptors to stimulate the activity of the enzyme adenylate cyclase. Foster and Perkins[81] showed that a specific glucocorticoid mechanism was responsible for potentiating this response to PGE_1 after exposure of cultured human astrocytoma cells to steroids. Later, Mano et al.[82] and Fraser and Venter[83] demonstrated an increase in β-receptor density in rat lung tissues and cultured human lung cells, respectively. An attractive hypothesis linking these findings is that the enhancement of adenylate cyclase activity in both instances is due to the ability of steroids to induce the synthesis of a peptide or protein which regulates receptor–adenylate cyclase coupling[84]. The implications of these findings in the context of β-adrenergic resistance in asthmatics is more fully discussed in Chapter 10.

Relevant to asthma

GENERAL

Although a considerable amount of knowledge has accumulated in the past six years, since the general mechanism of specific glucocorticoid action was established, there are still vast gaps to be filled. For example, it is only recently that human cells or tissues have been used, steroid receptors have not yet been demonstrated in many human cell types, it is not known whether the receptor or nuclear acceptor is the same in all tissues of one species, and in only one case has the specific protein resulting from steroid action been putatively identified. Combining these uncertainties with permutations of the complex events involved in acute and chronic inflammation and in the pathogenesis of asthma, does not allow firm statements to be made about how steroids work although they undoubtedly do suppress inflammation. Nonetheless, it is apparent that the pattern of response fits the general receptor-mediated glucocorticoid-specific mechanism of action.

Thus, free steroid concentrations of hydrocortisone or betamethasone needed to control severe asthma are about 3×10^{-7} M^{85} and 7×10^{-10} M^{53}, respectively, in the plasma, concentrations appropriate to the dissociation constant K_d of receptor for steroid. Although tissue concentrations may be higher, there is no evidence that the achievement of higher concentrations produces any qualitatively different response. The rank order of potencies of the steroids applies to asthma equally as well as to other conditions. The time lag in onset of response fits the biochemical events and can also be explained in physiological terms because of the time needed to effect some reduction in mucosal oedema. The prolongation of effect, beyond the maintenance of useful steroid concentrations, can be explained by the same mechanisms. The failure to protect against antigen challenge is matched by a failure to demonstrate inhibition of mediator release from mast cells. The reversal of β-adrenergic hyposensitivity or down-regulation can be explained by effects on receptor coupling. The possibility of loss of receptor number due to age or disease, or down-regulation of receptor binding[86,87], might explain why some patients need considerably higher doses of steroid than others.

'TOPICAL' AND 'SYSTEMIC' STEROIDS

The so-called topical steroids behave qualitatively in a similar manner to the systemic steroids. Clinically their beneficial effects are the same and their time course of action is also similar. Furthermore, as with oral steroids, inhaled steroids do not prevent the immediate bronchoconstrictor response but do prevent the late responses[88]. It is likely that local concentrations in the lung are in the submicromolar region. Receptor binding or displacement studies using human fibroblasts and epidermal cells have established that the glucocorticoid receptor has high affinity for the topical steroids[89,90]. The rank order of binding correlates with the rank order of potency when used by inhalation (*see* above and [91]). Whilst there are uncertainties about the effect of lipid solubility and bulky ester groupings on intracellular transport and binding, no overt differences in dose requirements or quality of response have been demonstrated solely on the basis of differences in lipid/water partition coefficient.

It therefore seems reasonable to conclude that 'topical' steroids work via the same mechanisms as the 'systemic' steroids. Differences between these two types of steroid in separation of wanted from unwanted effects are, however, considerable. An examination of their kinetic behaviour provides a logical explanation for this.

Most of an 'inhaled' dose is swallowed and possibly 10% or less reaches the lungs[92,93]. The theoretical ability of a more lipid-soluble drug to permeate better to its site of action once inhaled into the lung, is counterbalanced by a concommitantly poorer aqueous solubility, which might hinder transfer through mucoid secretions. Indeed, the higher lipid solubility of a 'topical' steroid should ensure more rapid absorption away from its site of action[94]. The absorption of beclomethasone dipropionate[95] and budesonide[96] from animal lungs is rapid, and the initial absorption of clobetasol propionate after aerosol delivery in man can be detected within a minute[93]. A further potential feature acting against the steroid esters is their liability to de-esterification within the lung[97], although hydrolysis of budesonide[96] and possibly other acetonides does not occur. Thus, on balance, there are no reasons to believe that the local kinetic behaviour of the 'topical' steroids in the lung is more advantageous than that of the 'systemic' steroids.

There are, however, considerable differences in systemic handling after gastrointestinal absorption which would account for the dissociation of wanted from unwanted effects (*Table 14.4*). It is apparent that the absorption of the systemic steroids is almost complete[98–102] as is absorption of beclomethasone dipropionate[97], flunisolide[103] and budesonide[104]. Once

TABLE 14.4. Some kinetic features of glucocorticoids in man

Steroid	Plasma half-life (h)	Volume of distribution (l)	Bio availability (%)	Biliary excretion (%)
'Systemic'				
Cortisol	1.5	40	80	10
Prednisolone	2.5	70	80	10
Dexamethasone	5.0	120	80	10
'Topical'				
Fluocortin butyl ester	2.5	*	*	45
Betamethasone valerate	*	*	*	*
Beclomethasone dipropionate	*	*	*	65
Clobetasol propionate	3.9	165	50	*
Flunisolide	1.6	125	20	40
Budesonide	2.8	300	10	30

* = Unknown.

absorbed, these drugs are exposed to the liver and subject to 'first-pass' metabolism. The bioavailability of prednisolone and dexamethasone, as assessed by ratio under the plasma level time curve, oral:intravenous dosing, is approximately 80%[98,99]; first-pass metabolism is therefore about 20%. This situation is reversed with the topical steroids: the bioavailability of flunisolide[103] and budesonide[105] averaged only 20% and 11%, respectively, in healthy volunteers. First-pass metabolism was therefore about 80%. Considerable first-pass metabolism can be inferred for beclomethasone dipropionate, since an oral dose of 4 mg was needed to produce cortisol suppression in comparison with 100 μg given intravenously[106].

In conjunction with this extensive first-pass effect goes biliary excretion, although this is probably a secondary effect only and related to the higher molecular weights of the substituted derivatives. Thus, whereas excretion of the systemic steroids is principally via the kidney (almost entirely as polar metabolites), about half the excretion of topical steroids and their metabolites after intravenous injection is in the bile: 64% for beclomethasone dipropionate[94], 40% for flunisolide[103], 30% for budesonide[105] and 44% for fluocortin butyl ester[107]. Furthermore, it is likely that the more lipid-soluble compounds have a larger apparent volume of distribution and, since their plasma half-lives are similar to those of the systemic steroids, this implies greater clearance of drug. Hence, it would appear that enhanced lipid solubility improves hepatic extraction in a manner as yet unidentified. Lastly, de-esterification of the steroid esters may be important in reducing systemic activity since their parent molecules are intrinsically less active[28].

The future

Will corticosteroids still be widely prescribed for the treatment of asthma in the year 2000? The answer must undoubtedly be 'yes', if only in global terms since oral prednisolone is an established, cheap and effective therapy. This view is reinforced by consideration of the mechanisms of action of these drugs, complex and incompletely understood as they are today. The hope that a single 'second messenger' could be identified to account for the anti-inflammatory actions, thus opening the way for a selective and safer alternative method of treatment, seems to have failed. Several key biochemical events involved in the inflammatory process appear to be inhibited or modified by steroids. It is, therefore, unlikely that a single drug, for example an enzyme or mediator blocker, could produce such profound effects. Until an entirely new approach to the treatment of asthma becomes available (such as an IgE synthesis blocker?) corticosteroids will be with us.

This raises the question of whether novel steroids can be developed to provide yet greater separation of beneficial from unwanted effects. This seems unlikely for the oral or parenteral forms and clearly the best separation of activity is achieved by dosing by the inhaled route. Improvements in the therapeutic ratio after dosing by this route may be achieved by (a) increasing the proportion of the dose delivered to the lungs, (b) reducing the bioavailability of the swallowed portion, or by (c) the selection of a steroid with a short plasma half-life. The first two of these aims have already been tackled by the introduction of applicators of improved design, which maximize delivery to the lungs whilst trapping larger particles and minimizing the total dose delivered to the patient[108,109]. Such applicators will no doubt be more widely used or improved upon in the future. Modifications such as these may limit the occurrence of oropharyngeal candidiasis, in addition to allowing higher doses of inhaled steroid to be given. Higher doses may also be given if the steroid is cleared rapidly and has a short plasma half-life. Whether the use of higher doses will result in worthwhile therapeutic improvements over those obtained with high-dose beclomethasone dipropionate[110] is less likely. There are still a number of patients who require supplementary oral steroids for reasons not fully understood, although probably related to ventilation inequalities and poor aerosol distribution.

Finally, the reasons for the failure of some patients to respond even to parenteral steroids may be elucidated in the next two decades and the question of whether to give steroids earlier in an attack[111] or not at all[112] may be resolved.

References

1. HENCH, P.S., KENDALL, E.C., SLOCUMB, C.H. and POLLEY, H.F. *Proceedings of the Staff Meeting of the Mayo Clinic*, **24**, 181 (1949)
2. BORDLEY, J.E., CAREY, R.A., HARVEY, A.M., HOWARD, J.E., KATTUS, A.A., NEWMAN, E.V. et al. *Bulletin of the Johns Hopkins Hospital*, **85**, 396 (1949)
3. CARRYER, H.M., KOELSCHE, G.A., PRICKMAN, L.E., MAYTUM, C.K., LAKE, C.F. and WILLIAMS, H.L. *Journal of Allergy*, **21**, 282 (1950)
4. GLYN, J.J. *Cortisone Therapy*. pp. 18–41. London: Heinemann (1957)
5. REEDER, W.H. and MacKEY, G.S. *Diseases of the Chest*, **18**, 528 (1950)
6. GELFAND, M.L. *New England Journal of Medicine*, **245**, 293 (1951)
7. RINGLER, I., WEST, K., DULIN, W.E. and BOLAND, E.W. *Metabolism*, **13**, 37 (1964)
8. POPPER, T.L. and WATNICK, A.S. *Antiinflammatory Agents*, **1**, 245 (1974)
9. JACOBSON, M.E. *Postgraduate Medicine*, **49** (2), 181 (1971)
10. FALLIERS, C.J., CHAI, H., MOLK, L., BANE, H. and CARDOSO, R.R. DE A. *Journal of Allergy and Clinical Immunology*, **49**, 156 (1972)

11. WILSON, C.G., SSENDAGIRE, R., MAY, C.S. and PATERSON, J.W. *British Journal of Clinical Pharmacology*, **2**, 321 (1975)
12. SWARTZ, S.L. and DLUHY, R.G. *Drugs*, **16**, 238 (1978)
13. DAVID, D.S., GRIECO, M.H. and CUSHMAN, P. *Journal of Chronic Diseases*, **22**, 637 (1970)
14. FOULDS, W.S., GREAVES, D.P., HERXHEIMER, H. and KINGDOM, L.G. *Lancet*, **i**, 234 (1955)
15. BROCKBANK, W. and PENGELLY, C.D.R. *Lancet*, **i**, 187 (1958)
16. HELM, W.H. and HEYWORTH, F. *British Medical Journal*, **2**, 765 (1958)
17. FRANK. L. and STRITZLER, C. *Archives of Dermatology*, **72**, 547 (1955)
18. FRANKLIN, W., LOWELL, F.C., MICHELSON, A.L. and SCHILLER, I.W. *Journal of Allergy*, **29**, 214 (1958)
19. ARBESMAN, C.E., BONSTEIN, H.S. and REISMAN, R.E. *Journal of Allergy*, **34**, 354 (1963)
20. BICKERMAN, H.A. and ITKIN, S.E. *Journal of the American Medical Association*, **184**, 533 (1963)
21. BROWN, H.M. *Lancet*, **ii**, 147 (1963)
22. BIEDERMAN, A. *Wiener Medizinische Wochenschrift*, **121**, 331 (1971)
23. TURIAF, J., GUEROT, C. and AMSEL, M. *Le Poumon et le Coeur*, **26**, 769 (1970)
24. LINDER, W.R. *Archives of Internal Medicine*, **113**, 655 (1964)
25. NOVEY, H.S. and BEALL, G. *Archives of Internal Medicine*, **115**, 602 (1965)
26. TOOGOOD, J.H. and LEFCOE, N.M. *Journal of Allergy*, **36**, 321 (1965)
27. SIEGEL, S.C., HEIMLICH, E.M., RICHARDS, W. and KELLEY, V.C. *Pediatrics*, **33**, 245 (1964)
28. PHILLIPPS, G.H. In *Mechanisms of Topical Corticosteroid Activity*. Eds L. Wilson and R. Marks. pp. 1–18. Edinburgh: Churchill Livingston (1976)
29. McKENZIE, A.W. and STOUGHTON, R.B. *Archives of Dermatology*, **86**, 608 (1962)
30. McKENZIE, A.W. *Archives of Dermatology*, **86**, 611 (1962)
31. McKENZIE, A.W. and ATKINSON, R.M. *Archives of Dermatology*, **89**, 741 (1964)
32. WILLIAMS, D.I., WILKINSON, D.S., OVERTON, J., MILNE, J.A., McKENNA, W.B., LYELL, A. *et al.* *Lancet*, **i**, 1177 (1964)
33. WILSON, L. *British Journal of Dermatology*, **94**, Suppl. 12, 33 (1976)
34. WILSON, L. *Postgraduate Medical Journal*, **50**, Suppl. 4, 7 (1974)
35. CHOO-KANG, Y.F.J., ROSCOE, P. and HORNE, N.W. *Postgraduate Medical Journal*, **50** Suppl. 4, 73 (1974)
36. ROSCOE, P., CHOO-KANG, Y.F.J. and HORNE, N.W. *British Journal of Diseases of the Chest*, **69**, 240 (1975)
37. GRANT, I.W.B., CROMPTON, G.K., MALONE, D.N.S. and CHOO-KANG, Y.F.J. *British Medical Journal*, **2**, 110 (1972)
38. SMITH, A.P., BOOTH, M. and DAVEY, A.J. *British Medical Journal*, **3**, 705 (1971)
39. BROWN, H.M., STOREY, G. and GEORGE, W.H.S. *British Medical Journal*, **1**, 585 (1972)
40. PROCEEDINGS OF A SYMPOSIUM. *Postgraduate Medical Journal*, **50**, Suppl. 4 (1974)
41. PROCEEDINGS OF A SYMPOSIUM. *Postgraduate Medical Journal*, **51**, Suppl. 4 (1975)
42. DORFMAN, R.I. *Vitamins and Hormones*, **10**, 331 (1952)
43. CLEVER, U. and KARLSON, P. *Experimental Cell Research*, **20**, 623 (1960)
44. GREENGARD, O. and ACS, G. *Biochimica et Biophysica Acta*, **61**, 652 (1962)
45. GARREN, L.D., HOWELL, R.R. and TOMKINS, G.M. *Journal of Molecular Biology*, **9**, 100 (1964)
46. ROUSSEAU, G.G. *Journal of Steroid Biochemistry*, **6**, 75 (1976)
47. BAXTER, J.D. *Pharmacology and Therapeutics*, Part B, **2**, 605 (1976)
48. MUNCK, A. and LEUNG, K. In *Receptors and Mechanism of Action of Steroid Hormones*. Part II. Ed. J.R. Pasqualini. pp. 311–397. New York: Marcel Dekker (1977)
49. BAXTER, J.D. and ROUSSEAU, G.G. In *Glucocorticoid Hormone Action*. Eds J.D. Baxter and G. Rousseau. Berlin: Springer-Verlag (1979)
50. YOUNG, J.M., WAGNER, B.M. and FISK, R.A. *British Journal of Dermatology*, **99**, 665 (1978)
51. MUNCK, A. *Journal of Biological Chemistry*, **243**, 1039 (1968)
52. HARDING, S.M. *Progress in Respiration Research*, **14**, 224 (1980)
53. HARDING, S.M. *Allergologie*, **3**, (4), S214 (1980)
54. SKIDMORE, I.F. *Molecular Aspects of Medicine*, **4**, 303 (1981)
55. MISHLER, J.M. *Experimental Haematology*, **5**, Suppl., 15 (1977)
56. BRAIDMAN, I.P., COLLINS, K., JONES, C., MORRIS, K. and JAYSON, M.I.V. *Agents and Actions*, Suppl. 7, 233 (1980)
57. GAUMER, H.R., SALVAGGIO, J.E., WESTON, W.L. and CLAMAN, H.N. *International Archives of Allergy*, **47**, 797 (1974)
58. WERB, Z., FOLEY, R. and MUNCK, A. *Journal of Immunology*, **124**, 115 (1978)

59. ROSA, M. DI and PERSICO, P. *British Journal of Pharmacology*, **66**, 161 (1979)
60. BONNEY, R.J., DAVIES, P., KUEHL, F. and HUMES, J.L. *European Journal of Rheumatology and Inflammation*, **1**, 308 (1978)
61. BRAY, M.A. and GORDON, D. *British Journal of Pharmacology*, **63**, 635 (1978)
62. PEARSON, C.M., CLEMENTS, P.J. and YU, D.T.Y. *European Journal of Rhematology and Inflammation*, **1**, 216 (1978)
63. LIPPMAN, M. and BARR, R. *Journal of Immunology*, **118**, 1977 (1981)
64. McMILLAN, R., LONGMIRE, R. and YELENOSKY, R. *Journal of Immunology*, **116**, 1592 (1976)
65. SHERMAN, N.A., SMITH, R.S. and MIDDLETON, E. *Journal of Allergy and Clinical Immunology*, **52**, 13 (1973)
66. YU, D.T.Y., RAMER, S.J. and CLEMENTS, P.J. *Transplantation*, **25**, 163 (1978)
67. BALOW, J.E., HURLEY, D.L. and FAUCI, A.S. *Journal of Immunology*, **114**, 1072 (1975)
68. KARIMAN, K. *Lung*, **158**, 41 (1980)
69. DAVIES, A.O. and LEFKOWITZ, R.J. *Journal of Clinical Endocrinology and Metabolism*, **51**, 599 (1980)
70. HILLS, A.G., FORSHAM, P.H. and FINCH, C.A. *Blood*, **3**, 755 (1948)
71. GAUDERER, C.A. and GLEICH, G.J. *Proceedings of the Society for Experimental Biology and Medicine*, **157**, 129 (1978)
72. HARDING, S.M. and FREEDMAN, S. *Thorax*, **33**, 214 (1978)
73. MORR, H. and BORNEMANN, G. *Allergologie*, 3(4), S237 (1980)
74. McCARTHY, D.S. and PEPYS, J. *Clinical Allergy*, **1**, 415 (1971)
75. CLAMAN, H.N. *Journal of Allergy and Clinical Immunology*, **55**, 145 (1977)
76. NIJKAMP, F.P., FLOWER, R.J., MONCADA, S. and VANE, J.R. *Nature*, **263**, 479 (1976)
77. BLACKWELL, G.J., FLOWER, R.J., NIJKAMP, F.P. and VANE, J.R. *British Journal of Pharmacology*, **62**, 79 (1978)
78. FLOWER, R.J. and BLACKWELL, G.J. *Nature*, **278**, 456 (1979)
79. BLACKWELL, G.J., CARNUCCIO, R., ROSA, M. DI, FLOWER, R.J., PARENTE, L. and PERSICO, P. *Nature*, **287**, 147 (1980)
80. FLOWER, R. *Trends in Pharmaceutical Sciences*, **7**, 186 (1981)
81. FOSTER, S.J. and PERKINS, J.P. *Proceedings of the National Academy of Sciences of the United States of America*, **74**, 4816 (1977)
82. MANO, K., AKBARZADEH, A. and TOWNLEY, R.G. *Life Sciences*, **25**, 1925 (1979)
83. FRASER, C.M. and VENTER, J.C. *Biochemical and Biophysical Research Communications*, **94**, 390 (1980)
84. DAVIES, A.O. and LEFKOWITZ, K.J. *Journal of Clinical Endocrinology and Metabolism*, **53**, 703 (1981)
85. COLLINS, J.V., CLARK, T.J.H., BROWN, D. and TOWNSEND, J. *Quarterly Journal of Medicine*, **174**, 259 (1975)
86. PRATT, W.B. *Journal of Investigative Dermatology*, **71**, 24 (1978)
87. HARRIS, A.W. and BAXTER, J.D. In: *Glucocorticoid Hormone Action*. Eds J.D. Baxter and G.G. Rousseau. pp. 424–448. Berlin: Springer-Verlag (1979)
88. PEPYS, J., DAVIES, R.J., BRESLIN, A.B.X., HENDRICK, D.J. and HUTCHCROFT, B.J. *Clinical Allergy*, **4**, 13 (1974)
89. PONEC, M., HASPER, I., VIANDEN, G.D.N.E. and BACHRA, B.N. *Archives of Dermatology Research*, **259**, 125 (1977)
90. PONEC, M., KEMPENAAR, J.A. and DE KLOET, E.R. *Journal of Investigative Dermatology*, **76**, 211 (1981)
91. HAHN, H.L. and HARDING, S.M. *Progress in Respiration Research*, **14**, 290 (1980)
92. DAVIES, D.S. *Evaluation of Bronchodilator Drugs*. Folkestone: F.J. Parsons Ltd (1975)
93. HARDING, S.M. In *Proceedings of the XIth International Congress of Allergology and Clinical Immunology*. Eds J.W. Kerr and M.A. Ganderton. pp. 517–522. Basingstoke: MacMillan Press (1983)
94. SALVATORE, E. and SCHANKER, L.J. *American Journal of Physiology*, **223**, 1227 (1972)
95. MARTIN, L.E., HARRISON, C. and TANNER, R.J.N. *Postgraduate Medical Journal*, **51**, Suppl. 4, 11 (1975)
96. BRATTSAND, R., KALLSTROM, L. NILSSON, E. RYRFELDT, A. and TONNESSON, M. *European Journal of Respiratory Diseases*, **63**, Suppl. 122, 263 (1982)
97. MARTIN, L.E., TANNER, R.J.N., CLARK, T.J.H. and COCHRANE, G.M. *Clinical Pharmacology and Therapeutics*, **15**, 267 (1974)
98. SANDBERG, A.A. and SLAUNWHITE, W.R. *Journal of Clinical Endocrinology*, **17**, 1040 (1957)

99. PETEREIT, L.B. and MEIKLE, A.W. *Clinical Pharmacology and Therapeutics*, **22,** 912 (1977)
100. DUGGAN, D.E., YEH, K.C., MATALIA, N., DITZLER, C.A. and McMAHON, F.G. *Clinical Pharmacology and Therapeutics*, **18,** 205 (1975)
101. HAACK, D., LICHTWALD, K. and VECSEI, P. *Acta Endocrinologica*, **96,** Suppl. 240, 64 (1981)
102. RAITH, L. ND KARL, H.J. *Klinische Wochenschrift*, **44,** 298 (1966)
103. CHAPLIN, M.D., ROOKS, W., SWENSON, E.W., COOPER, W.C., NERENBERG, C. and CHU, N.I. *Clinical Pharmacology and Therapeutics*, **27,** 402 (1980)
104. RYRFELDT, A., TONNESSON, M., NILSSON, E. and WIKBY, A. *Journal of Steroid Biochemistry*, **10,** 317 (1979)
105. RYRFLEDT, A., ANDERSSON, P., EDSBACKER, S., TONNESSON, M., DAVIES, D. and PAUWELS, R. *European Journal of Respiratory Diseases*, **63,** Suppl. 122, 86 (1982)
106. HARRIS, D.M. *Postgraduate Medical Journal*, **51,** Suppl. 4, 20 (1975)
107. MUETZEL, W. *Drug Research*, **27,** 2230 (1977)
108. BLOOMFIELD, P., CROMPTON, G.K. and WINSEY, N.J.P. *British Medical Journal*, **2,** 1479 (1978)
109. TOOGOOD, J.H., JENNINGS, B., BASKERVILLE, J. and JOHANSSON, S.A. *European Journal of Respiratory Diseases*, **63,** Suppl. 122, 100 (1982)
110. FRANCIS, R.S. *British Journal of Diseases of the Chest*, **73,** 424 (1979)
111. BRITISH THORACIC ASSOCIATION. *British Medical Journal*, **285,** 1251 (1982)
112. LUKSZA, A.R. *British Journal of Diseases of the Chest*, **76,** 15 (1982)

Chapter 15

Non-steroidal inhibitors of arachidonic acid metabolism

T.Y. Shen and A.N. Tischler

Introduction

Following the dramatic discovery of the anti-inflammatory effects of corticosteroids, the search for non-steroidal agents with similar activities but, hopefully, with less severe side-effects was launched in many laboratories. From an extensive chemical and pharmacological effort, a large family of non-steroidal anti-inflammatory–analgesic drugs, commonly known as NSAIDs, have emerged in the past two decades[1,2]. NSAIDs were developed mainly with the use of animal assays and their biochemical mechanism of action remained obscure for a number of years. The inhibition of prostaglandin biosynthesis by two NSAIDs, aspirin and indomethacin (1), first observed by Vane and coworkers in 1971[3], marked the beginning of an extensive biological study of the effects of NSAIDs on the metabolism of arachidonic acid. The availability of indomethacin as a research

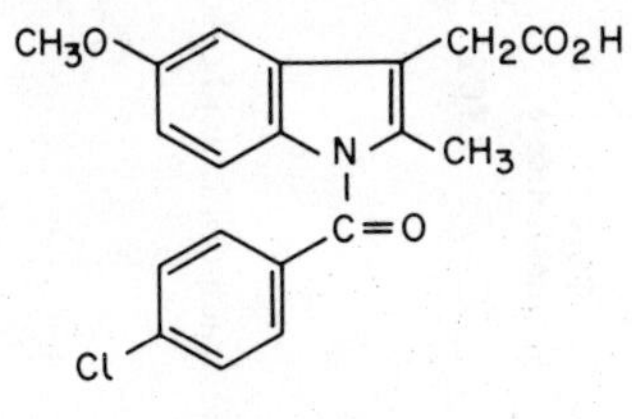

Indomethacin

(1)

tool both clarified the involvement of prostaglandins in many pathological conditions and facilitated the elucidation of other arachidonic acid pathways which produce a variety of oxygenated metabolites with potent biological activities.

315

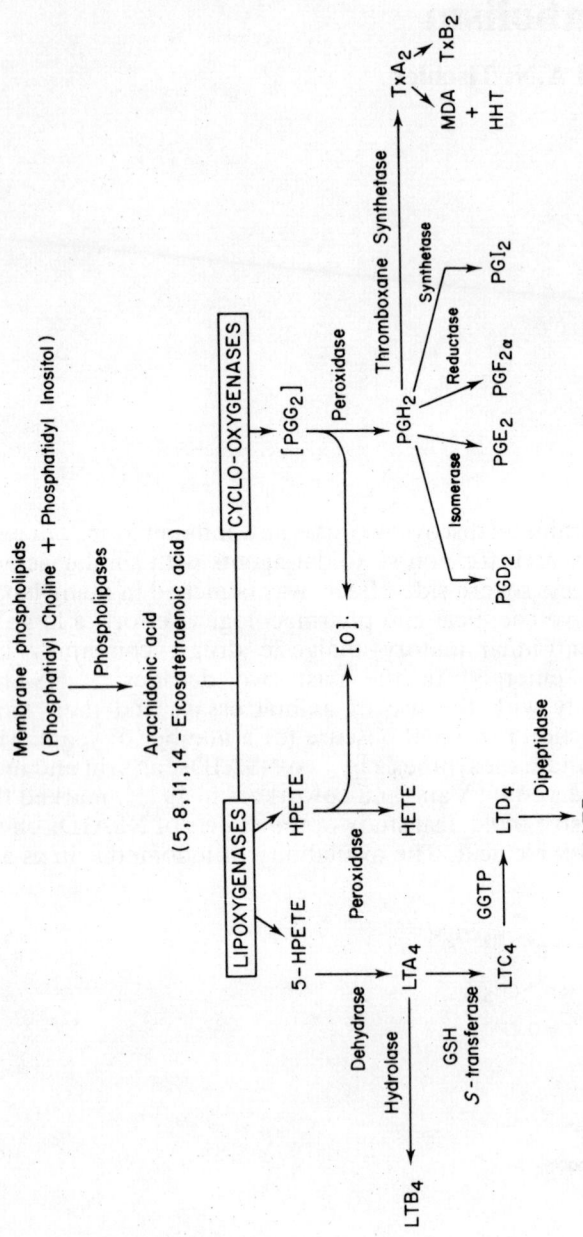

Figure 15.1 The arachidonic acid cascade. GSH = glutathione; MDA = malondialdehyde; HHT = 12-hydroxy-5,8,10-heptadecatrienoic acid.

As shown in *Figure 15.1*, the cyclo-oxygenase pathway, inhibitable by indomethacin, is now recognized as one of the two principal pathways in the expanding arachidonic acid cascade. The cyclo-oxygenase system converts arachidonic acid to prostaglandins, prostacyclin, thromboxanes, and other oxygenated products. The importance of the lipoxygenase pathway was realized a few years ago when it was shown that slow-reacting substance (SRS), of traditional interest in pulmonary research, was a mixture of several leukotrienes[4]. The interaction of the two pathways, e.g. the shunt of the common substrate arachidonic acid from one pathway to the other in the presence of selective inhibitors, and the activation of the cyclo-oxygenase pathway by lipoxygenase metabolites in several biological systems, has also been recognized. As the biological properties of these arachidonic acid metabolites are amply discussed in a previous chapter, their synthetic inhibitors will be discussed mainly in terms of their chemical and enzymatic characteristics.

The therapeutic potential of inhibitors of cyclo-oxygenase, thromboxane synthetase, lipoxygenases and scavengers of oxygen radicals have received much attention. In view of the very extensive literature on a variety of cyclo-oxygenase inhibitors as non-steroidal anti-inflammatory–analgesic agents, only a brief overview is given below. Various factors, such as enzyme and tissue selectivity and pharmacodynamics, which affect their overall *in vivo* efficacy, as well as side-effects, will be mentioned. Many inhibitors of other biosynthetic or catabolizing enzymes in this cascade have also been described, but in most cases their *in vivo* activities have not been well established. For further consideration, several potential therapeutic approaches, such as the inhibition of phospholipase A$_2$, the concomitant blockade of both cyclo-oxygenase and 5-lipoxygenase, the inhibition of other sites in the lipoxygenase pathway and the regulation of the platelet-activating factor, will also be described.

Inhibition of phospholipase A$_2$

The substrate, arachidonic acid, for both cyclo-oxygenase and lipoxygenase pathways is derived from membrane phospholipids, for example C$_2$-arachidonyl phosphatidyl choline can release arachidonic acid by the action of phospholipase A$_2$ upon the activation of an inflammatory stimulus. The anti-inflammatory and anti-asthmatic effects of corticosteroids may be, in part, attributable to their ability to induce the synthesis of a protein inhibitor, macrocortin (lipomodulin) of phospholipase A$_2$[5,6] (*Figure 15.2*). Non-steroidal anti-inflammatory–analgesic agents (NSAIDs) in general are very

TABLE 15.1. Inhibition of phospholipase A$_2$ by NSAIDs

NSAID	IC$_{50}$ (M) of	
	Rat PMN phospholipase A$_2$	*Rabbit platelet cyclo-oxygenase*
Indomethacin	>10^{-4}	10^{-7}
Naproxen	>10^{-4}	10^{-5}
Benoxaprofen	10^{-4}	3 × 10^{-5}
Aspirin	>10^{-4}	10^{-5}

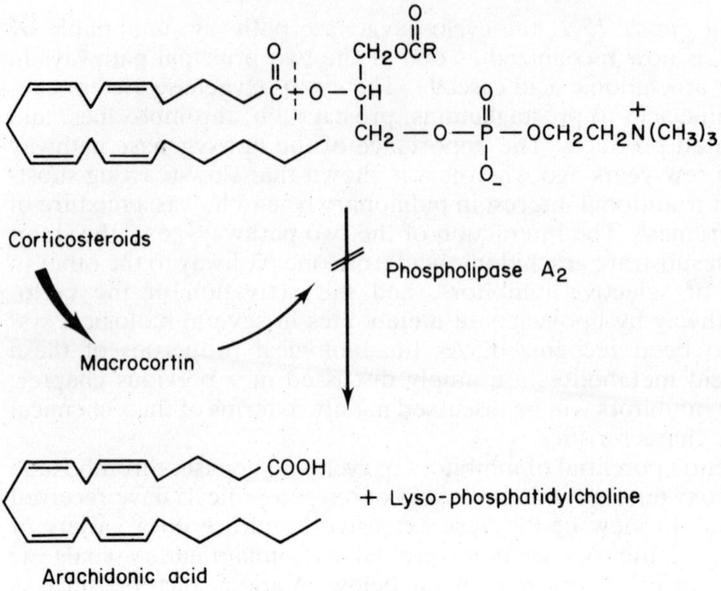

Figure 15.2 Phospholipase A_2 inhibition.

weak phospholipase A_2 inhibitors[7]. As shown in *Table 15.1*, the concentrations of these drugs needed for phospholipase A_2 inhibition are much higher than their cyclo-oxygenase inhibitory levels[8]. Experiments *in vivo* measuring either the efficacy or side-effects of these drugs also confirm their lack of systemic phospholipase A_2 inhibitory activities.

Inhibition of the cyclo-oxygenase pathway

NSAIDs as cyclo-oxygenase inhibitors

The arachidonic acid cyclo-oxygenase is a microsomal enzyme which converts arachidonic acid in the presence of oxygen to an unstable hydroperoxy-endoperoxide intermediate, PGG_2 (*Figure 15.1*). PGG_2 is readily converted to the corresponding hydroxy derivative, PGH_2, through the action of a peroxidase. Further transformation of PGH_2 yields thromboxane A_2 (TxA_2, as in platelets), PGI_2 (particularly in vascular endothelium) and other primary prostaglandins, e.g. PGD_2, PGE_2, $PGF_{2\alpha}$ etc., either enzymatically or chemically (*Figure 15.3*). The inhibition of the cyclo-oxygenase by aspirin, indomethacin and several other NSAIDs at their therapeutic concentrations provided a mechanistic explanation of their biological actions[3]. It also provided a biochemical approach for the development of similar agents. Cyclo-oxygenase preparations from sheep or bovine seminal vesicles and human platelets have been widely used *in vitro* to determine the prostaglandin synthesis inhibitory activity of many NSAIDs[9]. A few typical examples are shown in *Table 15.2*. In general, a semiquantitative correlation of their cyclo-oxygenase inhibition with their

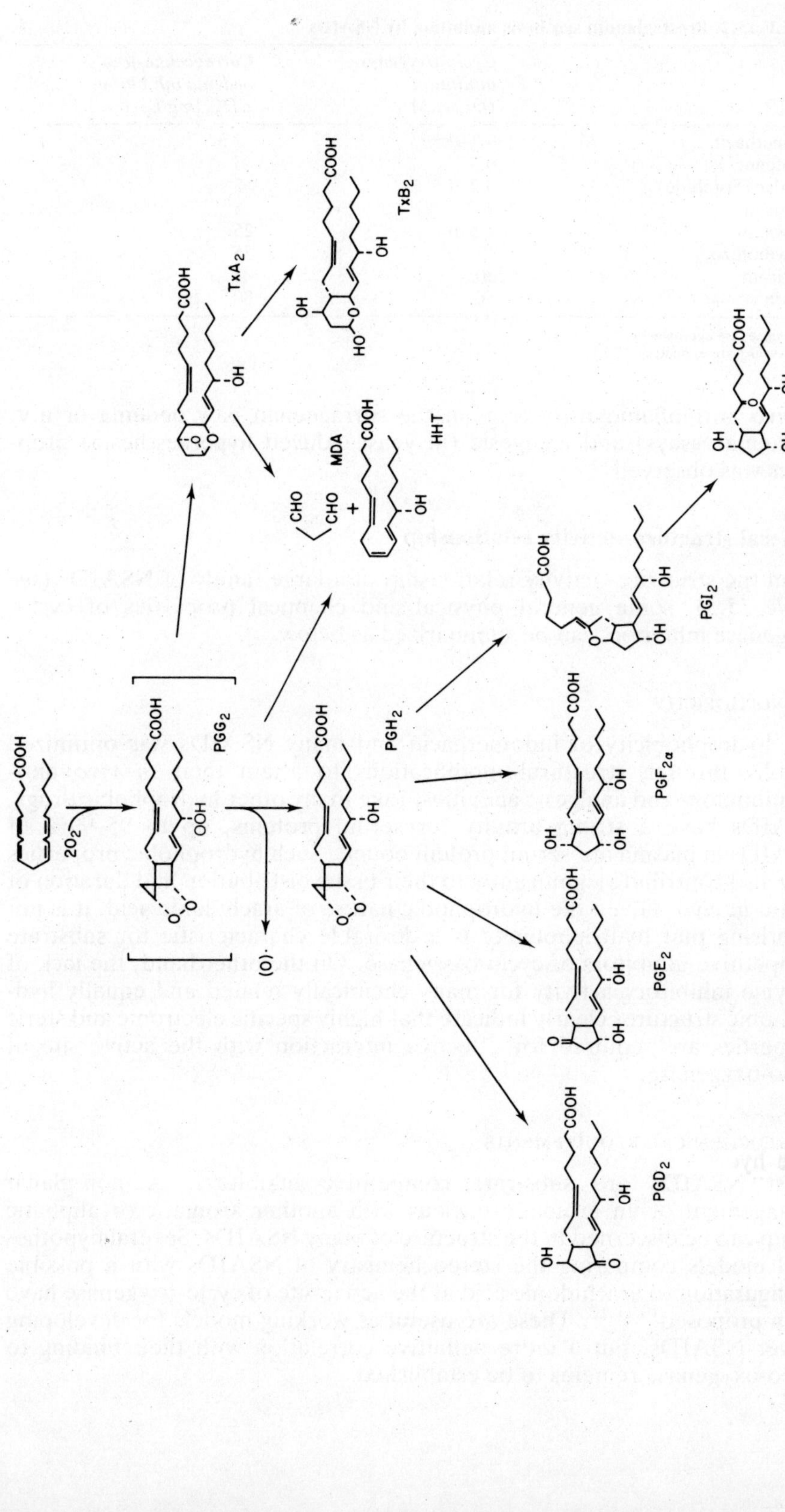

Figure 15.3 The cyclo-oxygenase pathway.

TABLE 15.2. Prostaglandin synthesis inhibition by NSAIDs

NSAID	Cyclo-oxygenase inhibition ID_{50} $(\mu M)^*$	Carrageenan-foot oedema inhibition ED_{50} $(mg/kg)^\dagger$
Indomethacin	0.1–0.5	2.3
Diclofenac	0.3	3
Sulindac (Sulphide)	0.2–0.5	2
Naproxen	1–2	5
Ibuprofen	1.5–6	25
Phenylbutazone	17–37	35
Piroxicam	20	3
Aspirin	50	80

* ID_{50} values are approximate.
† ED_{50} values are estimates.

in vivo anti-inflammatory (e.g. in the carrageenan paw oedema or u.v. erythema assays) and analgesic (in yeast-induced hyperaesthesia) properties was observed.

General structure–activity relationship

From the structure–activity relationship of a large family of NSAIDs (*see Table 15.3*), some general physical and chemical properties of cyclo-oxygenase inhibitors can be summarized as below.

HYDROPHOBICITY

The hydrophobicity of indomethacin and many NSAIDs was optimized initially through structural modifications to attain their *in vivo* anti-inflammatory and analgesic activities. Like many other hydrophobic drugs, NSAIDs have a strong affinity for serum proteins, up to 95–99% of NSAIDs in plasma are serum protein bound. Such hydrophobic properties may also contribute significantly to their tissue distribution and duration of action *in vivo*. Given the hydrophobic nature of arachidonic acid, it is not surprising that hydrophobicity is a desirable characteristic for substrate competitive inhibitors of cyclo-oxygenase. On the other hand, the lack of enzyme inhibitory activity for many chemically related and equally hydrophobic structures clearly indicate that highly specific electronic and steric properties are required for effective interaction with the active site of cyclo-oxygenase.

STEREOCHEMICAL REQUIREMENTS

Most NSAIDs are substrate competitive inhibitors. A non-planar arrangement of an aromatic nucleus with another aromatic or aliphatic group can be discerned in the structure of many NSAIDs. Several hypothetical models comparing the stereochemistry of NSAIDs with a possible configuration of arachidonic acid at the active site of cyclo-oxygenase have been proposed[10,11,12]. These are useful as working models for developing newer NSAIDs, but a more definitive correlation with their binding to cyclo-oxygenase remains to be established.

TABLE 15.3. Acidic cyclo-oxygenase inhibitors

Structural class
(1) *Salicylates*
Aspirin
Diflunisal
(2) *Fenamic acids*
Mefenamic acid
Meclofenamic acid
(3) *Aryl acetic acids*
Indomethacin
Sulindac (sulphide)
Tolmetin
Zomepirac
(4) *Phenyl acetic acids*
Diclofenac
Fenclofenac
(5) *Aryl propionic acids*
Ibuprofen
Naproxen
Fenoprofen
Ketoprofen
Flurbiprofen
Pirprofen
Carprofen
Benoxaprofen
Suprofen
Indoprofen
(6) *Aryl butyric acids*
Fenbufen
Furobufen
(7) *Acid enols*
Phenylbutazone
Oxyphenbutazone
Piroxicam
Isoxicam

For inhibitors of the aryl propionic acid type the stereochemistry of the chiral centre of the α-methyl acetic acid side chain was recognized early as being highly specific[13]. The $S(+)$ enantiomers are generally more active than the $R(-)$ enantiomers *in vitro* as well as *in vivo*. In some cases, for

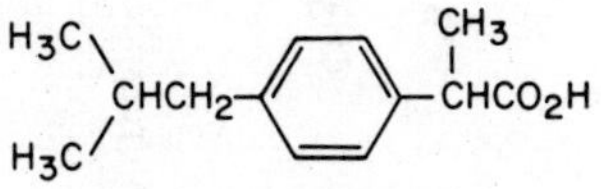

Ibuprofen

(2)

example, ibuprofen (2), naproxen (3), ketoprofen (4) and flurbiprofen (5), (*Figure 15.4*) such differences become less prominent *in vivo*, possibly due to a differential metabolism of the two enantiomers and/or racemization of the chiral centre.

322

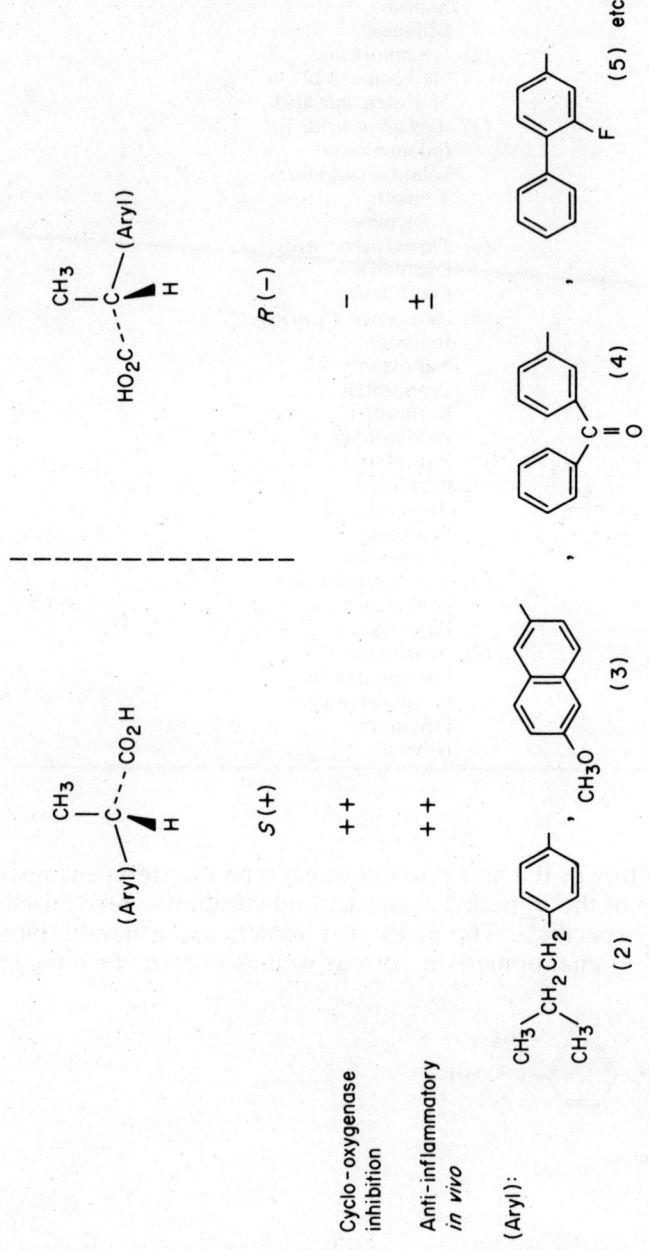

Figure 15.4 Stereospecificity of the chiral α-propionic acid side-chain.

ACIDIC FUNCTION

In the early study of NSAIDs, the presence of an acidic function, e.g. carboxyl, tetrazole, or an acidic enol, in substituted aryl or heteroaryl molecules was found to be highly desirable. The acidic group may compete with the carboxyl of arachidonic acid for enzyme binding, but no simple correlation with the acidity (pK_a) was observed. Later, it became apparent that the acidic function is not really essential for cyclo-oxygenase inhibition[14]. Non-acidic agents, for example, proquazone (6), tiflamizole (7)[15] and timegadine (8)[73] were found to be potent cyclo-oxygenase inhibitors *in vitro* and effective anti-inflammatory agents *in vivo* (*Table 15.4*). Furthermore,

TABLE 15.4. Non-acidic cyclo-oxygenase inhibitors

Compound	Cyclo-oxygenase inhibition ID_{50} (μM)*
Indoxol	1.5
Ciproquazone (6)	0.5
Timegadine (8)	0.05
Tiflamizole (7)	0.4
2-Aryl-oxazolopyridines	0.1–1
Thiabendazole	30

* ID_{50} values are approximate.

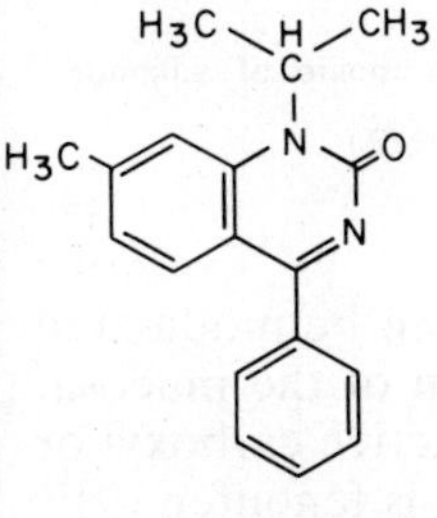

Proquazone
(6)

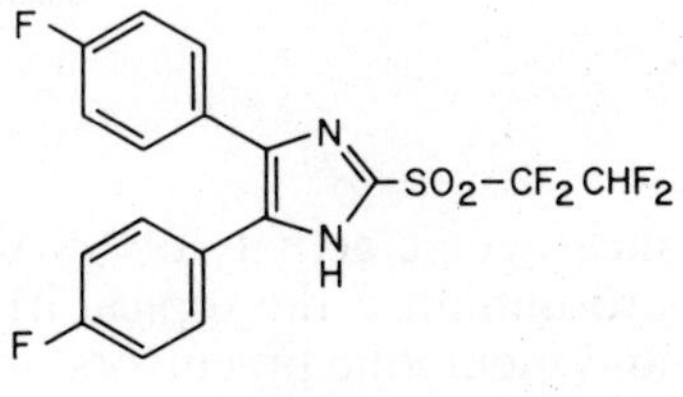

Tiflamizole
(7)

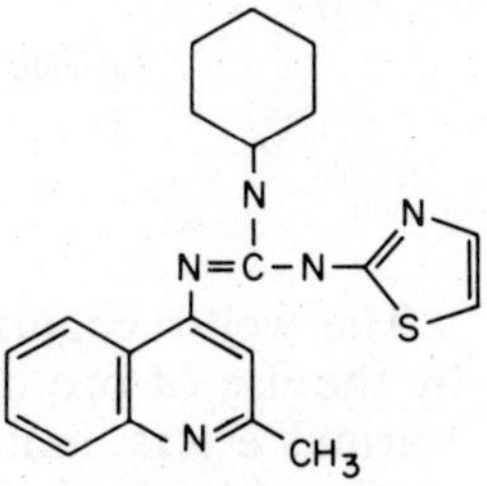

Timegadine
(8)

the non-acidic agents generally cause less gastrointestinal irritation in animal models. These molecules, unlike most acidic compounds, do not accumulate in the parietal cells and, presumably, cause less disturbance of prostaglandin synthesis in the mucosa[16]. Whether the altered *in vivo* distribution of non-acidic cyclo-oxygenase inhibitors will also change their potential side-effects in, for example aspirin-sensitive or renal-impaired, patients remains to be clarified.

Side-effects

Prostaglandins are involved in many physiological responses and excessive inhibition of prostaglandin synthesis by NSAIDs, especially in patients with gastric or renal impairment, may cause side-effects related to local prostaglandin deficiency. The well-known chronic side-effects of NSAIDs in man are listed in *Table 15.5*. It is of interest to note that some of these side-effects can be reversed or reduced by the administration of exogenous prostaglandins. For example, a combination of a stable PGE_2 analogue with indomethacin was shown to be much better tolerated in animal models and in man than indomethacin alone[17]. The potential renal side-effects of indomethacin in infants with patent ductus arteriosus can also be reduced by concomitant administration of prostaglandins.

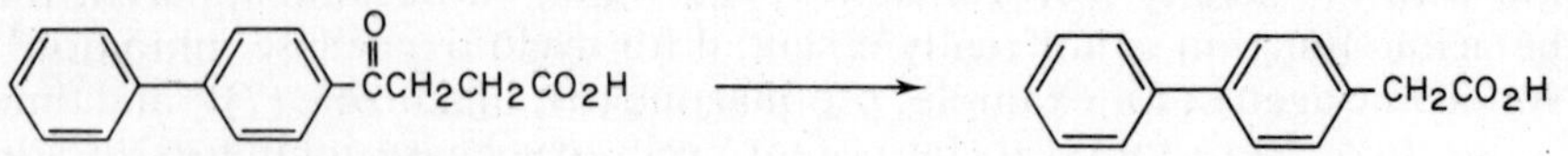

Fenbufen
(9)

Biphenylacetic acid
(10)

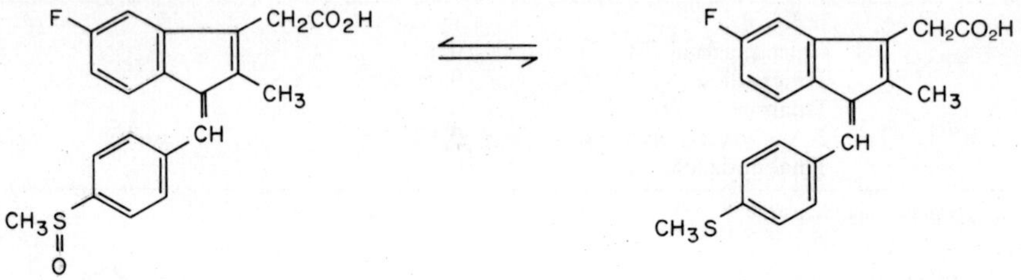

Sulindac
(11)

Sulphide metabolite of sulindac
(12)

The well-recognized ulcerogenic activity of NSAIDs can be modulated by the use of pro-drugs to minimize the topical irritation of the mucosa. Various esters, amides and metabolic precursors of the active carboxyl or acetic acid side-chain have been used[1]. A recent example is fenbufen (9)[18] which yields biphenyl acetic acid (10) as a major metabolite previously shown to be an active anti-inflammatory agent. A reversible pro-drug, sulindac (11), which is reversibly convertible to its active sulphide metabolite (12), is only half as irritating as the active metabolite in acute gastric haemorrhage models in rats[19]. In some patients, sulindac also appeared to have less effect on renal function,[20,21,21a], presumably attributable to the very low level of sulphide metabolite in some parts of the kidney.

TABLE 15.5. Chronic side-effects of NSAIDs

(1) Gastrointestinal irritation	
(a) Symptomatic: nausea, dyspepsia etc.	(10–20%)
(b) Ulcerogenic	(1–2%)
(2) Renal side-effects	
(a) Dysfunction: insufficiency, electrolyte abnormalities	
(b) Interstitial nephritis	(rare)
(3) Hepatic injury	
(a) Degeneration of hepatic parenchyma, hepatocellular jaundice	
(b) Cholestatic	(few)

Differential *in vivo* effects

An early finding was that, in cell-free systems, the relative inhibitory potency (as expressed by IC_{50}) of NSAIDs reported by different laboratories varied considerably[9]. Cyclo-oxygenase inhibition is generally dependent upon the tissue origin of the enzyme and the amount of substrate and cofactors present[22]. Extensive investigation with many NSAIDs further showed that several major factors may alter both the efficacy and safety of anti-inflammatory drugs *in vivo* (*Table 15.6*).

TABLE 15.6. Factors influencing differential inhibition of PG synthesis

(1) Characteristics of tissue enzymes
(*a*) Local levels of enzymes, cofactors
(*b*) Variation of enzyme sensitivity in different tissues
(2) Characteristics of inhibitors
(*a*) Reversibility
(*b*) Spectrum
(*c*) Pharmacodynamics

Aspirin is an irreversible inhibitor of cyclo-oxygenase acting by acetylating the terminal seryl hydroxyl group of the enzyme[23], whereas most NSAIDs, including the new salicylate analogue, diflunisal (13)[24], are substrate competitive reversible inhibitors. The susceptibility of cyclo-oxygenase prepared from different tissues to the inhibition by individual NSAIDs may vary. A notable example is the preferential inhibition of the brain enzyme by the analgesic acetaminophen[25]. On the other hand, for

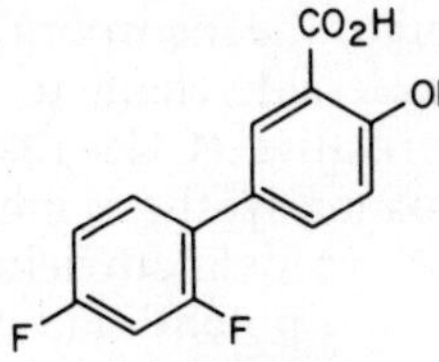

Diflunisal

(13)

many inhibitors such as indomethacin (1), ibuprofen (2), naproxen (3) etc., no tissue selectivity was observed. In other words, at their therapeutic anti-inflammatory dosage, these drugs will inhibit the biosynthesis of prostaglandins from platelets, gastric tissue, synovial tissue or other target tissues approximately to the same extent. In contrast, the platelet enzyme can be inactivated by a very small dose (5 mg/kg daily) of aspirin, at a level much lower than its usual anti-inflammatory dosage[26].

Another important factor contributing to the *in vivo* non-equivalence of NSAIDs is the pharmacodynamics of these drugs. Obviously, distribution of the drug in extracellular fluid and target cells and the gross *in vivo* pharmacokinetics will affect the local production of prostaglandins in different tissues. The differential distribution of sulindac (11) and its active sulphide metabolite (12) is an example. There is a greater tendency for the more hydrophilic sulindac to remain in the extracellular fluid and for the more lipophilic sulphide to accumulate inside the cells.

Thromboxane synthesis inhibitors

The principal metabolite derived from PGH_2 in platelets is thromboxane A_2, a potent and short-lived platelet-aggregating substance. Most cyclo-oxygenase inhibitors block the formation of PGG_2/PGH_2 and, consequently, all prostaglandins and thromboxanes. Low doses of aspirin have been shown to inhibit thromboxane production in platelets without affecting the prostacyclin synthesis by endothelial cells[26]. Prostacyclin is a potent inhibitor of platelet aggregation and is secreted by endothelial cells of the vasculature and attempts have been made, therefore, to produce inhibitors of thromboxane synthetase which do not inhibit prostaglandin production. In the past few years, several thromboxane synthesis inhibitors have been described (*see Table 15.7*). Several compounds have also been found to be thromboxane antagonists at the receptor level. The efficacy of imidazole and alkyl-substituted imidazoles was recognized early[27]. The potency was

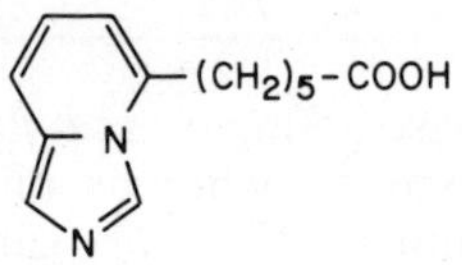

CGS 13080

(14)

then improved by optimizing the lipophilic moiety and/or the incorporation of an acidic function[28,29]. Cyclization of the aliphatic side-chain to the imidazole ring yielded an imidazo[1,5-*a*]pyridine derivative (CGS 13080) (14)[104] which is a highly selective and potent thromboxane synthesis inhibitor active at 3 μM *in vitro* and 1 mg/kg *in vivo*[30,61]. A pyridylmethylcinnamic acid analogue OKY-1581 (15) is also a selective and potent inhibitor. A group of synthetic analogues of prostaglandins and thromboxanes have been shown to be thromboxane synthesis inhibitors. The azoprostanoic acid(16)[31], and the carbo- (17) and pinane (18) analogues of TxA_2 also block TxA_2 receptors on human platelets[31]. Other analogues, such as (19), (20) and (21), are pure thromboxane receptor antagonists. The clinical efficacy of such inhibitors is still under active investigation. Dazoxiben (22) is orally active in man. It apparently reduces serum TxB_2 selectively, since there is a concomitant increase in the levels of 6-keto-$PGF_{1\alpha}$, the main metabolite of prostacyclin[32].

Catabolic enzyme inhibitors

The *in vivo* level of cyclo-oxygenase metabolites can obviously be regulated through inhibition of their catabolic enzymes. The principal routes of metabolic inactivation of prostaglandins are oxidation of the 15-OH group, saturation of the Δ^{13} double bond and degradative oxygenation of the two aliphatic side chains (*Figure 15.5*). Both PGE_2 and $PGF_{2\alpha}$ are initially inactivated by the prostaglandin 15-OH dehydrogenase followed

TABLE 15.7. Thromboxane synthesis inhibitors/antagonists

| Structure | Inhibition of Thromboxane A_2 | |
	Synthetase	Receptor
$N{=}\!\!<\!\!>\!\!N-(CH_2)_7CO_2H$	+	−
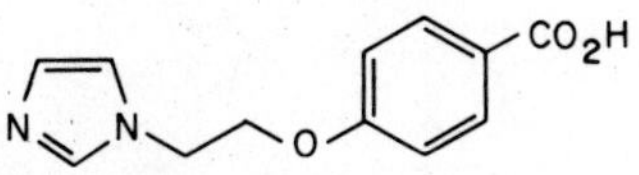 (Dazoxiben, UK 37248) (22) [imidazole–CH_2CH_2–O–phenyl–CO_2H]	+	+
(UK 34787) [imidazolylmethyl indole, iPr, N–H]	+	−
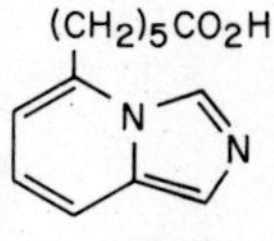 (CGS 13080) (14) [$(CH_2)_5CO_2H$ imidazopyridine]	+	−
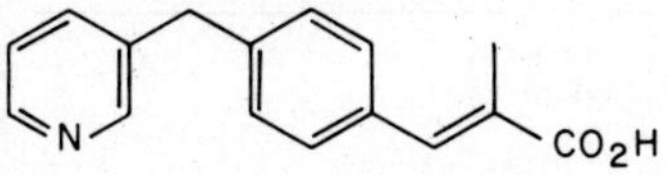 (OKY-1555, Na$^+$ salt OKY-1581) (15) [pyridine–CH_2–phenyl–CH=C(CH$_3$)CO_2H]	+	−
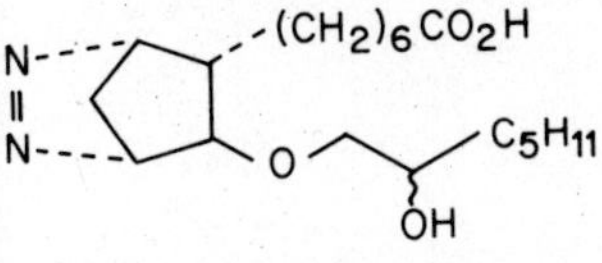 (16) [$(CH_2)_6CO_2H$, O–CH_2–CH(OH)–C_5H_{11}]	+	+
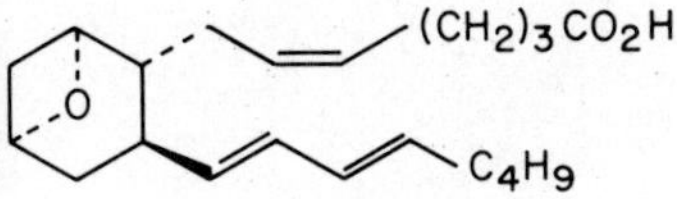 (17) [$(CH_2)_3CO_2H$, C_4H_9]	+	+
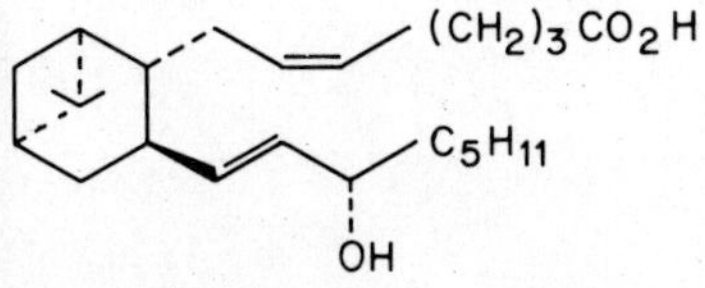 (18) [$(CH_2)_3CO_2H$, CH(OH)–C_5H_{11}]	+	+

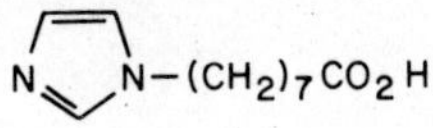

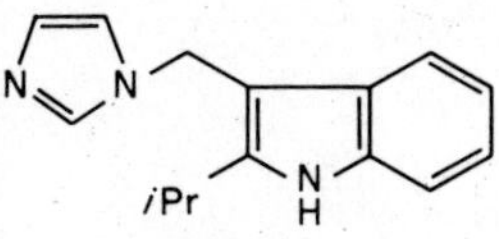

TABLE 15.7 (contd). Thromboxane synthesis inhibitors/antagonists

Structure		Inhibition of Thromboxane A_2	
		Synthetase	Receptor
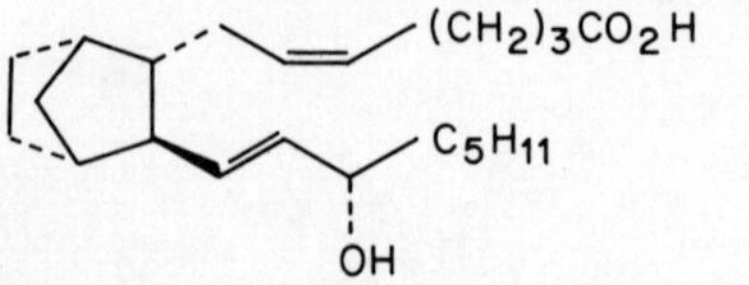	(19)	–	+
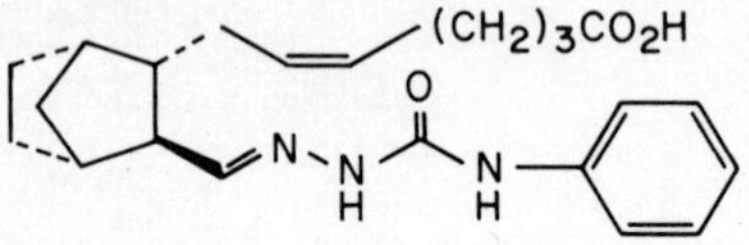	(20)	–	+
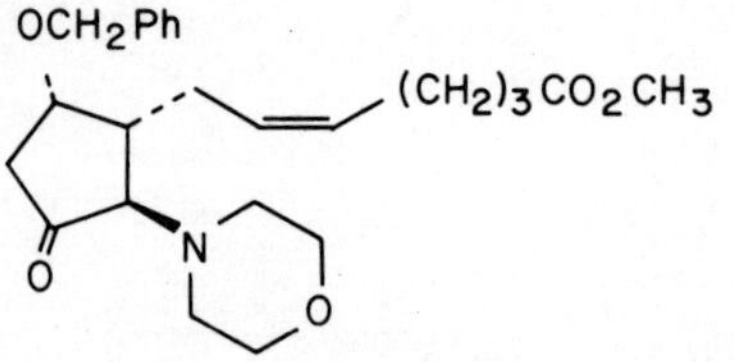	(21)	–	+

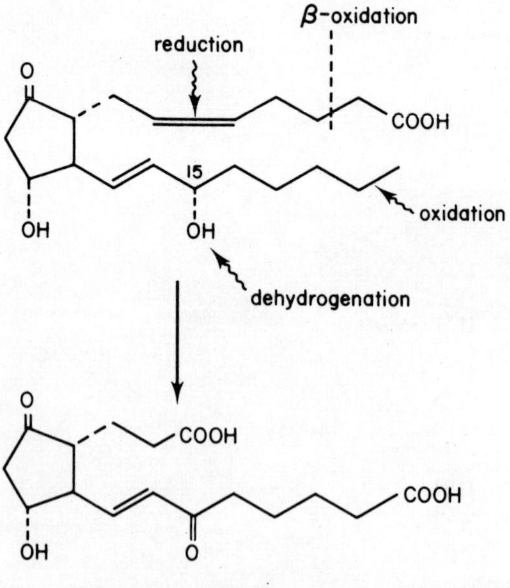

Figure 15.5 Common catabolic conversions of prostaglandins.

by further inactivating stages as in *Figure 15.5*. Anti-inflammatory agents, e.g. indomethacin (1) and meclofenamic acid, inhibit this enzyme only at the high concentration of 10^{-4} M[33]. The flavonoids, polyphosphoretin phosphate and diphloretin phosphate, can inhibit the pulmonary inactivation of PGE$_2$ and PGF$_{2\alpha}$ at 10^{-7} M[9].

Oxygen radicals

Biochemical background

The hydroperoxy intermediates (ROOH) formed in the cyclo-oxygenase and lipoxygenase pathways (e.g. PGG$_2$ and HPETE) are converted to the corresponding hydroxy compounds (e.g. PGH$_2$ and HETE) by peroxidases. The formation of these hydroxy metabolites is usually accompanied by the liberation of an oxygen species, probably of a radical nature[34] (*Figure 15.6*). Such radical oxidants or their derivatives are capable of degrading biopolymers, e.g. hyaluronic acid, proteins, and membrane components, and are generally pro-inflammatory. Recently it was shown that oxidant radicals can also affect the prostaglandin synthetic pathway in several ways. First, oxidant radicals can activate the pathway: 15-HETE

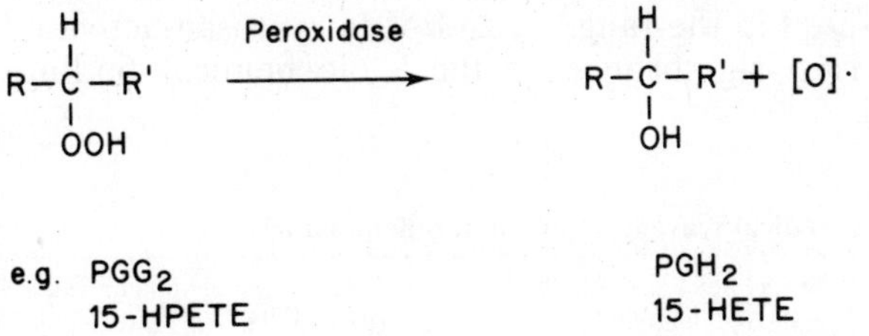

Figure 15.6 Liberation of an oxidant radical from hydroperoxy metabolites. 15-HPETE = 15-hydroperoxyeicosatetraenoic acid; 15-HETE = 15-hydroxyeicosatetraenoic acid.

and H$_2$O$_2$ produced by neutrophils can trigger the release of arachidonic acid and its metabolites from endothelial cells. Low levels of peroxides are required for the initiation and maintenance of cyclo-oxygenase as well as 5-lipoxygenase[34a]. On the other hand, oxidant radicals can selectively inactivate certain biosynthetic enzymes in the pathway. They can preferentially inactivate PGI$_2$ synthetase without affecting thromboxane synthetase and thus change the ratio of PGI$_2$ and TxA$_2$ levels[34b]. Scavengers of oxidant radicals, e.g. phenols and other reducing agents, at low levels can stimulate prostaglandin synthesis by protecting the enzyme from oxidant destruction, whereas at higher concentration they can prevent the oxidative release of arachidonic acid and its metabolites[35a]. Some of these reductants have shown anti-inflammatory activities *in vivo*. Due to their multiple effects on the arachidonic acid cascade, their overall activity *in vivo* may depend upon their distribution in different tissues and other enzymatic factors such as the availability of substrate and cofactors etc.

Radical scavengers

A variety of reducing agents have been observed to be radical scavengers *in vitro* and, in some cases, anti-inflammatories *in vivo* (*see Table 15.8*). Oxyphenbutazone (23) is known to be co-oxygenated by prostaglandin peroxidases[35b]. The active sulphide metabolite of sulindac (12) has also

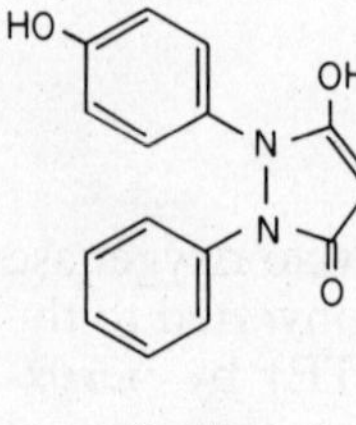

Oxyphenbutazone

(23)

been shown to be a highly effective acceptor of the oxygen radical generated in the peroxidase system. The transfer of ^{18}O from a hydroperoxy-arachidonic acid metabolite in the presence of a peroxidase to the sulphide metabolite is stoichiometric and stereospecific, leading to the formation of an optically active sulphoxide (sulindac) (11). The sulindac sulphide metabolite is also a moderately active 5-lipoxygenase inhibitor with a dose causing 50% inhibition (ID_{50}) in the range of 25 μM in zymosan-activated macrophages[36]. The *in vivo* significance of these biochemical findings remains to be established.

TABLE 15.8. Reducing agents as radical scavengers and anti-inflammatories

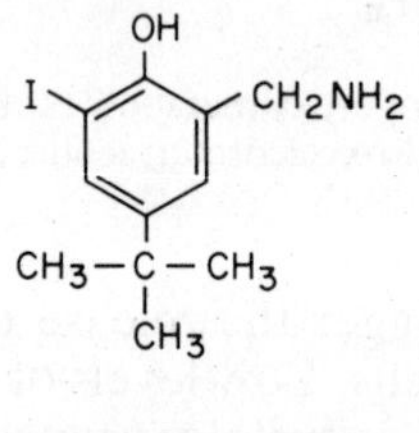

MK-447   (24) 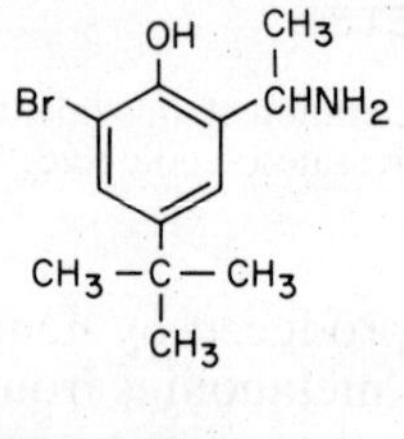   Isomer (+) >> (−)   (25)

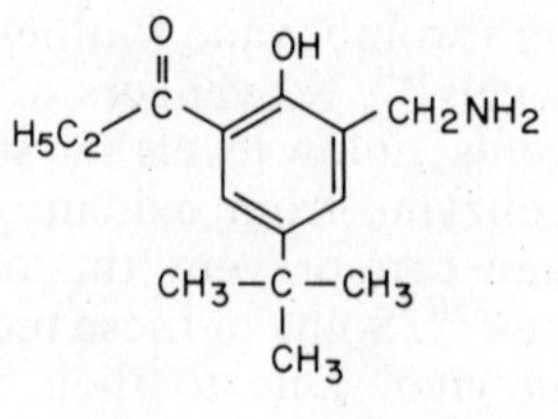

ONO-3144   (26) 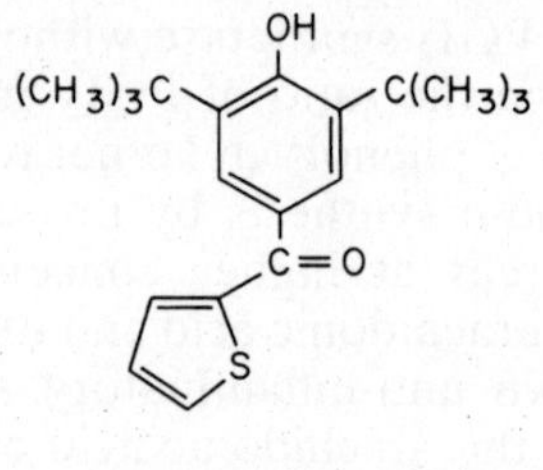   R-830   (27)

Among phenolic compounds, the new salicylate diflunisal (13) with its increased hydrophobicity is more potent than sodium salicylate as a radical scavenger[37]. MK-447 (24), a diuretic–anti-inflammatory agent, was first noted for its ability to promote the conversion of the hydroperoxy-PGG_2 to PGH_2, to protect cyclo-oxygenase and stimulate the biosynthesis of prostaglandins *in vitro*, possibly as a consequence of oxygen radical removal[38]. It was found to also have anti-inflammatory activity *in vivo*. A recent study showed that the anti-inflammatory actions of MK-447 and analogue (25) are stereospecific and apparently independent of their non-selective antioxidant activity[39]. These paradoxical observations can be rationalized by the assumption that some phenolic compounds can affect the cyclo-oxygenase pathway in two distinct manners: antagonizing the activation of cyclo-oxygenase by lipid hydroperoxides, and a stereospecific interference with substrate binding with cyclo-oxygenase[40]. As the former mechanism can be overcome by a higher level of hydroperoxides, phenolic agents such as paracetamol and MK-447 may be more effective in peripheral hyperalgesia or certain anti-inflammatory conditions where cellular peroxide levels are not greatly elevated.

In an effort to dissociate the diuretic activity of MK-447, the corresponding 6-propionyl analogue, ONO-3144 (26), was recently found to be an effective anti-inflammatory agent[41]. ONO-3144 does not inhibit, but stimulate, prostaglandin–hydroperoxidase activity, but it does inhibit thromboxane synthetase. Another related phenol, R-830 (27) is a potent cyclo-oxygenase inhibitor with a concentration producing 50% inhibition (IC_{50}) of 0.5 μM with moderate lipoxygenase inhibition (at 20 μM) and antioxidant properties. In addition to its anti-inflammatory action *in vivo*, it inhibits reverse passive cutaneous Arthus reaction contact sensitivity as well[42].

Inhibitors of the lipoxygenase pathway

The pathway

Arachidonic acid can be oxygenated by a number of different lipoxygenases to yield hydroperoxyeicosatetraenoic acids (HPETEs)[4]. The reactions of three of the most commonly encountered mammalian lipoxygenases, the 5, 12 and 15-lipoxygenases are outlined in *Figure 15.7*. These hydroperoxide products are readily reduced by appropriate peroxidases to the corresponding hydroxy acids (HETEs) as shown.

5-Lipoxygenase, and its subsequent pathway to the leukotrienes (*Figure 15.8*), has been the focus of the most intensive investigation. Interest in this pathway is derived from the leukotrienes C_4, D_4 and E_4 (collectively the slow-reacting substance of anaphylaxis, SRS-A), which are primary mediators in human asthma, and from leukotriene B_4, a potent chemotactic factor believed to play a role in chronic inflammation[4].

Upon stimulation, 5-lipoxygenase activity is detected in various leucocytes. The most frequently encountered sources of the enzyme are rat basophilic leukaemia (RBL) cells and polymorphonuclear leucocytes (PMNs) derived from man, rat, rabbit etc. These sources sometimes contain smaller amounts of 15-lipoxygenase. Platelets are rich in 12-lipoxygenase. The enzymes are usually studied either in whole cells or in

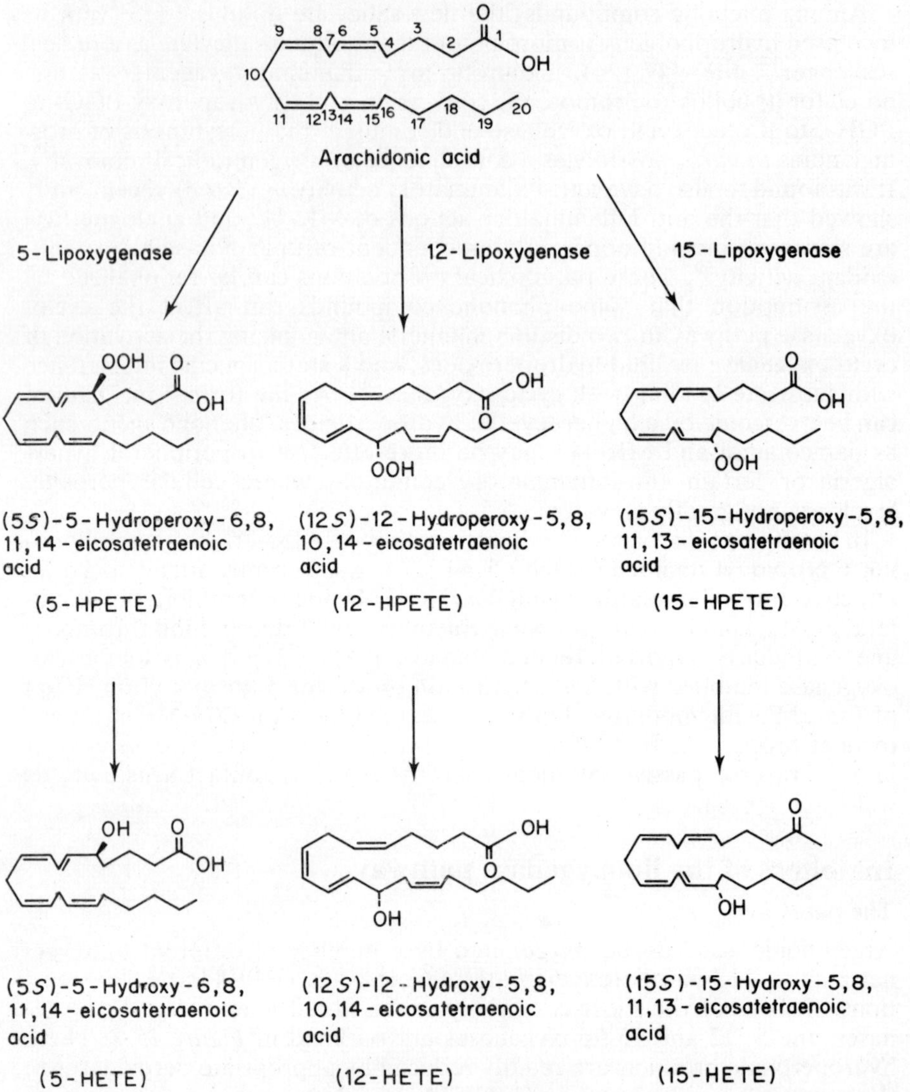

Figure 15.7 5-, 12- and 15-lipoxygenases.

partially purified cell extracts. Detailed characterization of physical properties and mechanism of action must await further investigation.

5-Lipoxygenase inhibitors

The development of mammalian lipoxygenase inhibitors is still in its infancy. The discovery of the link between 5-lipoxygenase and the leukotrienes dates back only to 1979. As in the case of cyclo-oxygenase inhibitors, due to a lack of uniformity in such factors as enzyme source, preparation and assay procedures, it is often very difficult to compare results from

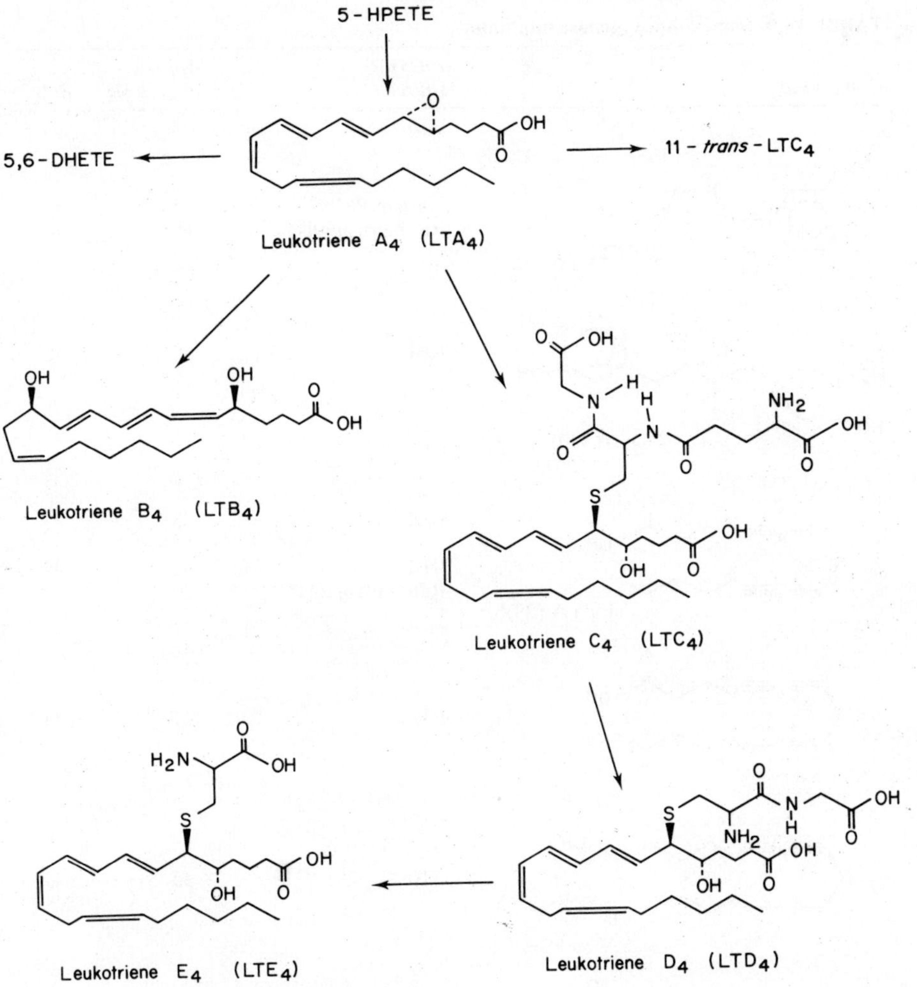

Figure 15.8 5-Lipoxygenase pathway.

different studies. For example, 5,8,11,14-eicosatetraynoic acid (ETYA, 28), one of the more widely studied inhibitors, is reported to be approximately 17 times more active against RBL cell 5-lipoxygenase when preincubated with intact cells, than against the partially purified RBL enzyme with no preincubation[43,44]. Others claim ETYA is not an inhibitor of 5-lipoxygenase at all[45]. Against human platelet 12-lipoxygenase, ETYA was found to be 100 times more active in the platelet cytoplasmic fraction than the intact platelet assay.

Products of the lipoxygenase pathway can, themselves, have a stimulatory or inhibitory effect on the activity of the 5-lipoxygenase enzyme. For example, 5-HETE, the product of 5-HPETE and peroxidase, has been shown to inhibit 5-lipoxygenase[46]. 15-HETE, produced in at least some leucocytes is also a potent inhibitor of 5-lipoxygenase[45,47]. PGE$_2$ and PGI$_2$ inhibit the production of leukotrienes by PMNs and macrophages. Thus there appears to be a complex feedback regulation of 5-lipoxygenase. The

TABLE 15.9. Some 5-lipoxygenase inhibitors

Compound	Enzyme source	Approx. IC_{50} (μM)	Ref.
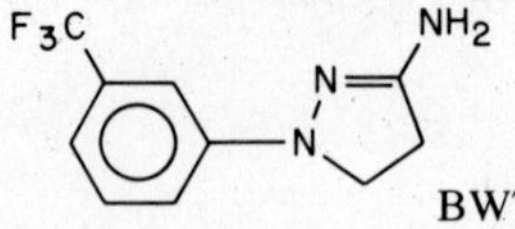 BW755c (29)	RBL	4	94
	Human PMN*	15	55
	Rat neutrophils*	60	71
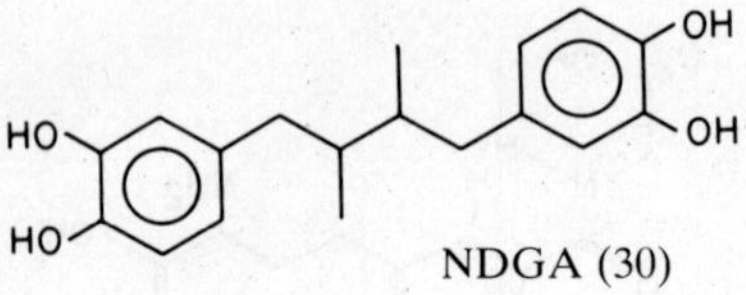 NDGA (30)	RBL*	2	43
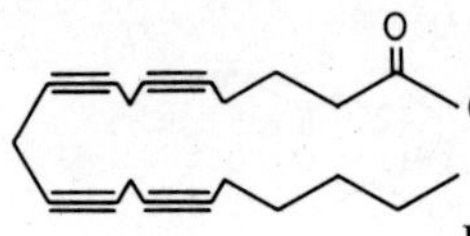 ETYA (28)	RBL*·†	3	43
	RBL	52	44
	Rat neutrophils*	20	50
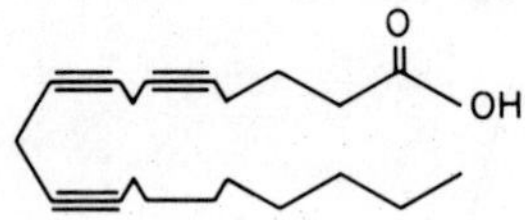	RBL	37	44
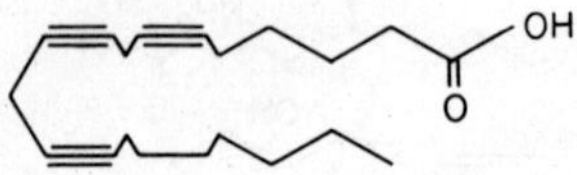	RBL	15	44
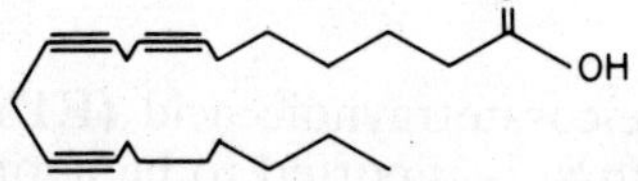	RBL	3	44
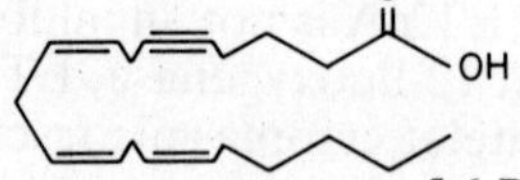 5,6-DHA (31)	RBL	0.5‡	51
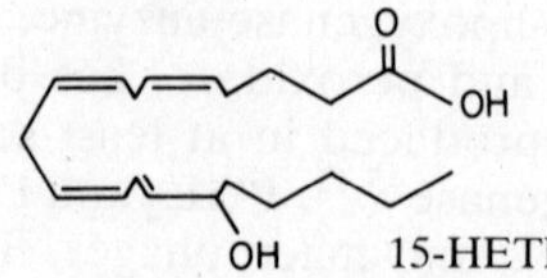 15-HETE	Rabbit PMN*	5.7	45
	Human T-lymphocytes*	9	47

TABLE 15.9 (contd). Some 5-lipoxygenase inhibitors

Compound	Enzyme source	Approx. IC$_{50}$ (μM)	Ref.
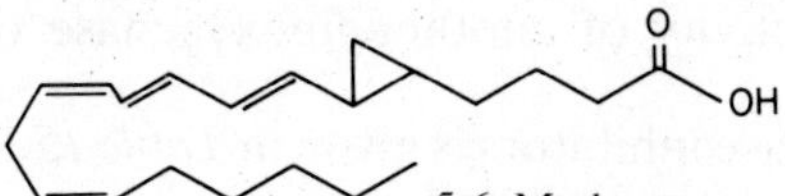 5,6–Methano-LTA$_4$ (32)	Mastocytoma P-815	31	52
	Guinea-pig PMN	3	46
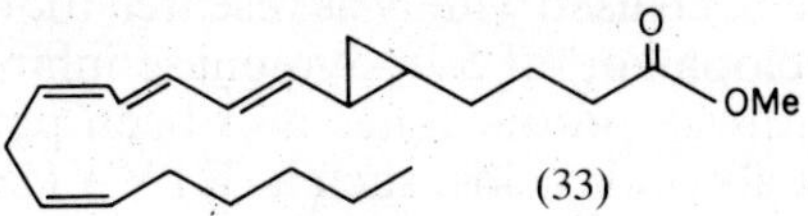 (33)	Mastocytoma P-815	6	52
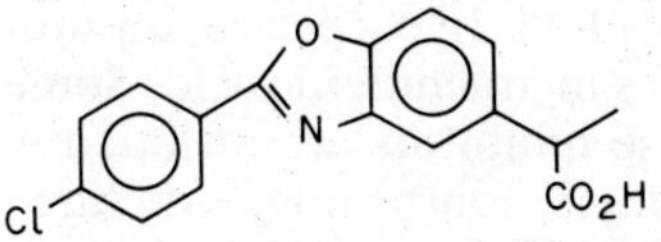 Benoxaprofen	Rabbit PMN*	100	72
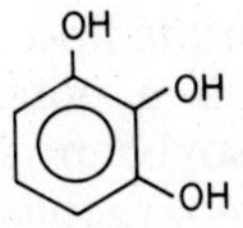 Pyrogallol	RBL*	4	43
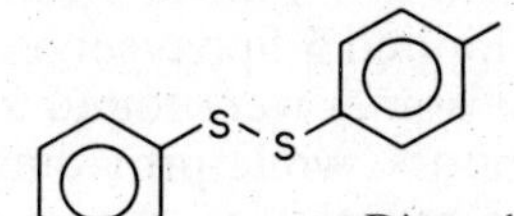 Di-p-tolyldisulphide	RBL	0.8	69
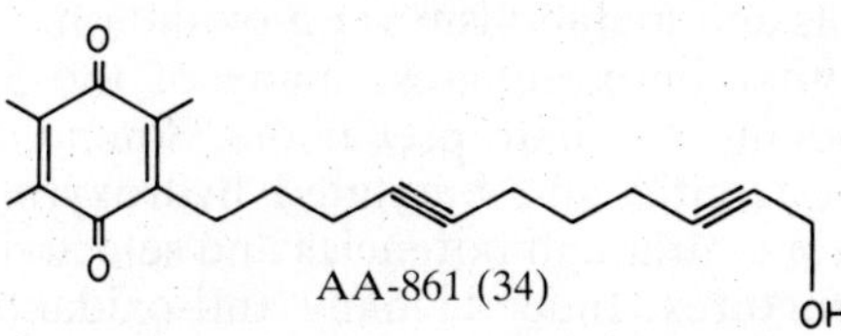 AA-861 (34)	Pig peritoneal PMN	0.8	53
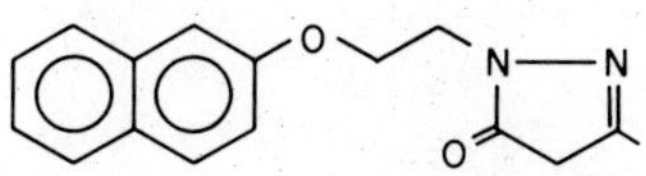 Nafazatrom	B16 amelanotic melanoma	3	76
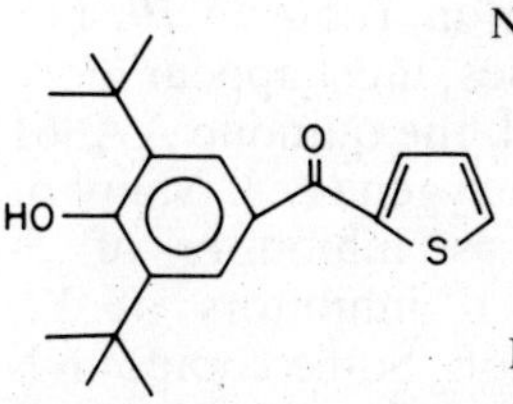 R-830 (27)	Guinea-pig lung	20	103

* Intact cells.
† 5 min preincubation.
‡ Time dependent, irreversible inhibition.

activity of lipoxygenases is further complicated by the possibility of arachidonic acid shunting. For example, any selective inhibition of cyclo-oxygenase can result in the increased processing of arachidonic acid via one or more of the lipoxygenases[48,49]. Likewise, selective inhibition of one lipoxygenase can result in increased activity of another lipoxygenase or cyclo-oxygenase.

A compilation of selected 5-lipoxygenase inhibitors is given in *Table 15.9*. Only IC_{50} values of 100 μM or less have been included.

The two prototype lipoxygenase inhibitors, BW 755c (29)[50] and nordihydroguaiaretic acid, NDGA (30), have been used widely as research tools. A considerable amount of 'logical development' of 5-lipoxygenase inhibitors based on arachidonic acid and pathway products has also been pursued. From early on, it was known that alkynoic acids, such as ETYA (28) inhibit lipoxygenases. In addition to these 5-alkynoic acids, a number of 4-alkynoic acids through 10-alkynoic acids, varying both in chain length and in the number of triple bonds, have also been studied. In each case, unsaturated bonds are separated by a methylene unit as in arachidonic acid. Some of the more potent alkynoic acid 5-lipoxygenase inhibitors are included in *Table 15.9*. Disappointingly, few generalizations concerning structure–activity can be drawn. A class of dehydroarachidonic acids functions as selective, time-dependent, irreversible inhibitors of the appropriate lipoxygenase. Thus 5,6-dehydroarachidonic acid (5,6-DHA) (31) is a potent irreversible inhibitor of RBL 5-lipoxygenase, but not of soybean 15-lipoxygenase. 5,6-DHA was found to be a substrate for cyclo-oxygenase, while 11,12-DHA inhibited cyclo-oxygenase irreversibly[51]. Two different groups prepared methano-LTA$_4$ (32) and found it inhibited 5-lipoxygenase (*Table 15.9*). Its methyl ester (33) and a double bond isomer were found to be even more potent[52]. All of these fatty acid inhibitors, while providing valuable tools for *in vitro* investigations, offer little promise as systemic therapeutic agents, due to such metabolic problems as tight binding to serum proteins, incorporation into lipid pools and metabolism via β-oxidation.

As is the case for inhibitors of other lipoxygenases, many of the 5-lipoxygenase inhibitors are anti-oxidants or their precursors. Phenolic compounds, such as α-tocopherol, quercitin and butylated hydroxytoluene, are known lipoxygenase inhibitors, although potencies and selectivities can vary widely according to structures. Indeed, many anti-oxidants are essentially void of inhibitory activity.

Inhibitors of other lipoxygenases

A selection of inhibitors of 12-lipoxygenases is given in *Table 15.10*. For those inhibitors that block both 5- and 12-lipoxygenases, most appear more selective for 12-lipoxygenase. At least one compound, the quinone AA861 (34) (*Table 15.9*) is reported to be specific for 5-lipoxygenase[53]. Many of the same alkynoic acids that were evaluated as inhibitors of 5-lipoxygenase, were evaluated broadly as potential inhibitors of 12-lipoxygenase, cyclo-oxygenase and platelet aggregation. Some compounds selectively inhibit either cyclo-oxygenase or 12-lipoxygenase, and others act as dual inhibitors. Suppression of platelet aggregation was found to correlate mainly with cyclo-oxygenase inhibition.

TABLE 15.10. Some 12-lipoxygenase inhibitors

Compound	Enzyme source	Approx. IC_{50} (μM)	Ref.
ETYA	Human platelet*	3–4	67, 70, 77
	Human platelet	0.03	77
BW755c	Horse platelet	7.4	65
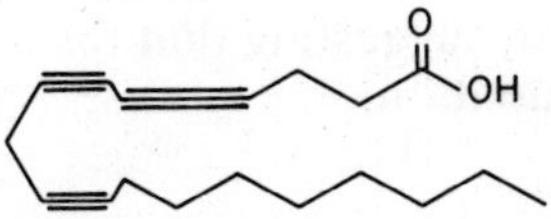	Human platelet*	8.3	67
	Murine mastocytoma	5	78
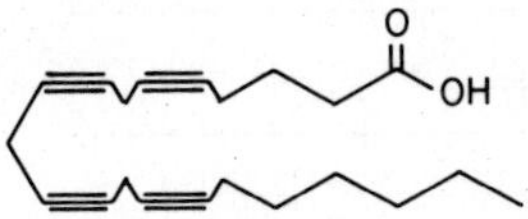	Human platelet*	1.7	67
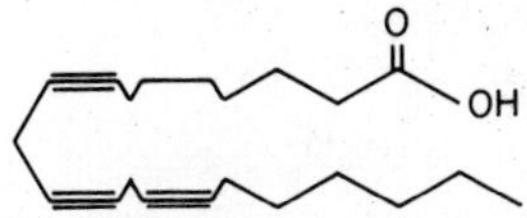	Human platelet*	4.2	67
15-HETE	Human platelet*	8.2	79
	Rabbit platelet*	0.34	45
15-HPETE	Human platelet*	2.5	79
	Human platelet*	20	80
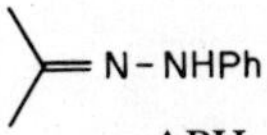 APH	Human platelet*	2	77
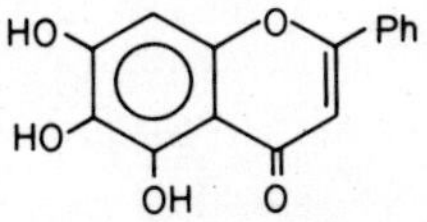 Baicalein	Rat platelet	0.12	68
Toluene-3,4-dithiol	Human platelet	5	81

* Intact platelets.

A somewhat limited study noted that human platelet lipoxygenase inhibition appears to correlate with the ferric ion chelating property of some inhibitors. Strong ferric ion chelators, toluene-3,4-dithiol and dithiazone, were potent 12-lipoxygenase inhibitors, while the weaker chelator, o-phenanthroline, was also a weaker inhibitor. Ferrous ion chelators, 2,2′-dipyridyl, bathophenanthroline and EDTA reportedly did not inhibit the enzyme.

Inhibitors of 15-lipoxygenases are given in *Table 15.11*. Most inhibitors reported are for the soybean 15-lipoxygenase which, although available commercially as a pure enzyme, is of uncertain value relative to mammalian enzymes. There is not yet enough inhibition data to compare soybean and leucocyte 15-lipoxygenase. Perhaps pertinent to this issue, BW755c is reported as a good soybean inhibitor[54], but not as an inhibitor of human

PMN 15-lipoxygenase, which it actually activates at lower concentrations[55]. *Table 15.11* includes only studies that used arachidonic acid as substrate.

14,15-DHA (35) is a potent irreversible inhibitor of soybean 15-lipoxygenase. Other related dehydroarachidonic acids have no effect on this enzyme. Through the use of a tritiated 14,15-DHA, it was demonstrated that the inhibitor becomes covalently bound to the enzyme. Irreversible inhibition was observed only in the presence of oxygen, suggesting that the inhibition is directly connected with the enzymatic oxidation.

TABLE 15.11. Some 15-lipoxygenase inhibitors

Compound	Enzyme source	Approx. IC_{50} (μM)	Ref.
BW755c	Human PMN	>300	55
	Soybean	11	54
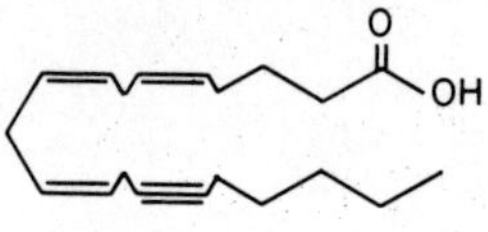 14,15-DHA (35)	Soybean	0.6*	98
15-HETE	Rabbit PMN	40	45
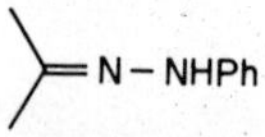 APH	Soybean	0.3–1	99, 100
1,5-Dihydroxynaphthalene	Soybean	20	101
	Soybean	117	99
NDGA (30)	Soybean	72–100	99, 102
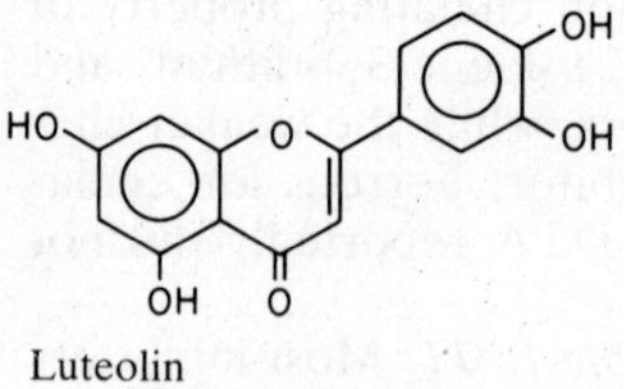 Luteolin	Soybean	30	101
BHT	Soybean	0.01	102
DL-α-Tocopherol	Soybean	0.4	102

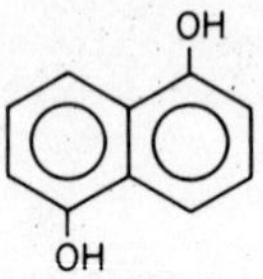

* Preincubation with inhibitor.

Effects of several pharmacological agents

So far, no clinical studies on the activity of potent and selective lipoxygenase inhibitors have been reported. However, several pharmacological agents previously developed in other biological systems have been shown to inhibit the formation or cellular release of SRS-A or lipoxygenase products.

An SRS antagonist, FPL 55712 (36), was found to be weakly active in man in preventing LTC_4 and LTD_4-induced bronchoconstriction[56]. It also blocks the formation of 5-HETE and 5,12-DHETE in RBL-1 cells[57].

The anti-allergic agent, RO 21-7634 (37), inhibits the antigen-induced release of SRS-A from guinea-pig lung tissue[58]. Similar to corticosteroids, its effect on histamine release is considerably less.

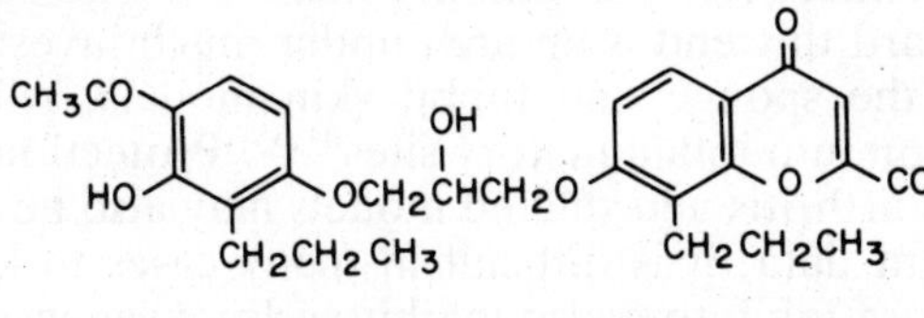

FPL 55712   (36)

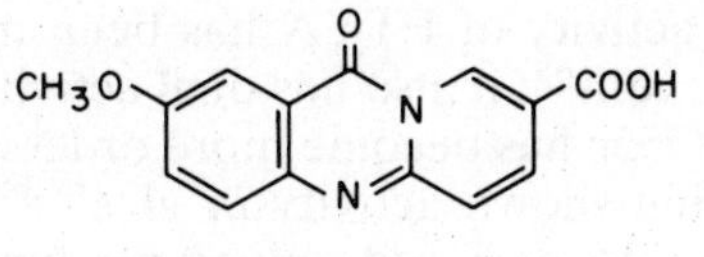

RO 21-7634   (37)

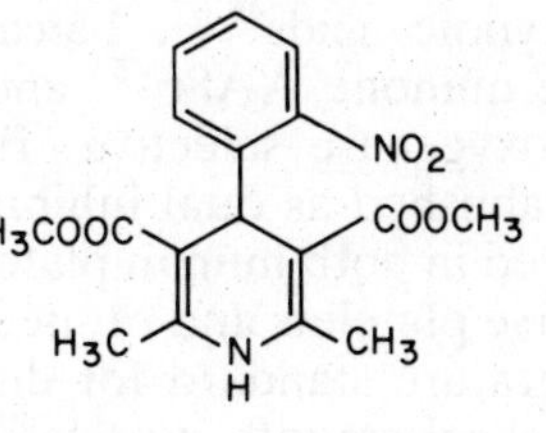

Nifedipine   (38)

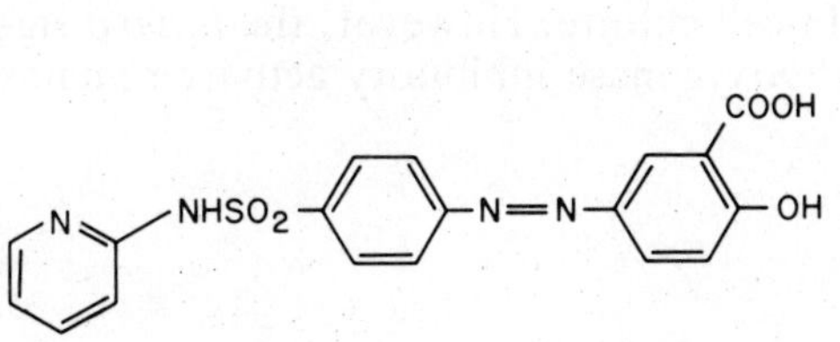

Sulfasalazine   (39)

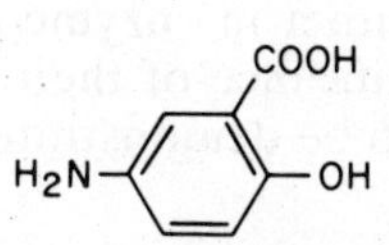

4 - Aminosalicylic acid

(40)

The calcium antagonist, nifedipine (38), inhibits the release of both SRS and, to a lesser extent, platelet-activating factor from human PMN, at $>10^{-6}$ M in a concentration-dependent manner[59].

Sulfasalazine (39), a drug used in ulcerative colitis, inhibits the synthesis of 5-HETE in human neutrophils[60]. It and its metabolite, 5-aminosalicylic acid (40), also block the synthesis of 5,12-DHETE in the same preparation. This suggests the possible use of a dual cyclo-oxygenase/lipoxygenase inhibitor in the treatment of this bowel inflammatory condition.

Lipoxygenase versus cyclo-oxygenase: selective versus dual inhibitors

It is possible that a systemically active 5-lipoxygenase inhibitor will be beneficial in the treatment of asthma and other immediate hypersensitivity disorders. The situation regarding the value of 5-lipoxygenase inhibition in the treatment of inflammatory disorders is less certain. While lipoxygenase products have been identified in inflammatory exudates, and LTB_4 is noted for its chemotactic properties, suitable animal models to demonstrate a significant anti-inflammatory effect of selective 5-lipoxygenase inhibitors are lacking[62,63]. One must also be concerned with the effect of 5-lipoxygenase inhibition on the cyclo-oxygenase pathway and, to a lesser extent, on other lipoxygenases. It is currently widely believed that a dual lipoxygenase–cyclo-oxygenase inhibitor would be of greater value in the treatment of inflammation than either selective inhibitor alone[4,64]. The development of animal models toward this end is an area under much investigation. Such models, including the sponge and rabbit skin models, will most likely involve cell migration into inflammatory sites[64,65]. Protection against bone erosion in adjuvant arthritis and related models may also be of value.

Due to insufficient data, it is difficult in many cases to know whether reported lipoxygenase inhibitors also inhibit cyclo-oxygenase. Particularly difficult to classify are the anti-oxidant inhibitors, since many anti-oxidants will inhibit cyclo-oxygenase *in vitro* under some assay conditions[66]. Some alkynoic acids[45,67], baicalein (12-lipoxygenase)[68], 5,6-methano-LTA_4[52], the quinone AA861[53] and diaryl disulphides[69] have all been reported as lipoxygenase selective. Both ETYA (28) and BW755c (29) have been established as dual inhibitors. The dual activity of ETYA has been measured in both human platelets[70] and RBL cells[68]; it also has dual activity in horse platelets and rat neutrophils[71]. BW755c has become more or less the literature standard for dual activity having shown activity *in vivo*[64,65] on tracheal smooth muscle[49], and on sensitized perfused guinea-pig lung[48]. Several anti-inflammatory agents, including sulindac sulphide[36], benoxaprofen[72] and timegadine[73] have been described as dual pathway inhibitors either in enzyme preparations or in cell culture. However, the *in vivo* significance of their relatively weak lipoxygenase inhibitory activity remains to be demonstrated.

Glutathione transferase

While 5-lipoxygenase remains the most likely target for blocking leukotriene synthesis, there are two other possible target steps: the conversion of 5-HPETE to LTA_4, and the glutathione transferase that converts LTA_4 to LTC_4. Very little is known about the dehydration step which, if blocked, would prevent the synthesis of all the leukotrienes. Inhibition of glutathione transferase, which prevents synthesis of SRS-A but not LTB_4, could possibly be of value in the treatment of asthma.

Recently, two types of inhibitors with some selectivity for glutathione transferase have been described. Several 4-alkynoic acids are effective inhibitors of the conversion of LTA_4 to LTC_4[44,74]. 4,7,10,13-Henicosatetraynoic acid inhibits SRS formation in RBL cells with an IC_{50}

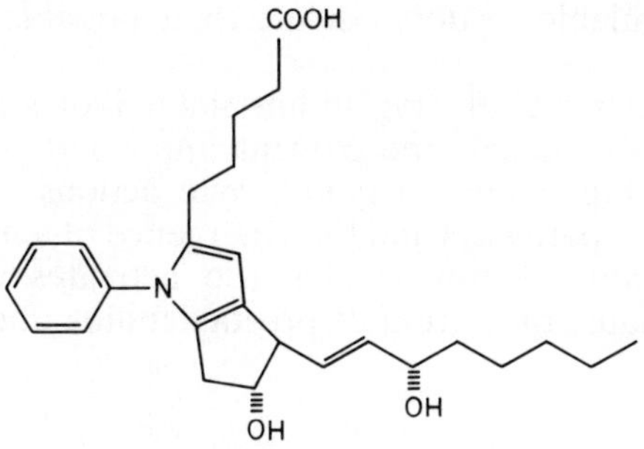

COOH

U – 60, 257   (41)

of 7 μM, while it has little or no effect on either 5-lipoxygenase or cyclo-oxygenase at 50 μM. A selective glutathione transferase inhibitor, U-60,257, (41) has also been reported[41,75]. This compound inhibits the formation of SRS-A in rat peritoneal mononuclear cells with an IC_{50} of 4.6 μM, and inhibits the glutathione transferase activity from RBL cells at 37 μM.

Future developments

The decade of cyclo-oxygenase inhibitors has brought forth a large family of NSAIDs which are clinically useful as anti-inflammatory–analgesic–antipyretic agents for the symptomatic relief of arthritic conditions. Their clinical applications have been extended to other prostaglandin-mediated disorders, such as patent ductus arteriosus, dysmenorrhea, Bartter's syndrome and hypercalcaemia secondary to neoplasia. Some progress has also been made in the synthesis of selective and long-acting prostaglandin antagonists for renal function disorders and in the development of thromboxane synthesis inhibitors and thromboxane antagonists for thrombosis. But the major emphasis in drug development appears to have shifted to the newer lipoxygenase arena.

The search for antagonists and biosynthesis inhibitors of leukotrienes has received a great deal of attention in the past few years. Undoubtedly, the clinical trials on these inhibitors of the lipoxygenase pathway will take place in the very near future. The inhibition of 5-lipoxygenase to block the formation of LTA_4 and, consequently, LTB_4, LTC_4, LTD_4 and LTE_4 for asthmatic conditions, appears to be well founded but the question regarding the consequence of modulating other lipoxygenases remains to be clarified. The biological roles of a variety of mono- and dihydroperoxy/hydroxy metabolites of arachidonic acid, either mediatory or regulatory, are still being defined in different target organs and in different species. Clearly a major effort, not unlike that devoted to the cyclo-oxygenase pathway metabolites in the past decade, may be needed to elucidate the significance of their biological actions and the merits of therapeutic interventions of a myriad of eicosanoids. The oxidant radicals, the ubiquitous by-product in the metabolism of hydroperoxyeicosanoids, are fundamental reactive species possibly affecting a wide range of biological targets. The radical scavenging effect of several redox agents, e.g. phenols and sulphides, can readily be demonstrated *in vitro*, but unfortunately no convenient animal models are available to demonstrate their possible *in vivo* benefits.

Compounding the biological scenario of prostaglandins and leukotrienes are three more recent developments: namely the growing appreciation of the feedback control role of prostaglandins on lymphocyte actions, the interaction of metabolites of the two pathways and the emergence of a new lipid mediator, the platelet-activating factor, which also activates the lipoxygenase pathway and potentiates the action of prostaglandins under certain experimental conditions.

Immunopharmacological activities of arachidonic acid metabolites

The immune-based chronic inflammation, the interactions of macrophages, T and B lymphocytes, lead to the elaboration of lymphokines, the formation of antigen–antibody complex and activation of neutrophils, macrophages and local cells to produce swelling, tissue proliferation and cartilage destruction. These immunological events are subject to modulation by prostaglandins. For example, PGE_2 activates T-suppressor cells[82], and increases the production of T-cell-derived suppressive factors (PITS) which can inhibit blastogenesis, mixed lymphocyte reactions and antibody response[83]. PGE_2 inhibits the production of lymphokines such as interleuken 2, which stimulates cellular proliferation and the cytotoxicity of natural killer (NK) cells[84]. Furthermore, PGE_2 can modulate neutrophil chemotaxis[85]. In considering the possible *in vivo* significance of these observations, it may be recalled that, in man, the cyclo-oxygenase inhibitor, indomethacin, was found to enhance the cellular immunity in some melanoma[86] and Hodgkin's disease[87] patients. Indomethacin can also restore the skin reaction to delayed hypersensitivity in allergic patients and to increase the secondary antibody response to influenza in immune-deficient patients[88]. Indomethacin and several other NSAIDs also inhibit the production of rheumatoid factor by lymphocytes from rheumatoid arthritis patients[88a]. With further delineation of these biochemical events involved in immune processes, the development of non-cytotoxic immunopharmacological agents should be facilitated.

Interaction of cyclo-oxygenase and lipoxygenase pathways

The possible shunting of the common substrate, arachidonic acid, from cyclo-oxygenase pathway to lipoxygenase pathway when the former is blocked by inhibitors like NSAIDs has been demonstrated. The extent of shunting, of course, depends upon the cellular compartmentation of the two enzymes. Recently, more complex interactions, both stimulatory and inhibitory, between the two pathways via their metabolites have also been noted. For example, LTB_4 can stimulate the cyclo-oxygenase pathway, possibly via its effect on phospholipase, to increase the availability of free arachidonic acid from membrane phospholipids. Conversely, PGE_2 and PGI_2 can inhibit the production of leukotrienes by human PMN and rat peritoneal macrophages[89]. PGI_2 may further inhibit the adhesion of PMN to endothelial cells after stimulation by LTB_4. Yet to be defined are the effects of other lipoxygenase products on the activation and regulation of various synthetic enzymes, as well as the responses of target cells to prostaglandins and leukotrienes[90]. The overall *in vivo* effect of inhibition of individual pathways in the arachidonic acid cascade is likely to be a highly complex and dynamic one.

Regulation of the platelet-activating factor

Prostaglandins and leukotrienes produced in the arachidonic acid cascade are only but one family of inflammatory mediators derived from membrane phospholipids (*Table 15.12*). The possible role of phosphatidic acid as an endogenous calcium ionophore has received some attention[90a]. An unusual

TABLE 15.12. Inflammatory lipid mediators

(1) Phospholipid Derivatives
PAF-acether
Phosphatidic acid (PA)
(2) Arachidonic acid metabolites
Prostaglandins PGE_2, PGI_2, TxA_2 etc.
Leukotrienes LTB_4, LTC_4 etc.
Hydroperoxy and hydroxy derivatives   HPETE, HETE etc.

phospholipid, the platelet-activating factor (PAF), was recognized recently as a very potent platelet-activating substance active at 10^{-11} M[91,92]. Since its structural elucidation and chemical synthesis, a growing list of its biological actions, such as bronchoconstriction, pulmonary and cardiac anaphylaxis, hypotension, hyperalgesia and oedema has been observed (*Table 15.13*). PAF induces leucocyte chemotaxis, neutrophil degranulation and an increase in vascular permeability[93]. Most recently a relationship between PAF and the arachidonic acid was demonstrated by its activation of the lipoxygenase pathway in human PMN and in isolated lung[94]. The 2-arachidonoyl analogue of PAF was also shown to be a significant source of both metabolizable arachidonic acid and PAF in rabbit neutrophils[95].

TABLE 15.13. Platelet-activating factor (PAF-acether)

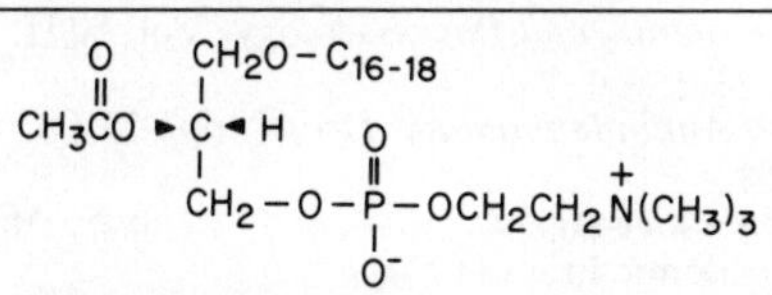

Cellular origins: macrophages, leucocytes, platelets
Biological actions:
● Platelet aggregation and release $<10^{-10}M$
● Bronchoconstriction with vasodilatation
● Anaphylactic actions
● Hypotensive
● Oedema/hyperalgesia ($\sim$PG)

A membrane receptor assay to measure the blockade of ^{3}H-labelled PAF-receptor binding has been developed[96]. For a group of inhibitors, receptor blockade was shown to be parallel with the inhibition of PAF-induced platelet aggregation. By using this assay modest dose-dependent inhibitory activity was seen with indomethacin at 50 μM. However, there is no correlation between PAF antagonism and anti-inflammatory activity for indomethacin analogues and many other NSAIDs[97]. In view of the current interest in PAF, the development of specific and effective PAF receptor antagonists and PAF biosynthesis inhibitors in the near future are to be expected.

In conclusion, starting from cyclo-oxygenase inhibition, a continued interest in the intervention of the arachidonic acid cascade has opened up a new era of research on inflammatory mediators with profound biomedical implications. Investigations to delineate the structural variations and potential roles of hydroxylated arachidonic acids and of phospholipid analogues are still at an early stage. The need for pertinent and specific *in vivo* models to verify some fascinating biochemical stipulations is keenly felt in many cases. Already novel inhibitors of the lipoxygense pathway and antagonists of PAF hold promise to be potentially useful in immediate hypersensitivity and chronic inflammatory disorders. The coming years should be an exciting period both for basic research and for drug discovery in this area.

References

1. SHEN, T.Y. *Burger's Medicinal Chemistry*, 4th ed. Part III. Chap. 62. New York: Wiley (1981)
2. SCHERRER, R.A. and WHITEHOUSE, M.W. *Antiinflammatory Agents, Medicinal Chemistry Monographs*. Vol. 13–1. New York: Academic Press (1974)
3. VANE, J.R. *Nature New Biology*, **231**, 232 (1971)
4. SAMUELSSON, B. *Science*, **220**, 568 (1983)
5. BLACKWELL, G.J., CARNUCCION, R., DIROSA, M., FLOWER, R.J., PARENTE, L. and PERSICO, P. *Nature*, **287**, 147 (1980)
6. HIRATA, F., SCHIFFMANN, E., VENKATASUBRAMANIAN, K., SALOMON, D. and AXELROD, J. *Proceedings of the National Academy of Sciences of the United States of America*, **77**, 2533 (1980)
7. KAPLAN-HARRIS, L. and ELBACH, P. *Biochimica et Biophysica Acta*, **618**, 318 (1980)
8. AHNFELT-RØNNE, I. and ARRIGONI-MARTELLI, E. *Biochemical Pharmacology*, **31**, 2619 (1982)
9. SHEN, T.Y. *Handbook of Experimental Pharmacology*. Vol. 50/II. Chap. 30. New York: Springer-Verlag (1979)
10. SHEN, T.Y. *Non-Steroidal Antiinflammatory Drugs*. pp. 13–20. New York: Excerpta Medica Foundation (1965)
11. SCHERRER, R.A. *Antiinflammatory Agents, Medicinal Chemistry Monographs*. Vol. 13–1. pp. 45–89. New York: Academic Press (1974)
12. SANKAWA, U., SHIBUYA, M., EBIZUKA, Y., NOGUCHI, H., KINOSHITA, T., ENDO, A. et al. *Prostaglandins*, **24**, 21 (1982)
13. SHEN, T.Y. *Angewandte Chemie International edition in English*, **11**, 460 (1972)
14. SHEN, T.Y. *Antiinflammatory Agents, Medicinal Chemistry Monographs*. Vol. 13–1. pp. 180–207. New York: Academic Press (1974)
15. HEWES, W.E., RAKESTRAW, D.C., WHITNEY, C.C. and VERNIER, V.G. *Pharmacologist*, **24**(3), 129 (1982)
16. BRUNE, K., RAINSFORD, K.D., WAGNER, K. and PESKAR, B.A. *Naunyn-Schmiedeberg's Archives of Pharmacology*, **315**, 269 (1981)
17. COHEN, M.M. and POLLETT, J.M. *Surgical Forum*, **21**, 400 (1976)
18. CHICCARELLI, F.S., EISNER, H.J. and VAN LEAR, G.E. *Arzneimittel-Forschung*, **30**, No. 4a, 707 (1980)
19. SHEN, T.Y. and WINTER, C.A. *Advances in Drug Research*. Vol. 12. pp. 89–246. New York: Academic Press (1977)

20. CINOTTI, G., MANZI, M., MENE, P., PIERUCCI, A., PUGLIESE, F., SIMONETTI, B.M. *et al. Clinical Research*, **30**, 445A (1982)

21. BUNNING, R.D. and BARTH, W.F. *Journal of the American Medical Association*, **248**(21), 2864 (1982)

21a. CIBATTONI, G., CINOTTI, G.A., PIERUCCI, A., SIMONETTI, B.M., MANZI, M., PUGLIESE, F. *et al. New England Journal of Medicine*, **310**, 279 (1984)

22. FLOWER, R.J., *Pharmacological Reviews*, **26**, 33 (1974)

23. ROTH, G.J., STANFORD, N. and MAJERUS, P.W. *Proceedings of the National Academy of Sciences of the United States of America*, **72**, 3073 (1975)

24. SHEN, T.Y. *Pharmacotherapy*, **3**, Part 2, 3S–8S (1983)

25. MAJERUS, P.R. and STANFORD, N. *British Journal of Clinical Pharmacology*, **4**, Suppl. 1, 15 (1977)

26. PATRIGNANI, P., FILABOZZI, P. and PATRONO, C. *Journal of Clinical Investigation*, **69**, 1366 (1982)

27. TAI, H.H. and YUAN, B. *Biochemical and Biophysical Research Communications*, **80**, 236 (1978)

28. YOSHIMOTO, T., YAMAMOTO, S. and HAYAISHI, O. *Prostaglandins*, **16**, 529 (1978)

29. HIROSE, T., AOKI, E., DOMAE, M., ISHIBASHI, M., IKEDA, T. and TANAKA, K. *Prostaglandins Leukotrienes and Medicine*, **10**, 187 (1983)

30. BURKE, S.E., DICOLA, G. and LEFER, A.M. *Federation Proceedings*, **42**, 633 (1983)

31. GORMAN, R.R., BUNDY, G.L., PETERSON, D.C., SUN, F.F., MILLER, O.V. and FITZPATRICK, F.A. *Proceedings of the National Academy of Sciences of the United States of America*, **74**, 4007 (1977)

32. CLARK, R.A., SZOT, S., VENKATASUBRAMANIAN, K. and SCHIFFMANN, E. *Journal of Immunology*, **124**, 2020 (1980)

33. HANSEN, H.S. *Prostaglandins*, **8**, 95 (1974)

34. KUEHL, F.A. and EGAN, R.W. *Science*, **210**, 978 (1980)

34a. KULMACZ, R.J. and LANDS, W.E.M. *Prostaglandins*, **25**, 531 (1983)

34b. HAM, E.A., EGAN, R.W., SODERMAN, D., GALE, P.H. and KUEHL, F.A. *Journal of Biological Chemistry*, **254**, 2191 (1979)

35a. EGAN, R.W., GALE, P.H., VANDENHEUVEL, W.J.A., BAPTISTA, E.M. and KUEHL, F.A. Jr *Journal of Biological Chemistry*, **255**, 323 (1980)

35b. MARNETT, L.J., WLODAWER, P. and SAMUELSSON, B. *Journal of Biological Chemistry*, **250**, 8510 (1975)

36. HUMES, J.L., SADOWSKI, S., GALAVAGE, M., GOLDENBERG, M., SUBERS, E., KUEHL, F.A. Jr *et al. Biochemical Pharmacology*, in press (1983)

37. KUEHL, F.A. Jr and EGAN, R.W. *Diflunisal in Clinical Practice*. pp. 13–20. Mt Kisco, New York: Futura Publishing Co. (1978)

38. KUEHL, F.A., HUMES, J.L., EGAN, R.W., HAM, E.A., BEVERIDGE, G.C. and VAN ARMAN, C.G. *Nature*, **265**, 170 (1977)

39. PAYNE, R.G., DERVALD, B., SIEGL, H., GUBLER, H.U., OTT, H. and BAGGIOLINI, M. *Nature*, **296**, 160 (1982)

40. LANDS, W.E.M. and HANEL, A.M. *Prostaglandins*, **24**, 271 (1982)

41. AISHITA, H., MORIMURA, T., OBATA, T., MIURA, Y., MIYAMOTO, T., TSUBOSHIMA, M. *et al. Archives Internationales de Pharmacodynamie et de Thérapie*, **261**, 316 (1983)

42. MOORE, G.G.I. and SWINGLE, K.F. *Agents and Actions*, **12**, 674 (1982)

43. FALKENHEIM, S.F., MacDONALD, H., HUBER, M.M., KOCH, D. and PARKER, C.W. *Journal of Immunology*, **125**, 163 (1980)

44. JAKSCHIK, B.A., DISANTIS, D.M., SANKARAPPA, S.K. and SPRECHER, H. *Advances in Prostaglandin, Thromboxane and Leukotriene Research*, Vol. 9. pp. 127–135. New York: Raven Press (1982)

45. VANDERHOEK, J.Y., BRYANT, R.W. and BAILEY, J.M. *Journal of Biological Chemistry*, **255**(21), 10 064 (1980)

46. ARAI, Y., SHIMOJI, K., KONNO, M., KONISHI, Y., OKUYAMA, S., IGUCHI, S. *et al. Journal of Medicinal Chemistry*, **26**, 72 (1983)

47. GOETZL, E.J. *Biochemical and Biophysical Research Communications*, **101**, 344 (1981)

48. NIJKAMP, F.P. and RAMAKERS, A.G.M. *European Journal of Pharmacology*, **62**, 121 (1980)

49. MITCHELL, H.W. *British Journal of Pharmacology*, **77**, 701 (1982)

50. WANNER, A. and ABRAHAM, W.M. *Lung*, **160**, 231 (1982)

51. COREY, E.J. and MUNROE, J.E. *Journal of the American Chemical Society*, **104**, 1752 (1982)

52. KOSHISHARA, Y., MUROTA, S., PETASIS, N.A. and NICOLAOU, K.C. *FEBS Letters*, **143**, 13 1982)

53. YOSHIMOTO, Y., YOKOYAMA, C., OCHI, K., YAMAMOTO, S., MAKI, Y., ASHIDA, Y. *et al. Biochimica et Biophysica Acta*, **713**, 470 (1982)
54. ROBAK, J. and DUNIEC, Z. *Biochemical Pharmacology*, **31**, 1955 (1982)
55. RADMARK, O., MALMSTEN, C. and SAMUELSSON, B. *FEBS Letters*, **110**, 213 (1980)
56. LEE, T.H., WALPORT, M.J., WILKINSON, A.H., TURNER, W.M. and KAY, A.B. *Lancet*, **ii**, 304 (1981)
57. CASEY, F.B., APPLEBY, B.J. and BUCK, D.C. *Federation Proceedings*, **41**, 820 (1981)
58. WELTON, A.F., HOPE, W.C., CROWLEY, H.J. and SALVADOR, R.A. *Agents and Actions*, **11**, 3345 (1981)
59. CERRINA, J., JOUVIN, E., DUROUX, P. and BENVENISTE, J. *American Review of Respiratory Diseases*, **123**, 44 (1981)
60. STENSON, W.F. and LOBOS, E. *Journal of Clinical Investigation*, **69**, 494 (1981)
61. KU, E.C., McPHERSON, S.E., SIGNOR, C., CHERTOCK, H. and CASH, W.D. *Biochemical and Biophysical Research Communications*, **112**, 899 (1983)
62. PALMER, R.M.J., STEPNEY, R.J., HIGGS, G.A. and EAKINS, K.E. *Prostaglandins*, **20**, 411 (1980)
63. FORD-HUTCHINSON, A.W., BRAY, M.A., DOIG, M.V., SHIPLEY, M.E. and SMITH, M.J.H. *Nature*, **286**, 264 (1980)
64. HIGGS, G.A., BAX, C.M.R. and MONCADA, S. *Leukotrienes and Other Lipoxygenase Products*. pp. 331–339. New York: Raven Press (1982)
65. HIGGS, G.A., FLOWER, R.J. and VANE, J.R. *Biochemical Pharmacology*, **28**, 1959 (1979)
66. EGAN, R.W., GALE, P.H., BEVERIDGE, G.C., MARNETT, L.J. and KUEHL, F.A. *Advances in Prostaglandin and Thromboxane Research*. Vol. 6. pp. 153–155. New York: Raven Press (1980)
67. SAMS, A.R., SPRECHER, H., SANKARAPPA, S.K. and NEEDLEMAN, P. *Leukotrienes and Other Lipoxygenase Products*. pp. 19–28. New York: Raven Press (1982)
68. SEKIYA, K. and OKUDA, H. *Biochemical and Biophysical Research Communications*, **105**, 1090 (1982)
69. EGAN, R.W., TISCHLER, A.N., BAPTISTA, E.M., HAM, E.A., SODERMAN, D.D. and GALE, P.H. *Advances in Prostaglandin, Thromboxane and Leukotriene Research*. Vol. 11. New York: Raven Press in press
70. HAMMARSTRÖM, S. *Biochimica et Biophysica Acta*, **487**, 517 (1977)
71. SIEGEL, M.I., McCONNELL, R.T., BONSER, R.W. and CUATRECASAS, P. *Prostaglandins*, **21**(1), 123 (1981)
72. HONN, K.V. and DUNN, J.R. *FEBS Letters*, **139**(1), 65–68 (1982)
73. AHNFELT-RØNNE, I. and ARRIGONI-MARTELLI, E. *Biochemical Pharmacology*, **29**, 3265 (1980)
74. JAKSCHIK, B.A., DISANTIS, D.M., SANKARAPPA, S.K. and SPRECHER, H. *Biochemical and Biophysical Research Communications*, **102**, 624 (1981)
75. BACH, M.K., BRASHLER, J.R., SMITH, H.W., FITZPATRICK, F.A., SUN, F.F. and McGUIRE, J.C. *Prostaglandins*, **23**, 759 (1982)
76. TISCHLER, A.N., EGAN, R.W. and BAPTISTA, E. Unpublished results
77. SUN, F.F., McGUIRE, J.C., WALLACH, D.P. and BROWN, V.R. *Advances in Prostaglandin and Thromboxane Research*. Vol. 6. pp. 111–113. New York: Raven Press (1980)
78. ORNING, L. and HAMMARSTRÖM, S. *Journal of Biological Chemistry*, **255**, 8023 (1980)
79. VANDERHOEK, J.Y., BRYANT, R.W. and BAILEY, J.M. *Journal of Biological Chemistry*, **255**, 5996 (1980)
80. VERICEL, E. and LAGARDE, M. *Lipids*, **15**, 472 (1980)
81. AHARONY, D., SMITH, J.B. and SILVER, M.J. *Prostaglandins, Leukotrienes and Medicine*, **6**, 237 (1981)
82. FISCHER, A., DURANDY, A. and GRISCELLI, C. *Journal of Immunology*, **126**, 1452 (1981)
83. ROGERS, T.J., CAMPBELL, L., CALHOUN, K., NOWOWIEJSKI, I. and WEBB, D.R. *Cellular Immunology*, **66**, 269 (1982)
84. WALKER, C., KRISTENSEN, F., BETTENS, F. and DEWECK, A.L. *Journal of Immunology*, **130**, 1770 (1983)
85. FANTONE, J.C., MARASCO, W.A., ELGAS, L.J. and WARD, P.A. *Journal of Immunology*, **130**, 1495 (1983)
86. TILDEN, A.B. and BALCH, C.N. *Surgery*, **90**, 77 (1982)
87. GOODWIN, J.S., MESSNER, R.P. and PEAKE, G.T. *Journal of Clinical Investigation*, **62**, 753 (1978)
88. GOODWIN, J.S., MURPHY, S., BANKHURST, A.D., SELINGER, D.S., MESSNER, R.P. and WILLIAMS, R.C. Jr *Journal of Clinical and Laboratory Immunology*, **1**, 197 (1978)

88a. GOODWIN, J.S., CEUPPENS, J.L. and GUALDE, N. *Advances in Inflammation Research*. Vol. 7. pp. 79–92. New York: Raven Press (1984)

89. HAM, E.A., SODERMAN, D.D., ZANETTI, M.E., DOUGHERTY, H.W., McCAULEY, E. and KUEHL, F.A. Jr *Proceedings of the National Academy of Sciences of the United States of America*, in press (1983)

90. BORGEAT, P., DELACLOS, B.F. and MACLOUF, J. *Biochemical Pharmacology*, **32**, 381 (1983)

90a. SHERHAN, C., ANDERSON, P., GOODMAN, E., DUNHAM, P. and WEISSMANN, G. *Journal of Biological Chemistry*, **256**, 2736 (1981)

91. DEMOPOULOS, C.A., PINCKARD, R.N. and HANAHAN, D.J. *Journal of Biological Chemistry*, **254**, 9355 (1979)

92. BEVENISTE, J., TENCE, M., VARENNE, P., BIDAULT, J., BOULLET, C. and POLONSKY, J. *Comptes Rendus des seances de L'Academie des Sciences (D) (Paris)*, **289**, 1037 (1979)

93. SNYDER, F. *Annual Reports in Medicinal Chemistry*, **17**, 243 (1982)

94. PIPER, P.J. and TEMPLE, D.M. *Journal of Pharmacy and Pharmacology*, **33**, 384 (1981)

95. SWEDSEN, C.L., ELLIS, J.M., CHILFON, III, F.H., O'FLAHERTY, J.T. and WYKLE, R.L. *Biochemical and Biophysical Research Communications*, **113**, 72 (1983)

96. HWANG, S.B., LEE, C.-S.C., CHEAH, M.J. and SHEN, T.Y. *Biochemistry*, in press (1983)

97. SHEN, T.Y., HWANG, S.B., CHEAH, M.J. and LEE, C.-S.C. *INSERM Symposia*. Vol. 23, *Platelet-Activating Factor and Structurally Related Ether-Lipids*. Amsterdam: North-Holland Biomedical Press/Elsevier. In press (1983)

98. COREY, E.J. and PARK, H. *Journal of the American Chemical Society*, **104**, 1750 (1982)

99. KNIPPEL, I., BAUMANN, J., BRUCHHAUSEN, F.V. and WURM, G. *Biochemical Pharmacology*, **30**(12), 1677 (1981)

100. BAUMANN, J. and WURM, G. *Agents and Actions*, **12**, 360 (1982)

101. BAUMANN, J., BRUCHHAUSEN, F.V. and WURM, G. *Prostaglandins*, **20**, 627 (1980)

102. PANGANAMALA, R.V., MILLER, J.S., GWEBU, E.T., SHARMA, H.M. and CORNWELL, D.G. *Prostaglandins*, **14**, 261 (1977)

103. MOORE, G.G.I. and SWINGLE, K.F. *Agents and Actions*, **12**, 674 (1982)

Section 4 Specific hyposensitization

Chapter 16

Specific hyposensitization

D.M. Moran and A.W. Wheeler

Introduction

Although hyposensitization therapy has been used in the management of allergic conditions for the greater part of this century, it is widely acknowledged that definitive evidence for the general clinical utility of the procedure has yet to be wholly established[1–4]. Reductions in symptoms of patients with seasonal allergic rhinitis have been formally demonstrated in a number of controlled studies[5,6], but for the more restricted application of extrinsic asthma, the position is somewhat more controversial[2,4,7]. Relatively fewer controlled investigations have been reported and, for those that are available, most have been compromised to some degree, either by the very complexities of the syndrome or by the general overall difficulties of the undertaking[7,8]. As a result, it is not surprising that application of hyposensitization therapy to extrinsic asthma has been subject to some criticism, particularly perhaps for certain indications, such as bacterial or mould allergies[2,6,9–11]. Together with the sometimes conflicting clinical literature, the use of ill-defined and relatively unstandardized allergen extracts, the attendant potential hazard of allergen administration, and the overall lack of a thorough-going rationale for a likely mechanism of therapeutic action, have all conspired to consolidate this body of adverse comment[1,2,4,12]. Nevertheless, despite these alleged limitations, large numbers of clinical allergists remain vehemently convinced of the value of the practice and, correspondingly, many patients appear to benefit from these oftentimes unformalized, but compelling, clinical convictions[13–15]. Accordingly, the subject continues to attract much attention and interest, and efforts to improve treatment procedures and methods of assessment continue to be intensively researched, as do attempts to elucidate a convincing basic mechanistic rationale.

Given this general position, how then is the role of hyposensitization therapy in relation to the treatment of allergic asthma to be viewed, and

349

what are the limitations of the procedure which are readily amenable to change and development? In this review, primary concern has been directed to these latter issues. No attempt has been made to assess and catalogue the intricate details of allergen vaccine treatments in asthma in anything like a comprehensive manner. Much of such data and analysis thereof has been the subject of many earlier excellent articles[2,9,12,15,16]. Rather, attention has been restricted predominantly to selected modern clinical and laboratory studies, in an attempt to delineate the established allergenic and immunological properties of important aeroallergen extracts, and to examine how these attributes have been and could be best exploited in order to contribute to therapeutic benefit in the allergic asthmatic.

Hyposensitization therapy—general comments

Hyposensitization therapy was introduced by Noon and Freeman in 1911 to treat seasonal pollinosis[17,18]; application to other allergic conditions, including asthma, followed rapidly[19]. Since those early studies, numerous investigations have been reported, many indicating favourable, albeit largely subjective, clinical impressions[5,12]. Unfortunately, in part perhaps due to the intrinsic complexities of the clinical conditions being treated and in part because of the relatively variable and unstandardized nature of the allergen extract preparations employed, much of this hard-won but predominantly empirical information has served as much to obscure, as to clarify, the basic issues of clinical utility and treatment rationale. The voluminous literature available on the subject of hyposensitization therapy is indeed difficult to collate and, in many instances, provides conflicting arguments. Nevertheless, in more recent times, the introduction of placebo-controlled studies has begun to provide firmer and more objective evidence in favour of the value of allergen injection regimes[15,16]. No concensus exists, however, supporting the general utility of the procedure; nor has it become clear in mechanistic terms as to what is being attempted or achieved by allergen injection treatments.

Indeed, ignorance of mechanisms of action has clearly limited opportunities to develop and improve hyposensitization vaccines. As a result, it is not perhaps too surprising, if not disappointing, that treatment regimens and practices have not changed fundamentally over the last half century or more[19]. At the root of this problem, of course, has been the lack of detailed knowledge about the underlying pathogenesis of allergic disease. Enormous advances have indeed been made in the understanding of the detailed biochemical events involved in acute allergic reactions[20,21]. The role of reaginic or IgE antibodies in the elaboration of anaphylactic mediators and in clinical allergy generally, is also well documented and appreciated[22,23]. However, despite these major developments, identification of objective parameters relating clinical sensitivity and severity of the disease to environmental allergen exposure remains obscure. For the case of asthmatic symptoms attributable to extrinsic agents, the situation is perhaps particularly uncertain. Asthma is a highly complex and multifactorial syndrome[24]. The importance of any one factor, therefore, is less likely to be of general relevance and may be expected to vary between sensitized individuals. Accordingly, the effectiveness of any treatment may also be anticipated to be largely patient dependent, again emphasizing the crucial need to establish appropriate diagnostic procedures and discerning selection critieria, such that only suitable patients are hyposensitized.

Immunological and mechanistic considerations

Traditionally, and perhaps not surprisingly, hyposensitization therapy has been tacitly assumed to achieve clinical benefit as a result of influences on the immune status of the treated individual[2]; the common use of the term immunotherapy to describe this form of treatment clearly illustrates this point. As is widely appreciated, it was the notion that pollen-associated toxins were responsible for eliciting the characteristic allergic symptoms of hay-fever which provided the first rational basis for allergen injection treatments[17,18]. Induction of neutralizing anti-toxin antibodies clearly offered itself in such a scheme as a reasonable and highly plausible therapeutic possibility. Later events, and in particular the finding that so-called reaginic antibodies were basically responsible for precipitating immediate allergic symptoms, showed this rationale to be unacceptable[25]. Nevertheless, this finding preserved the immunological connection and perhaps served to predispose attitudes even more to the view that allergic disease, being perceived essentially as an immunological dysfunction, should, therefore, be amenable to immunological manipulation. In more recent times, the discovery and establishment of the central role of IgE antibody in immediate, type I hypersensitivity conditions has consolidated this view still further, and opened up whole new opportunities for immunological studies in allergic disease[26,27]. Measurement of changes in these, and indeed other, immunological parameters following allergen injection treatment, have featured prominently in clinical study protocols[5,9]. Correspondingly, efforts to develop a mechanistic explanation for hyposensitization treatment based on these observations have also been pursued.

Blocking antibody concepts

Although the therapeutic relevance of anti-toxin antibodies has long since been excluded as an explanation for a likely mode of action following allergen injection treatments, the thought that administration of allergen extracts could induce the formation of protective antibodies has seemingly remained firmly entrenched in the minds of many allergists. This rather comfortable and intuitively appealing concept of a blocking antibody as a therapeutic parameter has indeed been regularly revamped under one pretext or another during intervening years since Noon's early experiments. The finding that the Prausnitz–Kustner reaction[25] could be inhibited effectively by sera from hyposensitized individuals clearly reinforced the view in the mid-1930s that an immunologically induced protective function was therapeutically relevant[28]. More recently, similar observations of the blocking effects of sera taken from treated patients on allergen-mediated histamine release from sensitized human basophils, again accorded with this expectation[29–31]. The therapeutic potential of passive transfer of allergen-specific IgG antibodies has also been evaluated[32,33]. Indeed, numerous studies have been carried out to study the induction of these so-called protective antibodies in both serum[34-37] and secretions[38-40] of treated allergic subjects, in an attempt to relate such parameters to therapeutic efficacy. However, few studies have in fact found convincing relationships between these changes in antibody levels and patient benefit[5]. For other applications, such as hymenoptera sensitivities, the protective function of IgG antibodies has been more surely established[41].

What then is the therapeutic relevance in respiratory allergies of blocking antibodies produced by conventional hyposensitization regimens, particularly serum antibodies? It has always been difficult to reconcile the expectation of serum antibodies providing a protective element for allergens entering via the nasal or bronchial routes. This conceptual anomaly has been further complicated by the finding that target mast cells, and possibly basophils, are in fact present in the lumen of the respiratory tract, and not merely sequestered in the submucosae[42-44]. To be effective, therefore, antibodies generated by conventional parenteral administration routes would be required to establish appropriate levels in the external secretion phases, and not merely within interstitial regions. Some evidence of small rises in allergen-specific antibodies in nasal secretions has indeed been observed[40,45], and encouraging protective responses to allergen bronchial challenges have been reported in sensitized dogs, following passive administration of allergen-specific IgG antibodies[46]. However, the overall apparent failure to furnish compelling evidence of a relationship between protection of sensitized individuals and antibody levels, suggests of itself that blocking antibodies are unlikely to be of general significance. For asthma, available data would appear to be particularly unconvincing[47-51].

Effects on IgE production

In conjunction with the well-documented studies on the increase of allergen-specific IgG antibodies following hyposensitization treatments, corresponding changes have also been observed with respect to IgE antibody levels.

In general, modest increases in serum levels of allergen-specific IgE have been observed immediately after hyposensitization treatments. Most studies have involved pollenosis patients[5,49], although data with house-dust mite[48,50,52,53], and animal dander[54] sensitive individuals are also available. Long-term treatments in pollenosis patients have been shown to effect a gradual fall in IgE levels[37,55]. Recently, Gleich et al.[56], have reported an overall reduction of some 73% over six seasons of treatments with ragweed pollen extracts. Evidence of ablation of rises in specific IgE antibodies due to seasonal pollen exposure has also been noted as a particular consequence of hyposensitization therapy[57-59], as has blunting of treatment-induced rises[36,58]. Explanations for these various changes have not been forthcoming, but such effects have been loosely ascribed as being indicative of therapeutic benefit[58]. The assertion would appear to be extremely tenuous. The relatively marginal differences observed in IgE antibody levels generally fail to provide convincing support for any firm relationship with clinical effectiveness[60]. Studies of IgE antibody changes involving patients with perennial asthma afford similarly unremarkable data[48,51,53].

Changes in cellular responsiveness

With the advent of improved procedures for monitoring lymphocyte function, various cellular changes have been measured following hyposensitization therapy. Attempts have also been made to identify these changes as potential therapeutic and mechanistic correlates. Particular attention has focused on the role of the T-lymphocyte, since dysfunction in this cell population has been implicated as a causal factor in atopy in general, as well as being specifically identified as a major underlying factor contributing to excessive reaginic antibody production[61–63].

Most investigations in this context have involved assessment of allergen or mitogen-induced lymphocyte transformation responses, using peripheral blood mononuclear cells from patients suffering from allergic rhinitis. Generally, however, measurements of allergen-induced effects have not proved to be of particular value as indices of allergic status or of therapeutic benefit following treatment. Relatively poor correlations have been found with clinical sensitivities and symptoms in both allergic rhinitics[64] and asthmatics[65,66], and although changes in lymphoproliferative responses have been reported following hyposensitization, usually depressive[60,65,67–70], the functional significance of these data has not been readily apparent. For example, Rocklin et al.[71] have demonstrated that lymphocytes manifest depressed proliferative responses in vitro after allergen injection treatment, as a direct result of T-suppressor cell induction. However, whether these same regulatory cells were capable of influencing other, perhaps more pertinent, immunological functions, such as inhibiting reaginic antibody production, was not clear; serological data were not presented in this study.

Similar ambiguities also remain for assessing the relevance of mitogen or histamine-induced T-suppressor cell effects in lymphoproliferative assays. Abnormal T-cell function has been reported in a number of studies using these systems with cells obtained from atopic subjects[72–77]. Unfortunately, only limited data are available relating such findings to possible therapeutic benefits. Indeed, no prospective investigations of the effect of hyposensitization therapy on these parameters have been described in asthmatic subjects, although Rivlin et al.[78], have suggested that concanavalin-A-inducible suppressor cells were within the normal range only in asthmatic children who had previously received allergen injection treatments; a second series of untreated children displayed markedly depressed responses. However, that prior hyposensitization treatment was the critical determinant in the observed differential immune status of these two asthmatic groups is questionable. Children not selected for allergen treatment in this study were rejected on the basis of positive criteria, namely the absence of demonstrable allergen sensitivities. Whether the two groups could be legitimately compared, therefore, remains open to some doubts. In any event, these findings appeared to be unrelated to the clinical status of the patients.

Some evidence for a possible mechanistic rationale of hyposensitization therapy has also been suggested from studies of T-cell phenotypic markers. Asthmatic[79–81] and atopic dermatitis patients[82–85], in particular, have been widely observed to exhibit imbalances in helper and suppressor T cells, with both groups typically displaying low proportions of cells with the T-suppressor phenotype. The consequence of these abnormalities has also been shown to manifest itself in possible disease-related terms, as illustrated by the demonstration of a negative correlation of serum IgE levels and reduced numbers of circulating T-supressor cells[83]. Importantly, however, these immunological parameters have been shown to be favourably influenced by hyposensitization therapy. Canonica et al.[86] have demonstrated in a small series of severe asthmatic patients that imbalances in the $T\gamma/T\mu$ (suppressor/helper) lymphocyte subpopulations were normalized following allergen injection treatment. Moreover, and most significantly, concomitant with these changes, symptom benefit was also achieved. Unfortunately, the clinical data substantiating this most important latter claim were not presented. Nevertheless, such findings provide much encouragement for the possibility of establishing objective treatment criteria and a credible rationalization for the mechanism of hyposensitization treatment. Restoration of observed imbalances in regulatory lymphocyte function clearly offers itself as a most plausible target for immunological intervention. Consequently, such potentially important observations obviously merit further consideration. Unfortunately, this has not been forthcoming as yet. Moreover, other studies have sounded a note of caution when interpreting such findings. Phenotypic expression and functional performance in lymphocyte populations have not always been shown to correlate[50,87]. This feature has been illustrated most clearly in experiments reported by Strannegard et al.[88]. In a recent investigation involving atopic dermatitis patients, imbalances in serologically defined OKT4 (T-helper) and OKT8 (T-suppressor) lymphocyte ratios were found to be readily normalized by short-term treatments with the thymic pentapeptide TP-5[89]. Nevertheless, despite this seemingly beneficial change, the typically elevated serum levels of reaginic antibody observed in these patients were not immediately influenced[90]; of course, longer treatments may have been more effective. Evidently other factors are also involved in the control of hyperproduction of IgE antibodies, possibly not represented in terms of phenotypic markers on circulating lymphocytes. Identification of these regulatory elements obviously awaits further research.

The impact of hyposensitization therapy on the expression of immunoglobulin Fc and complement receptors on monocytes and polymorphonuclear cells (PMN) has also been suggested as a mechanism possibly responsible for clinical effectiveness. Hsieh[91] has reported that asthmatic children display lower mean percentages of monocytes and PMNs bearing Fc and complement receptors than non-atopic subjects, and that these numbers decrease still further following exposure to allergen in vitro. Interestingly, injection treatments were found to ablate the sensitivity of these receptors on phagocytic cells to allergen challenge[50], possibly via histamine-mediated events[92]; similar results have also been observed with corresponding lymphocyte receptors[50,87,93]. Based on these and other complementary findings, Hsieh[91] has postulated that impaired receptor function of phagocytes, coupled with hyperpermeability of mucosa to macromolecules, could lead to abnormally prolonged persistence of allergen in the atopic subject, resulting finally in chronic immunological stimulation and augmented IgE production. Despite the fact that the linkage between these latter two phenomena was not explained, the influence of hyposensitization therapy was seen as mitigating this impaired allergen clearance function. Noticeably, however, no changes in allergen-specific serum antibodies were observed in treated children in these studies[50], suggesting that the cellular changes seen presumably related to an intrinsic defect not directly concerned with mechanisms controlling established, ongoing serological responses.

Desensitization

In addition to immunological considerations, direct tissue desensitization has also been considered as a possible mechanism of action in conventional hyposensitization treatment[94]. Much laboratory-based evidence, especially in older literature, has been accrued to show that refractory or tachyphylactic states of sensitized tissue can be achieved by repeated allergen exposure at levels suboptimal for receptor triggering[95,96]. Observation of reductions in reactivity of basophilic leucocytes[58,97], skin-tests[98,99] and bronchial sensitivity[100] to allergen challenge following injection therapy all accord with, although of course do not establish, the validity of such a phenomenon. Tolerant states induced over relatively short time intervals by accelerated 'rush-desensitization' treatment regimens have also provided clinical evidence consistent with such a process[98,101,102].

However, despite such findings and anecdotal clinical impressions that sensitivities to secondary allergens may decrease during hyposensitization to a major or perhaps seasonal allergen, the case for densensitization as a mechanistic explanation remains unfashionable. The difficulty of readily accommodating the more generally acknowledged allergen specificity of the treatment[103,104] and the fact that, in some instances, shock tissues appear to manifest increased sensitivities to challenge after therapy[105–107], possibly accounts for this view. Reports of the loss of peripheral basophilic sensitivities to both specific and unrelated allergens after hyposensitization, once considered as possible evidence for a more general non-specific desensitization phenomenon[108,109], have also been undermined by the finding that corresponding changes were not apparent in skin-test or bronchial provocation measurements[110].

Summary

It is evident that allergen injection treatments effect significant changes in both humoral and cellular immunological parameters. Also, clearly defined immunological characteristics and dysfunctions have been identified in atopic populations by a number of laboratory techniques, all of which offer the potential to evaluate the impact of hyposensitization on the immune status of treated individuals, incisively and relatively comprehensively. However, despite these developments, interpretation of much of these accrued data in relation to clinical status remains uncertain. None of these various immunological changes has been found to correlate consistently with symptom amelioration in asthmatic patients and, as a consequence, rationalization of such information in terms of possible modes of action cannot be other than speculative. Therefore, although affording interesting and possibly useful descriptive diagnostic data, measurements of immunological parameters have not as yet provided the much sought after objective index of likely therapeutic benefit with this form of therapy, nor has a basis for developing a comprehensive treatment rationale been established.

Clinical studies

Over the last decade alone, the number of communications reporting data relating to hyposensitization treatments has been vast. Clearly, enormous resources have been committed to this area of clinical medicine. Complementing these primary research articles, numerous reviews have also been published. Most of these have been concerned with appraisals of specific allergen treatments in the managment of allergic disease in general[1,3,5,10,16,112,113]. However, a number of authors have emphasized aspects applicable to asthma therapy; in particular diagnosis and efficacy[2,4,6,9,12,114,115], childhood asthma[15,116,117], mould allergies[118], study design[8], mechanisms[96,119], and controversial issues concerning the treatment practice[2,7,120,121], have all received detailed consideration. In this section, a brief summary of the more recent studies is outlined, considering first general issues relating to investigations of therapeutic performance and associated clinical parameters in hyposensitization therapy, and then subsequently, efficacy data derived predominantly from controlled studies.

General considerations

Asthma is an extremely complex condition. Not surprisingly, therefore, design and execution of appropriate clinical trial protocols employed to evaluate the effectiveness of hyposensitization therapy have often proved to be inadequate[4,7,8]. Establishing the generality of clinical findings has also been problematic. Variation in patient clinical status, sensitivity patterns, treatment regimens, extracts, assessment procedures and environmental factors are examples, among many, of parameters which commonly compromise, or even preclude, legitimate comparison between one study experience and another. Possibly the most difficult area for those attempting to compare the merits of different forms of treatment or elucidating underlying mechanistic considerations, has been the question of quantifying therapeutic assessments. In early literature, much emphasis was placed on clinical impression. Although generally favourable of hyposensitization treatments, this approach was often little more than anecdotal[5]. More recently, attempts have been made to introduce seemingly objective means of evaluating clinical performance, including the use of appropriate control patient groups. The latter innovation has, of course, given perspective to clinical studies. However, this development has produced other problems since satisfactory matching of patients, a critical feature of any controlled study design, is perhaps especially difficult with asthmatic subjects[12,122,123]. Patient selection criteria, based on extensive clinical characterization, are particularly crucial, therefore, if satisfactorily controlled studies are to be undertaken; long-term cross-over designs are also probably necessary if random bias is to be minimized. Few studies have been carried out in this manner.

Nevertheless, much progress has been made in study design and reports are available documenting patient symptom and medication scores, supplemented in many cases with measurements of various clinical parameters. Provocation of shock tissues with putative offending allergens, pulmonary function tests, attendant immunological changes and many miscellaneous parameters, such as levels of anaphylactic or suspected anaphylactic mediators, have all been monitored and correlated with symptomology. Unfortunately, little of the data reported in these various contexts to date enjoys universal approval. Indeed, much appears to be conflicting. For example, changes in bronchial sensitivity to allergen has been found to be reduced following allergen treatment in some instances[52,100,101,124–130], but not in others[110,131] and to be related to clinical benefit by some investigators[52,124,125] but not by others[100,126–128,131]. Warner et al.[130] found symptom amelioration was correlated only with ablation of the late reaction[132]. Corresponding variations in skin test sensitivity to allergen challenge have also been found[52,98,105,110,129,133]. Similarly, and in contradistinction to general expectations in allergic rhinitis[5], allergen-specific IgG antibodies have been reported as unchanged when efficacy was established[50,51], yet, almost perversely, modestly enhanced when therapeutic benefit was adjudged to be poor[49]. Doubtless, some of these discrepancies result primarily from differences in technical aspects of measurement procedures or data interpretation[131]. Even so, these inconsistencies have resulted in an overall impression of confusion, if not frustration[8].

A further feature of possible ambiguity in hyposensitization studies relates to the analytical aspects of expressing symptom and medication score data. As a result of the very nature of modern studies, vast amounts of data are often accumulated. Reduction of this information to manageable proportions inevitably means that subtle trends in individual patient responses may be sacrificed at times, in order to communicate general patient group effects. Group comparisons of this type naturally rely heavily on statistical methods to discern significance, which is clearly desirable. However, there is some concern that establishment of formal statistically significant differences between group responses in such studies may exaggerate or even obscure genuine clinical findings[8,134,135]. Symptom scores recorded in well-controlled investigations indeed illustrate that variation in responses within patient groups commonly exceeds that noted between groups[131]. Formal differences established between the two groups in this context, therefore, inevitably relate primarily to trends and gross probabilities of benefit, rather than to genuine expectation of individual patient improvement. Also, it is evident that absolute, as well as relative, therapeutic benefit are clearly most important, a feature not always apparent in unqualified statistical analyses. As a consequence, this approach has been subject to criticism[7].

Clearly, there is not a concensus for conducting and evaluating efficacy studies in allergic disease. At the present time, and in the absence of wholly reliable disease-related indices, it would seem that reliance must still be placed on enlightened combination of both clinical judgement and available objective parameters. The former of course is not amenable to quantitiative analysis; the latter have perhaps been subject to over-analysis. It is against this rather uncertain background that clinical data collected in support of hyposensitization therapy have to be evaluated.

Parenteral studies

As has been indicated, early hyposensitization studies were conducted largely on an empirical basis, with assessment of performance being predominantly the product of subjective clinical impressions. Authoritative and comprehensive reviews of these early data have been reported by a number of pioneering contributors to the field[136,137]. Since the late 1940s, however, serious efforts have been made to establish more formal evidence of efficacy. A number of controlled studies has been undertaken and attempts have been made to introduce various objective assessment procedures amenable to quantitative analysis.

A list of controlled investigations reported for the treatment of house-dust asthma is collected in *Table 16.1*; corresponding data for studies applied to other allergic sensitivities are given in *Table 16.2*. As is apparent, the majority of controlled hyposensitization studies as yet reported have been concerned with patients manifesting asthmatic symptoms to house-dust; pollen and bacterial allergen-induced asthma have also received considerable attention.

Much controversy has arisen over the utility of bacterial vaccines[2,138]. Despite continuing claims that hyposensitization with bacterial extracts contribute effectively to the management of so-called infective asthma[139–142], little formal evidence has accrued to support this view. Of six controlled studies reported, five were unable to demonstrate more benefit in actively treated patients compared with placebo[143–147], including one investigation using autogenous vaccines[143]. In the remaining study[148], trends to improvement were indeed noted in treated subjects, although only one of the parameters monitored, inhaler prescriptions, achieved a level of statistical significance. These findings, taken together with the attendant possibilities of adverse reactions with such materials[2] and the disputed aetiology of infective asthma[149,150], have persuaded many authorities to recommend this practice to be contraindicated[2,10,117,151]. Emphatic opposition to this view, however, remains in some quarters[142].

Support for hyposensitization treatment of asthma secondary to house-dust sensitivities has also been uncertain, but generally more favourable. Controlled studies in Britain during the 1960s[152,153] failed to confirm the extremely satisfactory therapeutic claims reported in an earlier investigation by Bruun[154]. However, Aas[126], in what is widely recognized to be a pivotal paediatric study in this context, involving some 80 asthmatic children, subsequently provided firmer evidence that clinical benefits could be achieved with this form of therapy. Using perennial treatments with house-dust extract injections over a three-year period, significant symptomatic improvements were recorded, and increases in bronchial tolerance were demonstrated in 73% of treated patients, compared with 31% in the placebo group. Although changes in bronchial sensitivities appeared to be generally associated with symptom amelioration, a close correlation adequate for predictive purposes was not established.

TABLE 16.1. Controlled studies of hyposensitization with house-dust

Allergens used	Patient group	Dosage form	Number of patients		Response	Date	Ref.
			Treated	Placebo			
Dust	Not stated	Aq/not stated	100	89	Favourable	1949	154
Dust	Mixed	Aq/short-term	33	37	Unfavourable	1968	153
Dust	Children	Aq/perennial	52	28	Favourable	1971	126
Mite (Dpt)*	Mixed	Aq/short-term	11	11	Favourable	1971	164
Mite (Dpt)*	Mixed	Aq/short-term	45	46	Favourable	1973	47
Mite (Dpt)*	Adults	Tyrosine/perennial	20	25	Unfavourable	1976	168
Mite (Df)†	Adults	Alum/perennial	7	7‡	Unfavourable	1978	128
Mite (Dpt)*	Children	Tyrosine/perennial	27	24	Favourable	1978	130
Mite (Dpt)	Adults	Tyrosine/perennial short-term	16	12	Favourable	1978	169
Mite (Dpt)*	Adults	Aq/perennial	29	17	Unfavourable	1979	166
Mite (Dpt)*	Adults	Tyrosine/perennial	31	14	Unfavourable§	1981	170
Mite (Dpt)	Children	Aq/oral perennial	17	15	Unfavourable	1982	167

* *D. pteronyssinus.*
† *D. farinae.*
‡ Placebo received aqueous injections.
§ High placebo response.
Aq = aqueous vehicle.

TABLE 16.2. Controlled studies of hyposensitization with allergens other than house-dust

Allergens used	Patient group	Dosage form	Number of patients		Response	Date	Ref.
			Treated	Placebo			
Mixed (grasses/ moulds/dust)	Children	Aq/perennial	10	5†	Unfavourable	1973	127
Bacteria	Mixed	Aq/perennial	100	84	Unfavourable	1955	143
Bacteria	Children	Aq/perennial	60	58	Unfavourable	1959	145
Bacteria	Mixed	Aq/variable	77	79	Unfavourable	1959	144
Bacteria	Children	Aq/perennial	15	10	Unfavourable	1963	146
Bacteria	Mixed	Aq/perennial	22	22	Favourable	1965	148
Bacteria	Children	Aq/perennial	15	15	Unfavourable	1965	147
Dander (cat)	Adults	Aq/short-term	5	5	Favourable	1978	129
Grass	Mixed	Aq/Preseason	31	26	Favourable	1954	178
Grass	Adults	Alum/perennial	11	4	Favourable	1982	180
Grass	Children	Aq/perennial*	11	9	Unfavourable	1982	49
Ragweed	Children	Aq/perennial	58	14	Favourable	1957	179
Ragweed	Adults	Aq/perennial†	13	17	Unfavourable	1977	131

* 'Rush' desensitization regimen used.
† Low-dose placebo group.
Aq = aqueous vehicle.

All other placebo-controlled investigations with house-dust sensitive asthmatic patients have been undertaken with extracts of house-dust mites. House-dust extracts are inevitably highly variable and complex mixtures. Diagnostic and therapeutic properties of materials derived from such ill-defined sources can be expected to differ widely, therefore, and this feature alone has probably been responsible for much of the variation seen in clinical performance. Consequently, the findings by Voorhoorst and coworkers[155], that the house-dust mite was the primary source of major allergens in house-dust, marked a potentially crucial phase in the development of more appropriate vaccine preparations for this indication. Subsequent studies by several groups have indeed confirmed the important role of the house-dust mite in extrinsic asthma[156,157] and, more recently, these observations have been consolidated and extended by others[158–161].

Of the controlled studies reported with house-dust mite preparations (*Table 16.1*), most have been carried out in UK centres, using extracts of *Dermatophagoides pteronyssinus* or *Dermatophagoides farinae*. The former has been shown to be the predominant species found in Europe, whereas *D.farinae* appears to be more common in the USA[155]. Partial immunological cross-reactivity has been demonstrated, however, between these two important mite species[162,163]. Early clinical studies with these extracts employed conventional aqueous presentations[47,52,164–167]; recently, alum[128] and L-tyrosine adsorbate vaccines[168–170] have also been used.

Despite the potential advantages offered by using house-dust mite extracts of more consistent composition, results obtained in the available controlled clinical studies have again been variable. Possibly the most encouraging data obtained to date is that recorded by Warner and coworkers[130] who investigated the effects of hyposensitization to *D. pteronyssinus* in well-managed, and carefully selected, asthmatic children. Reduction in medication requirements of treated children compared with controls in this investigation was particularly impressive, and a novel correlation of bronchial sensitivities to allergen challenge and symptoms was also established. No consistent relationship was found between immediate responses and symptom benefit but, remarkably, ablation of late reaction responses occurred in those children who showed most improvements in clinical status. This latter observation accords with earlier findings by Warner[132] who demonstrated a close relationship between the severity of the clinical condition of asthmatic subjects and the pattern of bronchial response to allergen challenge. It is of interest to note, however, that associations of late bronchial responsiveness and serum IgG_4 subclass antibody levels have been reported by Gwynn and coworkers[171,172]. Since long-term immunization[173], including some hyposensitization treatments[174,175], are known to induce IgG_4 antibodies preferentially, inhibition of late responses by such therapy would appear to be mutually inconsistent. Hopefully, further work will clarify these observations and provide the basis for developing a truly reliable index of likely therapeutic benefit. Satisfactory results, assessed predominantly in terms of medication records, have also been reported in a double-blind study of perennial asthmatic adult subjects by Marques and Avila[169]. Both these studies employed *D.pteronyssinus* extracts adsorbed to L-tyrosine.

Other placebo-controlled studies, however, have recorded either equivocal or relatively unsatisfactory findings. For example, Taylor et al.[165] found growth characteristics of certain children treated with an extract described as house-dust fortified with D.farinae to be improved compared with placebo-treated controls, but no advantages were evident in clinical parameters. Whether the apparent benefits observed were indeed treatment related was not clear either, however, since the treated group in this study seemingly contained a disproportionate number of children displaying pubertal growth spurts. In earlier studies, Smith[164] and D'Souza et al.[47] also provided evidence of clinical improvements in adult patients receiving D.pteronyssinus hyposensitization, but the levels of benefit attained were relatively moderate. Similar doubts were expressed by the coordinators of a multicentre study sponsored by the British Thoracic Association[166], who concluded that the marginal beneficial effects observed in this investigation were unlikely to be of clinical importance. Wholly negative findings have also been reported by other investigators using both D.pteronyssinus adsorbed to L-tryosine[168,170] and D.farinae adsorbed to alum[128]. Perhaps, significantly, all these latter unfavourable studies involved predominantly adult asthmatic patients.

Consideration of these results suggests that the innovation of house-dust mite extract has consolidated, rather than dramatically improved, therapeutic prospects for house-dust-sensitive asthmatics. The inconsistencies in the data recorded by different investigators preclude the possibility of establishing definitive conclusions, but clearly the overall value of house-dust mite injection treatment for asthma management remains uncertain. No obvious major causal differences were evident in trial designs between groups of studies reporting favourable or unfavourable clinical performance, although it is worthy of note that all these investigations employed a relatively limited treatment period, usually less than 12 months. Only the multicentre study organized by the British Thoracic Association continued therapy for a longer duration, although here, in fact, no benefit was observed by extending treatment from 18 weeks to 18 months[166]. Nevertheless, general clinical experience with hyposensitization therapy suggests that several years of treatment is often necessary to achieve significant levels of symptomatic relief. Longer-term treatment regimens for house-dust-sensitive asthmatics may therefore be necessary to ensure consistent beneficial effects. Chu et al.[176] have recently illustrated that progressive clinical improvements are indeed evident in patients treated with multiple courses of D.farinae extract over a four-year period. Others have also stressed the advantage of extended treatment regimens with house-dust mite vaccine[51,177].

Controlled studies with other major aeroallergens implicated in extrinsic asthma have also afforded conflicting findings. Several studies have been reported dealing with pollen-induced asthma[49,131,178–180], another with a mixture of allergens, including moulds[145], and more recently, Taylor and coworkers[129] have reported an elegant double-blind evaluation of hyposensitization therapy in cat-induced asthma. Initially, clinical advantage in this latter study was limited to the demonstration of treatment-related reductions in bronchial sensitivities. Most encouragingly, however, follow-up studies have illustrated that benefit was also evident in treated patients subject to natural cat exposure[181].

Early controlled studies of hyposensitization therapy in pollen-induced asthma generally afforded highly favourable clinical results. Frankland and Augustin[178] first demonstrated some 30 years ago that seasonal asthmatic symptoms precipitated by grass pollen could be significantly relieved by preseasonal allergen injections; 29 of 31 (98%) subjects were said to report good or excellent results after therapy whereas only 8 of 26 (34%) control patients were in this category. Although patients maintained diary cards, no formal analysis of the data nor other objective measurements were presented to support these encouraging observations. In a subsequent study from the same centre, however, extremely favourable clinical results were again reported and, in this instance, 12 of 13 patients were also found to display falls in bronchial sensitivity, whereas no consistent changes were evident in 5 untreated control subjects[124]. In another early controlled study, Johnstone[179], using a long-term perennial treatment regimen, was able to demonstrate impressive clinical results in children displaying seasonal asthmatic symptoms to ragweed pollen. The importance of allergen dosage for effective treatment was particularly evident in this investigation. More recently, further support for the effectiveness of hyposensitization in seasonal pollen asthma has been reported by Osterballe et al.[180]. Studying a small subseries of adult patients with grass pollen asthma within a larger group of pollenosis subjects, no changes in asthmatic symptoms between active and placebo-treated groups were initially observed following a primary 12-week preseasonal course of injections. However, further preseasonal treatments were shown to effect benefit during subsequent grass pollen seasons; 4 of 4 placebo-treated subjects continued to experience asthmatic episodes whereas 9 of the 11 treated patients were asymptomatic. Both these latter studies clearly provide supportive evidence for the value of protracted treatments.

In contrast with these favourable experiences, other investigators have recorded less optimistic findings. In a series of carefully diagnosed and monitored adults with asthmatic sensitivities secondary to ragweed pollen, Bruce et al.[131] reported unsatisfactory clinical results with preseasonal injection therapy. More recently, Hill and coworkers[49] were also unable to demonstrate any clinical advantage of grass pollen hyposensitization in a particularly well-controlled paediatric study. Both these studies, however, used relatively low dosages of extract and only one preseasonal course of treatment. Interestingly, the ragweed study also demonstrated that approximately half the patient study group manifested symptoms which failed to correspond to the ragweed pollen count, unlike most rhinitis patient responses[5]. Moreover, symptom scores registered by the asthmatic subjects appeared to be markedly reduced compared with typical rhinitis counterparts, a feature which possibly contributed to the difficulty of differentiating treatment-induced effects.

With regard to the therapeutic use of other allergens involved in allergic respiratory disease, the clinical literature would appear to be relatively fragmented. Differing views exist over the use of moulds and animal danders, for example, and although recent studies have demonstrated the potential therapeutic utility of cat allergens, others have suggested such applications to be questionable; avoidance is recommended as the treat-

ment of choice with dander allergens[6,182]. No placebo-controlled studies
have been reported with mould extracts and the possibility of provoking
adverse reactions has resulted in extreme caution being advocated in this
context also[11,118,183]. The use of food allergens for hyposensitization is not
widely recommended[4,184].

Oral administration studies

As with conventional parenteral hyposensitization, allergen administration
via the oral route also has a long tradition of use in the treatment of
respiratory allergic disease. Although regarded as being of questionable
significance by some[121,151], this approach continues to command support,
particularly in Europe[14,185,186]. Moreover, it has been claimed that oral
administration of allergen is especially successful for asthma as compared
to allergic rhinitis[187]. Application of the treatment practice for paediatric
use has also been strongly recommended[14].

Unfortunately, few controlled studies of oral hyposensitization are available, although as long ago as 1940 a multicentre study in the USA showed
the approach to be comparable only to placebo and less effective than
parenteral administration[188]. More recently, further formal study data
have been reported comparing the performance of oral and parenteral
applications in an open study format. Additionally, placebo-controlled
investigations have been reported. In a preliminary account of a double-
blind paediatric study, Lorn-Shore and Weinberg[189] indicated that appropriately diagnosed asthmatic children, treated orally with a mixture of grass
pollen and house-dust mite extracts (*D.pteronyssinus*), fared better than
corresponding placebo-treated controls. Assessments were apparently
made using a range of objective measurements supported by parent and
patient symptom record cards. The authors concluded that the results were
sufficiently meaningful to merit further study. Morrow-Brown[190] has also
described a series of single-blind cross-over placebo-controlled studies in
pollenosis patients using an adaptation of the oral hyposensitization procedure, involving daily sublingual applications. Although only preliminary
data were reported, results were claimed to be most encouraging. More
recently, however, Urbanek and Gehl[167] have reported findings from a
double-blind study of oral hyposensitization with *D.pteronyssinus* extract
in 32 asthmatic children; patients were treated weekly for 42 weeks. Following this therapy the investigators could find no advantage of active
treatment over placebo. Both subjective symptomatic assessments and
various airways function tests confirmed these observations.

This unfavourable view of oral treatment has also been partially sub-
stantiated by comparative studies with parenteral allergen administrations.
Von Rebien et al.[191] studied the immunological and clinical efficacy of preseasonal oral and subcutaneous hyposensitization in 40 children with allergies to grass pollen. Interestingly, symptom indices for orally treated
patients appeared to parallel the grass pollen count for asthma as well as
conjunctivitis and rhinitis; this contrasts somewhat with the findings of
Bruce et al.[131]. Nevertheless, although no differences could be discerned
between the two treatment regimens for rhinitis and conjunctivitis symptoms, it was evident that asthmatic episodes were reduced significantly

more effectively by injection of allergen. In the absence of a placebo group, however, it was not possible to deduce whether the orally treated group achieved any absolute benefit.

At present, therefore, it must be concluded that the evidence available from controlled studies, fails to provide a compelling case for oral administration. As has been noted by several authors, however, the treatment offers many potential attractions in terms of convenience and seeming lack of adverse reactions. It is of particular interest to note that studies using oral administration have involved patient self-administration[14]. The apparent absence of high incidences of reactions under such conditions attests to the evident safety of the procedure. If further evidence of therapeutic activity could be obtained, such an approach may find important applications, especially for paediatric use. The favourable impressions reported by some investigators would appear to merit additional definitive studies being attempted in this area.

Summary

In summarising the clinical data, it is evident that the one most striking feature of the literature dealing with allergen injection therapy in bronchial asthma is inconsistency. Few aspects of the treatment practice appear to enjoy universal concensus and the gradual, but ever-increasing, list of available controlled clinical studies has failed to influence the situation conclusively. As a consequence, the value of specific allergen treatments for general therapeutic use remains uncertain and, given the nature of the subject, it would seem that this situation is unlikely to change in the immediate future. For those with positive clinical experiences of hyposensitization treatments, the question of effectiveness and utility has long since been a sterile debate; for the uncommitted, the formal clinical trial data are likely to remain unconvincing. Nevertheless, despite this overall equivocal position, it is clear that evidence of clinical benefit is available in controlled studies for each of the major aeroallergens. Irrespective of counterbalancing negative findings, therefore, the treatment has been demonstrated to be effective. Whether these favourable results are perceived as being clinically relevant, however, is a matter for the individual judgement of the responsible physician. Unfortunately, what obscures the clinical assessment in many of these formal studies is the high placebo response, commonly reaching 30–40% of patients, and indeed the converse situation, namely the corresponding relatively high failure rate of many individuals to benefit from treatment, even when group trends indicate a favourable clinical outcome. These findings suggest that patient populations studied are often markedly heterogeneous, and raise questions both about selection criteria commonly employed and assessment procedures. Evidently, diagnostic methods and examination of treatment failures require even more careful scrutiny. Means to identify patients who are and are not likely to benefit from such treatments clearly continues to represent a major challenge in this area.

In this context, and based on formal controlled study data, it would generally seem that a stronger case could be made for hyposensitization therapy with carefully diagnosed asthmatic children; the case for adults is perhaps less compelling. Taken together, the results reported by Aas[126], Warner *et al.*[51,130], and the slightly more contentious data of Taylor and coworkers[165], provide a seemingly sound base for the application of allergen injection therapy in appropriately selected asthmatic children, with sensitivities to house-dust. This view accords also with the optimistic prognosis advanced by Johnstone[15] and others[14] for asthmatic children receiving hyposensitization therapy in childhood. The markedly reduced incidence of adolescent asthma demonstrated by Johnstone and Dutton[192] of 30% to 70% in the now classic prospective study of allergen treated and untreated children, respectively, also remains striking data. However, dissenting views exist even on this point. Tabachnik and Levison[117], quoting recent follow-up reports of young adults who had asthma in childhood[193,194], conclude that no evidence exists to support the view that any treatment will influence prognosis in the longer term. The position is therefore confusing and unsatisfactory. It is disappointing also to note that the only double-blind controlled study reported to date in full and using orally administered allergen, has shown the treatment to be ineffective[167]. Removal of the trauma of parenteral injection therapy is clearly a desirable objective for paediatric use which, if achieved, could possibly facilitate the application of hyposensitization treatments in younger patients.

Developments in conventional hyposensitization treatments

Allergen extract standardization

As has been mentioned, without the establishment of a convincing mechanistic rationale for hyposensitization therapy, it is not surprising to find that currently employed treatment regimens and practices have not changed radically in over half a century[19]. Moreover, given the complexity of the asthmatic syndrome and this lack of understanding of the therapeutic process, it would not be too unexpected if fundamental advances in the performance of conventional allergen vaccines failed to occur in the immediate future. However, improvements in the quality and consistency of allergen extracts destined for diagnostic and therapeutic use would seem to be a realizable short-term goal and are generally agreed to be an urgent requirement[10,12,16,113].

During the last decade or so, considerable efforts have been devoted to establishing procedures for standardizing allergenic extracts[195], particularly by Scandanavian workers[196–198]. However, naturally occurring aeroallergens, such as those usually implicated in respiratory allergic disease, are commonly composed of highly heterogeneous mixtures of macromolecular materials[199]. As a consequence, allergic subjects manifest highly variable response profiles to these putatively offending allergens[200,201]. The concept of a standardized extract in such circumstances, therefore, raises formidable philosphical as well as practical difficulties. Standardized with respect to which property or to achieve which function are clearly crucial questions. Inevitably the use of crude and relatively uncharacterized allergenic extracts for diagnostic or therapeutic purposes is intuitively unacceptable and generally receives universal condemnation[4,12,202]; conversely, obtention of definable materials enjoy widescale support. Definition of practicable target parameters for standardization is, however, perhaps less clear than is often recognized or admitted.

For diagnostic purposes, it seems apparent that extracts should contain all allergens characteristic of the primary putative aeroallergen source, such that a definitive response can be consistently expected in appropriately diagnosed individuals. Such developments are indeed well advanced for the more common aeroallergens, and primary standard extracts are becoming available under the auspices of various national and international regulatory agencies[203,204]. These innovations have also been complemented by the isolation and purification of a number of major allergenic components derived from these various extracts. However, for therapeutic use, the question of standardization clearly requires more subtle considerations, since the concept of allergen vaccine potency presupposes knowledge of mechanism of action and, as has been discussed, this largely remains obscure. At the present time, therefore, it would seem that this position is essentially intractable at a truly fundamental level, and that only pragmatic solutions are possible. Consistency in allergen content and activity, as defined in terms of approved allergen extract standards, appears to be the most expedient and practicable compromise. Unfortunately, this measure does not preclude the on-going acceptance of extraneous, nonallergenic materials, nor is the problem circumvented of exposing atopic individuals to allergenic components to which they do not happen to be sensitized. Happily, although it is known that sensitization of non-atopic subjects can be affected by allergen injection treatments[199], the weight of available evidence suggests that *de novo* sensitization occurs rarely following hyposensitization[200,205–207].

It remains to be seen whether the implementation of more rigorous allergen standardization procedures, as currently conceived, contributes to improvements in hyposensitization therapy, but the prospects are clearly optimistic.

Allergen vaccine presentation forms

Traditional hyposensitization therapy has generally involved a series of subcutaneous injections of aqueous solutions of allergen extract of progressively increasing concentrations. Such regimens are often protracted ranging from some 15 to 40 injections for preseasonal allergen extract courses, to perennial treatments continuing perhaps over several years.

Aside from the question of patient and clinician convenience with extended treatment courses, the potential problems of adverse reactions with aqueous allergen extract injection have always caused concern[19], and have possibly limited wider application of the practice. As a result of these considerations, and the general concensus that efficacy of hyposensitization therapy is related closely to the allergenic load administered[5,6,16], various attempts have been made to reconcile these two opposing features of the treatment.

Most efforts in this regard have been centred on reducing the bioavailability of the allergenic material, either by sequestration within hydrophobic oily vehicles[208,209], adsorption to insoluble carriers, such as alum[210] or, more recently, the amino acid L-tyrosine[211,212]. All these sustained-release preparations have proved to be generally effective and well received[152,213], although some controversies have arisen over pyridine-extracted ragweed extracts adsorbed to alum[214]. Mineral oil vehicles have also fallen from favour, largely due to the tendency to produce nodule formation and concerns about potential local toxicity problems[5]. Nevertheless, despite providing a viable means of increasing tolerance to allergen dose, the presence of native allergen in these preparations has still been considered to be limiting for some applications, such as pollenosis[5]. For this reason, efforts to reduce the intrinsic allergenic activity of therapeutic extracts by other means, such as chemical modification, and thereby improve the safety of the material, have also been investigated.

Attempts to achieve acceptable chemically modified hyposensitization vaccines were conducted as early as the mid-1930s; an early US patent describing formaldehyde-modified extract granted to Carter in 1935[215], and other reports from the laboratory of Cooke and coworkers[216], attest to these endeavours. In more recent times, renewed efforts to produce improved allergen vaccines via this approach have been undertaken in several laboratories. Marsh and coworkers, for example, have demonstrated that rye[217], mixed-grass[218], and ragweed pollen extracts[219] react with formaldehyde to produce materials which display a reduced capacity to interact with cell-bound reagins, yet seemingly retain the ability to induce an allergen-specific blocking or IgG antibody response. The term allergoid has been used to describe these preparations. Others have achieved similar results using glutaraldehyde[220–225], or selective photoxidation[226,227]; recently, covalently linked alginate preparations of grass pollen extract have also been employed[228].

The development of these modified allergoid-type preparations has been evidently predicated on the supposed clinical relevance of selectively retaining the capacity to induce allergen-specific blocking antibodies. Without detailed knowledge of mechanisms of action, however, it is clear that the prospective clinical effectiveness of such processed allergens cannot be assumed and, as has been noted previously, allergen-specific antibody induction is of doubtful relevance in asthma therapy. For the treatment of allergic rhinitis, a number of clinically successful studies with chemically modified pollen extracts have indeed been reported[223,229,230]. For the case of asthma treatments, however, these modified materials have been used seemingly rarely and no double-blind controlled studies have been reported. Only the photoxidized form of house-dust has been used specifically for the treatment of perennial asthma to date, and results were assessed as being comparable with a commercially available alum-adsorbed preparation[231]. More modest benefits have been claimed for pollenosis patients. Summarizing a multicentre open study with grass pollen sensitive individuals treated preseasonally with allergoid materials, Von Schreyer[232] has recently reported that seasonal asthma appeared to be notably less well controlled than rhinitis. Although it is clearly premature to judge the impact of allergoid-like vaccines for hyposensitization treatment in asthma generally, it would appear that developments towards intrinsically safer and, if possible, more convenient vaccine forms of this type, are highly desirable. Whether this objective can be achieved by empirical chemical modification approaches remains to be seen. The evidence available from the treatment of allergic rhinitis would seem to augur well although, as has been noted, the asthmatic syndrome is considerably more complex and, in order to achieve clinical benefit, may require wholly different biological properties of the modified extract. Hopefully, however, such materials will become available for evaluation in the near future. Speculative opportunities are discussed subsequently.

Aside from the developments of relatively simple sustained-release vaccine presentations, and empirically derived chemically or physically modified forms of allergen extracts, advances in physicochemical separation technology has also provided for the possibility of examining the therapeutic utility of a number of purified allergens. Major allergens of ragweed pollen have been available for almost two decades and corresponding materials from grass pollen have also been identified over a similar time-span[199]. More recently, other clinically important components of pollens[233,234], house-dust mite[161,235], danders[236,237] and alternaria[238], amongst others, have been prepared in purified form. The availability of such materials clearly provides the opportunity of examining whether improved clinical benefit could be achieved if such purified materials were used in place of crude whole extracts. Of course, it is possible that the multicomponent allergen sensitivity profiles of most patients to complex aeroallergens will dictate that broad-spectrum whole extract treatments are always required. Clearly such questions reach to the heart of the debate surrounding specificity of treatment in hyposensitization therapy and impinge on the whole range of issues relating to the evolution of appropriate specifications for allergen standardization. It is of interest to note, in this context, that, despite the widescale tacit acceptance of the importance of allergen specificity, the clinical evidence available to support this view is relatively limited. Aside from the controlled studies of Lowell and Franklin[103] with ragweed pollenosis patients and, more recently, the elegant studies of Norman and Lichtenstein[104], who followed symptoms of patients sensitive to ragweed and grass pollen throughout both pollen seasons, having treated half the group with ragweed only, evidence is lacking. Indeed, no such data are available for asthma treatments.

Evidence of the therapeutic utility of purified allergen components for asthma treatment is also unavailable, but studies have been reported in allergic rhinitis. In the much-quoted experiments comparing whole ragweed extract with ragweed antigen E, Norman et al.[239] were unable to find differences in the therapeutic performance of either material in patients displaying seasonal allergic symptoms to ragweed pollen. More recently, somewhat different results have been observed with grass pollen sensitive patients. Using a mixture of two major allergens of temperate grasses, termed Ag 19 and Ag 25 on the basis of cross-immunoelectrophoresis designations[240], Osterballe[180] reported that patients treated only with these purified components fared less well than other patients receiving whole grass pollen extracts. Importantly, however, both treated groups were improved compared with placebo treatment. Conversely, others have found that partially purified extracts were clinically superior to standard whole grass extracts[241-243]; in these latter instances, however, quantitiative rather than qualitative effects were probably being recorded.

Doubtless, apparent inconsistencies in these types of experiments are almost inevitable and are likely to relate to the selection criteria employed for patient inclusion and the diagnostic facilities available to characterize the sensitivity pattern of the various individuals being tested. Without discerning diagnostic tests, it is perhaps reasonable to anticipate that patients manifesting a particular sensitivity pattern to a number of components of an aeroallergen extract, such as grass pollen extract, will manage less well if treated only with restricted purified components. Alternatively, patients with limited allergenic sensitivities will possibly be compromised if treated with a mixture of redundant components, which perhaps merely serve to dilute the effectiveness of allergen activities relevant to their condition. Resolution of these problems will only be achieved when more comprehensive diagnostic tests, together with the corresponding purified extract components, become more readily available. Fortunately, a number of relatively practicable procedures for obtaining improved and more discerning diagnostic information about individual patient allergen sensitivity patterns have been developed. Based primarly on a combination of radioimmunoassay and electrophoretic techniques, profiles of patient allergenic responses can now be obtained relatively easily, without necessitating prior allergen purification. Data in *Figure 16.1* shows typical IgG antibody response patterns to major components of rye grass pollen extract using an immunoprecipitation technique with ^{125}I-labelled whole rye extract, followed by sodium dodecylsulphate (SDS)-gel electrophoresis. Variations in the individual patient response patterns to the different extract components are clearly evident. Routinely, responses to some 10–14 different components of grass pollen extracts can be discerned by this method[244]. Employing other procedures, even more subtle resolution of allergenic responses can be obtained[201,245]. Such techniques obviously offer considerable potential for evaluating the immunological impact of hyposensitization therapy more thoroughly, as well as providing more powerful diagnostic capability. Hopefully, these methods will be employed more widely in future, as a necessary complement to the development of improved extracts, be they purified or partially purified. Already indications are available to suggest that these methods are likely to find useful application in hyposensitization therapy[246].

Summary

In recent years, much attention has been focused on establishing practicable methodologies appropriate for the characterization and standardization of allergen extracts. Progress has been considerable. As a consequence, opportunities to develop higher quality and more consistent allergenic reagents have become available. Hopefully, these developments will result in the rapid improvement in the standards of commercially available products. However, it would seem unrealistic to anticipate that these relatively straight-forward innovations will necessarily influence the effectiveness of the more important aeroallergen extracts used in asthma hyposensitization therapy in a truly profound manner. Already, good quality materials have been employed in many experimental clinical studies and the results obtained, good or poor, presumably reflect the order of intrinsic efficacy of the treatment. Moreover, the therapeutic attributes of allerge-

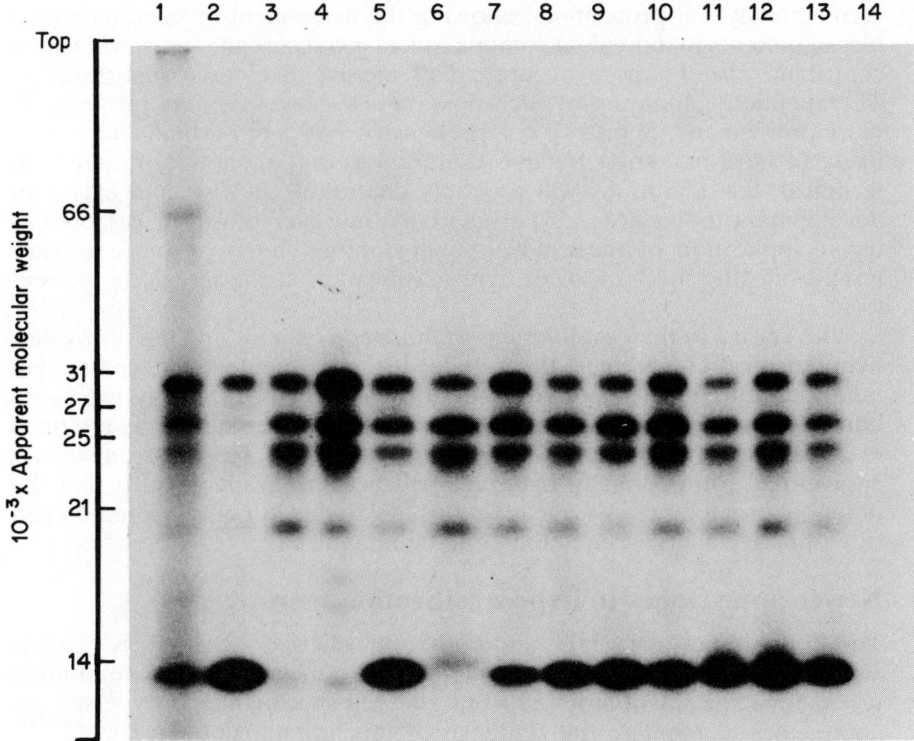

Figure 16.1 Electrophoretic profiles of ^{125}I-labelled rye pollen components following immunoprecipitation by serum IgG antibodies obtained from pollen-sensitive patients. Each gel track shows the profile of ^{125}I-labelled rye pollen extract components after incubation with patients' serum (except track 1), immunoprecipitation with protein A–Sepharose, reduction with mecaptoethanol and electrophoresis in a flat-bed sodium dodecylsulphate/polyacrylamide gel system (tracks 2–12); a pool of all these sera (track 13); a normal human serum control obtained from a non-atopic individual (track 14), or the ^{125}I-radiolabelled rye extract alone (track 1). The whole gel was fixed and stained, dried on a Bio-Rad slab gel dryer and autoradiography was performed by exposing the dried gels to X-ray film (*see* [244]). For each sample, similar levels of radioactivity were loaded to the gel.

nic extracts have not been identified. Generally, allergenic activity is assumed to be closely related to or to be the active principle, but is it? The claimed therapeutic effectiveness of allergoids with markedly reduced allergenic properties, could be said to argue against this view, at least for rhinitis treatments. More reasonable would seem the expectation that such standardized materials would display a greater degree of uniformity of activity, including well-defined stability characteristics. For diagnostic purposes, however, the position woudl appear to be significantly clearer. Appropriate diagnostic properties of given allergenic extracts can be delineated in experimentally accessible terms. Here allergenic activity is the crucial parameter and both quantitation and spectrum of activities can be measured satisfactorily with available immunochemical procedures. It would seem reasonable to assume, therefore, that substantial improvements can be expected with diagnostic reagents. Application of more discerning analytical procedures, allowing the assessment of sensitivity profiles of patients to individual components of given aeroallergens, will surely contribute also to more accurate and incisive diagnosis opportunities. Therapeutic exploitation of such possibilities, however, may prove to be more problematic. Supply of comprehensive assays of purified allergens is likely to be a non-cost-effective exercise, so that economic, rather than technical, considerations will probably determine the rate and extent of development in this area. Experimentally, however, it will be disappointing if application of these newer opportunities fails to provide greater insight into the mechanism of hyposensitization at the individual patient level.

With regard to the development of more convenient, and possibly safer, hyposensitization vaccines, the data for asthma treatments are sparse, but mildly encouraging. Adsorbate preparations have been widely used with house-dust mite extracts to some effect, but available chemically modified extracts remain, as yet, unproven for asthma therapy. Hopefully, however, appropriate forms of such materials will become available such that the potential problems of adverse reactions, a variable but not uncommon feature of native allergen injections, can be minimized.

Newer approaches to hyposensitization therapy

The importance of IgE antibody in allergic disease is widely established[61,63]. As a result, considerable resources have been committed to examine the possibilities of both allergen-specific and isotype-specific approaches to regulate the synthesis of this immunoglobulin class[247,248]. Delineation of conditions, both intrinsic[249,250] and environmental[251,252], which predispose to the induction of reaginic antibody induction have also been evaluated.

Within the asthmatic population, surveys have shown that the majority of patients are sensitive to extrinsic allergens, as determined by history and immediate responses to skin-test challenges[253]. Moreover, most asthmatic individuals, although not all, manifest elevated serum IgE levels[253]. The relevance of IgE in the pathogenesis of the asthmatic syndrome, as well as other allergic disease in general, would appear, therefore, to be beyond doubt. Aside from IgE, however, no other parameter has been identified as being an obvious disease-related therapeutic target which may be amenable to immunological intervention. Consequently, all other approaches are inevitably speculative and ultimately require clinical experimentation to validate even the therapeutic relevance of the proposed manoeuvre. Nevertheless, some interesting opportunities exist. In this section, approaches to IgE suppression and elaboration of other possible developments are briefly considered. Emphasis has been focused predominantly on the practicability of translating principles established in the laboratory to clinical implementation, rather than details of underlying immunology. Numerous authoritative reviews have dealt with the latter issues[248,254,255].

Allergen-specific IgE suppression

Following the discovery of IgE and the recognition of its central role in atopic disease, strenuous efforts have been made to elucidate underlying mechanisms regulating the synthesis of this antibody class[256]. Much of this work has been undertaken in convenient small animal models, mainly murine systems[257], but, more recently, data have also been obtained with human cells using *in vitro* culture techniques[258,259]. As a result, a number of systems have been developed to study IgE synthesis and enormous advances in understanding of basic cellular processes involved in the control of IgE production have been established[260,261]. In particular, the marked sensitivity of reaginic antibody synthesis to T-cell control has been confirmed as a characteristic feature of the process[260].

Development of these various model systems has obviously provided opportunities for investigating the impact of various regulatory manoeuvres. A number of materials has been produced which display potentially interesting activities in test systems, including the capacity to suppress antigen-specific IgE antibody responses in an isotype-selective manner. Several different categories of suppressive reagents have in fact been developed, but most have been based on allergen poorly immunogenic macromolecular conjugate systems, involving, for example, amino acid polymers[262–265], polyethylene glycols and simple derivatives[262,266–268], poly(N-vinyl-pyrrolidone)[269], various polysaccharides[270,271], bacterial derivatives[272], and isologous proteins[273]. Certain denatured proteins, including those derived from important aeroallergens, such as house-dust[274] and pollen extracts[275], have also been found to display similar properties. Likewise, low-molecular-weight constituents and enzyme degradation products of allergen extracts have been claimed to suppress IgE antibody production with the specificity of the whole native extract[276–280]. Many of these various materials have also been shown to exhibit the clinically appealing attribute of low residual allergenic activity.

Other more subtle approaches to allergen-specific isotype suppression have also been developed, based on idiotypic network manipulation[281]. De Weck and coworkers[282,283] have demonstrated, in an elegant series of studies in guinea-pigs for example, that both passive and active induction of anti-idiotypic antibodies can contribute to the regulation of IgE synthesis. Malley *et al.*[284] have reported similar findings with timothy pollen allergen-specific idiotypic responses in mice. Implementation of such idiotypic regulatory procedures have not been progressed to clinical studies and, for the case of complex allergen responses, would appear to present formidable practical difficulties. However, the potential relevance of idiotypic network regulation has been illustrated in humans[285–287] and Roitt *et al.*[288] have proposed a scheme to produce practical amounts of appropriate anti-idiotypic antibody reagents using monoclonal antibody technology.

Several modified allergen preparations with IgE suppressive activities have been progressed to clinical study. Experiences with the poly(D-glutamic acid-D-lysine) ragweed pollen extract conjugates, a system which has been widely evaluated in animals[263,264] have been reported by Butterfield *et al.*[289] and others[290–292]. Surprisingly, in contrast to the expected decrease in IgE antibodies, serum levels of both IgE and IgG antibodies to ragweed were found to increase, following a single preseasonal treatment regime. Preliminary data reported with polyethyleneglycol, ragweed allergen derivatives after two year treatments, would seem to concur with these observations also[293,294]. Both these preparations, therefore, appeared to behave similarly to conventional ragweed hyposensitization treatments. The clinical performance of urea-denatured ragweed antigen E has also been studied by Norman and coworkers[295]. In this case, the treatment course extended over eighteen months with a two-weekly injection schedule. As with the conjugate preparations, modest increases in both IgE and IgG serum antibodies to ragweed were observed initially and, thereafter, unremarkable changes were noted; no evidence of marked antibody suppression was recorded. Interestingly, antigen E-specific lymphocyte proliferation responses were suppressed. These results are clearly disappointing and raise doubts about the therapeutic potential of this approach and the relevance of the supporting laboratory data. Many of these polymer–allergen conjugates in particular have been shown to afford highly suppressive properties in animal models[264,266,269–271]. However, opportunities for clinical assessment have not been exhausted and appropriate treatment schedules or different routes of administration from those used to date may yet provide a basis for establishing improved responses. Further work is clearly required.

Notwithstanding possibilities for future success, the apparent discrepancy between suppressive attributes of these variously modified allergen extracts in animal and human studies is of concern, and serves to highlight the more general problem of developing novel and relatively sophisticated immunoregulatory treatments in allergic disease. Such an issue is inevitably exacerbated by the very complex and heterogeneous nature of aeroallergen extracts, both with respect to controlling and characterizing the processed allergenic materials satisfactorily, and monitoring the conferred immunological properties comprehensively. However, these problems will surely require resolution if appropriate allergen-specific reagents are to be developed. Explanations for the relatively disappointing performance of the putatively IgE-suppressive materials seen to date remain obscure, but almost certainly reflect, in large measure, the inadequacies of current laboratory models. IgE antibody production has been widely studied in murine systems employing relatively immature and adjuvant-induced responses[264]. Unrealistically high doses of suppressive reagents and clinically impractical routes of administration have also been commonly used to achieve appropriate effects and often only pure proteins have been studied in detail[264,296]. Such conditions have questionable relevance to suppressing antibody synthesis in mature and complex immune responses, as is the case with IgE production in the human atopic state. Established responses are well known to be substantially more resistant to perturbation[262]. The use of non-discriminating antibody assay procedures, such as passive cutaneous anaphylaxis, have possibly served to obscure more subtle limitations of animal models also. Response patterns of experimental animals to complex allergens are not necessarily equivalent to those in humans and, importantly, may be deficient with regard to some components. Several mouse strains commonly used in such studies, for example, have been shown to respond notably poorly to so-called major allergen components of temperate grass pollen extracts[244]. Failure to take account of such considerations may clearly provide a distorted view of the true activity profile of a supposedly broad-spectrum allergen-extract-specific suppressive preparation. This presumably becomes a particularly important factor when dealing with chemically modified allergen extracts, since the various constituent proteins could be expected to be influenced differently by the reaction process. Under such circumstances, some components may display suppressive activities while others could remain immunogenic. Evidently, more clinically relevant animal models, and possibly more sophisticated analyses of the immunological and immunochemical attributes of proposed immunoregulatory allergenic reagents, are required if a comprehensive assessment of the therapeutic potential of such materials is to be satisfactorily achieved.

Isotype suppression

Recent studies from several groups have demonstrated that soluble factors from T cells appear to be capable of selectively suppressing IgE production in an antigen-independent fashion[297–300]. Most of these findings have been restricted to rodent responses although, encouragingly, Katz and coworkers[301] have also demonstrated that factors derived from human mixed lymphocyte reactions, suppressor factor of allergy (SFA), display the capacity to inhibit, seemingly selectively, pokeweed mitogen-induced IgE production in human tissue culture systems. IgG responses were found to be unaffected or even slightly enhanced in such experiments, although it should be added that the influence of SFA in cultures containing absolutely equivalent numbers of IgG and IgE-producing lymphocytes have not been reported. It is possible, therefore, that the selectivity observed, may reflect a quantitative effect. In earlier studies, this human SFA material, and an analogous murine suppressive factor, were also shown to afford similar suppressive properties in an *in vivo* mouse model[302]. Further indirect evidence of the role of these factors in IgE systems has been obtained in studies of IgE receptors (FcεR) on lymphocytes. FcεR-positive cells have been shown to be involved in the regulation of reaginic antibody production *in vitro* with both human peripheral cells and cord blood cells[303,304]. Recently, suppressive factors have been shown to inhibit the induction of FcεR expression[305]. Interestingly, FcεR-positive cells have been shown to occur at generally higher frequency in allergic donors and increase during active disease[306].

Identification of putative IgE suppressor factors obviously offers important opportunities for treatment of allergic conditions. However, it is not wholly clear how such material could be used. Katz has speculated that the normal damping mechanism of IgE synthesis, mediated possibly by such materials, may be a dominant influence preventing the induction of allergic sensitivities[307]. Sensitization at the time of temporary imbalance of this normal regulatory IgE-suppressive activity was suggested to be a likely scenario for the so-called 'allergic breakthrough', thereafter effecting permanent sensitization in the already genetically predisposed individual. Various environmental pressures were considered as possible precipitants of this susceptible period, including viral infections[308]. As yet, however, evidence is lacking to show that individuals producing high levels of IgE antibody are in fact deficient in so-called SFA-type activities. Moreover, in relation to prospective therapeutic possibilities, the suppressive data available relates to the inductive aspect of IgE systems rather than inhibition of on-going responses. Consequently, whether stimulation of endogenous factors or direct replacement from exogenous sources, produced perhaps via hybridoma technology[309–312], are viable treatment alternatives, have not yet been confirmed. Biochemical characterization data currently available suggest that the suppressive factors are likely to be high-molecular-weight moieties in excess of 10000 daltons[248]. Administration of such macromolecular components, possibly on an on-going basis, raises a number of reservations. Practically, it would seem that induction of the biosynthesis of these materials, if appropriate, would be therapeutically more appealing.

Induction of murine suppressive factors has been achieved by mycobacterial adjuvants[313,314] and allogenic stimuli[315]. Kishomoto and coworkers[248,316] have also shown in rodents that T cells are activated by antigens conjugated to mycobacteria or N-acetylmuramyl-dipeptide (MDP) derivatives to produce IgE class-specific suppressive factors which are antigen independent. These authors have suggested that allergens coupled to MDP, the moiety shown by Lederer and colleagues to be the minimum adjuvant-active structure derived from bacterial cell-walls[317], may offer great potential in this context as a means for the treatment of allergic disease. IgE responses to ovalbumin (OA) have indeed been shown to be suppressed, albeit only partially, by pretreatment with OA–MTP (lysyl derivative of MDP) in mice[318]. These activities have not been reproduced, however, with conjugates of MDP and grass pollen allergens using similar systems[319]. Nevertheless, possible approaches for inducing IgE-suppressive factors have been identified. It remains to establish whether such manipulations can be achieved in a clinically acceptable manner. Exploitation of allergen-adjuvant conjugate stimulants for this purpose represents one such possibility.

Speculative approaches

As has been noted earlier, relatively little evidence is available to show that the largely expected immunological changes attendant upon hyposensitization therapy are directly related to perceived clinical benefits. Moreover, as only reaginic antibody production stands out as an overt disease-related parameter, approaches directed to ends other than IgE regulation are inevitably speculative. Given this situation, opportunities for further exploitation of allergen injection therapy would appear to be limited to essentially empirical exercises of developing forms of allergen extracts which affect the native-allergen-specific elements of the immune system in a prescribed, but differential, fashion. Allergoids, as discussed earlier, have already been produced with the objective of maintaining the capacity to induce allergen-specific IgG antibody. More recently, attention has been directed at materials which display a retained ability to activate allergen-specific T cells. In both these areas, supposedly exploitable immunological attributes have been maintained at the expense of allergenic activity. Clearly, any such allergen-derived agent which, for whatever reason, could sustain current levels of clinical performance without manifesting allergenic activity, would represent a significant advance.

Although it is intuitively evident that the functional consequences of

activating allergen-specific T cells in a selective manner are not predictable, the availability of such allergen-derived materials does offer the possibility of establishing the potential value of such a manipulation on an
empirical basis. Much evidence is available to show that T-cells orchestrate
and regulate the whole range of immunological functions[320]. The capacity
to modulate the level of activation of these cells selectively, therefore, is
obviously appealing. Whether, of course, different functional activities of
these lymphocytes could be stimulated preferentially by what is essentially
a simple change in antigen presentation remains unclear. It would seem
unlikely, although data exists to suggest that T-suppressor cells may be less
dependent upon accessory cell involvement than so-called T-helper
cells[321,322]. Modified allergens which by-pass accessory cell processing and
presentation pathways could be considered as potential candidates for such
a differential purpose.

Not unexpectedly, modified forms of allergen obtained to date with
these differential antigenic attributes have been considered largely as a
means of activating regulatory T-cell functions, primarily with IgE suppression in mind. The urea-denatured ragweed antigen E preparations
described by Ishizaka et al.[275] were developed and exploited for this purpose. Malley et al.[323] have also produced photo-oxidized forms of grass pollen extract and considered them in this potentially suppressive therapeutic
role. Enzyme-derived fragments and low-molecular-weight allergen fractions have been similarly categorized[278,324]. However, suppression of antibody production is not an exclusive possibility for such T-cell-selective
materials. The crucial question arises, therefore, as to how else could such
properties be exploited for hyposensitization-type treatments? One possibility noted recently by Platts-Mills[3], would seem to be in relation to the
control of inflammatory cell trafficking. Recent evidence in pollenosis
patients has demonstrated that basophils and mast cells are recruited into
nasal tissue at the time of the pollen season[42,43]. A relationship between
this recruitment phenomenon and increased sensitivity of the tissue to
allergen challenge has also been indicated[325]. Additionally, Okuda[326] has
suggested that symptomatic benefits conferred by hyposensitization treatment correlate with the inhibition of seasonal infiltration of basophilic
cells, indicating an association between cellular influx and clinical status.
Based on the assumption that these observations have general validity,
therefore, control of basophil or mast cell recruitment into shock tissue
areas by immunological intervention would seem to be worthy of further
study. The particular relevance of T-cell activity in this context is somewhat tenuous, but relates to the possibility that basophil chemotactic phenomena observed in nasal tissue may be subject to similar regulatory processes found in basophil cutaneous anaphylactic lesions[327]. In the guinea-
pig, at least, these late skin reactions have been shown to be under T-cell
control[328]. Although underlying mechanisms controlling late respiratory
responses to allergen provocation are unknown, it is also of interest to note
that successful hyposensitization treatment in asthmatic children has been
associated with an ablation of this type of reaction[130]. At the risk of making
falsely syllogistic comparisons, it is tempting, therefore, to speculate that
treatment of carefully selected asthmatic patients with allergen preparations displaying the capacity to modulate inflammatory cell recruitment

into respiratory tissue, provides an attractive therapeutic rationale. Modified allergens with negligible allergenic activity, yet a retained capacity to activate native allergen-specific T cells, offer themselves as appropriate candidates for this purpose. The rabbit model developed by Shampain *et al.*[329] of biphasic respiratory responses mediated via IgE antibody affords a convenient means of studying such possibilities.

Approaches other than the production of allergen-derived differential T-cell active materials have been limited. Recently, however, the possibility of producing allergen-specific clonal deletion has been indicated by results obtained with tetanus–toxoid–ricin conjugates in tissue culture. Volkman *et al.*[330] showed that human lymphocytes exposed to such materials were selectively deprived of cells producing tetanus-toxoid antibodies. Exploitation of this type of approach could obviously have merit for suppressing allergen-specific immune responses, if indeed such an effect can be achieved *in vivo*.

Summary

Attempts to develop newer approaches to hyposensitization therapy continues to be an extremely active research area. Progress, however, has been restricted to some degree by the lack of defined therapeutic targets and the complexity of aeroallergen extracts. Inevitably, the majority of effort in this area has been directed to devising approaches to suppress IgE antibody production. Various materials have been produced which display seemingly impressive allergen-specific IgE-suppressive properties in animal models, but, as yet, these attributes have not been confirmed in clinical studies. These somewhat discordant results suggest that the laboratory systems employed to select these suppressive reagents require refinement. The task of achieving a broad-spectrum allergen-specific IgE-suppressive reagent is obviously a formidable one, and the practical difficulties of simulating an established human IgE response directed to a wider range of allergen extract components, possibly accounts for some of these limitations. Ultimate success in this context will perhaps depend as much upon solving the problems of translating immunoregulatory principles devised within idealized laboratory environments into the clinical situation, as to the establishment of more novel immunological manoeuvres. These comments apply particularly perhaps to the possibilities offered by idiotype–anti-idiotype manipulations. Although such approaches have been elaborated, the heterogeneity of immune responses to aeroallergens probably render these considerations impractical.

Identification of various factors with selective IgE isotype suppressive activity has afforded yet another approach to attempt control of reaginic antibody synthesis. These materials have not as yet progressed to the stage of clinical evaluation, but activity in human tissue culture systems has been reported. The attraction of a suppressive reagent, independent of specificity and used either directly as a replacement therapy or induced *in situ*, is obviously considerable. Further developments in this area are awaited with great interest, although it should be noted that the relevance of such materials in the mature atopic individual has as yet to be established.

Approaches other than those indicated above have been relatively limited and have been focused predominantly on the possibilities offered by allergen-derived materials which display differential immunological characteristics. Reagents with retained allergen-specific T-cell activity without the capacity to interact with allergen-specific IgE antibody have attracted most attention. The consequences of perturbing the immune system selectively with T-cell probes are unpredictable, but offer potentially interesting therapeutic opportunities. The possibility of influencing inflammatory cell trafficking by such a means has been conjectured. Such reagents also provide for the opportunity of examining mechanistic aspects of hyposensitization therapy more incisively. The fact that commonly used aeroallergens provoke a multitude of immune response phenomena concomitantly, has undoubtedly contributed in the past to the difficulty of relating therapeutic performance and immunological changes.

Overall summary

Hyposensitization therapy has featured prominently in the treatment of allergic disease, including extrinsic asthma, for over seventy years. Significantly, however, and despite much dedicated work, clinical practices and understanding of the therapeutic processes involved in the therapy have advanced little since the earliest studies. The procedure remains essentially an empirical phenomenon. Moreover, because the claimed clinical benefits in asthma are adjudged to be of questionable value by some, and because the potential of serious immediate adverse reactions cannot be wholly excluded with this form of treatment, the procedure also remains controversial.

Given this position, and the fact that pharmacological programmes for asthma management have improved markedly in recent times, what then is the prospectus for specific hyposensitization treatments? Firstly, it should be noted that significant developments can be anticipated. Advances in allergen standardization and improvements in vaccine presentation forms are likely to mitigate some of the mechanical disadvantages and inconveniences of current allergen preparations, particularly in terms of consistency of performance. Greater confidence in the diagnostic accuracy of improved allergen extracts can also be expected. Additionally, improvements in the sophistication of immunological investigations are likely to provide more cogent information about the changes effected in the immune systems of hyposensitized individuals. All these developments will serve to characterize and optimize traditional allergen injection treatments more appropriately. However, it would be surprising if these innovations were able to influence the therapeutic potential of the therapy fundamentally. It would seem more reasonable to conclude that the clinical literature currently available, although limited in some respects, especially in terms of numbers of appropriately controlled studies, has, nevertheless, probably defined the range of likely performance which could be routinely anticipated if clinically heterogeneous populations of asthmatic patients were treated. Consequently, expectations of dramatic progress with conventional specific allergen treatments would appear to be unrealistic. More apposite, perhaps, is the prospect of more effective application of the therapy to patients designated as being more likely to benefit. Such an approach is obviously predicated on the availability of more discerning diagnostic techniques and, although appropriate procedures have not as yet been developed, evidence of interesting possibilities has been reported. Without such developments, or unless more basic approaches to treatment are evolved, it is difficult to conceive that the current patterns of hyposensitization therapy in asthma will change markedly.

One of the attractive attributes of hyposensitization therapy has been the implicit expectation that the treatment was capable of influencing the natural course of the disease state, rather than merely affecting symptoms. In practice, this hope has not always been realized; cures are relatively rare and, as indicated previously, the claim that the prognosis for hyposensitized asthmatic children was markedly enhanced, has also been seriously challenged. Nevertheless, if the treatment practice is to move forward and compliment pharmacological symptomatic treatment programmes even more effectively, it would seem to be essential that therapeutic targets are identified which are amenable to manipulation by allergen injections and perceived to be relevant to the allergic condition. Subject to these criteria, the obvious target is IgE antibody synthesis. Not surprisingly, therefore, much work has been undertaken to devise immunoregulatory procedures, based primarily on empirically derived tolerogenic forms of allergen presentation, which have been shown to suppress IgE antibody production effectively in animal systems. More recently, this approach has been extended to consider IgE isotype suppression. Both these approaches clearly offer significant therapeutic potential. To date, however, the clinical evidence obtained with supposedly allergen-specific suppressive reagents has not been encouraging, largely perhaps because of the inevitable difficulties of translating complex immunological manoeuvres, appropriate to relatively artificial animal model systems, into the clinical environment. Realistic appraisal of the situation would also suggest that the demands of allergen-specific suppression, possibly involving some tens or even hundreds of different antibody specificities, is asking much of the relatively crude allergen reagents as yet developed. Further clinical work with such materials is needed to resolve these uncertainties. Possibly more appealing is the prospect of isotype-specific suppression. The disadvantage of the multiplicity of allergenic specificities commonly encountered with atopic individuals would be circumvented by this approach, and there is no evidence to indicate that unexpected problems are likely if such a manoeuvre was successful. The beneficial biological role of IgE, at least in modern Western man, is largely unknown. Whether isotype suppression would indeed involve allergen injections, possibly acting as a carrier for inducers of so-called suppressive factors, remains to be seen. As yet, developments in this area have not progressed from the laboratory stage. Aside from these possibilities, it would seem that only speculative options exist, based primarily on empirical manipulations of the immune response. Doubtless, therapeutically useful innovations of this type will ultimately occur. Better appreciation of environment and even genetic factors predisposing to the allergic state may also provide opportunities for avoiding or mitigating the likelihood of inducing allergenic sensitivities. However, for the present, it would seem that consolidation and optimization of current clinical practices, supplemented by the availability of better characterized and standardized allergen extracts, are likely to be the more probable immediate tangible developments.

Overall, it is evident that hyposensitization therapy in asthma continues to be something of an enigma. The procedure has a long tradition of clinical use and still commands widescale support. Conversely, however, the subject also attracts criticism and controversy. Unless a thorough-going treatment rationale is developed, it is difficult to believe that this situation will ever be resolved. Given the complex nature of both allergic asthma and aeroallergen extracts, the prospects for such an outcome would not appear to be overly optimistic for the immediate future. Nevertheless, as in the past, the therapeutic aspirations of many atopic individuals will doubtless continue to be satisfied by conventional allergen injection treatments and, as such, hyposensitization will continue to make a significant contribution to the management of respiratory allergic disease.

References

1. ROSE, B. *Medical Clinics of North America*, **58**, 127 (1974)
2. LICHTENSTEIN, L.M. *American Review of Respiratory Disease*, **117**, 191 (1978)
3. PLATTS-MILLS, T.A.E. *Immunology Today*, **2**, 35 (1981)
4. WARNER, J.O. *Journal of the Royal Society of Medicine*, **74**, 60 (1981)
5. NORMAN, P.S. *Allergy*, **33**, 62 (1978)
6. PATTERSON, R. *Journal of Allergy and Clinical Immunology*, **64**, 155 (1979)
7. MAY, C.D. *Pediatric Clinics of North America*, **22**, 221 (1975)
8. AAS, K. *Allergy*, **37**, 1 (1982)
9. ROSENTHAL, R.R. and LICHTENSTEIN, L.M. In *Bronchial Asthma, Mechanisms and Therapeutics*. Chapter 57. p. 837. Boston: Little Brown and Co. (1976)
10. NORMAN, P.S. *Annual Reviews of Medicine*, **26**, 337 (1975)
11. KAAD, P.H. and OSTERGAARD, P.A. *Clinical Allergy*, **12**, 317 (1982)
12. AAS, K. In *Asthma*. Chapter 24. p. 385. London: Academic Press (1976)
13. NIAZAMI, R.M. and COLLINS-WILLIAMS, C. *Annals of Allergy*, **35**, 296 (1975)
14. WORTMANN, F. *Allergologia et Immunopathologia*, **5**, 15 (1977)
15. JOHNSTONE, D.E. *Annals of Allergy*, **46**, 59 (1981)
16. ZEIGLER, R.S. and SCHATZ, M. *Pediatric Clinics of North America*, **65**, 987 (1981)
17. NOON, L. *Lancet*, **i**, 1572 (1911)
18. FREEMAN, J. and NOON, L. *Lancet*, **ii**, 814 (1911)
19. COOKE, R.A. *New York Medical Journal*, **107**, 579 (1918)
20. BECKER, E.L., SIMON, A.S. and AUSTEN, K.F. (eds) In *Biochemistry of the Acute Allergic Reaction*. Vol. 14. New York: Alan R. Liss Inc. (1981)
21. STANWORTH, D.R. *Immediate Hypersensitivity, Frontiers of Biology*. Vol. 28. London: North-Holland (1973)
22. ISHIZAKA, T. *Annals of Allergy*, **48**, 313 (1982)
23. JOHANNSON, S.G.O. and BENNICH, H.H. *Annals of Allergy*, **48**, 325 (1982)
24. REED, C.E. and TOWNLEY, R.G. *Allergy Principles and Practice*. Eds E. Middleton Jr, C.E. Reed and E.F. Ellis. Vol. 2. Chapter 36. St. Louis: C.V. Mosby Co. (1978)
25. PRAUZNITZ, C. and KUSTNER, H. *Centralblatt für Bacteriologie*, **86**, 160 (1921)
26. MOLLER, G. *Immunological Reviews*, Vol. 41. Copenhagen: Munksgaard (1978)
27. ISHIZAKA, K. (Ed.) *Progress in Allergy*, **32**. Basel: Karger (1982)
28. COOKE, R.A., BARNARD, J.H., HEBALD, S. and STULL, A. *Journal of Experimental Medicine*, **62**, 733 (1935)
29. LICHTENSTEIN, L.M. and OSLER, A.G. *Journal of Immunology*, **96**, 169 (1966)
30. STARR, M.S. and WEINSTOCK, M. *International Archives of Allergy and Applied Immunology*, **38**, 514 (1970)

31. STAHL-SKOV, P. and NORN, S. *Acta Allergologica*, **32,** 170 (1977)
32. RUBENSTEIN, E., FUIJA, Y., OKAZAKI, T., TRIPODI, D., REISMAN, R. and ARBESMAN, C.E. *Journal of Allergy and Clinical Immunology*, **57,** 335 (1976)
33. BERNSTEIN, I.L., MICHAEL, J.G., MALKIEL, S., SWEET, L.C. and BRACKETT, R.G. *International Archives of Allergy and Applied Immunology*, **58,** 30 (1979)
34. LICHTENSTEIN, L.M., NORMAN, P.S. and WINKENWERDER, W.L. *American Journal of Medicine*, **44,** 514 (1968)
35. YUNGINGER, J.W. and GLEICH, G.J. *Journal of Clinical Investigation*, **52,** 1268 (1973)
36. JOHANNSON, S.G.O., MILLER, A.C.L.M., OVERELL, B.G. and WHEELER, A.W. *Clinical Allergy*, **4,** 57 (1974)
37. IRONS, J.S., PRUZANSKY, J.J., PATTERSON, R. and ZEISS, C.R. *Journal of Allergy and Clinical Immunology*, **59,** 190 (1977)
38. TSE, K.S., WICHER, K. and ARBESMAN, C.E. *Journal of Allergy and Clinical Immunology*, **51,** 208 (1973)
39. DEUSCHL, H., JOHANSSON, S.G.O. and FAGERBERG, E. *Clinical Allergy*, **7,** 315 (1977)
40. PLATTS-MILLS, T.A.E. *Journal of Immunology*, **122,** 2218 (1979)
41. LESSOF, M.H., SOBOTKA, A.K. and LICHTENSTEIN, L.M. *Johns Hopkins Medical Journal*, **142,** 1 (1978)
42. HASTIE, R., HEROY, J.H. and LEVY, D.A. *Laboratory Investigation*, **40,** 554 (1978)
43. OKUDA, M., KAWABORI, S. and OHTSUKA, H. *Archives of Otorhinolaryngology*, **221,** 215 (1978)
44. PATTERSON, R., SUSKO, I.M. and HARRIS, K.E. *Journal of Clinical Investigation*, **62,** 519 (1978)
45. PLATTS-MILLS, T.A.E., VON MAUR, R.K., ISHIZAKA, K., NORMAN, P.S. and LICHTENSTEIN, L.M. *Journal of Clinical Investigation*, **57,** 1041 (1976)
46. FAITH, R., HESLER, S.R. and SMALL, P.A. *International Archives of Allergy and Applied Immunology*, **53,** 530 (1977)
47. D'SOUZA, M.F., PEPYS, J., TAI, E., PALMER, F., OVERELL, B.G., McGRATH, I.T. *et al. Clinical Allergy*, **3,** 177 (1973)
48. CHAPMAN, M.D., PLATTS-MILLS, T.A.E., GABRIEL, M., NG, H.K., ALLAN, W.G.L., HILL, L.E. *et al. International Archives of Allergy and Applied Immunology*, **61,** 431 (1980)
49. HILL, D.G., HOSKING, C.S., SHELTON, M.J. and TURNER, M.W. *British Medical Journal*, **1,** 306 (1982)
50. HSEIH, K.H. *Annals of Allergy*, **48,** 25 (1982)
51. WARNER, J.O., PRICE, J.C., HELMS, P., TURNER, M.W., PLATTS-MILLS, T.A.E., SOOTHILL, J.F. and HEY, E. *XIth International Congress of Allergology and Clinical Immunology*. London (1982)
52. ASSEM, E.S.K. and McALLEN, M.K. *Clinical Allergy*, **3,** 161 (1973)
53. HANNEUSE, Y., PINTENS, H. and DELESPESSE, G. *Allergologia et Immunopathologia*, **10,** 289 (1982)
54. LEITERMANN, K.M., FINDLAY, M.D. and OHMAN, M.D. *Journal of Allergy and Clinical Immunology*, **71,** (Suppl.) 91 (1983)
55. LICHTENSTEIN, L.M., ISHIZAKA, T., NORMAN, P.S., SOBOTKA, A.K. and HILL, B.M. *Journal of Clinical Investigation*, **52,** 472 (1973)
56. GLEICH, G.J., ZIMMERMANN, E.M., HENDERSON, L.L. and YUNGINGER, J.W. *Journal of Allergy and Clinical Immunology*, **70,** 261 (1982)
57. LEVY, D.A. and OSLER, A.G. *Journal of Immunology*, **99,** 1068 (1967)
58. LEVY, D.A., LICHTENSTEIN, L.M., GOLDSTEIN, E.O. and ISHIZAKA, K. *Journal of Clinical Investigation*, **50,** 360 (1971)
59. GLEICH, G.J., JACOBS, G.L. and YUNGINGER, J.W. *Journal of Allergy and Clinical Immunology*, **60,** 188 (1977)
60. EVANS, R., PENCE, H., KAPLAN, H. and ROCKLIN, R.E. *Journal of Clinical Investigation*, **57,** 1378 (1976)
61. BUCKLEY, R.H. and BECKER, W.G. *Immunological Reviews*, **41,** 288 (1978)
62. STRANNEGAARD, O. and STRANNEGAARD, I.L. *Immunological Reviews*, **41,** 149 (1978)
63. STRANNEGAARD, I.L. and STRANNEGAARD, O. *Acta Dermatovener, Stockholm*, **95,** (Suppl.) 20 (1978)
64. ROCKLIN, R., PEARCE, H., KAPLAN, H. and EVANS, R. *Journal of Clinical Investigation*, **53,** 735 (1974)
65. HIRATANI, M., MINTO, K., OSHIDA, Y., ITO, S. and KASEI, M. *Journal of Allergy and Clinical Immunology*, **68,** 205 (1981)

66. HILL, D.J., SMART, I.J. and HOSKING, C.S. *Clinical Allergy*, **12**, 83 (1982)
67. ANDERSON, J.A., LANE, S.R., HOWARD, W.A., LEIKEN, S. and OPENHEIM, J.J. *Cellular Immunology*, **10**, 441 (1974)
68. BROSTOFF, J. *International Archives of Allergy and Applied Immunology*, **45**, 162 (1974)
69. GATIEN, J.G., MERLER, E. and COLLEN, H.R. *Clinical Immunology and Immunopathology*, **4**, 32 (1975)
70. ROMAGNANI, S., BILIOTTI, G. and RICCI, M. *Clinical and Experimental Immunology*, **19**, 83 (1975)
71. ROCKLIN, R.E., SHEFFER, A.L., GREINEDER, D.K. and MELMON, K.L. *New England Journal of Medicine*, **302**, 1213 (1980)
72. STRANNEGAARD, I.C. and STRANNEGAARD, O. *Scandinavian Journal of Immunology*, **6**, 1225 (1977)
73. WANG, S.R. and ZWEIMAN, B. *Cellular Immunology*, **36**, 28 (1978)
74. OGDEN, B.E., KRUEGGER, G.G. and HILL, H.R. *Clinical and Experimental Immunology*, **35**, 269 (1979)
75. MARTINEZ, J.D., SANTOS, J., SCHECHSCHULTE, D.J. and ABDOU, N.I. *Journal of Allergy and Clinical Immunology*, **64**, 485 (1979)
76. ROLA-PLESZCZYNSKI, M. and BLANCHARD, R. *International Archives of Allergy and Applied Immunology*, **64**, 361 (1981)
77. BEER, J., OSBARD, D.E., McCAFREY, R.P., SOTER, N.A. and ROCKLIN, R.E. *New England Journal of Medicine*, **306**, 454 (1982)
78. RIVLIN, J., JUPERMAN, O., FREIER, S. and GODFREY, S. *Clinical Allergy*, **11**, 353 (1981)
79. GROVE, D.I., BURSTON, T.O., WELLBY, M.L., MUNRO-FORD, R. and FORBES, I.J. *Journal of Allergy and Clinical Immunology*, **55**, 152 (1975)
80. KHAN, A. *Annals of Allergy*, **37**, 267 (1976)
81. PERELMUTTER, L. and POTVIN, L. *Annals of Allergy*, **45**, 18 (1980)
82. McKREEDY, S.J. and BUCKLEY, R.H. *Journal of Allergy and Clinical Immunology*, **53**, 72 (1974)
83. COOPER, K.D., WUEPPER, K.D. and HANIFIN, J.M. *Clinical Research*, **28**, 566 (1980)
84. SCHUSTER, D.L., BONGIOVANNI, B.A., PIERON, D.L., BARBARO, J.F., WONG, D.T. and LEVINSON, A.I. *Journal of Immunology*, **124**, 1662 (1980)
85. FAURE, M.R., GAUCHERAND, M.A., THIVOLET, J., CZERNIDEWSK, J.M. and NICOLAS, J.F. *Clinical and Experimental Dermatology*, **7**, 513 (1982)
86. CANONICA, G.W., MINGARI, M.C., MELIOLO, G., COLOMBATTI, M. and MORETTA, L. *Journal of Immunology*, **123**, 2669 (1979)
87. VELA, C., GARCIA, R., TRICAS, L., PLATAS, C. and LAHOT, C. *Clinical and Experimental Immunology*, **46**, 621 (1981)
88. STRANNEGAARD, O., STRANNEGAARD, I.L., KUNG, K. and HANIFEN, J. *XIth International Congress of Allergology and Clinical Immunology*. London (1982)
89. GOLDSTEIN, G., SCHEID, M.P., BOYSE, F.A., SCHLESINGER, D.H. and VAN-WAUVE, J. *Science*, **204**, 1309 (1979)
90. STRANNEGAARD, O., STRANNEGAARD, I.L., KUNG, K., COOPER, D.K. and HANIFIN, J.M. *International Archives of Allergy and Applied Immunology*, **69**, 238 (1982)
91. HSIEH, K.H. *Annals of Allergy*, **44**, 313 (1980)
92. HSIEH, K.H. *Annals of Allergy*, **47**, 48 (1981)
93. ONG, K.S. and GRIECO, M.H. *Clinical Allergy*, **11**, 515 (1981)
94. SWINEFORD, O. *Annals of Allergy*, **30**, 464 (1972)
95. BRONFENBRENNER, J. *Annals of Allergy*, **2**, 472 (1944)
96. BURDON, K.L. *Annals of Allergy*, **25**, 483 (1968)
97. PRUZANSKY, J.J. and PATTERSON, R. *Journal of Allergy*, **39**, 44 (1967)
98. FREEMAN, J. *Lancet*, **ii**, 744 (1930)
99. CONNELL, J.T. and SHERMAN, W.B. *Journal of Allergy*, **43**, 22 (1969)
100. HERXHEIMER, H. and PRIOR, F.W. *International Archives of Allergy and Applied Immunology*, **3**, 189 (1952)
101. GOLDSTEIN, G.L. and CHAI, H. *Annals of Allergy*, **47**, 33 (1981)
102. KJELLMAN, N.I.M. and LANNER, A. *Allergy*, **35**, 323 (1980)
103. LOWELL, F.C. and FRANKLIN, W.A. *New England Journal of Medicine*, **273**, 675 (1963)
104. NORMAN, P.S. and LICHTENSTEIN, L.M. *Journal of Allergy and Clinical Immunology*, **61**, 370 (1978)
105. CONNELL, J.T. *New York Journal of Medicine*, **70**, 1751 (1970)

106. MATTHEWS, K.P., BAYRE, N.K. and BANAS, J.M. *Journal of Allergy and Clinical Immunology*, **65**, 191 (1980)
107. NICHELSEN, J.A., GOLDSTEIN, S., MUELLER, O., WYPCH, J., REISMAN, R.E. and ARBESMAN, C.E. *Journal of Allergy and Clinical Immunology*, **68**, 33 (1981)
108. LICHTENSTEIN, L.M. and LEVY, D.A. *International Archives of Allergy and Applied Immunology*, **42**, 615 (1972)
109. MAY, C.D., SCHUMACHER, M.J. and WILLIAMS, C.S. *Journal of Allergy and Clinical Immunology*, **50**, 99 (1972)
110. SCHUMACHER, M.J. and MAY, C.D. *Clinical Allergy*, **2**, 345 (1972)
111. MAY, C.D. and WILLIAMS, C.S. *Clinical Allergy*, **3**, 319 (1973)
112. NORMAN, P.S. *Medical Clinics of North America*, **58**, 111 (1974)
113. SOLLEY, G.O. *Southern Medical Journal*, **72**, 183 (1979)
114. LICHTENSTEIN, L.M., NORMAN, P.S., BRUCE, C.A. and ROSENTHAL, R.R. In *New Directions in Asthma*. Ed. M. Stein. p. 457. Illinois: Park Ridge (1975)
115. LOCKEY, R.F. and BUKANTZ, S.C. In *Bronchial Asthma*. Eds E.D.Weiss and M.S. Segal. p. 613. Boston: Little Brown and Co. (1976)
116. LEFFERT, F. *Medical Progress*, **97**, 875 (1980)
117. TABACHNIK, E. and LEVISON, H. *Journal of Allergy and Clinical Immunology*, **67**, 339 (1981)
118. SALVAGGIO, J. and AUKRUST, L. *Journal of Allergy and Clinical Immunology*, **68**, 327 (1981)
119. STEINBERG, A.D. and KIRKPATRICK, C.H. In *Bronchial Asthma*. Eds E.B. Weiss and M.S. Segal. p. 847. Boston: Little Brown and Co. (1976)
120. JOHNSTONE, D.E. *Pediatric Clinics of North America*, **22**, 230 (1975)
121. GOLDBERT, T.M. *Journal of Allergy and Clinical Immunology*, **56**, 170 (1975)
122. BRUCE, C.A., NORMAN, P.S., ROSENTHAL, R.R. and LICHTENSTEIN, L.M. *Journal of Allergy and Clinical Immunology*, **53**, 230 (1974)
123. OSTERBALLE, O., MORGAN, H.J. and WEEKE, B. *Allergy*, **34**, 175 (1979)
124. CITRON, K.M., FRANKLAND, A.W. and SINCLAIR, J.D. *Thorax*, **13**, 229 (1958)
125. McALLEN, M.K., HEAF, P.J.D. and McINROY, P. *British Medical Journal*, **1**, 22 (1967)
126. AAS, K. *Acta Paediatrica Scandinavica*, **60**, 264 (1971)
127. TUCHINDA, M. and CHAI, H. *Journal of Allergy and Clinical Immunology*, **51**, 131 (1973)
128. NEWTON, D.A.G., MAYBERLEY, D.J. and WILSON, R. *British Journal of Diseases of the Chest*, **72**, 21 (1978)
129. TAYLOR, W.W., OHMAN, J.L. and LOWELL, F.C. *Journal of Allergy and Clinical Immunology*, **61**, 283 (1978)
130. WARNER, J.O., PRICE, J.F. and HEY, E.N. *Lancet*, **ii**, 912 (1978)
131. BRUCE, C.A., NORMAN, P.S., ROSENTHAL, R.R. and LICHTENSTEIN, L.M. *Journal of Allergy and Clinical Immunology*, **59**, 449 (1977)
132. WARNER, J.O. *Archives of Diseases in Childhood*, **51**, 905 (1976)
133. VON KROIDL, R. *Allergologie*, **5**, 278 (1982)
134. EDITORIAL, *Lancet*, **i**, 534 (1979)
135. RENNIE, D. *New England Journal of Medicine*, **229**, 128 (1978)
136. COOKE, R.A. *Allergy in Theory and Practice*. Philadelphia: W.B. Saunders (1947)
137. FITZGERALD, J.D.L. and SHERMAN, W.B. *Journal of Allergy*, **20**, 286 (1949)
138. COLLINS-WILLIAMS, C. *Annals of Allergy*, **39**, 87 (1977)
139. BLATT, H. *Annals of Allergy*, **19**, 1198 (1961)
140. BLATT, H. *Annals of Allergy*, **19**, 1318 (1961)
141. BLATT, H. *Annals of Allergy*, **20**, 134 (1962)
142. OEHLING, A., BAENA-CAGNANI, C.E. and NEFFEN, H. *Allergologia et Immunopathologia*, **8**, 177 (1980)
143. FRANKLAND, A.W., HUGHES, W.H. and GORRILL, R.H. *British Medical Journal*, **2**, 941 (1955)
144. HELANDER, E. *Acta Allergologica*, **13**, 47 (1959)
145. JOHNSTONE, D.E. *Pediatrics*, **24**, 427 (1959)
146. AAS, K., BERDEL, P., HENRIKSEN, S.D. and GARDBORG, O. *Acta Paediatrica Scandinavica*, **52**, 338 (1963)
147. FONTANA, V.J., SALANITRO, A.S., WOLFE, H.I. and MORENO, F. *Journal of the American Medical Association*, **193**, 123 (1965)
148. BARR, S.E., BROWN, H., FUCHS, M., ORRIS, H., CONNOR, A., MURRAY, F.J. *et al. Journal of Allergy*, **36**, 47 (1965)

149. McINTOSH, K., ELLIS, E.F., HOFFMAN, L.S., LYBASS, T.G., ELLER, J.J. and FULGINITI, V.A. *Chest*, **63**, (Suppl.) 43s (1973)
150. HUDGEL, D.W., LANGSTON, L., SELMER, J.C. and McINTOSH, K. *American Review of Respiratory Disease*, **120**, 393 (1979)
151. REISMAN, R.E. *Journal of Allergy and Clinical Immunology*, **68**, 1 (1981)
152. McALLEN, M.K. *Thorax*, **16**, 30 (1961)
153. BRITISH TUBERCULOSIS ASSOCIATION REPORT. *British Medical Journal*, **3**, 774 (1968)
154. BRUUN, E. *Acta Allergologica*, **2**, 122 (1949)
155. VOORHOORST, R.M.I.A., SPIEKSMA-BOEZEMAN and SPIEKSMA, F.TH,M. *Allergie und Asthma*, **10**, 329 (1964)
156. MAUNSELL, K., HUGHES, A.M. and WRAITH, D.C. *The Practioner*, **205**, 779 (1970)
157. McALLEN, M.K., ASSEM, E.S.K. and MAUNSELL, K. *British Medical Journal*, **2**, 501 (1970)
158. KABASAWA, Y., ISHII, A., MURATA, H. and TABAOKU, M. *Acta Allergologica*, **31**, 442 (1976)
159. VIRCHOW, CHR., ROTH, A. and MOLLER, E. *Clinical Allergy*, **6**, 147 (1976)
160. TOVEY, E.R., CHAPMAN, M.D. and PLATTS-MILLS, T.A.E. *Nature*, **289**, 592 (1981)
161. DANDEU, J.P., LEMAO, J., LUX, M., RABBILLOU, J. and DAVID, B. *Immunology*, **46**, 679 (1982)
162. MIYAMOTO, T., OSHIMA, S., MIZUNO, K., SASA, M. and ISHIZAKA, T. *Journal of Allergy*, **44**, 228 (1969)
163. YAGO, A., ISHII, A., TAKAOKA, M., MATUHASI, T. and WODA, K. *Japanese Journal of Experimental Medicine*, **50**, 407 (1980)
164. SMITH, A.P. *British Medical Journal*, **4**, 204 (1971)
165. TAYLOR, B., SAUNDERS, S.S. and NORMAN, A.P. *Clinical Allergy*, **4**, 35 (1974)
166. BRITISH THORACIC ASSOCIATION REPORT. *British Journal of Diseases of the Chest*, **73**, 260 (1979)
167. URBANEK, R. and GEHL, R. *Monatsschrift für Kinderheilkunde*, **130**, 150 (1982)
168. GADDIE, J., STEINER, C. and PALMER, K.N.V. *British Medical Journal*, **2**, 561 (1976)
169. MARQUES, R.A. and AVILA, R. *Allergologia et Immunopathologia*, **6**, 231 (1978)
170. BUCHANAN, D.J., HILLIS, A. and WILLIAMS, P.N. *Medical Journal of Zambia*, **15**, 14 (1981)
171. GWYNN, C.M., ALMOUSAWI, T. and STANWORTH, D.R. *Clinical Allergy*, **12**, 459 (1982)
172. GWYNN, C.M., INGRAM, J., ALMOUSAWI, T. and STANWORTH, D.R. *Lancet*, **i**, 254 (1982)
173. AALBERSE, R., VAN DER GAAG, R. and VAN LEEUWEN, J. *Journal of Immunology*, **130**, 722 (1983)
174. DEVEY, M.E., WILSON, D.V. and WHEELER, A.W. *Clinical Allergy*, **6**, 227 (1976)
175. VAN DER GIESSEN, M., HOMAN, W.L., VAN KERNEBEEK, G., AALBERSE, R.C. and DIEGES, P.H. *International Archives of Allergy and Applied Immunology*, **50**, 625 (1976)
176. CHU, J.C.L., WUN, T.H. and CHEN, X.J. *Annals of Allergy*, **47**, 107 (1981)
177. DEICHMANN, B. and SHREYER, H. *Allergologie*, **5**, 11 (1982)
178. FRANKLAND, A.W. and AUGUSTIN, R. *Lancet*, **ii**, 1055 (1954)
179. JOHNSTONE, D.E. *American Journal of Diseases of Children*, **94**, 1 (1957)
180. OSTERBALLE, O. *Allergy*, **37**, 379 (1982)
181. OHMAN, J.L. *Journal of Allergy and Clinical Immunology*, **71**, (Suppl.), 91 (1983)
182. BROWN, F.R. and WOLFE, H.I. *Annals of Allergy*, **26**, 305 (1968)
183. NORMAN, P.S. *Journal of Allergy and Clinical Immunology*, **61**, 281 (1978)
184. PATTERSON, R., LIEBERMAN, P., IRONS, J.S., PRUZANSKY, J.J., MELAM, H.L., METZGER, W.J. *et al.* In *Allergy Principles and Practice*. Eds E. Middleton, Jr and C.E. Reed. Vol. 2, p. 877. St Louis: C.V. Mosby Co. (1978)
185. CERNELC, D., BOHINJEC, M. and CERNELC, P. *Monatsschrift für Kinderheilkunde*, **124**, 250 (1976)
186. WAHN, U., MAIER, H. and GEIGER, H. *Monatsschrift für Kinderheilkunde*, **124**, 245 (1976)
187. LAETSCH, C. and WUTHRICH, B. *Schweizerische Medizinische Wochenschrift*, **103**, 342 (1973)
188. FEINBERG, S.M., FORAN, F.L., LICHTENSTEIN, M.R., PADMOS, E., RAPPAPORT, B.Z., SHELDON, J. *et al. Journal of American Medical Association*, **115**, 23 (1940)
189. LORN-SHORE and WEINBERG, E. *Allergologia et Immunopathologia*, **8**, 288 (1980)
190. MORROW-BROWN, H., BORGE, P.A. and SU, S. *Allergologia et Immunopathologia*, **8**, 350 (1980)
191. VON REBIEN, W., WAHN, U., PUTTONEN, E. and MAASCH, H.J. *Allergologie*, **3**, 101 (1980)
192. JOHNSTONE, D.E. and DUTTON, A. *Pediatrics*, **42**, 793 (1968)
193. BLAIR, H. *Archives of Disease in Childhood*, **52**, 613 (1977)

194. MARTIN, J.A., LANDAU, L.I. and PHELAN, P.D. *American Review of Respiratory Disease*, **122**, 609 (1980)
195. BALBO, B.A., KRILIS, S. and BASTEN, A. *Contemporary Topics in Molecular Immunology*, **8**, 41 (1981)
196. CESKA, M., ERIKSSON, R. and VARGA, J.M. *Journal of Allergy*, **49**, 1 (1972)
197. LOWENSTEIN, H. *Progress in Allergy*, **25**, 1 (1978)
198. WEEKE, B., LOWENSTEIN, H. and NIELSON, L. *Acta Allergologica,* **29**, 402 (1974)
199. MARSH, D.G. In *The Antigens III.* Ed. M. Sela. p. 271. London: Academic Press (1975)
200. MORAN, D.M. *Clinical Allergy*, **11**, 199 (1981)
201. PELTRE, G., LEPEYRE, J. and DAVID, B. *Immunology Letters*, **5**, 127 (1982)
202. NORMAN, P.S. *Journal of Allergy and Clinical Immunology*, **69**, 1 (1982)
203. WHO and IABS Symposium. *Journal of Biological Standardisation*, **3**, 113 (1975)
204. *FDA Panel on Review of Allergenic Extracts.* Bureau of Biologics (1981)
205. PLATTS-MILLS, T.A.E., CHAPMAN, M.D. and MARSH, D.G. *Journal of Allergy and Clinical Immunology*, **67**, 129 (1981)
206. MARSH, D.G., MEYERS, D.A., FREIDHOFF, L.R., EHRLICH-KAUTZKY, E., ROEBBER, M., NORMAN, P.S. *et al. Journal of Experimental Medicine*, **155**, 1452 (1982)
207. OSTERBALLE, O., IPSEN, H., WEEKE, B. and LOWENSTEIN, H. *Journal of Allergy and Clinical Immunology*, **71**, 40 (1983)
208. LOVELESS, M.H. *American Journal of Medical Science*, **214**, 559 (1947)
209. BROWN, E.A. *Annals of Allergy*, **15**, 499 (1957)
210. SLEDGE, R.F. *US Naval Medical Bulletin*, **36**, 18 (1938)
211. MILLER, A.C.L.M. and TEES, A.C. *Clinical Allergy*, **4**, 49 (1974)
212. WHEELER, A.W., MORAN, D.M., ROBINS, B.E. and DRISCOLL, A. *International Archives of Allergy and Applied Immunology*, **69**, 113 (1982)
213. NORMAN, P.S. and LICHTENSTEIN, L.M. *Journal of Allergy and Clinical Immunology*, **61**, 384 (1978)
214. GOODMAN, D.H. and HARRIS, J.H. *Annals of Allergy*, **35**, 17 (1975)
215. CARTER, E.B., US Patent 2019808 (1936)
216. STULL, A., COOKE, R.A., SHERMAN, W.B., HEBALD, S. and HAMPTON, S.F. *Journal of Allergy*, **11**, 439 (1940)
217. MARSH, D.G., LICHTENSTEIN, L.M. and CAMPBELL, D.H. *Journal of Allergy*, **43**, 179 (1969)
218. HADDAD, Z.H., MARSH, D.G. and CAMPBELL, D.H. *Journal of Allergy and Clinical Immunology*, **49**, 197 (1972)
219. MARSH, D.G., NORMAN, P.S., ROEBBER, M. and LICHTENSTEIN, L.M. *Journal of Allergy and Clinical Immunology*, **61**, 449 (1981)
220. PATTERSON, R., SUSZKO, I.M. and McINTIRE, F.C. *Journal of Immunology*, **110**, 1402 (1973)
221. MORAN, D.M., WHEELER, A.W., OVERELL, B.G. and WORONIECKI, S.R. *International Archives of Allergy and Applied Immunology*, **54**, 315 (1977)
222. VON-SCHREYER, H. *Allergologie*, **3**, 92 (1980)
223. METZGER, W.J., DORMINEZ, H.C., RICHERSON, H.B., WEILER, J.M., DONNELLY, A. and MORAN, D.M. *Journal of Allergy and Clinical Immunology*, **68**, 442 (1981)
224. PATTERSON, R. *Journal of Allergy and Clinical Immunology*, **68**, 85 (1981)
225. HENDRIX, S.G., PATTERSON, R., ZEISS, C.R. and SUSZKO, I.M. *Journal of Clinical Immunology*, **2**, 10 (1982)
226. BERRENS, L., HENOCQ, E. and RADEMACKER, M. *Clinical Allergy*, **3**, 449 (1973)
227. MALLEY, A., DEPPE, L.B. and BRANDT, C.J. *International Archives of Allergy and Applied Immunology*, **65**, 129 (1981)
228. TAYLOR, W.A., SHELDON, D. and SPICER, J.W. *Immunology*, **44**, 41 (1981)
229. NORMAN, P.S., LICHTENSTEIN, L.M. and MARSH, D.G. *Journal of Allergy and Clinical Immunology*, **68**, 460 (1981)
230. GRAMMER, L.C., ZEISS, C.R., SUSZKO, I.M., SHAUGHNESSY, M.A. and PATTERSON, R. *Journal of Allergy and Clinical Immunology*, **69**, 494 (1982)
231. HENOCQ, E., GARCELON, M. and BERRENS, L. *Clinical Allergy*, **3**, 461 (1973)
232. VON-SCHREYER, H. *Allergologie*, **3**, 92 (1982)
233. LOWENSTEIN, H. In *Immunological Proceedings of the International Congress of Allergology.* Eds A. Oehling, E. Mathov and I. Glazer. p. 505. Oxford: Pergamon Press (1980)
234. HUSSAIN, R., NORMAN, P.S. and MARSH, D.G. *Journal of Allergy and Clinical Immunology*, **67**, 217 (1981)
235. CHAPMAN, M.D. and PLATTS-MILLS, T.A.E. *Journal of Immunology*, **125**, 587 (1980)

236. BRANDT, R. and YMAN, L. *International Archives of Allergy and Applied Immunology*, **61,** 361 (1980)
237. PRAHL, P. and NEXOV, E. *Allergy*, **37,** 49 (1982)
238. YUNGINGER, J.W., JONES, R.T., NESHEIM, M.E. and GELLER, M. *Journal of Allergy and Clinical Immunology*, **66,** 138 (1980)
239. NORMAN, P.S., WINKENWERDER, W.L. and LICHTENSTEIN, L.M. *Journal of Allergy*, **42,** 93 (1968)
240. LOWENSTEIN, H. *International Archives of Allergy and Applied Immunology*, **57,** 379 (1978)
241. FROSTAD, A.B., GRIMMER, O., SANDVIK, L. and ASS, K. *Allergy*, **35,** 81 (1980)
242. KJELLMAN, N.I.M. and LANNER, A. *Allergy*, **35,** 323 (1980)
243. NORDVALL, S.L., BERG, T., JOHANSSON, S.G. and LANNER, A. *International Archives of Allergy and Applied Immunology*, **67,** 132 (1982)
244. MORAN, D.M., STANDRING, R. and HENDERSON, D.C. *International Archives of Allergy and Applied Immunology*, **69,** 120 (1982)
245. NORDVALL, S.L., GRIMMER, O., KARLSSON, T. and BJORKSTEN, B. *Allergy*, **37,** 259 (1982)
246. OSTERBALLE, O., LOWENSTEIN, H., MALLING, H.J., PETERSON, B.N. and WEEKE, B. *International Archives of Allergy and Applied Immunology*, **68,** 286 (1982)
247. SEHON, A.H. *Progress in Allergy*, **32,** 161 (1982)
248. KISHIMOTO, T. *Progress in Allergy*, **32,** 265 (1982)
249. BIAS, W.B., MARSH, D.G. and PLATTS-MILLS, T.A.E. In *Genetic Determinants of Pulmonary Disease*. Ed. S.D. Litwin. New York: Mariel Dekker Inc. (1978)
250. MENDELL, N.P., AMOS, D.B., BLUMENTHAL, M.N. and GLEICH, G.J. *Human Immunology*, **4,** 63 (1982)
251. FRICK, O.L., GERMAN, D.F. and MILLS, J. *Journal of Allergy and Clinical Immunology*, **63,** 228 (1979)
252. FRICK, O.L. and BROOKS, D. *American Journal of Veterinary Research*, **44,** 440 (1983)
253. KUZCZYCKI, J. *Journal of Allergy and Clinical Immunology*, **68,** 5 (1981)
254. TADA, T. *Progress in Allergy*, **19,** 122 (1975)
255. OVARY, Z., ITAYA, T., WATANABE, N. and KOJIIMA, S. *Immunological Reviews*, **41,** 26 (1978)
256. KATZ, D.H. *Immunology*, **41,** 1 (1980)
257. LEHRER, S.B. and BOZELKA, B.E. *Progress in Allergy*, **32,** 8 (1982)
258. GEHA, R.S., SCHNEEBERGER, E., ROSEN, F.S. and MERLER, E. *Journal of Clinical Investigation*, **56,** 386 (1975)
259. ZURAW, B.L., NONAKA, M., O'HAIR, C.H. and KATZ, D.H. *Journal of Immunology*, **127,** 1169 (1981)
260. HAMAOKA, T., KATZ, D.H. and BENACERRAF, B. *Journal of Experimental Medicine*, **138,** 538 (1973)
261. ISHIZAKA, K. *Advances in Immunology*, **23,** 1 (1976)
262. KING, T.P., KOCHOUMIAN, L. and CHIORAZZI, N. *Journal of Experimental Medicine*, **149,** 424 (1979)
263. LIU, F.T., BOGOWITZ, C.A., BARGALZE, R.F., ZINNECKER, M., KATZ, L.R. and KATZ, D.H. *Journal of Immunology*, **123,** 2456 (1979)
264. LIU, F.T. and KATZ, D.H. *Proceedings of the National Academy of Sciences of the United States of America*, **76,** 1430 (1979)
265. MALLEY, A. and DEPPE, L. *International Archives of Allergy and Applied Immunology*, **63,** 113 (1980)
266. LEE, W.Y. and SEHON, A.H. *International Archives of Allergy and Applied Immunology*, **56,** 159 (1978)
267. LEE, W.Y. and SEHON, A.H. *International Archives of Allergy and Applied Immunology*, **56,** 193 (1978)
268. WIE, S.I., WIE, C.H., LEE, W.Y., FILION, L.G., SEHON, A.H. and AKERBLOM, E. *International Archives of Allergy and Applied Immunology*, **64,** 84 (1981)
269. SMORODINSKY, N., VON-SPECHT, B.Y., CESLA, R. and SHALTIEL, S. *Immunology Letters*, **2,** 305 (1981)
270. USUI, M. and MATUHASI, T. *Journal of Immunology*, **122,** 1266 (1979)
271. CARTER, B.G. *International Archives of Allergy and Applied Immunology*, **62,** 241 (1980)
272. KISHIMOTO, T., HIRAI, Y., NAKANISHI, K., AZUMA, I., ATSUO, N. and YAMAMURA, Y. *Journal of Immunology*, **123,** 6 (1979)
273. FILION, L.G., LEE, W.Y. and SELLON, A.H. *Cellular Immunology*, **54,** 115 (1980)

274. KUDO, K., OKUDAIRA, H., MIYAMOTO, T., NAKAGAWA, T. and HORIUCHI, Y. *Journal of Allergy and Clinical Immunology*, **61**, 1 (1978)
275. ISHIZAKA, K., OKUDAIRA, H. and KING, T.P. *Journal of Immunology*, **114**, 110 (1975)
276. MALLEY, A. and PERLMAN, F. *Journal of Allergy*, **45**, 14 (1970)
277. MUCKERHEIDE, A., PESCE, A.J. and MICHAEL, J.G. *Journal of Immunology*, **119**, 1340 (1977)
278. MICHAEL, J.G. and PESCE, A.J. United States Patent 4338297 (1982)
279. MUCKERHEIDE, A., PESCE, A.J. and MICHAEL, J.G. *Cellular Immunology*, **59**, 392 (1981)
280. PELTRE, G., MECHERI, S. and DAVID, B. *Journal of Allergy and Clinical Immunology*, **71** (Suppl.) 45 (1983)
281. GEHA, R.S. *New England Journal of Medicine*, **305**, 25 (1981)
282. GECZY, A.F., DE WECK, A.L., GECZY, C.L. and TOFFLER, O. *Journal of Allergy and Clinical Immunology*, **62**, 261 (1978)
283. BLASER, K., NAKAGAWA, T. and DE WECK,A.L. *International Archives of Allergy and Applied Immunology*, **64**, 42 (1981)
284. MALLEY, A. and DRESSER, D.W. *Immunology*, **46**, 653 (1982)
285. GEHA, R.S. and WEINBERG, R.P. *Journal of Immunology*, **121**, 1518 (1981)
286. MUDAWAR, F., JIRJUS, A. and KALLOGHLIAN, A. *Immunology Letters*, **4**, 125 (1982)
287. GEHA, R.S. and COMMUNALE, M. *Journal of Clinical Investigation*, **71**, 46 (1983)
288. ROITT, I.M., MALE, D.K., GUARNOTTA, G., DE CARVALHO, L.P., COOKE, A., HAY, F.C. *et al.* *Lancet*, **ii**, 1041 (1981)
289. BUTTERFIELD, J.H., GLEICH, G.J., YUNGINGER, J.W., ZIMMERMAN, E.M. and REED, C.E. *Journal of Allergy and Clinical Immunology*, **67**, 272 (1981)
290. BERNSTEIN, I.L. *Journal of Allergy and Clinical Immunology*, **65** (Suppl.), 165 (1980)
291. BUTTERFIELD, J., REED, C.E., YUNGINGER, J.W., ZIMMERMAN, E. M. and GLEICH, G.J. *Journal of Allergy and Clinical Immunology*, **65** (Suppl.), 165 (1980)
292. GOLDSTEIN, S., MUELLER, U. and WYPYCH, J. *Journal of Allergy and Clinical Immunology*, **65** (Suppl.), 164 (1980)
293. NORMAN, P.S. *Progress in Allergy*, **32**, 318 (1982)
294. JUNIPER, E.E., O'CONNER, J., ROBERTS, R.S. and HARGREAVE, F.E. *Journal of Allergy and Clinical Immunology*, **71** (Suppl.), 119 (1983)
295. NORMAN, P.S., ISHIZAKA, K., LICHTENSTEIN, L.M. and ADKINSON, N.F. *Journal of Allergy and Clinical Immunology*, **66**, 336 (1980)
296. KINGS, M.L., NAKAGAWA, T. and DE WECK, A.L. *Allergologia et Immunopathologia*, **8**, 253 (1980)
297. WATANABE, N. and OVARY, Z. *Journal of Experimental Medicine*, **145**, 1501 (1977)
298. SUEMURA, M., SHIHO, O., DEGUCHI, H., YAMAMURA, Y., BOTTCHER, I. and KISHIMOTO, T. *Journal of Immunology*, **127**, 465 (1980)
299. KATZ, D.H. *Immunology*, **41**, 1 (1980)
300. ISHIZAKA, K., SUEMURA, M., YODOI, J. and HIRASHIMA, M. *Federation Proceedings*, **40**, 2162 (1981)
301. ZURAW, B.L., NONAKA, M., O'HAIR, C. and KATZ, D.H. *Journal of Immunology*, **127**, 1169 (1981)
302. KATZ, D.H., BARGATE, R.F., BOGOWITZ, C.A. and KATZ, L.R. *Journal of Immunology*, **124**, 819 (1980)
303. PLUMMER, J.M., SIMON, R.A., ZEIGER, R.S. and SPIEGELBERG, H.L. *Federation Proceedings*, **41**, 967 (1982)
304. DELESPESSE, G.J.T., COLLET, H. and SEHON, A.H. *Federation Proceedings*, **41**, 967 (1982)
305. KATZ, D.H. *Progress in Allergy*, **32**, 105 (1982)
306. SPIEGELBERG, H.L. *Federation Proceedings*, **42**, 122 (1983)
307. KATZ, D.H. *Immunological Reviews*, **41**, 77 (1978)
308. KATZ, D.H., BARGATE, R.F., BOGOWITZ, C.A. and KATZ, L.R. *Journal of Immunology*, **122**, 2191 (1979)
309. WATANABE, T., KIMOTO, M., MARUYAMA, S. and KISHIMOTO, T. *Journal of Immunology*, **121**, 2113 (1978)
310. WATANABE, T., KIMOTO, M., NAKANISHI, T., MARUYAME, S., KISHIMOTO, T. and YAMAMURA, Y. *Transplantation Proceedings*, **XII**, 432 (1980)
311. HUFF, T.F., UEDE, T. and ISHIZAKA, K. *Journal of Immunology*, **129**, 509 (1982)
312. SUGIMURA, K., NAKANISHI, K., MAEDA, K., KASHIWAMURA, S.I., SUEMURA, M., SHIKO, O. *et al.* *Journal of Immunology*, **128**, 1637 (1982)
313. TUNG, A.S., CHIORAZZI, N. and KATZ, D.H. *Journal of Immunology*, **120**, 2050 (1978)
314. HIRASHIMA, M., YODOI, J. and ISHIZAKA, K. *Journal of Immunology*, **125**, 2154 (1980)

315. KATZ, D.H. *Journal of Experimental Medicine*, **149,** 539 (1979)
316. SUEMURA, M., KISHIMOTO, T., HIRAI, Y. and YAMAMURA, Y. *Journal of Immunology*, **119,** 149 (1977)
317. ELLOUZ, F., and ADAM, A., CIOBARA, R. and LEDERER, E. *Biochemical and Biophysical Research Communications*, **59,** 1317 (1974)
318. KISHIMOTO, T., HIRAI, Y., NAKANISHI, K., NAGAMATZU, A. and YAMAMURA, Y. *Journal of Immunology*, **123,** 2709 (1979)
319. MORAN, D.M., HENDERSON, D.C. and WHEELER, A.W. Unpublished observations (1982)
320. *Regulatory T Lymphocytes, P and S, Biomedical Sciences Symposia*. Eds B. Pernis and H.J. Vogel. London: Academic Press Inc. (1980)
321. SKIDMORE, B.J. and KATZ, D.H. *Journal of Immunology*, **119,** 694 (1977)
322. TAKATSU, K. and ISHIZAKA, K. *Journal of Immunology*, **118,** 151 (1977)
323. MALLEY, A., BAGLEY, D. and FORSHAM, A. *Molecular Immunology*, **16,** 929 (1979)
324. EKRAMODDOULLAH, A.K.M., KISIL, F.T. and SEHON, A.H. *International Archives of Allergy and Applied Immunology*, **64,** 277 (1981)
325. OHTSUKA, H., OKUDA, M. and KAWABORI, S. *Japanese Journal of Ophthalmology*, **83,** 543 (1980)
326. OKUDA, M. *Mechanisms in Nasal Allergy*, Parts I and II. ORL Digest. Vol. 39, pp. 22 and 31 (1977)
327. GLEICH, G.J. *Journal of Allergy and Clinical Immunology*, **70,** 160 (1982)
328. ASKENASE, P.W. *Journal of Allergy and Clinical Immunology*, **63,** 79 (1979)
329. SHAMPAIN, M.P., BEHRENS, B.L., LARSEN, G.L. and HENSON, P.M. *American Review of Respiratory Disease*, **126,** 493 (1982)
330. VOLKMAN, D.J., AHMAD, A., FAUCHI, A.S. and NEVILLE, Jr D.M. *Journal of Experimental Medicine*, **156,** 634 (1982)

Index